Physical Rehabilitation for Veterinary Technicians and Nurses

Physical Rehabilitation for Veterinary Technicians and Nurses

Second Edition

Edited by

Mary Ellen Goldberg
Veterinary Technician Specialist- lab animal medicine (Research anesthesia-retired), Veterinary Technician Specialist- (physical rehabilitation-retired)
Veterinary Technician Specialist- (anesthesia & analgesia) – H
Veterinary Medical Technologist, Surgical Research Anesthetist-retired
Certified Canine Rehabilitation Veterinary Nurse, Certified Veterinary
Pain Practitioner

and

Julia E. Tomlinson
Diplomate, American College of Veterinary Sports Medicine &
Rehabilitation (Specialist)
Twin Cities Animal Rehabilitation & Sports Medicine Clinic
VROMP | Veterinary Rehabilitation & Orthopedic Medicine Partners practice
12010 Riverwood Dr, Burnsville
MN, USA

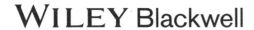 WILEY Blackwell

Published by John Wiley & Sons, Inc., Hoboken, New Jersey.
Published simultaneously in Canada.

For general information on our other products and services or for technical support, please contact our
Customer Care Department within the United States at (800) 762-2974, outside the United States at
(317) 572-3993 or fax (317) 572-4002.

Wiley also publishes its books in a variety of electronic formats. Some content that appears in print may
not be available in electronic formats. For more information about Wiley products, visit our web site at
www.wiley.com.

Library of Congress Cataloging-in-Publication Data
Names: Goldberg, Mary Ellen, editor. | Tomlinson, Julia, 1972– editor.
Title: Physical rehabilitation for veterinary technicians and nurses /
   edited by Mary Ellen Goldberg and Julia E. Tomlinson.
Description: Second edition. | Hoboken, New Jersey : Wiley-Blackwell,
   [2024] | Includes bibliographical references and index.
Identifiers: LCCN 2023048979 (print) | LCCN 2023048980 (ebook) | ISBN
   9781119892410 (paperback) | ISBN 9781119892427 (adobe pdf) | ISBN
   9781119892434 (epub)
Subjects: MESH: Physical Therapy Modalities–veterinary | Animal
   Technicians
Classification: LCC SF925 (print) | LCC SF925 (ebook) | NLM SF 925 | DDC
   636.089/5822–dc23/eng/20240102
LC record available at https://lccn.loc.gov/2023048979
LC ebook record available at https://lccn.loc.gov/2023048980

Cover Design: Wiley
Cover Images: Courtesy of Julia E. Tomlinson, Steve Adair, Mary Ellen Goldberg and Wendy Davies

Set in 9.5/12.5pt STIXTwoText by Straive, Pondicherry, India

SKY10067217_021524

Dedication

This book is dedicated to my granddaddy and my mother.

My paternal grandfather, John G. Richardson Sr, taught me about loving animals. When I was a little girl, I followed granddaddy everywhere. We went on walks to feed horses, mules, dogs, cats, squirrels, ducks, and birds. He told me about animals he had owned. Granddaddy died on August 9, 1970. I was 13 years old. I wish he could have seen how his influence affected me.

My mother, Eleanor Straub Richardson, was a nurse during WWII. She used her GI bill to get degrees in nursing education so she could teach. My mother was the kindest, most loving person I have ever known. I could never even hope to provide care that mother did for her patients, but I could have no better role model of what a nurse provides and advocates for her charges. Her students loved her and told me over the years that mother represented all the traits a nurse embodies. I hope in some small measure, I would have made her proud.

Mary Ellen Goldberg

This book is dedicated to the amazing team of veterinary technicians that I work with both in my own clinic, and those I have collaborated with in writing, teaching, and case discussion. The founding members of the veterinary technician specialty (VTS) in rehabilitation hold a dear place in my heart and I am so grateful to them for sharing their knowledge and expanding the skills of veterinary technicians worldwide.

Julia E. Tomlinson

Contents

21 Therapeutic Exercises Part 2: Hydrotherapy (Aquatic Therapy) *381*

Pádraig Egan

List of Contributors

Steve Adair
Equine Performance and
Rehabilitation Center
University of Tennessee
Veterinary Medical Center
Knoxville, TN
USA

Jessy Bale
Essex Animal Hospital
Essex, Ontario
Canada

Kara M. Burns
Academy of Veterinary Nutrition
Technicians
Independent Nutritional Consultant
Lafayette, IN
USA

Deana Cappucci
West Delray Veterinary
Delray Beach, FL
USA

Tracy A. Darling
Director of Canine Operations
National Disaster Search Dog Foundation
Santa Paula, CA
USA

Jacqueline R. Davidson (she/her/hers)
Clinical Professor
Small Animal Clinical Sciences, College
of Veterinary Medicine & Biomedical
Sciences
Texas A&M University
College Station, TX
USA

Wendy Davies
Rehabilitation and Regenerative Medicine
University of Florida
Gainesville, FL
USA

Robin Downing
The Downing Center for Animal Pain
Management, LLC
Windsor, CO
USA
and
Affiliate Faculty
Colorado State University College of
Veterinary Medicine
Fort Collins, CO
USA

Pádraig Egan
East Neuk Veterinary Clinic
Scotland

Mary Ellen Goldberg
Veterinary Technician
Specialist- lab animal medicine
(Research anesthesia-retired)
Veterinary Technician Specialist-
(physical rehabilitation-retired)
Veterinary Technician Specialist-
(anesthesia & analgesia) - H
Veterinary Medical Technologist
Surgical Research Anesthetist-retired
Certified Canine Rehabilitation
Veterinary Nurse
Certified Veterinary Pain Practitioner

Amie Lamoreaux Hesbach
EmpowerPhysio
Maynard, MA
USA

Janice L. Huntingford
Essex Animal Hospital
Essex, Ontario
Canada
and
Assistant Professor
Chi University
Reddick, FL
USA

Sherri Jerzyk
Small Animal Clinical Sciences, College
of Veterinary Medicine & Biomedical
Sciences
Texas A&M University
College Station, TX
USA

Stephanie Kube
Neurologist/neurosurgeon
Advanced Veterinary Specialty Center of
New England
Walpole, MA
USA

Carolina Medina
Elanco Animal Health
Fort Lauderdale, FL
USA

Darryl Millis
The College of Veterinary Medicine
University of Tennessee
Knoxville, TN
USA

Megan Nelson
Twin Cities Animal Rehabilitation &
Sports Medicine Clinic
Burnsville, MN
USA

Evelyn Orenbuch
Orenbuch Veterinary Rehabilitation
Marietta, GA
USA

Cynthia M. Otto
Director, Penn Vet Working Dog Center
Professor of Working Dog Sciences &
Sports Medicine
University of Pennsylvania
School of Veterinary Medicine
Philadelphia, PA
USA

Dawn Phillips
University of Tennessee
College of Veterinary Medicine
Knoxville, TN
USA

Dawn Rector
The College of Veterinary Medicine
University of Tennessee
Knoxville, TN
USA

Megan Ridley
Integrative Pet Care
Chicago, IL
USA

Angela Stramel
Advanced Care Veterinary Services
Carrollton, TX
USA

Douglas Stramel
Advanced Care Veterinary Services
Carrollton, TX
USA

Julia E. Tomlinson
Twin Cities Animal Rehabilitation &
Sports Medicine Clinic
Burnsville, MN
USA
and
Veterinary Rehabilitation and Orthopedic
Medicine Partners
San Clemente, CA
USA

Elizabeth E. Waalk
Twin Cities Animal Rehabilitation &
Sports Medicine Clinic
Burnsville, MN
USA

Sam Warren
Twin Cities Animal Rehabilitation &
Sports Medicine Clinic
Burnsville, MN
USA

Melissa Weber
Twin Cities Animal Rehabilitation &
Sports Medicine Clinic
Burnsville, MN
USA

Erin White
SportVet Canine Rehabilitation and
Sports Medicine
Tallahassee, FL
USA

Renée Yacoub
Integrative Pet Care
Chicago, IL
USA

Acknowledgments

The completion of this text would not have been possible without the talents of many people who need to be thanked.

Atul Ignatius David, Dr. Rituparna Bose, and Susan Engelken, all of John Wiley & Sons, Inc. need to be thanked for their help and advice to produce this book.

All our contributing authors and providers of images have contributed their time and knowledge beyond the "call of duty." This text is truly a joint effort that would not have been possible without each of our colleagues' efforts. Thank you for sharing your knowledge and experience.

We wish to thank the Academy of Physical Rehabilitation Veterinary Technicians (APRVT), which has elevated the role of veterinary technicians in physical rehabilitation practice. Many of our authors are members of APRVT.

Finally, to veterinarians performing physical rehabilitation and schools that certify veterinary technicians and nurses in physical rehabilitation, we wish to say thank you for your work and for improving the lives of our veterinary patients.

The Editors

About the Companion Website

This book is accompanied by a companion website:

www.wiley.com/go/goldberg/physicalrehabilitationvettechsandnurses

The website includes videos.

1

Introduction to Physical Rehabilitation for Veterinary Technicians/Nurses

Mary Ellen Goldberg

Veterinary Technician Specialist- lab animal medicine (Research anesthesia-retired), Veterinary Technician Specialist-
(physical rehabilitation-retired), Veterinary Technician Specialist- (anesthesia & analgesia) – H, Veterinary Medical Technologist,
Surgical Research Anesthetist-retired, Certified Canine Rehabilitation Veterinary Nurse, Certified Veterinary Pain Practitioner

As veterinary technicians, we vow to further our knowledge and competence through a commitment to lifelong learning (NAVTA, 1987). Over the past 15–20 years, awareness of animal physical rehabilitation has increased, and rehabilitation has become a rapidly growing service within veterinary specialty hospitals, referral centers, and primary care practices. Every day, we hear about laser therapy and underwater treadmills, equipment that was not traditionally covered in the veterinary technician's college curriculum. Learning more about rehabilitation enables the veterinary technician to better assist the supervising veterinarian when physical rehabilitation therapies are recommended. This chapter aims to answer some questions about rehabilitation for veterinary technicians and nurses.

What Is Rehabilitation?

Physical rehabilitation is the treatment of injury or illness to decrease pain and restore function (American Association of

Physical Rehabilitation for Veterinary Technicians and Nurses, Second Edition.
Edited by Mary Ellen Goldberg and Julia E. Tomlinson.
© 2024 John Wiley & Sons, Inc. Published 2024 by John Wiley & Sons, Inc.
Companion website: www.wiley.com/go/goldberg/physicalrehabilitationvettechsandnurses

Table 1.1 Sample conditions benefiting from physical rehabilitation.

Orthopedic	Neurological	General
Post-operative rehabilitation (e.g., stifle or hip surgery, arthrodesis, amputation, and ligament/tendon repair)	Post-operative rehabilitation (e.g., decompressive surgery and reconstructive surgery)	Pain management
Acute and chronic soft tissue injuries, involving muscle and fascia, tendon, joint capsule, or ligament (limbs or trunk)	Central or peripheral nerve injuries	Athletic/working dogs (performance problems, improving strength and endurance)
Arthritis (long-term management)	Fibrocartilaginous embolism, spinal shock	Obesity
Developmental orthopedic diseases (e.g., hip dysplasia, elbow dysplasia)	Degenerative nerve disease (e.g., myelopathy, polyneuropathies)	Depression
Trauma and wound care	Balance/vestibular problems	Senior care
	Nervous system trauma	

Source: Adapted from Sharp (2008).

Rehabilitation Veterinarians, 2023). Rehabilitation is used to address acute injuries and chronic injuries or diseases. Rest alone after injury usually does not relieve the problems caused by inflammation and spasm; for example, a muscle in spasm may not have adequate blood supply to heal. Protective mechanisms in place in the body following injury alter movement of the whole musculoskeletal system and increase strain in other areas. Physical rehabilitation should commence as soon as is possible for the patient and caregiver (Table 1.1).

History of Human Physical Therapy

International (Physiosite, 2015)

Physicians like Hippocrates and later Galenus are believed to have been the first practitioners of physical therapy, advocating massage, manual therapy techniques, and hydrotherapy. In 460 BC, Hector practiced *hydrotherapy* – which is Greek for water treatment. In 1894, Great Britain recognized physiotherapy as a specialized branch of nursing regulated by the Chartered Society of Physiotherapy. The first emergence of physiotherapy as a specialist discipline was in Sweden in 1913, when Per Henrik Ling founded the Royal Central Institute of Gymnastics (RCIG) for massage, manipulation, and exercise. In the following two decades, formal physiotherapy programs were established in other countries, led by the School of Physiotherapy at the University of Otago in New Zealand (1913). From 1950, chiropractic manipulations were also introduced, this was initially most common in Great Britain. A subspecialty of orthopedics, within physiotherapy, also emerged at about the same time.

United States of America (APTA, 2015; Moffat, 2003)

Physical therapists formed their first professional association in 1921, called the American Women's Physical Therapeutic Association. In 1922, the association changed its name to the American Physiotherapy Association (APA). In the 1930s, APA introduced its first "Code of Ethics," men were admitted, and membership grew to just under 1,000. With the advent of World War II and a nationwide polio epidemic during the 1940s and 1950s, physical therapists were in great demand. The association's membership grew to 8,000. By the late 1940s, the association had changed its name to the American Physical Therapy Association (APTA). APTA represents more than 90,000 members throughout the United States. A national professional organization, APTA's goal is to foster advancements in physical therapy practice, research, and education. Currently, 213 institutions offer physical therapy education programs, and 309 institutions offer physical therapist assistant education programs in the United States.

History of Veterinary Physical Rehabilitation

Physical rehabilitation for animals has been practiced since the 1980s. In biomedical research, the use of animal models in treatment protocols is common, and this includes research in the field of physical rehabilitation. From the late 1980s and throughout the 1990s, several groups helped to increase interest in canine and equine physical rehabilitation. These groups include the American Veterinary Medical Association (AVMA), the American College of Veterinary Surgeons (ACVS), and the formation of the Animal Physical Therapist Special Interest Group (APT-SIG) within the APTA. Success with human patients receiving post-operative physical therapy has galvanized the veterinary community into developing physical rehabilitation techniques that can be implemented for animal patients (McGonagle et al., 2014). In June 1993, the APTA issued a position statement that "endorses the position that physical therapists may establish collaborative, collegial relationships with veterinarians for the purposes of providing physical therapy services or consultation (APTA, 1993)." In 1996, "Guidelines for Alternative and Complementary Veterinary Medicine" were adopted by the AVMA House of Delegates (AVMA, 2000). New guidelines were adopted by the AVMA House of Delegates in 2001 (AVMA, 2001). Training in animal physical rehabilitation was established by a group at the University of Tennessee (McGonagle et al., 2014). This training and certification course was, and still is, provided for veterinarians, veterinary technicians, physical therapists, and physical therapy assistants (see below).

The International Association of Veterinary Rehabilitation and Physical Therapy (www.iavrpt.org) became an official association in July 2008 and is a collaborative association of veterinarians, technicians, physical therapists, and other allied health professionals. Veterinarians interested in rehabilitation in the United States are encouraged to join the American Association of Rehabilitation Veterinarians, founded in 2007 (www.rehabvets.org). Veterinary technicians can become members of the AARV as associate members, as can other allied health professionals.

In 2010, the American College of Veterinary Sports Medicine and Rehabilitation (ACVSMR) was approved by the American Association of Specialty Veterinary Boards (AASVB) to establish and maintain credentialing and specialty status for veterinarians who excel in sports medicine and rehabilitation. A veterinarian can become board-certified in either canine or equine specialties under this college; more details can be found at their website, www.vsmr.org.

Veterinary technicians can take one of several certification courses in animal rehabilitation. For those technicians who are already certified in physical rehabilitation, a veterinary technician specialty group has been formed. This group is under the umbrella and direction of the National Association of Veterinary Technicians in America (NAVTA) and is called the Academy of Physical Rehabilitation Veterinary Technicians. This specialty certification will allow veterinary technicians and nurses to possess the credential for VTS-physical rehabilitation. The Mission Statement of the Academy is, "We are credentialed rehabilitation veterinary technicians providing assistance in physical rehabilitation, encouraging veterinary technicians to further education, while improving the quality of animals' lives."

Specifics About Veterinary Physical Rehabilitation

The American Association of Rehabilitation Veterinarians produced a model set of guiding principles for the ideal practice of veterinary physical rehabilitative medicine (AARV, 2014). These model standards state:

- Patient care in the rehabilitation facility should be under the authority, supervision, or approval of a licensed veterinarian certified in rehabilitation therapy.
- Initial examination and diagnosis should be determined by a licensed veterinarian with rehabilitation certification.
- The rehabilitation treatment plan should be formulated and the case managed by a licensed veterinarian with rehabilitation certification, or a combination of these veterinarians, in consultation with an appropriately licensed physical therapist certified in animal rehabilitation.
- No technician/assistant (certified or otherwise) shall manage a rehabilitation patient.
- There shall be a formal policy in place to monitor and evaluate patient responses to care.
- The practice shall use individualized rehabilitation and therapy plans, including fitness plans.
- For patients with concurrent conditions, clients shall be advised early during care of the opportunity to request a second opinion or referral to a specialist for treatment of these conditions.
- The rehabilitation practice shall regularly update the patient's primary care veterinarian as well as any other veterinarian involved with the patient's current care.
- A summary of the initial rehabilitation evaluation findings should be sent to the referring veterinarian at the earliest opportunity, preferably within 24 hours of the evaluation.
- The patient shall be discharged back into the care of the primary veterinarian once therapy is complete.
- When referring a patient for additional workup, appropriate referral communication (such as a letter, email, or phone conversation) shall occur and should be properly documented in the patient's record.
- Evaluation for pain shall be part of every patient visit.
- Practice team members shall be trained to recognize pain and work in collaboration with the veterinarian to provide appropriate pain management, including physical and pharmaceutical modalities.
- Since medical and emergent issues may arise during treatment, and pain management monitoring needs to be addressed by a veterinarian, having the rehabilitation veterinarian on site is ideal. A plan must be in place to address emergent care medical issues and pain management in the absence of direct (on-site) veterinary supervision.
- Practice team members should be trained to identify causes of pain, levels of pain, medications, and physical methods used to control pain.
- Pain scores should be documented in the medical record at each visit.
- Pain management techniques should be used when the presence of pain in a patient is uncertain.

- Clients should be adequately educated to recognize pain in their pets.
- Clients should be adequately educated about the possible effects of any dispensed analgesic, including adverse events.
- Tentative diagnoses and medical plans, or their subsequent revisions, shall be communicated to clients at the earliest reasonable opportunity.
- A rehabilitation veterinarian should have current knowledge of veterinary-approved diets, nutraceuticals, supplements, as well as knowledge and skills in weight loss and weight-management programs.
- Nutritional assessment and counseling should be part of routine care.
- Recommended continuing education requirements:
  - Each veterinarian should have a minimum of 15 hours of continuing education every 2 years, specifically in veterinary rehabilitation topics.
  - Each veterinarian should have a minimum of 20 hours per year of documented continuing education in the field of veterinary medicine.
  - Each veterinary technician should have a minimum of 10 hours of documented continuing education in the field of veterinary rehabilitation every 2 years.
  - Each veterinary technician should have a minimum of 10 hours of documented continuing education in the field of veterinary technology every 2 years.
  - Each physical therapist should have a minimum of 15 hours of documented continuing education in the field of veterinary rehabilitation every 2 years.
  - Each physical therapist should complete continuing education in their own field as recommended by their governing state board.

How Do Veterinary Technicians and Nurses Fit In?

Veterinary technicians must complete either a 2- or 4-year program in the United States. Veterinary nurses are the primary para-veterinary workers in the United Kingdom. They assist vets in their work and have a scope of autonomous practice within which they can act for the animals they treat, which can include minor surgery. Registered veterinary nurses (RVNs) are bound by a code of professional conduct and are obliged to maintain their professional knowledge and skills through ongoing continuing professional development (RCVS, 2023). In the United States, in approximately 40 states, veterinary technicians are certified, registered, or licensed (Levine *et al.*, 2014). Veterinary technician programs do not include extensive coursework in physical rehabilitation.

Most continuing education courses offered at international, national, and local meetings offer physical rehabilitation lectures and hands-on laboratories. The AARV provides a full day of lectures at the North American Veterinary Conference, and the ACVSMR offers lectures (canine and equine) at this conference and a program in conjunction with the ACVS annual symposium.

Where Can I Become a Certified Rehabilitation Veterinary Technician?

The greatest asset for effective physical rehabilitation is an educated veterinary team (Sprague, 2013). A rehabilitation technician is a certified, licensed, or registered veterinary technician who has completed a prescribed curriculum to receive the title of Certified Canine Rehabilitation

Veterinary Nurse (CCRVN), Certified Canine Rehabilitation Practitioner (CCRP), or Certified Veterinary Massage and Rehabilitation Therapist (CVMRT). There are currently five certification programs available for veterinary technicians in the United States that offer the respective titles.

The Canine Rehabilitation Institute offers the Certified Canine Rehabilitation Assistant (CCRA) program for veterinary assistants or those who do not possess a license as a credentialed veterinary technician; CCRVN for those who are a credentialed veterinary technician; and the Certified Canine Rehabilitation Therapist (CCRT) program for veterinarians and physical therapists at training facilities in Missouri and Colorado (http://www.caninerehabinstitute.com).

Northeast Seminars offers the Certification in Companion Animal Therapy (CCAT) for veterinarians, licensed veterinary technicians, physical therapists, physical therapist assistants, and occupational therapists at North Carolina State University (https://www.ncsuvetce.com/canine-rehab-ccat/).

University of Tennessee offers the CCRP, or Certified Equine Rehabilitation Practitioner (CERP), for veterinarians, physical therapists, and veterinary technicians at The University of Tennessee (https://www.u-tenn.org/ccrp/ and https://vahl.vet/).

Healing Oasis offers the CVMRT program for licensed veterinarians, licensed or certified veterinary technicians, licensed physical therapists, licensed nurses, and/or licensed/certified massage therapists at their facility in Wisconsin (http://www.healingoasis.edu/VMRT-program).

Animal Rehabilitation Institute offers Certified Equine Rehabilitation Assistant (CERA) offered to Veterinary Technicians and Physical Therapist Assistants (https://animalrehabinstitute.com/open-enrollment-2/).

What Is Involved in Becoming a CCRA, CCRVN, CCAT, CCRP, CVMRT or CERA, CERP?

Formal educational courses and wet labs are involved in all the certification courses. Each school has its own curriculum. The cost is relatively expensive for a veterinary technician, but this certification may allow the veterinary technician to command a higher salary. You must be an LVT, CVT, and RVT to attend most of the courses. The best way to investigate the programs is to visit the webpages listed below:

1) http://www.caninerehabinstitute.com
2) https://www.ncsuvetce.com/
3) https://www.u-tenn.org/ccrp/ and https://vahl.vet/
4) http://healingoasis.edu/veterinary-massage-rehabilitation-therapy-program
5) https://animalrehabinstitute.com/about-ari/

Practice Regulations for Veterinary Technicians

Candidates for certified, registered, or licensed veterinary technician are tested for competency through an examination which may include oral, written, and practical portions. Every state is unique and maintains its own regulations with respect to the practice of veterinary medicine. Practice acts, legislated by states and provinces, often define the responsibilities of the veterinary technician. These responsibilities and duties are dependent in part on the type of employment the individual chooses. The current standards include obtaining an associate or bachelor's degree from a program accredited by the AVMA's Committee on Veterinary Technology and Education Activities (CVTEA), a passing score on the veterinary technician national examination by the American Association of Veterinary State Boards (AAVSB), and a varying number of continuing education hours within the renewal process.

A rehabilitation veterinary technician should be working under the direct supervision of a credentialed rehabilitation veterinarian who directs therapy. The larger team may be made up of a credentialed physical therapist, the referring veterinarian, a veterinary specialist (surgeon, neurologist, etc.), a veterinary chiropractor, acupuncturist, hospital support staff, the owner, and other trained veterinary professionals.

Working in the Physical Rehabilitation Field

The duties of the rehabilitation veterinary technician include assisting their supervising veterinarian in evaluations and in performing therapies. Therapies that the technician can provide include application of prescribed physical modalities and therapeutic exercises. Part of patient care is ensuring patient records are up-to-date and accurate. Proper documentation of treatments should be completed each day. Any member of the rehabilitation team should be able to refer to the record and understand the needs and past treatments of each patient. Clear client communication and education are also necessary. Chapter 2: Joining a Rehabilitation Team goes into detail about the role of each team member.

Pain plays a role in any patient's willingness and motivation. A patient's pain score should be assessed and documented in the medical record during each visit (AARV, 2014). A detailed history should indicate the degree of pain and the disability (Davies, 2014). How does the patient cope with the disability? If changes in a patient's pain level are noted, the supervising veterinarian should be notified. It is very important for the rehabilitation veterinary technician to remain in open communication with their supervisor about anything abnormal or any changes in progress. Chapter 3 will address pain management through physical rehabilitation.

Much of the certified veterinary rehabilitation technician's day is like any other LVT, RVT, or CVT. Animal patients are admitted, housed appropriately, and kept clean. Often during the day, patients are taken outside so they can relieve themselves. Records are pulled for the therapist (veterinarian or physical therapist). Patient forms must be in order, records sent from the referring veterinarian are available, and equipment is clean, orderly, and ready for use. Assisting the therapist with their patients and listening to them is all part of the routine. At this point, any veterinary technician could fill this position. What sets the veterinary technician apart who is certified in rehabilitation?

Therapeutic Exercises

Therapeutic exercises are a daily part of the veterinary technician's routine. The owner/handler must be well educated on the exercise program, especially the home exercise program (HEP). The supervising veterinarian chooses the exercises, and the technician carries them out. Exercises target proprioception and balance, specific muscle groups, overall pattern of gait, and overall strength and endurance. Therapeutic exercise equipment includes physioballs, cavaletti rails, balance blocks and discs, weights, tunnels, rocker boards, wobble boards, treadmills, air mattresses, and planks (Coates, 2013). Patient considerations such as motivation, footing, assistive devices, and leash/harness control must be assessed prior to beginning any exercise program, and therapist/handler body mechanics must be monitored to prevent injury. Exercises are designed to address specific impairments, and each is described with a goal, a technique, and a progression (McCauley and Van Dyke, 2013). In order to fully understand the therapies, certification at one of the rehabilitation schools is necessary.

Manual Techniques

Specialized manual techniques are used in evaluating and treating the patient. Types of techniques the technician is trained in are:

1) "Massage – Effleurage consists of long, slow strokes, generally light to moderate pressure, usually parallel to the direction of the muscle fibers. Petrissage involves short, brisk strokes with moderate to deep pressure, parallel, perpendicular, or diagonally across the direction of the muscle fibers. It may include kneading, wringing, or skin rolling. Tapotement is rhythmic, brisk percussion often administered with the tips of the fingers, primarily used as a stimulating stroke to facilitate a weak muscle, and cross-friction massage involves applying moderate pressure perpendicularly across the desired tissue. Pressure is maintained in such a way that the finger does not slide across the skin, but rather takes the skin with it" (Coates, 2013).
2) Normal range of motion (ROM) is the full motion that a joint may be moved through. Passive range of motion (PROM) motion of a joint that is performed without muscle contraction within the available ROM, using an external force to move the joint (Millis and Levine, 2014a, b).

   Stretching techniques are often performed in conjunction with ROM exercises to improve flexibility of the joints and extensibility of periarticular tissues, muscles, and tendons (Millis and Levine, 2014a, b).

Physical Modalities

Physical modalities are often used as part of the patient's treatment plan. Physical modalities are used as tools to manage pain, weak muscles, inflexibility, limited joint range of motion, and aiding in tissue healing (Niebaum, 2013). The modalities mentioned are not presented in detail.

Physical modalities include:

1) *Superficial thermal agents* – hot (thermotherapy) and cold (cryotherapy).
2) *Neuromuscular electrical stimulation (NMES)* – usually used to address muscular weakness.
3) *Transcutaneous electrical nerve stimulation (TENS)* – used for pain relief.
4) *Therapeutic ultrasound* – a deep heating technique used for rehabilitating musculoskeletal conditions (Levine and Watson, 2014).
5) *Photobiomodulation* – (not surgical lasers) is used to accelerate wound healing, promote muscle regeneration, treat acute and chronic pain, chronic and acute edema, and neurologic conditions (Millis and Saunders, 2014).
6) *Extracorporeal shock wave therapy (ESWT)* – benefits include increased bone, tendon, and ligament healing, accelerated wound healing, antibacterial properties, and pain relief (Niebaum, 2013).
7) *Pulsed electromagnetic field therapy (PEMF)* – can induce biological currents in the tissue. The Food and Drug Administration (FDA) has approved it as safe and effective for the treatment of fractures and their sequelae (Rosso *et al.*, 2015). The main therapeutic purpose is for enhancement of bone or tissue healing and pain control (Millis and Levine, 2014a, b).

   Additional areas of education include topics such as aquatic therapy, canine orthotics and prosthetics, rehabilitation of the orthopedic and neurologic patient, canine sports medicine, pain management, nutrition, and geriatric patients.

Conditions That Can Benefit from Physical Rehabilitation

A range of therapies are used to achieve one or more of the following functional goals:

- Speed recovery from injury or surgery
- Increase mobility and flexibility
- Improve endurance and agility
- Decrease pain
- Maintain function and prevent further problems
- Enhance quality of life (QoL)

Physical rehabilitation helps an individual who has had an illness or injury to achieve the highest level of function, independence, and QoL as possible (Sharp, 2008). The success or otherwise of any surgery is as much down to the rehabilitation carried out as to the surgical technique performed.

Rehabilitation offers numerous physiological benefits to patients, including:

- Increased blood flow and lymphatic drainage to the injured area
- Reduction of pain, swelling, and complications
- Increased production of collagen
- Prevention of contractions and adhesions
- Promotion of normal joint biomechanics
- Prevention of other injuries
- Prevention of or reduction in muscle atrophy
- Improved function and quality of movement

Conclusion

A rehabilitation veterinary technician's job is complex and fulfilling. There are advancements in veterinary medicine daily, and animal physical rehabilitation is on the cutting edge. Specialized rehabilitation equipment is helpful, but much can be achieved without it. Physical rehabilitation is rewarding even with minimal equipment; all you need is a rehabilitation team.

Resources

Romich, J.A. (2021). *Anesthesia, Analgesia, and Pain Management for Veterinary Technicians*, 1e. Boston, MA, USA: Cengage Learning.

Albi, M., Holden, J., Ensign, S. et al. (2020). *Anesthesia and Pain Management for Veterinary Nurses and Technicians*, 1e. Florence, OR: Teton NewMedia.

Bockstahler, B., Levine, D., Maierl, J. et al. (2019). *Essential Facts of Physical Medicine, Rehabilitation and Sports Medicine in Companion Animals*, 1e. VBS GmbH.

References

American Association of Rehabilitation Veterinarians (2014) *Model Standards for Veterinary Physical Rehabilitation Practice*. Updated February 2014; originally published February 7, 2011. (retrieved January 09, 2023) http://www.rehabvets.org/model-standards.lasso (being updated on website).

American Association of Rehabilitation Veterinarians (2023) http://www.rehabvets.org/.

American Physical Therapy Association History (2015) http://www.apta.org/History/ (retrieved April 22, 2015).

APTA (1993). Position on physical therapists in collaborative relationships with veterinarians. *Am Phys Ther Assoc House Delegates* 06-93-20-36 (Program 32).

AVMA (2000). Guidelines for alternative and complementary veterinary medicine. In:

AVMA Directory. Schaumburg, IL: American Veterinary Medical Association.

AVMA (2001). Guidelines for complementary and alternative veterinary medicine. In: *AVMA Policy Statements and Guidelines*. Schaumberg, IL: American Veterinary Medical Association.

Coates, J. (2013). Chapter 6: Manual therapy. In: *Canine Sports Medicine and Rehabilitation*, 1ste (ed. M.C. Zink and J.B. Van Dyke), 100. Ames, IA: John Wiley & Sons, Inc.

Davies, L. (2014). Chapter 11: Canine rehabilitation. In: *Pain Management in Veterinary Practice*, 1ste (ed. C.M. Egger, L. Love, and T. Doherty), 134. Ames, IA: John Wiley & Sons, Inc.

Levine, D. and Watson, T. (2014). Chapter 19: Therapeutic ultrasound. In: *Canine Rehabilitation and Physical Therapy*, 2nde (ed. D.L. Millis and D. Levine), 328–339. Philadelphia, PA: Elsevier.

Levine, D., Adamson, C.P., and Bergh, A. (2014). Chapter 3: Conceptual overview of physical therapy, veterinary medicine, and canine physical rehabilitation. In: *Canine Rehabilitation and Physical Therapy*, 2nde (ed. D.L. Millis and D. Levine), 18. Philadelphia, PA: Elsevier.

McCauley, L. and Van Dyke, J.B. (2013). Chapter 8: Therapeutic exercise. In: *Canine Sports Medicine and Rehabilitation*, 1ste (ed. M.C. Zink and J.B. Van Dyke), 132–156. Ames, IA: John Wiley & Sons, Inc.

McGonagle L, Blythe L, and Levine D (2014) Chapter 1: History of canine physical rehabilitation. In *Canine Rehabilitation and Physical Therapy*, 2nd edn (eds. DL Millis and D Levine). Elsevier, Philadelphia, PA, pp. 1–7.

Millis, D. and Levine, D. (2014a). Chapter 23: Other modalities in veterinary rehabilitation. In: *Canine Rehabilitation and Physical Therapy*, 2nde (ed. D.L. Millis and D. Levine), 393–400. Philadelphia, PA: Elsevier.

Millis, D.L. and Levine, D. (2014b). Chapter 25: Range of motion and stretching exercises. In: *Canine Rehabilitation and Physical Therapy*, 2nde (ed. D.L. Millis and D. Levine), 431–446. Philadelphia, PA: Elsevier.

Millis, D.L. and Saunders, D.G. (2014). Chapter 14: Laser therapy in canine rehabilitation. In: *Canine Rehabilitation and Physical Therapy*, 2nde (ed. D.L. Millis and D. Levine), 359–378. Philadelphia, PA: Elsevier.

Moffat, M. (2003). The history of physical therapy practice in the United States. *J Phys Ther Educ* 17: 5–25.

NAVTA (1987) Veterinary Technician Code of Ethics https://www.navta.net/about-navta/about (accessed September 10, 2014).

Niebaum, K. (2013). Chapter 7: Rehabilitation physical modalities. In: *Canine Sports Medicine and Rehabilitation*, 1ste (ed. M.C. Zink and J.B. Van Dyke), 115–128. Ames, IA: John Wiley & Sons, Inc.

RCVS (2023) Veterinary qualifications: Registered veterinary nurse: RVN. Royal College of Veterinary Surgeons. https://www.rcvs.org.uk/registration/applications-veterinary-nurses/uk-qualified-veterinary-nurses/ (retrieved January 09, 2023).

Rosso, F., Bonasia, D.E., Marmotti, A. et al. (2015). Mechanical stimulation (pulsed electromagnetic fields "PEMF" and extracorporeal shock wave therapy "ESWT") and tendon regeneration: A possible alternative. *Front Aging Neurosci* 9 (7): 211. https://doi.org/10.3389/fnagi.2015.00211.eCollection 2015.

Sharp, B. (2008). Physiotherapy in small animal practice. *In Practice* 30: 190–199.

Sprague, S. (2013). Introduction to canine rehabilitation. In: *Canine Sports Medicine and Rehabilitation*, 1ste (ed. M. Christine Zink and J.B. Van Dyke), 83. Ames, IA: John Wiley & Sons.

2

Joining a Rehabilitation Team

Julia E. Tomlinson[1,2]

[1] *Veterinary Rehabilitation & Orthopedic Medicine Partners, San Clemente, CA, USA*
[2] *Twin Cities Animal Rehabilitation and Sports Medicine Clinic, Burnsville, MN, USA*

Introduction

People Who Work in a Veterinary Rehabilitation Facility

A veterinary rehabilitation facility, like any veterinary clinic or hospital, relies on a team of people working together with a common goal. The common goal in a veterinary rehabilitation facility is to improve the quality of life of patients by improving the ability of the animal to perform the activities of daily living necessary for life to be fulfilling. Activities of daily living are daily self-care activities in the patient's home.

A useful approach to explaining who works in a veterinary rehabilitation facility is to look at it from the point of view of the patient and caregiver (client) entering the facility for the first time.

The patient and caregiver will be greeted and welcomed by a receptionist or client care representative in most cases; however, in some cases, it will be you, the veterinary nurse or technician, greeting them. The patient and caregiver will then either be directed to take a seat in the waiting room or be guided to an examination room, where any intake forms not completed online (and treats) will be handed out.

The receptionist's responsibilities are answering the phone, scheduling, admitting, and discharging patients, and facilitating the flow of traffic in the building. They may also explain treatment plans and

Physical Rehabilitation for Veterinary Technicians and Nurses, Second Edition.
Edited by Mary Ellen Goldberg and Julia E. Tomlinson.
© 2024 John Wiley & Sons, Inc. Published 2024 by John Wiley & Sons, Inc.
Companion website: www.wiley.com/go/goldberg/physicalrehabilitationvettechsandnurses

estimates. This person should have a good knowledge of the process of veterinary rehabilitation and the flow of the facility.

For most patients, the rehabilitation technician will be the first to enter the examination room and will put the patient and client/caregiver at ease. This is particularly important for nervous patients. History taking may be performed by the technician or the rehabilitation veterinarian. Once a complete and detailed history has been taken, the physical and observational examination begins.

The rehabilitation veterinarian (along with any other professionals) will make functional and physical diagnoses; using this information they will develop a treatment plan. This plan will likely include both at-home and in-clinic therapy. The rehabilitation technician will take part in explaining the at-home and in-clinic therapy plan to the client/caregiver in an easy-to-understand way and will teach home exercises to the client and to the patient.

In-clinic therapies will be performed by a combination of the rehabilitation veterinarian, rehabilitation veterinary technician, physical therapist, and other professionals, such as a veterinary acupuncturist, animal chiropractor, or massage therapist. The person performing the therapy depends on the therapy recommended and on that person's skill set. Many rehabilitation veterinarians have additional training in manual therapies (including manipulations) and in acupuncture. Both physical therapists and chiropractors are trained in human medicine to be manual therapists and to work in the veterinary world will need to have additional training and certification in working with animal patients.

Team Members

The Rehabilitation Veterinarian

The rehabilitation-trained veterinarian will examine the patient and assess pain level, injured tissues, concurrent disease, and functional limitations. If further diagnostics are needed, they will be performed for an exact diagnosis to be made. The treatment plan must be guided by an accurate diagnosis when one is possible. The rehabilitation veterinarian will develop a treatment plan including at-home and in-clinic therapy, medications, and recommended nursing care. Other professionals, if present, will contribute to this plan. The rehabilitation veterinarian may be a Diplomate of the American College of Veterinary Sports Medicine and Rehabilitation (DACVSMR) or be certified in rehabilitation.

The Rehabilitation Veterinary Technician

The rehabilitation technician will assist with the examination. The technician will assist in handling the patient, and with taking and recording measurements and observations, such as vital signs and pain scoring. The rehabilitation technician will take part in educating the client and explaining the home care and in-clinic therapy plan. The rehabilitation technician will also take part in in-clinic therapies under the supervision of the rehabilitation veterinarian. The rehabilitation technician should have received specific certification in veterinary rehabilitation.

The Physical Therapist

A physical therapist, trained in animal rehabilitation, can evaluate the animal patient with the rehabilitation veterinarian. A specific diagnosis needs to be made by a veterinarian. Together with the rehabilitation veterinarian, the physical therapist will develop and institute the treatment plan. Physical therapists who work in animal rehabilitation should be certified in veterinary rehabilitation.

The Physical Therapist Assistant

The physical therapist assistant works under the supervision and direction of the physical therapist and does not evaluate but is able to perform many therapeutic treatments. Physical therapist assistants who work in animal rehabilitation should be trained and certified in animal rehabilitation.

Adjunct Team Members

Other team members can include veterinarians who are trained in acupuncture or spinal manipulative therapy (veterinary term for chiropractic) and other veterinarians including specialists (surgeon, oncologist, neurologist, primary care veterinarian, and pain specialists). Chiropractors who have received additional training and certification in animal chiropractic along with massage therapists may be involved in care of the rehabilitation patient.

Becoming a Rehabilitation Technician (Nurse)

A rehabilitation veterinary technician or nurse is a skilled individual who has devoted time, study, and energy into training in the art and science of veterinary rehabilitation. A rehabilitation technician or nurse will be instrumental in the execution of the rehabilitation therapy plan and will often be the first line in noting a change in patient status and advocating for them. Before becoming a rehabilitation veterinary technician an individual will qualify as a veterinary technician or nurse.

According to the National Association of Veterinary Technicians in America (NAVTA):

> Veterinary technicians obtain 2–4 years of post-high school education and have an Associate's or Bachelor's degree in veterinary technology. (The AVMA accredits veterinary technology programs throughout the United States and Canada through their Committee on Veterinary Technician Education and Activities.) Veterinary technicians must pass a credentialing examination and keep up to date with continuing education to be credentialed. The credentialing term varies from state to state, with some known as "licensed," (LVT and LVMT), others as "registered," (RVT), and others as "certified" (CVT). In a growing number of arenas, veterinary technicians are called veterinary nurses, as this term alleviates the confusion of the various credentialing terms and more accurately describes the level and types of work these professionals handle every day, while a veterinary technician can perform a wide variety of tasks, they cannot diagnose, prescribe, perform surgery, or engage in any activity prohibited by a state's veterinary practice act.

More information is available on the website of the NAVTA (https://www.navta.net/membership).

This training includes education in veterinary anatomy and physiology, pathology, pharmacology, and disease processes. All this information is essential for someone working in the field of veterinary rehabilitation.

Becoming a veterinary nurse in the United Kingdom involves either taking vocational training or a degree course. More resources and information can be found on the website of the Royal College of Veterinary Surgeons (RCVS) at (www.rcvs.org.uk) and the website of the British Veterinary Nurses Association (www.bvna.org.uk).

Each country will have its own regulating body and contacting the main veterinarian-regulating body of your country will be the best initial approach to finding out more.

Training in veterinary rehabilitation is available at several educational facilities in the United States (Northeast Seminars partnering with the University of Tennessee, Canine Rehabilitation Institute, Equine Rehabilitation Institute, and Healing Oasis Education Center). For more information, see Chapter 1. Healing Oasis Education Center and Canine Rehabilitation Institute also run courses in other countries (e.g., Canada, Switzerland, the United Kingdom, Australia, and Brazil). These courses average 121 hours of education in the format of didactic (lecture) teaching in person and online along with interactive, practical training. This training is followed by a certification examination. It is important to note that these certification courses are self-regulating and may differ in content. There is no overseeing body ensuring that information is correct and applicable. Some courses have sought approval from state educational boards (Healing Oasis, for example).

After certification, the technician/nurse candidate gains a certificate in canine rehabilitation: Certified Canine Rehabilitation Veterinary Nurse (CCRVN), Certified Canine Rehabilitation Practitioner (CCRP), or Certified Veterinary Massage and Rehabilitation Therapist (CVMRT). These courses are available to veterinarians, veterinary technicians, physical therapists, physical therapy assistants, and, in some cases, chiropractors, massage therapists, and veterinary assistants. The certification gained from these courses should always be interpreted in the light of the individual's other qualifications and degrees and does not provide a blanket qualification to practice rehabilitation medicine, or to make a diagnosis and to prescribe therapy.

Completion of the certification process and emerging as a certified rehabilitation technician is only the beginning of the journey into this rewarding and fulfilling field of veterinary medicine. The next steps are on-the-job training and continuing education. Continuing education lectures, laboratories, and seminars on this subject are currently available at many major veterinary conferences. There are also stand-alone meetings entirely devoted to rehabilitation, such as the International Association of Veterinary Rehabilitation and Physical Therapy meeting (www.iavrpt.org) which occurs every two years and alternates between European and American locations.

Veterinary technicians can specialize in a certain area in the United States. Specialization in rehabilitation is guided by the Academy of Physical Rehabilitation Veterinary Technicians, visit www.aprvt.com for more details.

The Rehabilitation Patient

Surgical Patients

Surgical patients often make up a large proportion of cases in an animal rehabilitation facility. Many rehabilitation facilities are housed in, or adjacent to veterinary surgical facilities. The surgical patient may be seen by the rehabilitation technician/nurse and the supervising rehabilitation veterinarian both before and after surgery. A patient may need to lose weight before undergoing anesthesia or the surgeon may have advised some pre-surgical strengthening. Most surgical patients that are referred for rehabilitation will have already had orthopedic surgery or surgery aimed to improve neurologic dysfunction. Simple rehabilitation techniques (cryotherapy and range of motion) are also applicable for hospitalized patients, even those in a critical care setting.

The aim of rehabilitation therapy for post-surgical patients is to assist in recovery of strength and function; function includes flexibility and coordination. The specialist surgeon will give input to the rehabilitation therapist about restrictions in activity relative to stability of the surgical repair/procedure. The surgeon will give a unique perspective as they have seen the full extent of tissue damage and the relative success (or struggle) in repairing and minimizing the effects of that damage. The surgeon will be principally concerned about healing of the surgical site and may want to be more conservative than the rehabilitation team. Understanding the surgeon's point of view and acting with collegiate respect is important; however, the surgeon may need to be enlightened about the process of rehabilitation and the appropriate qualifications of the people he or she is working with pertinence to case management. Restricting activity and motion of the affected area unduly can transform the detrimental effects of immobilization from a temporary to a permanent one. In human medicine, mobilization of a patient after repair of a complex spinal fracture begins immediately post-operatively (J Yeater RN, EMT, personal communication, 2022). A rehabilitation veterinarian should be the person to govern communications with the surgeon.

The Injured Non-surgical Patient

These are patients with a physical injury or disease affecting mobility and comfort for which surgery is not indicated, or in some cases not possible for reasons such as the risks of anesthesia. Many soft tissue injuries are treated this way. Having a specific diagnosis of tissue pathology as well as a diagnosis of functional limitations is of paramount importance. An exact diagnosis still needs to be reached to formulate an appropriate rehabilitation plan. Lame patients referred for "strengthening" should be carefully evaluated and diagnosed by the veterinarian before the onset of rehabilitation therapy; for example, exercising a patient with a severely damaged tendon can cause further pathology.

The aim of rehabilitation therapy for the injured patient is to manage pain and restore maximal function.

Patients with Chronic Degenerative Disease

Chronic degenerative diseases (e.g., osteoarthritis, immune-mediated polyarthritis, degenerative myelopathy, spinal stenosis, and obesity) all affect mobility and strength and many of them will slowly progress causing a steady decline in status. The aim of rehabilitation therapy for these patients is to improve function in the light of their disability, to manage pain, and to improve quality of life. Even an unstable neurologic patient with permanent nerve damage can improve gait with improved strength because they can overcome the forces of motion while ataxic and improve forward momentum and stabilization if their muscles are working well. Balance and proprioceptive exercises can result in a relative improvement in overall stability.

Geriatric Patients

As individuals age, they lose muscle (this muscle loss is termed sarcopenia) and fine motor control/balance along with strength. The relatively immobile patient is also prone to obesity. Aging is not a disease process, but the incidence of systemic disease does increase with age. The aim of rehabilitation therapy for these patients is to improve their quality of life through pain management, improvements in mobility, and regaining the ability to perform the activities of daily living – even if this requires the use of assistive devices (see Chapter 13). Concurrent morbidity (e.g., bladder infections from incomplete emptying in the weak patient) must be considered and, of all the rehabilitation patient populations, this aged one needs the most frequent veterinary intervention.

The Canine Athlete/Working Dog

Working with canine athletes is an extremely rewarding process. Trainers/caregivers are motivated and generally knowledgeable. These patients cannot self-advocate and yet they have the drive of a human professional athlete; injuries are common. The aim of rehabilitation therapy for these patients is to return to sport or work. A survey of agility owners found the injury rate of agility dogs to be 32% at the time of survey (Cullen *et al.*, 2013). Injury rates in young human athletes vary from 12% to 28% depending on sport. This is of great concern to doctors because conditioned adult athletes have only a 2–3% injury rate (AOSSM, 2009; Ganse *et al.*, 2014). Part of the problem for young human athletes is their open growth plates when training; part is thought to be due to inadequate conditioning and relative overload. Conditioning plans have the potential to reduce injury rates in sporting dogs along with maintenance therapies (usually manual therapies and acupuncture, possibly therapeutic modalities). The goal of conditioning is to optimize the performance of the athlete and minimize the risk of injury and illness. Training adaptations are specific to the nature of the exercise (e.g., muscle contraction type and mechanics) and so conditioning should be appropriate for the demands of the sport (Tomlinson and Nelson, 2022). For example, long periods of trotting or walking exercises are an inappropriate conditioning plan for a sprinting athlete.

Your Team Role as Rehabilitation Veterinary Technician

Being a Patient Advocate

As a rehabilitation veterinary technician/nurse, you will be one of the team members who interacts most with both patient and client/caregiver. As you provide veterinarian-prescribed therapies, the time that you spend with the patient and client/caregiver will give you a unique insight into the personalities of both, and this will help you to quickly recognize changes in patient status.

When you encounter a patient for the first time, there will need to be an immediate assessment of patient demeanor (people experienced with working on animals tend to do this automatically) and an understanding of how this patient may respond to novel situations and touch. Clients may not be immediately forthcoming or even honest with themselves about how their loved one reacts to unfamiliar situations. Taking time to put the patient at ease, no matter how long that takes, is crucial to enable a full examination and functional assessment. The rehabilitation examination is extensive and relies on a lot of touch, including physically moving the patient around. If pain is an issue, the patient may react in an aggressive manner. It is, therefore, paramount that proper pain management be included in the final analysis. A relatively relaxed patient is easier to examine from the point of view of compliance but also from the point of view of identifying areas of discomfort. Understanding animal behaviors, including signs of stress and fear, and having fundamental training skills will go a long way toward enabling an easy examination and a low-stress process. Animal behavior is a branch of veterinary medicine that extends into everything we do. If we can put our patients at ease, future therapy visits will go well.

History taking may be performed by the technician or the rehabilitation veterinarian. History taking is often a lengthy process and includes questioning the client about the exact home environment (e.g., flooring and stairs in the home, pain scoring using home behaviors, patient activity level, and number of walks each day), timeline of the problem, any current or previous treatments and medications, other concurrent diseases, and activity level before the issue (owner expectations of return to normalcy). The examination is a full physical and functional assessment. Once a complete and detailed history has been taken, the physical and observational examination begins. The rehabilitation examination looks for areas of dysfunction and pain. The examination includes subjective and objective observations. Examples of subjective observations include conformation and posture, stance and sit position, transitions between postures, ability to hold posture, and response to palpation (both static palpation and palpation during movement of a joint, stretch of a muscle, etc.). Objective observations are those that can be measured, for example, measurement of thigh girth with a spring-weighted tape measure, using a stance analyzer to assess the weight put through each paw and gait analysis. As rehabilitation technician, you will assist the rehabilitation veterinarian and any adjunct professionals with their examination. The rehabilitation technician assists in handling the patient, applying restraint, if needed, using a minimal restraint approach. The technician may also be responsible for taking and recording measurements and observations, pain scoring the patient, and charting. The rehabilitation examination takes longer than a routine clinical examination and keeping the patient and client relaxed and focused can be a challenge.

The rehabilitation veterinarian will make a physical diagnosis and a functional assessment. Using this information, they will develop a treatment plan. This plan will include at-home and in-clinic therapy. The rehabilitation technician will take part in explaining the home and in-clinic therapy plan to the client/caregiver in an easy-to-understand way. Communication skills and empathy are essential parts of being a rehabilitation veterinary technician, just as they are for a veterinary technician or nurse working in general practice. The technician is often the translator of words from medical terminology to accessible terms and can repeat an explanation of the diagnosis in a different way. In many cases, the visit to the rehabilitation veterinarian is the last in a long list of visits to several veterinarians, so clients may be frustrated with the long process and need time and a sympathetic ear to vent these frustrations. Part of the skill of communication is the ability to listen without interrupting and to help the client feel heard before moving on with a full explanation of the treatment plan which engages the client as part of the therapy team.

The rehabilitation technician will go over the recommended plan with the client/caregiver using a step-by-step approach. This will include a financial estimate for the in-clinic plan, explaining the in-clinic therapy plan along with prescribed medications and supplements, and then covering the home therapy plan. The client/caregiver should gain a thorough understanding of the initial plan, therapeutic goals, and the potential for changes in the plan. They should be educated about the time-consuming nature of therapy, along with understanding reasonable benchmarks for improvement (expectations) and how long it can take for even small improvements to occur.

Any questions that arise from the client/caregiver can be addressed directly by you or conveyed to the rehabilitation veterinarian. Finally, mediating the checkout at reception by scheduling a set of therapy visits before the client leaves can help to improve compliance. As one of the main people communicating with the client, the rehabilitation technician should make sure that the client knows how to contact the clinic with any follow-up questions prior to next visit – the large amount of information generated from the first visit often takes time to digest and questions can come up later.

Talking casually with clients/caregivers during therapy sessions and asking gentle questions about home progress can often reveal potential pitfalls in the home care plan and other red flags: "Fluffy doesn't chase squirrels in the back yard so I decided he needed some off leash time." You are also uniquely situated to address concerns and to notice early and subtle changes in patient status: "Sam is not getting any better, I am worried that therapy isn't working" and "We had a great Christmas thanks for asking, apart from Sam did get on the kitchen counter and stole a ham; he hasn't done that in years!" Information revealed during conversations can be used to gently counsel and guide the client/caregiver regarding small positive or negative changes. Any issues of potential concern can then be discussed with the client/caregiver and with your supervising veterinarian so that you can implement any change in therapy plan. Plan changes should then be explained to the client/caregiver.

The special relationship that develops during therapy between you and a client/caregiver means that you are uniquely situated as an ally and confidant, more so than the veterinarian or other professional. You may be the only person able to gently point out to a client/caregiver that they are being non-compliant, without seeming judgmental or negative. Sometimes the technicians that Dr. Julia works with will use an indirect approach and "tell the dog" that they cannot go off leash yet, and even though they feel better, it does not mean that they are fully healed. The rehabilitation veterinary technician also can gently remind the supervising veterinarian of issues. For example, the enthusiastic home plan with 15 separate exercises devised by the veterinarian may be overwhelming to an otherwise compliant client/caregiver. Perhaps the client/caregiver has downplayed a physical issue that they themselves have, which restricts their ability to implement the home plan. It may be that the owner is at risk of getting bitten and did not want to admit that to the rehabilitation veterinarian.

Observing a patient for a relatively long period during therapeutic visits may also highlight an issue that was not noted during the initial examination. The rehabilitation technician can become a skilled observer of gait and function and use this information to alert the veterinarian of the need for reassessment.

Many patients in rehabilitation are at risk of or are already suffering from concurrent disease, this can be as simple as a mild gastrointestinal upset, a medication reaction/interaction, or it may be a more complex systemic issue (diabetes and chronic kidney disease), or even an acute crisis such as a gastrointestinal bleed. The veterinary technician's skill set extends beyond rehabilitation and using your other skills and knowledge of medicine will be needed daily. You will need to be able to differentiate important issues, which require a halt in therapy and immediate veterinary attention, from mild issues that can be monitored.

Working with clients over the phone is another important part of the rehabilitation technician's job. Questions about therapy, the rehabilitation process, and other medical questions can often be answered immediately, the rehabilitation veterinarian is involved only on an as-needed basis. This "gatekeeping and educating" job is very much a part of a rehabilitation technician's role and should not be undervalued.

Providing the Prescribed Therapies

Learning how to provide therapy takes time and teaching by an experienced rehabilitation team. Introduction to modalities and therapeutic exercises is provided in the rehabilitation courses. Most of your skills, however, will be gained on the job under supervision. Knowing when to apply therapy appropriate for the diagnosis is the job of the supervising rehabilitation veterinarian; a physical therapist trained in animal rehabilitation may also provide a therapy plan once a veterinary diagnosis has been made. Complex manual therapies are not provided by the veterinary technician and require additional training before they can be provided by a veterinarian. Physical therapists learn manual therapy techniques during their years in school, but still need additional training in specifics of animal anatomy and biomechanics before applying their skills (quadrupeds are very different from bipeds, and horses are very different from dogs). Your supervisor will advise and teach you appropriate light manual therapies such as massage and stretches, you can also gain additional training such as massage. Your knowledge of veterinary anatomy and physiology will help you to understand and apply therapy to the appropriate site; for example, knowing the specific origin and insertion of a muscle and the direction of the fibers can help you to apply therapeutic ultrasound and follow it with cross fiber massage. During therapy, you will note any response from the patient. The subtlest signs of discomfort can be identified by a skilled veterinary technician/nurse. Signs of discomfort need to be differentiated from signs of general stress or restlessness. Halting the therapy for a moment and noting whether the patient then relaxes while still being restrained is a simple method of differentiating discomfort due to therapy from discomfort due to restraint so that you can alert your veterinarian when appropriate for a change in plan.

Bribery goes a long way during treatment sessions, high-value treats (and a variety of treats, from immediate rewards to those needing some work to eat) help to ease patient tension and improve compliance. In Twin Cities Animal Rehabilitation and Sports Medicine, we often ask that owners refrain from buying the same treats that we use in clinic. That way the patients happily visit for "special treat time." Most of our patients come into a therapy room and point their noses straight at the treat bucket.

Assessing pain level is a part of each therapy visit. Question the owners about home behaviors and note in-clinic behaviors and responses to palpation. For example, when we provide laser therapy, we can palpate the treatment area before and after therapy and note whether we get some immediate pain relief.

Client/Caregiver Education

Education of the client extends from helping them to gain an understanding of the disease process or injury to help them to be part of the rehabilitation team for their pet. The rehabilitation technician will need to teach the owner the therapeutic exercises that will be performed at home. Teaching is a skilled job, and your team will have developed strategies, including handouts with pictures, online video demonstrations, and step-by-step instructions to aid you (Figure 2.1. Insert link to teaching video here). First demonstrating the exercise slowly to the owner, then watching them perform the exercise and giving gentle hints and tips is advised. Every person learns in a different way so providing a demonstration, hands-on practice, and reminders to be used later is a good way of ensuring that everyone is on the same page. Short videos posted online (password protected) work well, or the client can record you demonstrating the exercise in the room. A review of home exercises should occur at regular intervals (for example, weekly) during in-clinic therapy visits and, as the patient progresses, new exercises will need to be demonstrated. When teaching a home exercise, remember to consider the fact that there may be multiple members of the household responsible for therapy and that not all clients will be skilled at teaching

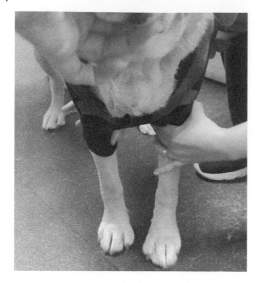

Figure 2.1 Your team will have developed strategies for teaching, including handouts with pictures, posters, models, videos, and step-by-step instructions. Explain and demonstrate the exercise, then it is time for the client to practice.

other household members. Clients also need to be taught to watch for postural decompensations and "cheating" during specific exercises.

Nursing Care

Part of nursing care is patient advocacy as described earlier in this chapter. Physically caring for a patient in clinic involves, for example, addressing discomfort, identifying areas at risk for pressure (bed) sores, and making sure elimination is occurring adequately at home and that the patient is clean. Having the necessary skills to express a bladder, pass a urinary catheter, and evacuate a rectum manually or via enema is part of a veterinary technician's training. Pain management involves the use of pharmaceuticals, manual therapies, and modalities and the protocol for each patient may need to be adjusted at each visit. Grooming to remove excess hair from paws to improve traction, nail trimming, and removing excess hair from the perineum is important for patients with disabilities. Counseling owners about the home environment, home modifications, assistive devices, and home nursing care is time-consuming, and adequate time needs to be devoted to this. For more on nursing the disabled patient, see Chapter 14.

Working Under Supervision

Working with a Diagnosis and Prescribed Therapies

A veterinary technician is legally obligated to work in veterinary medicine under the supervision of a veterinarian. The veterinarian is responsible for the diagnosis and for the therapeutic plan. Adjunct professionals may contribute to this plan; however, they are not suitable supervisors for veterinary technicians. Both the veterinarian and veterinary technician have skills that complement each other and so make up a team. It is sometimes the belief of general practitioners that veterinary rehabilitation is solely the practice of therapeutic exercise and that any person can quickly become skilled in veterinary rehabilitation ("there is not much to it"). This is very far from the truth. The rehabilitation examination is one of the most extensive examinations that a veterinary patient undergoes. Patients arriving with an existing diagnosis are not an exception to this, just as a neurologic examination is different from an orthopedic examination despite some overlap, so a rehabilitation examination is very different. Patients undergo a thorough assessment of function, including pain level, muscle tone, strength, and mobility with objective measurements. The whole body is examined not just the injured area. Compensatory issues are identified and a treatment plan covers all issues, including any systemic disease, endocrine issues, nutritional status, body condition, and body

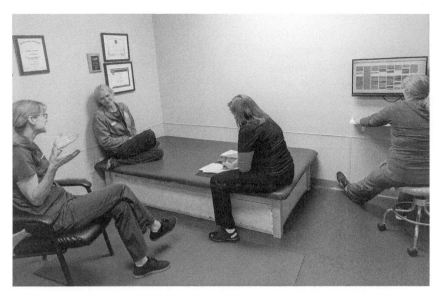

Figure 2.2 Daily medical rounds are recommended. Parameters are set and recorded for the therapy when to change the plan, and when it is necessary to consult your supervisor.

composition. Any rehabilitation patient who is not examined this way is done a disservice. Therapeutic approach changes frequently as patient status changes, if patient compliance is a challenge, or if inadequate progress is being made. The rehabilitation veterinarian and technician will be in constant communication. Daily medical rounds are recommended. Rehabilitation technicians will apply and assist with therapies and are therefore closely monitoring a patient just as a technician would monitor a hospitalized patient; parameters are set for when to change the plan and when it is necessary to consult your supervisor (Figure 2.2). The same protocol of communication with the veterinarian applies to all aspects of veterinary medicine.

Approaching a Change in Patient Status

A sudden decline in patient status is always a reason to alert the attending veterinarian. Subtle changes may take additional time to recognize. As rehabilitation veterinary technician/nurse, you will become very familiar with observing a patient's gait and behaviors. Patient status can decline due to pain, relative overload (exercise was increased too rapidly, patient jumped on and off the couch at home), infection (e.g., implant infection and urinary tract infection), systemic disease, and many other reasons. Unmasking of a previously unrecognized systemic disease can sometimes occur. For example, as we slowly increase demands on a patient's respiratory system, early laryngeal paresis may be identified by increased breath sounds and increased panting. The supervising veterinarian will then need to outline necessary precautions and change the therapeutic plan accordingly. In the case of laryngeal changes, the team will need to avoid thoracic compression during hydrotherapy and provide frequent rest breaks while avoiding overheating.

It is important to remember and use every one of your skills, including general medicine. We use general medicine in our clinic every day, even though we are a stand-alone specialty rehabilitation clinic. Every clinic should have a list of red flags – signs that all therapists know are important indicators of a decline in patient status. Signs that indicate an emergency may not always be obvious to adjunct professionals (distended abdomen in an already obese patient, cardiovascular changes, hydration status, and cool extremities), and a large rehabilitation team needs every individual to be on task in order to catch signs early (see Boxes 2.1–2.5).

Also, team members need to be aware of their own limitations in training, pay close attention to the patient throughout therapy (even during conversing with the client), and understand that it is better to alert their supervisor than to overlook potential issues.

Box 2.1   Red flags – alert the veterinarian of these changes

- Any worsening symptoms from previous sessions
- New lameness or gait changes
- Sudden muscle atrophy/weakness
- Postural changes – head tilt, etc.
- Changes to balance/coordination
- Change in mentation
- Tremors, clonus, seizures
- Other neurologic changes – circling, falling, etc.
- Change in temperament
- Ocular changes
- Head shaking
- Broken nails, pad changes
- Swelling
- Pale mucous membranes
- Distended abdomen
- Increased respiratory effort
- Change in urine color or odor
- Changes in stool color or consistency
- Incontinence or change in frequency of elimination
- Gastrointestinal disturbance
- Change in skin/hair coat

Box 2.2   Red flags for skin and coat

Skin
- Signs of pressure/friction
- Self-mutilation (e.g., lick granuloma)
- Wounds
- Urine scald
- Bruising
- Discharge

Coat
- Thinning/alopecia
- Thicker, coarse
- Dryness/flaking
- Pruritus

Box 2.3   Red flags to listen for

- Popping
- Clicking
- Scraping
- Vocalizing in pain
- Change in pitch of vocalization
- Breathing – stertor (heavy snoring or gasping)/stridor
- Cough
- Change in heart rate/rhythm

Box 2.4   Red flags to feel for

- Local temperature change
- Masses
- Enlarged lymph nodes
- Change in pulse
- Joint swelling (effusion)
- Edema
- Localized muscle atrophy
- Change in end feel on passive motioning
- Crepitus
- Flinch and aversion
- Bony and/or soft tissue asymmetry
- Joint displacement

Box 2.5   Red flag odors
• Ears
• Mouth
• Urine
• Wounds
• Skin/coat

Legal Issues

Working with a rehabilitation-trained veterinarian is necessary because only a veterinarian can legally make a diagnosis and prescribe treatment. A veterinary technician must work under veterinary supervision by law in the United States, so from a legal standpoint, a rehabilitation veterinary technician must have a supervising veterinarian. Working with a primary care veterinarian with no formal training in physical rehabilitation is not recommended, veterinary schools teach little to no physical rehabilitation at this time. Working for a surgeon managing post-operative rehabilitation cases without a rehabilitation veterinarian is also not ideal, as even specialty surgery training does not generally include training in rehabilitation therapy (or sports medicine). The challenge comes due to the relative scarcity of veterinarians trained in rehabilitation in the United States; however, as this branch of veterinary medicine grows, more facilities will house appropriately trained personnel. A rehabilitation veterinarian will often have other qualifications, for example, manipulative therapies, myofascial dry needling, and acupuncture. Specialists in veterinary rehabilitation and sports medicine are veterinarians who have completed residency training in the subject, experienced a large clinical caseload and have published scientific research and passed a specialty examination; they are given the qualification DACVSMR. In Europe, the equivalent qualification is DECVSMR with the E standing for European. The formulation of the therapy plan may involve consultation with veterinary specialists (e.g., neurologists, nutritionists, oncologists, surgeons, and pain practitioners), and with other professionals (e.g., animal chiropractors and physical therapists). The rehabilitation veterinary technician will be part of a small or large team whose direct supervisor is the veterinarian. Different states (and countries) will have different laws. Be aware of the law in your region and the specifics of required veterinary supervision for a technician or nurse.

Future Directions for the Rehabilitation Technician

Cutting Edge of Rehabilitation Medicine

Rehabilitation medicine continues to grow and expand in both availability and complexity. As part of the veterinary rehabilitation team, you will be at the forefront of an exciting and expanding branch of veterinary medicine. Joining a team of trained individuals will expand your knowledge base and experience. Setting up a rehabilitation department with no other qualified individuals in regular veterinary practice is more of a challenge and less than ideal. Rehabilitation medicine should not be an adjunct to a regular veterinary practice, rather it is its own entity, with its own skill set, like surgery or oncology. We need to recognize the high level that rehabilitation practice can achieve and to avoid limiting ourselves to low-level therapeutic exercises and laser therapy. Focusing on best practices in veterinary rehabilitation will expand and further the field, allowing us to act in the patients' best interests and improve outcomes. Best practices are outlined in the American Association of Rehabilitation Veterinarians Ideal Standards listed in Chapter 1.

Regenerative Therapies

Regenerative medicine (stem cells and growth factors used to stimulate healing and grow new tissue) is still in its infancy. There is a large amount of ongoing research into the effects of regenerative techniques, and results are promising. As rehabilitation technician, you will need to be familiar with these procedures, from harvesting tissue and blood to extracting cells and then administering the therapy (usually by injection). You will assist with these procedures. Basic principles of collection and sterile technique are used, with the same techniques as for all sterile procedures. Stem cells and blood products are usually taken from the patient they are returned to, but research and early clinical trials are starting to use allogenic (same species, different individual) stem cells and there may eventually be "off the shelf" products available (Parker and Katz, 2006; Black *et al.*, 2007). Your supervising veterinarian will train you in sample handling, harvesting, and administration procedures. It is helpful to write protocols for your clinic so that all team members understand set-up and protocol. Companies such as Vet-Stem Biopharma (www.vet-stem.com) provide complete instructions for harvesting, processing, and injection of the processed cells. Platelet rich plasma (PRP) can be processed at an outside facility, or there are in-clinic systems available. It is imperative that the rehabilitation veterinarian is the one making any decisions about this therapy as different preparation methods yield very different products.

Nuclear Medicine

In addition to bone scans for diagnosis, radioisotopes are used for therapy in veterinary medicine. Commonly, radioactive iodine for thyroid disease in cats.

Radiosynoviorthesis is the local application of a radioactive agent to reduce joint inflammation and restore synovial function in production of synovial fluid. It is used in patients with osteoarthritis. The radioisotope Tin117m is used for elbow arthritis by licensed veterinarians in the United States who have additional State licensing for the procedure. Veterinary technicians assist in the technique and in the safe handling protocols for the procedure including weekly wipe tests and daily closeout reports, package receiving, and waste handling.

Orthotics and Prosthetics

In recent years, the field of veterinary orthotics and prosthetics has grown and continues to grow. It is no longer always routine to treat an amputee with the view that they will cope well throughout life; gait analysis studies actually show evidence to the contrary (Hogy *et al.*, 2013; Jarvis *et al.*, 2013). A patient with a missing limb also has minimal ability to compensate for an injury to the remaining limbs. When considering a prosthesis, the planning needs to be made preoperatively, prior to amputation. As patient advocate you will ensure that communications and planning between all veterinarians involved and with the owner go smoothly.

A patient with a limb deformity is no longer resigned to limited motion. Sophisticated devices allow for good movement at all gaits and speeds. Orthoses, braces, and prostheses are veterinary medical devices and need to be prescribed by a suitably trained veterinarian. These devices are complex and fit is custom. High-tech materials ensure close fit, minimal motion between device and limb, and low friction. This minimizes the risk of complications such as skin irritation. These devices can store the energy of motion to assist forward movement, just as the elastic tissues of the body do. Chapter XXX goes into detail about these devices.

Hospice

Hospice care is providing nursing care to a patient in the final stages of life or a disease process that will end in loss of life. Home hospice care is a relatively new field of veterinary medicine, there are mobile veterinarians that provide home-based care and many of these veterinarians have equipment for home-based hospice (e.g., intravenous fluids and injectable analgesics). The International Association of Animal and Hospice Care (www.iaahpc.org) is an excellent resource. As rehabilitation therapists, we work with a lot of aged patients and patients with high levels of morbidity, and so hospice care is relevant to the field. Providing caregivers access to home visits and understanding the limitations and patient needs in the home is part of the scope of all veterinary medicine.

Respite care (temporary hospitalization or boarding of a high-need patient) is provided in human medicine and involves temporary institutionalized care for disabled patients and rest for their caregivers. A similar need is present, but little is currently provided in veterinary medicine. Many rehabilitation clinics provide daycare or have facilities for hospitalization and extended rehabilitation stays.

Specific Organizations for Veterinarians and Veterinary Technicians

The Academy of Physical Rehabilitation Veterinary Technicians is an organization that is under the NAVTA Committee on Veterinary Technician Specialties (CVTS) (www.aprvt.com). The American Association of Rehabilitation Veterinarians (www.rehabvets.org) is an advocacy group that provides membership, continuing education, and other resources for veterinarians and technicians. The International Veterinary Academy of Pain Management (IVAPM) is an organization of veterinarians and veterinary technicians/nurses who have a special interest in the study of analgesia and pain management. There is a certification offered to both the veterinarian and veterinary nurse. Certified Veterinary Pain Practitioner (CVPP) is a credential that requires continuing education credit hours, written case studies, and a qualifying examination (http://ivapm.org/for-professionals/certification/).

Conclusions

Being part of a rehabilitation team is a highly rewarding experience. Working as a rehabilitation technician expands your horizons and gives you an avenue to explore and gain skills beyond your veterinary technician certification or degree. Along with your new skills, you will use your veterinary technician training and practice conventional veterinary care every day, even in a practice that focuses only on physical rehabilitation. You will have the opportunity to work closely with patients on a relatively long-term basis, often one-on-one, and with some autonomy. You and your team will progress a case all the way to completion of care. Seeing your patient make a full recovery, or markedly improving their quality of life is immensely fulfilling. You end each work day knowing that you and your team are making a huge difference in your patients' quality of life and, therefore, making a difference to their whole families.

References

AOSSM (American Orthopedic Society of Sports Medicine) (2009) Preserving the Future of Sport: From Prevention to Treatment of Youth Overuse Sports Injuries. 2009 Annual Meeting Pre-Conference Program, Keystone, Colorado.

Black, L.L., Gaynor, J., Gehring, D. et al. (2007). Effect of adipose-derived mesenchymal stem and regenerative cells on lameness in dogs with chronic osteoarthritis of coxofemoral joints: A randomized, double-blinded, multicenter, controlled trial. *Vet Ther* 8 (4): 272–284.

Cullen, K.L., Dickey, J.P., Bent, L.R. et al. (2013). Survey-based analysis of risk factors for injury among dogs participating in agility training and competition events. *J Am Vet Med Assoc* 243 (7): 1019–1024.

Ganse, B., Degens, H., Drey, M. et al. (2014). Impact of age, performance and athletic event on injury rates in master athletics – First results from an ongoing prospective study. *J Musculoskelet Neuronal Interact* 14 (2): 148–154.

Hogy, S.M., Worley, D.R., Jarvis, S.L. et al. (2013). Kinematic and kinetic analysis of dogs during trotting after amputation of a pelvic limb. *Am J Vet Res* 74 (9): 1164–1171.

Jarvis, S.L., Worley, D.R., Hogy, S.M. et al. (2013). Kinematic and kinetic analysis of dogs during trotting after amputation of a thoracic limb. *Am J Vet Res* 74 (9): 1155–1163.

Parker, A. and Katz, A. (2006). Adipose-derived stem cells for the regeneration of damaged tissues. *Expert Opin Biol Ther* 6 (6): 567–578.

Tomlinson, J. and Nelson, M. (2022). Conditioning dogs for an active lifestyle. *Vet Clin North Am Small Anim Pract* 52 (4): 1043–1058. https://doi.org/10.1016/j.cvsm.2022.03.008.

3

Physical Rehabilitation Pain Management and the Veterinary Technician

Mary Ellen Goldberg

Veterinary Technician Specialist- lab animal medicine (Research anesthesia-retired), Veterinary Technician Specialist- (physical rehabilitation-retired), Veterinary Technician Specialist- (anesthesia & analgesia) – H, Veterinary Medical Technologist, Surgical Research Anesthetist-retired, Certified Canine Rehabilitation Veterinary Nurse, Certified Veterinary Pain Practitioner

Introduction

The ability to experience pain is universally shared by all mammals and other vertebrates including fish, birds, reptiles, and amphibians. Physiological and behavioral observations show that animals experience the sensory aspect of pain but also the unpleasantness, averseness, and negative emotions attached to that experience (Monteiro *et al.*, 2022) (see Box 3.1). Animal sentience refers to the capacity of animals to feel both positive and negative emotions and is observed by animals seeking pleasure and avoiding suffering. Animal sentience is now legally recognized in numerous countries and jurisdictions.

Pain for the typical physical rehabilitation patient can occur during post-operative recovery, post-injury, because of a disease state, or because of the aging process. It is beyond the scope of this chapter to provide in-depth information about the neurophysiology of pain, neuropharmacology, and most drug doses.

Physical Rehabilitation for Veterinary Technicians and Nurses, Second Edition.
Edited by Mary Ellen Goldberg and Julia E. Tomlinson.
© 2024 John Wiley & Sons, Inc. Published 2024 by John Wiley & Sons, Inc.
Companion website: www.wiley.com/go/goldberg/physicalrehabilitationvettechsandnurses

---

Box 3.1   2022 WSAVA global pain management guidelines tenets of pain

- Pain is an illness that can be recognized and effectively managed in most cases.
- Pain is the fourth vital sign and should be incorporated into the temperature, pulse, and respiration (TPR) assessment of every patient.
- Preventive and multi-modal analgesia should always be considered.
- Perioperative pain can extend for several days and should be managed accordingly, including managing pain in the "home environment."
- Pain perception is influenced by numerous internal and external factors including the social and physical environment.
- Treatment of pain should always include pharmacological and non-pharmacological therapies.

Source: Adapted from WSAVA Guidelines (2022).

__Remember that the credentialed physical rehabilitation veterinary technician is not to diagnose, prescribe, or perform procedures that are the practice of veterinary medicine and will obey all individual state and regional laws and regulations pertaining to the field of veterinary physical rehabilitation (NAVTA North American Veterinary Technician Association webpage 2023, https://navta.net/faqs/). The credentialed physical rehabilitation veterinary technician will report to their supervising rehabilitation veterinarian on initial visit, during treatments, and on all follow-up visits.__

Exercise and Rehabilitation Therapy

The undeniable health benefits of movement and exercise are well established in human medicine, including the benefits of exercise in reducing and controlling pain (Gruen *et al.*, 2022). The terms physiotherapy and physical therapy refer to the treatment of humans. In veterinary medicine, the best-applied term is rehabilitation therapy.

Rehabilitation therapy broadly encompasses the use of varied manual techniques (joint mobilization, passive range of motion, stretching, massage, and myofascial release, to name a few), treatment modalities (therapeutic ultrasound, photobiomodulation-laser therapy, extracorporeal shock wave therapy, neuromuscular electrical stimulation, and thermal modification of tissue), and therapeutic exercises including hydrotherapy.

Physical Rehabilitation Benefits

- Reduce pain (Sharp, 2008; Flaherty, 2019)
- Increase and maintain muscle strength and flexibility (Millis and Ciuperca, 2015)
- Joint mobility (Millis and Ciuperca, 2015)
- Promote and restore normal movement patterns (Millis and Ciuperca, 2015)
- Increase cardiovascular fitness (Millis and Ciuperca, 2015)
- Combat acute and chronic inflammatory processes (Riviere, 2007; Petersen and Pedersen, 1985)
- Improve blood perfusion and consequently tissue repair (Millis and Ciuperca, 2015)
- Prevent adhesions, fibrosis, and tissue retraction (Millis and Ciuperca, 2015)
- Stimulate the nervous system and prevent neurapraxia (temporary loss of motor and sensory function due to blockage of nerve conduction) (Frank and Roynard, 2018)
- Promote the healing process (Neal Webb *et al.*, 2020)

Patients that are seen for rehabilitation therapy are reluctant to move. One of the major factors contributing to this reluctance is pain. It is necessary that pain be controlled prior to initiation of physical rehabilitation. The credentialed rehabilitation veterinarian (CCRT/CCRP/CVMRT/CCAT) will be gathering information that will influence the treatment choices for individual patients. Patients experiencing acute pain following orthopedic surgery have different needs than the elderly dog experiencing chronic maladaptive pain associated with long-standing osteoarthritis. Patients may present already being administered various pain medications that the rehabilitation veterinarian may consider changing. If it is at all possible the rehabilitation veterinarian should be in contact with the surgeon or primary care veterinarian before a patient is referred for rehabilitation so that they are aware of the treatment or perioperative pain management plan.

Pain plays a role in any patient's willingness and motivation. A patient's pain score should be assessed and documented in the medical record during each visit. A detailed history should indicate the degree of pain and disability. How does the patient cope with the disability? If changes in a patient's pain level are noted, the supervising veterinarian should be notified immediately. It is vital for the rehabilitation veterinary technician/nurse to remain in open communication with their supervisor about anything abnormal or any changes in progress.

Recognition and Assessment of Pain

The International Association for the Study of Pain (IASP) has revised its definition of pain for the first time since 1979 (IASP, 2023). The new definition states that pain is "An unpleasant sensory and emotional experience associated with, or resembling that associated with, actual or potential tissue damage." The definition has been expanded to include:

- Pain is always a personal experience that is influenced to varying degrees by biological, psychological, and social factors.
- Pain and nociception are different phenomena. Pain cannot be inferred solely from activity in sensory neurons.
- Through their life experiences, individuals learn the concept of pain.
- A person's report of an experience of pain should be respected.
- Although pain usually serves an adaptive role, it may have adverse effects on function and social and psychological well-being.
- Verbal description is only one of several behaviors to express pain; inability to communicate does not negate the possibility that a human or a non-human animal experiences pain (see Table 3.1).

Categories of Pain

Adaptive (acute) pain serves a protective role by enabling healing and tissue repair and usually is considered to end within three months (Muir and Woolf, 2001).

Maladaptive (chronic) pain serves no biological function and can become a disease. Chronic pain induces biochemical and phenotypic changes in the nervous system that escalate and alter sensory inputs, resulting in physiologic, metabolic, and immunologic alterations that threaten homeostasis and contribute to illness and death (Maier and Watkins, 1998).

Types of Pain

A) *Inflammatory pain* – acute postoperative pain until the wound has healed. There is a rapid onset and in general, its intensity and duration are related directly to the severity and duration of tissue damage. The pain results from the activity of inflammatory and immune cells and the products of tissue damage (WSAVA, 2023).
B) *Neuropathic pain* – is a maladaptive phenomenon caused by pathologic neuroplasticity and can become a disease of

Table 3.1 Signs of pain in dogs and cats.

Dogs	Cats
Decreased social interaction	Hiding
Increased sleeping	Reduced activity
Anxious expression	Changes in litterbox habits
Reluctance to move	Hissing, spitting, screaming
Whimpering, groaning, yelping	Lack of agility or jumping
Panting when resting	Excessive licking or grooming
Lameness or limping	Stops grooming; fur is matted
Not going up and down stairs	Stiff posture or gait
Lack of interest in food or play	Tail flicking
Sudden behavior changes (growling, aggression, biting)	Loss of appetite, weight loss
Arched or hunched back	Changes in facial expressions – squinting eyes, ears pointing outward, tense muzzle
Excessively chewing or licking a particular area of the body	

the neurologic system by persisting beyond resolution of an inciting cause (von Hehn *et al.*, 2012).

C) *Dysfunctional pain* – A state where the nervous system is grossly normal (i.e., there is no physical damage) but the functioning of the CNS is abnormal. Abnormal central processing results from repeated input to the CNS (WSAVA, 2023).

Physiologic Signs of Pain

- Increased heart rate
- Increased blood pressure
- Increased respiratory rate
- Vocalization

It is now accepted that the most accurate method for evaluating pain in animals is not by physiological parameters but by observations of behavior. Pain assessment should be a routine component of every physical examination, and a pain score is considered **the fourth vital sign**, after temperature, pulse, and respiration (*Gruen et al.*, 2022; Richmond, 2016; Bucknoff, 2019).

Behavioral Keys to Look for with Pain

What normal behaviors are maintained?
What normal behaviors are lost?
What new behaviors have developed?

The most common approach to pain assessment is the use of charts and scales. Pain scales should be used in conjunction with a thorough physical exam and history to assess every patient (see Box 3.2). Recognize that all pain scales have limitations. Individual patient behavior may indicate that prompt pain relief is needed, regardless of the pain score. Caregivers should strive for low pain scores in a comfortable-appearing patient. Neonates and geriatric animals may not express their pain as plainly as other animals. Choose one system to be used by the entire veterinary team. There are scales for acute and chronic pain. Pain scales should be practical, user-friendly, and easy to implement, independent of who is assessing (technician/nurse, veterinarian, student, or individual under training).

Box 3.2   Practical assessment and recognition of acute pain in cats and dogs (WSAVA Guidelines, 2022)

1) Observe the animal from a distance in its cage/bed/kennel (observe posture, facial expressions, attention to the wound, interest in surroundings, listen to the type of, or absence of vocalization). If the animal is clearly sleeping in a comfortable, relaxed position, do not disturb it.

2) Approach the animal calmly and open the cage/kennel while observing the animal's response.

3) Interact with the animal by calling its name using a gentle voice and petting and/or playing while observing the animal's response. If the animal shows no interest in interacting, do not force the issue, and give the animal space.

4) If possible, while already touching the animal, slide your hand closer to the painful area. First, attempt to touch it, then apply gentle pressure. Stop approaching, touching, or pressing as soon as the animal shows a behavioral response (e.g., lip licking, swallowing, turning the head towards your hand, flinching, guarding, growling, snapping, attempting to bite, crying).

5) Use a pain scale to score the animal's level of pain based on your observations.

Unidimensional Pain Scales are subjective such as visual analog scales (VAS); numerical rating scales (NRS); and simple descriptive scales (SDS). VAS – a line with no markings is used, numbers are at each end 0 being no pain and 100 being worst. NRS – a number line with individual numerical markings (1–10) which are chosen as the score. SDS – numbers used to assign to descriptions that categorize different levels of pain intensity. The Colorado State University Acute (canine and feline) are numeric and categoric, convenient pain scales that are easy to use in a clinical setting (see Figures 3.1–3.3). A pain scale should ideally be multidimensional, in that several aspects of pain intensity and pain-related disability are included and questioned, especially the dynamic aspects (see Table 3.2).

Pain scales can be objective such as the Glasgow composite pain scale. "A pain scale that considers the various dimensions of pain is thought to be more useful in indicating how much the pain" meant "to the animal, but VAS, NRS, and SDS scales are unidimensional. A pain scale should ideally be multidimensional, in that several aspects of pain intensity & pain related disability are included and question especially the dynamic aspects. The Glasgow CPS is thought to be Multidimensional" (Karas, 2011; see Figures 3.4 and 3.5; Table 3.3).

The Feline Grimace Scale (FGS) (© Université de Montréal 2019) is a valid, fast, reliable, and easy-to-use tool that can help with pain assessment. Based on the scores of the Feline Grimace Scale, it is possible to know if the administration of analgesics (i.e., painkillers) is required to help veterinarians with clinical decisions in pain management https://www.felinegrimacescale.com/. The Steagall Laboratory is a team of veterinarians at the Faculté de Médecine Vétérinaire, Université de Montréal, working together to better understand and treat pain in animals. They study naturally occurring, spontaneous pain in animals with a particular focus on cats (see Figure 3.6). Visiting the website will provide downloads and a training manual for the Feline Grimace Scale.

Colorado State University
✠ VETERINARY TEACHING HOSPITAL

How We Assess Your Canine's Pain Level

The Anesthesia and Pain Management team tailors all of their anesthesia and pain management services to the individual needs of your pet, and use the following scale to score the level of your pet's pain. This score helps us determine how to best make your pet's experience the most comfortable possible.

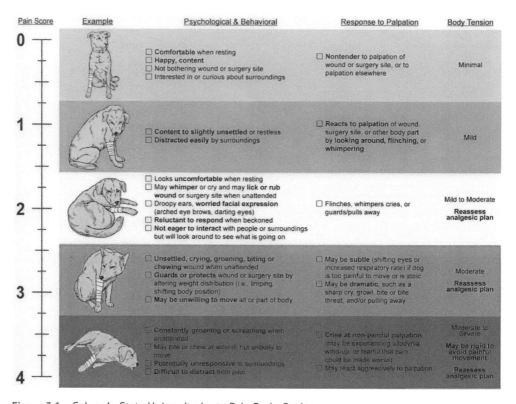

Figure 3.1 Colorado State University Acute Pain Scale Canine.

Clinical Metrology Instruments

When designing a clinical measurement system, there are only two potential aims: measurement for selection or measurement for improvement. The majority of the standardized clinical metrology instruments in use have been developed for owners to complete. These instruments are designed to detect and monitor chronic pain. These instruments ask owners to rate their pets ability to perform behaviors known to be affected by chronic musculoskeletal pain. They are simple to use and have good reproducibility and generate a score that can be tracked over time

Colorado State University
VETERINARY TEACHING HOSPITAL

How We Assess Your Feline's Pain Level

The Anesthesia and Pain Management team tailors all of their anesthesia and pain management services to the individual needs of your pet, and use the following scale to score the level of your pet's pain. This score helps us determine how to best make your pet's experience the most comfortable possible.

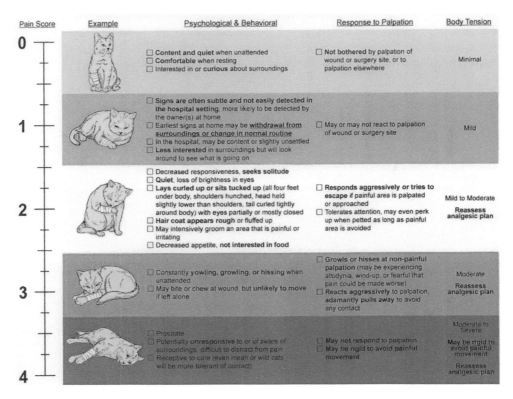

Pain Score	Example	Psychological & Behavioral	Response to Palpation	Body Tension
0		☐ Content and quiet when unattended ☐ Comfortable when resting ☐ Interested in or curious about surroundings	☐ Not bothered by palpation of wound or surgery site, or to palpation elsewhere	Minimal
1		☐ Signs are often subtle and not easily detected in the hospital setting; more likely to be detected by the owner(s) at home ☐ Earliest signs at home may be withdrawal from surroundings or change in normal routine ☐ In the hospital, may be content or slightly unsettled ☐ Less interested in surroundings but will look around to see what is going on	☐ May or may not react to palpation of wound or surgery site	Mild
2		☐ Decreased responsiveness, seeks solitude ☐ Quiet, loss of brightness in eyes ☐ Lays curled up or sits tucked up (all four feet under body, shoulders hunched, head held slightly lower than shoulders, tail curled tightly around body) with eyes partially or mostly closed ☐ Hair coat appears rough or fluffed up ☐ May intensively groom an area that is painful or irritating ☐ Decreased appetite, not interested in food	☐ Responds aggressively or tries to escape if painful area is palpated or approached ☐ Tolerates attention, may even perk up when petted as long as painful area is avoided	Mild to Moderate **Reassess analgesic plan**
3		☐ Constantly yowling, growling, or hissing when unattended ☐ May bite or chew at wound, but unlikely to move if left alone	☐ Growls or hisses at non-painful palpation (may be experiencing allodynia, wind-up, or fearful that pain could be made worse) ☐ Reacts aggressively to palpation, adamantly pulls away to avoid any contact	Moderate **Reassess analgesic plan**
4		☐ Prostrate ☐ Potentially unresponsive to or unaware of surroundings, difficult to distract from pain ☐ Receptive to care (even mean or wild cats will be more tolerant of contact)	☐ May not respond to palpation ☐ May be rigid to avoid painful movement	Moderate to Severe May be rigid to avoid painful movement **Reassess analgesic plan**

Figure 3.2 CSU Acute Pain Scale Feline.

(Gruen *et al.*, 2022). The instruments can be divided into those specific for dogs and those specific for cats.

Dog Specific CMIs

- *Helsinki chronic pain index (HCPI)* – (Hielm-Björkman *et al.*, 2009) 10 questions for owner

- *Canine brief pain index (CBPI)* – (Brown *et al.*, 2008; Essner *et al.*, 2017) 11-point scale
- *Cincinnati orthopedic disability index (CODI)* – (Gingerich and Strobel, 2003) three domains and essay
- *Health-related quality of life (HRQL)* – (Wiseman-Orr *et al.*, 2006) 12 questions

Colorado State University
VETERINARY TEACHING HOSPITAL

How We Assess Your Horse's Pain Level

The Anesthesia and Pain Management team tailors all of their anesthesia and pain management services to the individual needs of your animl, and use the following scale to score the level of your horse's pain. This score helps us determine how to best make your horse's experience the most comfortable possible.

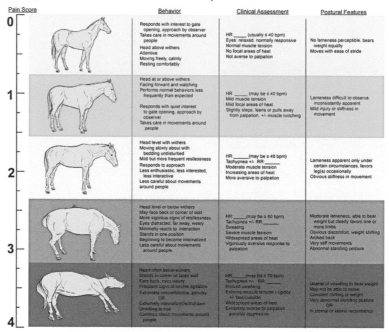

Pain Score		Behavior	Clinical Assessment	Postural Features
0		Responds with interest to gate opening, approach by observer Takes care in movements around people Head above withers Attentive Moving freely, calmly Resting comfortably	HR:_____ (usually ≤ 40 bpm) Eyes: relaxed, normally responsive Normal muscle tension No focal areas of heat Not averse to palpation	No lameness perceptible, bears weight equally Moves with ease of stride
1		Head at or above withers Facing forward and watching Performs normal behaviors less frequently than expected Responds with quiet interest to gate opening, approach by observer Takes care in movements around people	HR:_____ (may be ≤ 40 bpm) Mild muscle tension Mild focal areas of heat Slightly steps, leans or pulls away from palpation, +/- muscle twitching	Lameness difficult to observe, inconsistently apparent Mild injury or stiffness in movement
2		Head level with withers Moving slowly about with bedding undisturbed Mild but more frequent restlessness Responds to approach Less enthusiastic, less interested, less interactive Less careful about movements around people	HR:_____ (may be ≥ 48 bpm) Tachypnea +/- RR:_____ Moderate muscle tension Increasing areas of heat More aversive to palpation	Lameness apparent only under certain circumstances, favors leg(s) occasionally Obvious stiffness in movement
3		Head level or below withers May face back or corner of stall More vigorous signs of restlessness Eyes distracted, far away, weary Minimally reacts to interaction Stands in one position Beginning to become internalized Less careful about movements around people	HR:_____ (may be ≥ 60 bpm) Tachypnea +/- RR:_____ Sweating Severe muscle tension Widespread areas of heat Vigorously aversive response to palpation	Moderate lameness, able to bear weight but clearly favors one or more limbs Obvious discomfort, weight shifting Arched back Very stiff movements Abnormal standing posture
4		Head often below withers Stands in corner or faces wall Ears back, eyes weary Frequent signs of severe agitation Extremely uncomfortable, panicky OR Extremely internalized/withdrawn Unwilling to rise Careless about movements around people	HR:_____ (may be ≥ 70 bpm) Tachypnea +/- RR:_____ Profuse sweating Extreme muscle tension / rigidity +/- fasciculation Widespread areas of heat Extremely averse to palpation, possibly aggressive	Unable or unwilling to bear weight May not be able to move Constant shifting of weight Very abnormal standing posture OR In sternal or lateral recumbency

List of Behavioral Descriptors

General
- Pawing
- Stamping
- Tail switching w/o insects or other stimulus
- Circling in stall
- Flaring nostrils frequently
- Frequent head shaking w/o obvious reason
- Repetetive behaviors: Examples can include rubbing, pacing
- Getting up and laying down frequently
- Rocking to and fro on limbs
- Grunting
- Difficult to get settled down

Musculoskeletal-specific
- Frequent weight shifting
- Rocking to and fro on limbs
- "Grimacing" (assoc. w/ laminitis)
- Stamping
- Frequent weight shifting

Abdomen-specific
- Rolling on ground
- Pawing
- Flank watching
- Flank biting
- Teeth grinding
- Kicking at abdomen
- Grunting
- Thrashing

Palpation Reactions
Averse reaction to palpation may manifest as:
- Splinting
- Muscle twitching
- Biting
- Striking
- Kicking
- Hyperalgesia

Figure 3.3   CSU Acute Pain Scale Equine.

Table 3.2 Tools for assessing acute pain in cats.

Tool	Type	Condition	Reference
Feline Grimace Scale	Facial Expressions	Any surgical or medical pain including cats with oral disease and those undergoing dental extractions	Evangelista *et al.* (2019, 2020), Watanabe *et al.* (2020a), and Evangelista *et al.* (2021)
Unesp-Botucatu Feline Pain Scale	Behavior and facial expression	Any surgical or medical pain	Belli *et al.* (2021), Luna *et al.* (2022), and Brondani *et al.* (2013)
Glasgow composite measure pain scale-Feline	Behavior and facial expressions	Any surgical or medical pain	Reid *et al.* (2017) and Holden *et al.* (2014)

- *Liverpool osteoarthritis in dogs (LOAD)* – (Walton *et al.*, 2013) 3 domains; 23 questions
- *Canine osteoarthritis staging tool (COAST)* – (Cachon *et al.*, 2018) grades the dog and the joint by various questions

Cat Specific CMIs

Feline Musculoskeletal Pain Index (Enomoto *et al.*, 2022)

Client Specific Outcome Measures (Lascelles *et al.*, 2007)

Montreal Instrument for Cat Arthritis Testing for use by caretaker (MI-CAT(C)) (Klinck *et al.*, 2012)

Montreal Instrument for Cat Arthritis Testing for use by veterinarian (MI-CAT(V)) (Klinck *et al.*, 2018a, b)

How Can You Use Pain Scoring Effectively?

- Have same person evaluate the patient
- Place the VAS readings on the treatment/flow sheet as a chart
- Assess behavior
- Assess body posture, activity, and position in cage
- Evaluate response to approach
- Interact with patient
- Palpation of surgical site
- Ask patient to ambulate, if appropriate
- Ask patient to eat, if appropriate

To Summarize

No single pain scoring system is right for all practices or facilities. It is not as important which system you choose as it is to simply choose one system to be used by the entire team. Once a pain scoring system is chosen, apply it! At every single visit, assess the animal for pain and record the finding in the medical record, even if the finding is zero. Each individual pain assessment is important; for a patient with chronic pain, trends are even more important because they tell us whether the patient's pain is improving or worsening. Similarly, surgical patients with acute pain need to be assessed at regular intervals (possibly every 1–2 hours immediately post-operatively) and thereafter twice daily with the results recorded in the medical record. Trends allow the team to understand the success of a perioperative pain management plan. Owners should be educated and taught how to pain score their pets. Encourage the owner to take videos of their pet so you can see firsthand how the patient is progressing. The veterinary technician/nurse plays a primary role in educating the client.

SHORT FORM OF THE GLASGOW COMPOSITE PAIN SCALE

Dog's name _____

Hospital Number _____ Date / / Time

Surgery Yes/No (delete as appropriate)

Procedure or Condition _____

_____

In the sections below please circle the appropriate score in each list and sum these to give the total score.

A. Look at dog in Kennel

Is the dog?

(i)
Quiet	0
Crying or whimpering	1
Groaning	2
Screaming	3

(ii)
Ignoring any wound or painful area	0
Looking at wound or painful area	1
Licking wound or painful area	2
Rubbing wound or painful area	3
Chewing wound or painful area	4

> In the case of spinal, pelvic or multiple limb fractures, or where assistance is required to aid locomotion do not carry out section B and proceed to C
> *Please tick if this is the case* ☐ then proceed to C.

B. Put lead on dog and lead out of the kennel.

When the dog rises/walks is it?

(iii)
Normal	0
Lame	1
Slow or reluctant	2
Stiff	3
It refuses to move	4

C. If it has a wound or painful area including abdomen, apply gentle pressure 2 inches round the site.

Does it?

(iv)
Do nothing	0
Look round	1
Flinch	2
Growl or guard area	3
Snap	4
Cry	5

D. Overall

Is the dog?

(v)
Happy and content or happy and bouncy	0
Quiet	1
Indifferent or non-responsive to surroundings	2
Nervous or anxious or fearful	3
Depressed or no-responsive to stimulation	4

Is the dog?

(vi)
Comfortable	0
Unsettled	1
Restless	2
Hunched or tense	3
Rigid	4

© University of Glasgow

Total Score (i+ii+iii+iv+v+vi) = _____

Figure 3.4 Glasgow Composite Pain Scale Canine Short Form.

Glasgow Feline Composite Measure Pain Scale: CMPS - Feline

Choose the most appropriate expression from each section and total the scores to calculate the pain score for the cat. If more than one expression applies choose the higher score

LOOK AT THE CAT IN ITS CAGE:

Is it?
Question 1

Silent / purring / meowing	0
Crying/growling / groaning	1

Question 2

Relaxed	0
Licking lips	1
Restless/cowering at back of cage	2
Tense/crouched	3
Rigid/hunched	4

Question 3

Ignoring any wound or painful area	0
Attention to wound	1

Question 4

   a) Look at the following caricatures. Circle the drawing which best depicts the cat's ear position?

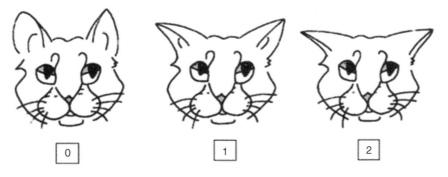

   b) Look at the shape of the muzzle in the following caricatures. Circle the drawing which appears most like that of the cat?

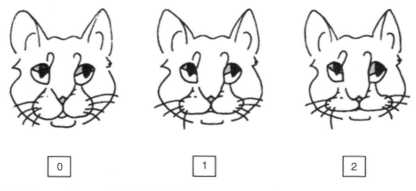

Figure 3.5 Glasgow Composite Pain Scale Feline.

Table 3.3 Tools for assessing acute pain in dogs.

Tool	Type	Condition	Reference
Glasgow composite measure pain scale-short-form	Behavior	Any surgical or medical pain	Holton *et al.* (2001), Reid *et al.* (2007), and Murrell *et al.* (2008)
French Association for Animal Anaesthesia and Analgesia pain scoring system (4A-Vet)	Behavior	Orthopaedic surgery	Rialland *et al.* (2012)
University of Melbourne Pain Scale	Behavior and physiologic data	Ovariohysterectomy	Firth and Haldane (1999)

Rehabilitation as a Treatment of Pain

The physical rehabilitation interventions aim to treat pain through techniques or modalities that:

1) Treat the cause of pain
2) Mask, hide, or modify the symptoms of pain

Treatment of the Cause of Pain

Chemical Pain

Inflammation as a Pain Cause

Aim: Promote resolution of inflammatory phase of healing (Veenman and Watson, 2008)
Methods:

- *Modalities* – ultrasound/laser/Pulsed Short Wave
- Diathermy (pulsed shortwave diathermy or PSWD) (Braid-Lewis, 2002)
- Cold

Ischemia as a Pain Cause

Aim: Improve blood flow (Veenman and Watson, 2008)
Methods:

- *Modalities* – ultrasound/PSWD/heat
- Active muscle contraction (manual techniques/muscle stimulation/exercise therapy)
- Manual techniques (example: lymphatic drainage)

Mechanical Pain

Aim: Alleviate abnormal force on normal tissue (Veenman and Watson, 2008)
Methods:

- Alleviate muscle spasms through medications or massage and acupressure
- Alleviate postural faults/muscle imbalance/compensatory movement patterns through therapeutic exercises

Aim: Restore normal mechanical properties to damaged tissue (Veenman and Watson, 2008)
Methods:

- Active and passive stretching
- Joint mobilization
- Rehabilitative exercise therapy

Neurogenic Pain

Aim: Alleviate adverse mechanical tension on nerves (Veenman and Watson, 2008)
Methods:

- Relieve muscle spasms through medications or massage and acupressure
- Mobilize connective tissue component of neural tissue where restricted

Treatment to Alter Pain Perception

Maximizing A-Beta Sensory Stimulation to Close the Pain Gate

Involves physiological manipulation of pathways involved in transmission and perception of painful sensations to mask, hide,

FELINE GRIMACE SCALE FACT SHEET

Evangelista et al. Facial expressions of pain in cats: the development and validation of a Feline Grimace Scale. Sci Rep 9, 19128 (2019)

WHY?

- Pain-induced behavioral changes are unique in cats and can be subtle

WHO?

- The instrument has been developed and validated to be used by veterinarians
- It is currently under testing for use by other veterinary care professionals

WHAT?

- The Feline Grimace Scale (FGS) is a simple method of acute pain assessment. It is based on changes in facial expressions and can be easily and quickly performed in the clinical setting
- It differentiates painful and non-painful cats and response to analgesic treatment

WHEN?

- The FGS is used for acute pain assessment in cats with medical, surgical or oral pain, etc.
- Pain assessment should be performed as often as needed and on a case-by-case basis

HOW?

- There are five action units (AU): ear position, orbital tightening, muzzle tension, whiskers position and head position
- Each AU is scored: 0 (absent), 1 (moderately present) or 2 (present)
- The final score is calculated by the sum of scores divided by the maximum possible scores
- Analgesic treatment is suggested when the final score is ≥4/10 or 0.4/1.0

0 = AU is absent

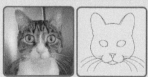

- Ears facing forward
- Eyes opened
- Muzzle relaxed (round shape)
- Whiskers loose and curved
- Head above the shoulder line

1 = AU is moderately present*

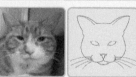

- Ears slightly pulled apart
- Eyes partially opened
- Muzzle mildly tense
- Whiskers slightly curved or straight
- Head aligned with the shoulder line

*The score of 1 can be also given when there is uncertainty over the presence or absence of the AU

2 = AU is markedly present

- Ears flattened and rotated outwards
- Squinted eyes
- Muzzle tense (elliptical shape)
- Whiskers straight and moving forward
- Head below the shoulder line or tilted down (chin towards the chest)

Steagall laboratory
felinegrimacescale@umontreal.ca

Faculté de médecine vétérinaire
Université de Montréal

Access the training manual
bit.ly/FGSmanual

Access the video
bit.ly/FGSvideo

Acknowledgement

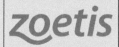

Figure 3.6 Feline Grimace Scale chart.

or modify the perception of pain (Veenman and Watson, 2008).

- The use of analgesics to alter pain perception
- Transcutaneous electrical stimulation (TENS): A-beta fiber stimulation to close the pain gate
- Massage
- Joint mobilization
- Manipulation
- Heat
- Cold

Stimulating the Production of Endogenous Opioids

- *TENS and endogenous opioid production* – Thirty minutes of low-frequency TENS (frequency 2–5 Hz, pulse width 200–250 μs) has been shown to raise opioid levels in spinal cord cerebrospinal fluid (CSF) by 400% in humans. Levels can remain elevated for up to six hours. High-frequency TENS results in no significant change in opioid levels (Han *et al.*, 1991).
- Electroacupuncture has been shown to increase β endorphin levels in dogs in dogs after ovariohysterectomy (Groppetti *et al.*, 2011) and to be equal to or better than phenylbutazone for treatment of chronic thoracolumbar pain in horses (Xie *et al.*, 2005).
- Manual techniques that may have a stimulatory effect on A-delta pathways leading to endogenous opiate release:
  - *Acupressure* – in a study on rats, acupressure raised the threshold to painful stimulus, and this was reversed by naloxone, an opioid inhibitor, implying the effect was through opioids (Trentini *et al.*, 2005).
  - *Trigger point release* – dry needling of trigger points in rabbits has been found to increase levels of endorphins (Hsieh *et al.*, 2012).
  - *Deep friction massage* – in a small number of human volunteers, deep tissue massage was found to release endorphins (Kaada and Torsteinbø, 1989).

Canine Rehabilitation

When Should Your Patient Be Assessed for Pain?

New patients should have a detailed history to correctly identify the animal's degree of pain and disability. Identifying how the patient copes with daily living activities creates a realistic picture of the patient's disability. Information regarding the following should be gathered (Davies, 2014a, b):

- Ability to ascend and descend stairs
- Ability to enter and exit vehicles
- Ability to cope with difficult surfaces such as wooden or tiled floors
- Ability to remain standing while eating
- Willingness to exercise and exercise tolerance
- Ability to remain squatting while defecating
- Ability to posture for urination
- Inappropriate elimination
- Willingness to play
- Change in demeanor
- Response to grooming
- Response or lack thereof to medication
- Effect of exercise on the lameness/pain
- Effect of rest on the lameness/pain
- Duration and intensity of the lameness/pain
- Changes in sleep patterns

One of the first questions you should ask the client (whether new or long-standing) is "has your pet appeared painful?" If the pet is on pain medication, then you should ask what medications these are and the dosages. Each time the patient is seen the client should be asked about any changes to medications or stoppage of a specific type of medication. Good communication will improve outcomes, and recent studies have shown that the relationship between the clinician and the patient and owner is of primary importance in successful management of chronic pain (Davies, 2014a, b).

During the certified rehabilitation veterinarian's clinical evaluation, several items will be assessed:

A) *Posture* – Assessment of posture during various positions (looking for kyphosis, lordosis, etc.), including transitions between those positions, for example, sit to down to stand. Postural adaptations may be due to pain, stiffness, weakness, or a combination.

B) *Objective measurements* – for example, goniometry to assess joint range of motion and compare for symmetry, muscle circumference measurements using a spring-weighted (Gulick) tape measure, and weight distribution using standing pressure platforms or scales.

C) *Response to palpation* – Palpation detects pain, muscle tone, resistance during passive motioning, and asymmetry (atrophy, swelling, fibrosis, etc.). Animals respond to a painful stimulus in a variety of ways, with a grimace or blink being a mild reaction, to flinch and aversion, to vocalization and aggression. This includes response during measurements taken. The aim of the diagnosing veterinarian is to begin with light digital pressure, sometimes using the hand to try to spread the load, this progresses to palpating more deeply to feel texture of the tissue and identify focal painful spots (tender and trigger points). A skilled veterinarian understands animal behavior and can recognize the difference between anxiety in response to touch and a pain response.

D) *Gait assessment* – This portion of the assessment allows grading of the severity of the lameness, localization of the lameness, and description of the gait in terms of cranial and caudal phases, arc of flight, and linearity of the movement.

E) *Neurological examination* – A neurological examination should always be part of the assessment to help differentiate poor motion due to stiffness and pain, from ataxia due to neurologic disease. Though neurologic disease is often painful, each has different rehabilitation requirements and prognosis.

The credentialed rehabilitation veterinary technician/nurse will be assisting with various aspects of these assessments.

Commonly used rehabilitation techniques that aid with pain management are:

- Cryotherapy
- Thermotherapy
- Therapeutic exercises
- Transcutaneous electrical nerve stimulation (TENS) or neuromuscular electrical stimulation (NMES)
- Low-level laser therapy (LLLT)
- Pulsed electromagnetic field therapy (PEMF)
- Extracorporeal shock wave treatment (ESWT)
- Acupuncture
- Manual therapies – massage, mobilizations, manipulations

(These therapies will be addressed in individual chapters for this textbook.)

Recognize the Link Between Pain and Weakness

Weakness is defined as reduced strength in one or more muscles (Medline Plus, 2023). Weakness may be caused by diseases or conditions affecting many different body

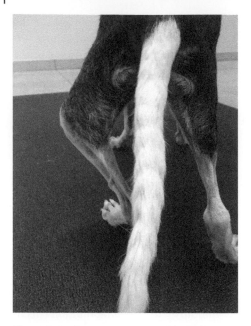

Figure 3.7 Severe osteoarthritis deformity rear view. *Source:* With permission from MEG.

systems. It is generally accepted that muscle weakness in osteoarthritis (OA) is due to its atrophy, which is believed to be secondary to joint pain (arthrogenic muscle inhibition) (Valderrabano and Steiger, 2010) (see Figure 3.7). Persons with chronic hip joint pain have weakness in the hip rotator and hip abductor muscles (Harris-Hayes *et al.*, 2014). It has been determined that both muscle and joint pain are associated with reductions in quality of life (Vasiliadis *et al.*, 2002). In cats with lumbosacral intervertebral disk disease, clinical signs included reluctance to jump, low tail carriage, elimination outside the litter box, reluctance to ambulate, pelvic-limb paresis, urinary incontinence, and constipation (Harris and Dhupa, 2008). Canine and feline muscle contracture is reported to affect several different muscles. The clinical signs include lameness, pain, weakness, decreased range of motion, a firmness noted throughout the entire muscle, and usually a characteristic gait. Pre-disposing factors for muscle contracture include

compartment syndrome, infection, trauma, repetitive strains, fractures, infectious diseases, immune-mediated diseases, neoplasia, and ischemia (Taylor and Tangner, 2007). From the studies in humans and animals, it appears that muscle weakness can occur because of pain. Therefore, be sure to look at patients that have muscle atrophy. Bring this to the attention of the rehabilitation veterinarian and be sure to question the client about a decline in activity to determine how much pain is involved. A trial of pain medication can help to differentiate weakness due principally to pain, from other causes.

Environmental Modifications

By having a conversation with the client, you can help to determine if some simple modifications to the home environment will aid mobility and reduce pain. Slippery floors are detrimental to the aging patient. Non-skid area rugs, flooring used in children's play areas, and rubber-backed mats are examples of how the owner can make the home more comfortable for a painful patient. Raising the water and food bowl off the floor and standing on a non-skid surface makes mealtime more comfortable. Ramps can be utilized for getting into and out of vehicles. Child restraint gates may be useful at the top and bottom of stairs. Memory foam or eggshell foam may help make sleeping more comfortable. Slings and assistive devices may be helpful.

Owners should be asked questions such as:

- Is the pet an indoor or outdoor pet?
- If the pet is indoors, does the home have steps that the pet must navigate?
- Does the pet sleep in the owner's bed?
- Does the pet travel in the car?
- What type of flooring is in the house, and what type of terrain is outside?

Questionnaires regarding mobility and activities of daily living will help determine how much care the pet may need to maintain quality of life (Shearer, 2011). Facilitating a referral to a specialist in pet rehabilitation or pain management is highly recommended to ensure that the pet owner is aware of all aspects of care that may improve a pets quality of life. Many pets benefit from physical rehabilitation and pain management. A veterinarian should look for facilities that have certified rehabilitation veterinarians for advanced care for mobility-impaired pets. Pain is often associated with mobility challenges and should be treated immediately or anticipated and prevented. For a pet with hard-to-manage pain, referral to a specialist may be critical. One remedy for caring for a pet that is experiencing pain is to give pain medications one or two hours before coming to the rehabilitation session (Millis *et al.*, 2014). Signs of pain when performing everyday care or care at the rehabilitation session include biting, scratching, whimpering, crying out, moaning, wiggling, struggling, reluctance to move, and resisting the care (Shearer, 2011; Box 3.3).

Box 3.3   Mobility questionnaire – Does your pet have signs of pain?

Pet's name_____ Owner's name_____
Breed_____ Age_____

In general, how do you rate your pet's health?
___Excellent ___Very Good ___Good ___Fair ___Poor

Has your pet ever seen a veterinarian because of joint pain, stiffness, or limping?
___Yes, Details_____
___No

Living in pain can lead to changes in behavior. This can be hard to read in a pet. On average, would you say your pet is: (Choose one)
___Completely uninterested in their surroundings and sleep all the time
___Will show interest, but no longer comes to greet you
___Mostly interested in life and food, but reluctant to play
___Plays only when encouraged and not for long
___Has had no change in personality

Has your pet's activity level changed?
___Seeks more affection than usual   ___Trembling
___Reluctant to move   ___Circling
___Difficulty getting up from a laying position   ___ Lying very still
___Repetitively gets up and lays down   ___Becomes restless

Has your pet's appetite/thirst changed?
___Yes   ___No

Does your pet have trouble in areas he never used to need assistance?
___Stairs
   ___cannot manage any steps without assistance
   ___cannot manage a full flight of steps (only 2-4 steps alone)
   ___manages a full flight of steps, but has difficulty
   ___Can only go upstairs without assistance
   ___Can only go downstairs without assistance
   ___No problems on stairs
___Jumping
   ___Cannot jump onto the furniture without assistance
   ___Cannot get into your vehicle without assistance
   ___Has no problem jumping

Has your pet become protective of himself?
___Protects hurt body part   ___Hides
___Doesn't put weight on a limb   ___Limps
___Doesn't want to be held or picked up
Does your pet have pain, swelling, warmth, or stiffness in one or more legs?
___Yes, only one joint   ___Very rarely
___Yes, in a few joints   ___Never
___Yes, in many joints

How long can your pet walk without getting tired, limping, or stopping?
___ Less than 5 minutes
___10 to 20 minutes
___more than 30 minutes/ my pet doesn't get tired or sore
___He does not show signs until after he is done walking and rests for a while (he will stiffen up)

Does your pet favor one side of his body more than the other?
___Yes, Describe_____
___No

Did your pet's signs begin slowly or suddenly?
___Slowly, over the course of a few months
___Suddenly, within days or a few weeks

Has the joint pain suddenly gotten worse?
___Within the past few days
___Within the past few weeks
___No

In the morning, are the affected areas stiff for more than half an hour?
___Yes ___No ___There is no morning stiffness

Has your pet had a joint/bone injury or surgery?
___Yes, Details_____
___No
___Unsure (Adopted)

Which of the following methods do you use to manage the pain, swelling, or stiffness? (Check all that apply.)
___Physical activity/exercise
___Nutritional supplements (fish oils, vitamins)
___Weight management
___Physical therapy/chiropractic/massage
___Cold or heat treatment
___medication
___Other_____
___None of the above

Which medication and/or joint supplements do you currently use? (Check all that apply.)
___Prescription medication from veterinarian_____
___Over-the-counter medication_____
___Aspirin
___Glucosamine human medication(brand)_____
___Veterinary joint supplement (brand) _____
___Herbal supplement (brand) _____
___Other_____
___None of the above

Does your pet have any of the following conditions? (Check all that apply.)
___Kidney disease   ___Skin disease
___Liver disease   ___Active infection
___Lung disease   ___Bladder problems
___Cardiovascular disease   ___Other

Is there anything else we should know about your pet? _____
_____
_____

Questionnaire Created by Dr. Julia Tomlinson

Painful Mobility Issues in Geriatrics

Dr. Julia Tomlinson DACVSMR (https://www.vetromp.com/) states that in her practice she sees two types of geriatric pets with painful mobility issues: the aging, often overweight pet with little systemic disease and varying amounts of physical disability; and the extremely frail, geriatric pet with reduced appetite, weight loss, concurrent diseases, and more extreme loss of strength and mobility (Tomlinson, 2012). Pain needs to be well controlled before strengthening begins so first she works on improving pain and flexibility. Very simple techniques such as range of motion (ROM) exercises and stretching can be taught to clients. Handouts with pictures are very helpful and can be referred to when the therapist is not there to give advice. **The exercises MUST be demonstrated for the client and then the client repeat the exercise back to the demonstrator to ensure it is being performed properly.** "Pain during the motion must be avoided as much as possible and the fine art of adequate pressure, but not too much is a difficult one to teach." It is not until several weeks of this therapy have been completed that Dr. Tomlinson will move on to strengthening and balance exercises.

Feline Physical Rehabilitation

Feline physical rehabilitation involves the diagnosis and management of painful or functionally limiting conditions. The goals are to treat injury or illness, decrease pain, restore function, and achieve the highest level of independence, function, and quality of life for the patient (Goldberg, 2022). Cats are most often referred to rehabilitation facilities for osteoarthritis, fractures, neurologic conditions, femoral head and neck excision, and weight reduction (Goldberg, 2016).

10 Things to Know for Cat Pain and Physical Rehabilitation

1) Videos of a cats activity, prior to each appointment, can be instructive for the veterinary team when deciding which rehabilitation therapies to provide.
2) Administration of gabapentin (25–100 mg/cat orally) two hours prior to the visit could lessen stress (reduced dose for cats with chronic kidney disease [CKD]).

3) Identify a quiet, secure room for the cat to explore before therapy is begun. Use pheromone diffusers in the room, and towels or sprays prior to each session.
4) Have equipment already placed in the room for the cat to view and smell?
5) Behavioral knowledge of cats and an understanding of how to adjust to each cat is imperative.
6) Knowledge about how cats act when in pain is a requirement.
7) Prioritize which therapies for pain are most important and utilize those first even if the session is kept short until subsequent sessions when pain is less.
8) Keep exercises fun resembling play time or hunting prey.
9) Hydrotherapy should be introduced slowly. Allow the cat to adjust to the tank and learn about the movement of the treadmill prior to filling it with water.
10) Above all else, be flexible with the rehabilitation plan. Plans may be made ahead of time but rethinking the plan for each session may be needed. Never try to force a cat to perform an activity that they are unwilling to do on a specific day.

Cats show pain by changes in their behavior, activity, and personality (see Table 3.4). Our ability to point out these behavioral changes to caregivers can encourage them to watch for these pain-related behaviors at home. This is especially important for cats, as the most common cause of chronic pain in this species is degenerative joint disease, which in the cat most commonly includes osteoarthritis and spondylosis deformans of the intervertebral disc. It presents primarily as behavioral changes which caregivers are best positioned to detect (Gruen et al., 2022).

Cats often make willing patients, but rehabilitation sessions should be kept short and interesting and should be undertaken in a

Table 3.4 Changes in cats indicating pain.

Changes in mobility	Changes in behavior
More hesitant or less able to jump up and/or down	Increased hiding
More hesitant or less able to go up and/or downstairs	House-soiling
More hesitant or less able to run	Increased or decreased grooming
Less active or willing to play	Increased aggression
Changes in posture while playing	Changes in temperament
	Sensitive to touch
	Decreased appetite

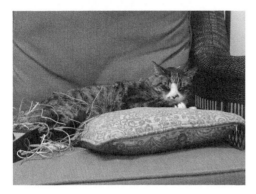

Figure 3.8 Calvin on a couch electroacupuncture. *Source:* With permission from Dr. Sheilah Robertson.

quiet, relaxed environment (Goldberg, 2016). Setting up for feline rehabilitation therapy requires prioritization of what therapies are most important for the cats pain (e.g., underwater treadmill, acupuncture, photobiomodulation, therapeutic exercises). Acupuncture is a recommended option early in the treatment regime for any patient that is painful, especially until such time as balanced analgesia is achieved with other multimodal options (Goldberg, 2022). Acupuncture may be one of a few treatments, or the sole option for analgesia, especially if the patient has kidney or liver disease limiting the analgesic drugs that can be used (see Figure 3.8). Some patients benefit from ongoing acupuncture treatment. Therapeutic lasers (photobiomodulation) could be used along with acupuncture in these patients to help with pain.

After several sessions of acupuncture in the senior patient, movement maybe not so painful, and therapeutic exercise can be initiated.

Heat therapy is used to help relax tissues, sometimes prior to other forms of treatment and to decrease pain and improve blood flow, which aids healing. It can be used to improve muscle and soft tissue movement and to help with joint range (Halkett and Romano, 2018). Cold therapy can sometimes be applied in the first few days following trauma and is most effective in the first 72 hours. It can be used longer term after exercise where inflammation may occur. Cold packs provide pain relief, reduce inflammation and swelling, and help control bleeding (Halkett and Romano, 2018).

The rehabilitation technician or nurse should be prepared to instruct the owner in a home exercise program for the cat. It is best to provide written and verbal instructions and hands-on demonstrations for clients, then have the clients perform the exercises while still in the facility to ensure they understand the instructions and are performing the exercises correctly (Goldberg, 2016).

The owner should be encouraged to interact with the cat and engage it in play for several minutes at least three times a day (or according to the preference of the individual cat) to encourage exercise and

> **Box 3.4   Home modifications to help cats with osteoarthritis**
>
> - Secure hiding places
> - Stairs or ramps to alleviate sore joints
> - Litterboxes that have easy access (cutout section or lower sides)
> - Scratching posts that are horizontal instead of vertical for patients with abnormal joint motion
> - Raised food and water bowls for patients with stiffness in elbows, shoulders, or spine
> - Padded, comfortable bedding
> - Non-slip flooring (e.g., yoga mats)

mental stimulation. Using different toys or alternating play techniques and locations is likewise helpful. Some cats may even be amenable to outdoor exercise on a leash or harness. Simple home modifications that can help cats with osteoarthritis are listed in Box 3.4.

Physical rehabilitation for cats differs from rehabilitation for dogs. The plan must be creative, fun, easy to follow, and composed of short sessions to reduce the risk of causing anxiety or frustration. Ultimately, feline patients will benefit from a rehabilitation program just like any patient. It is all a matter of learning to speak "cat."

Equine Rehabilitation

Equitation involves close contact between horse and rider. Most presenting horses are athletes of some form; thus, the rider expects a full return to function. Because of this, the Certified Equine Rehabilitation Practitioner (CERP) or Diplomate of the American College of Veterinary Sports Medicine and Rehabilitation must evaluate the horse, the farrier, the saddle fit, and the role of the rider in causing or magnifying the lameness (Davies, 2014a, b). The rider may need to undergo their own rehabilitation program if problems are caused by the rider's posture and balance, collaboration with a physical therapist or chiropractor treating the rider is beneficial. An entire chapter in this text is devoted to equine rehabilitation (see Chapter 23).

Pain Assessment for Horses

Behavioral changes that are associated with pain in the horse may include kicking or biting when the tender area is touched, generalized restlessness, sweating, frequent movement of the painful limb, or continuous shifting of weight from one limb to another (Davies, 2014a, b). Changes associated with back pain, such as poor performance, poor appetite, and slight changes in demeanor may be very subtle initially. These may progress to tail swishing or holding the tail to one side, bruxism, head shaking, resistance to saddling and grooming, loss of flexibility, stumbling, bucking, and rearing (Marks, 2000; Paulekas and Haussler, 2009). The horse may be withdrawn, and the abdomen may have tight abdominal muscles or appear to be "tucked-up." The horse's breed and temperament must also be assessed.

Objective measurements of pain in the horse that may be of assistance in diagnosing and treating pain include heart rate (not consistently increased in pain), respiratory rate, pressure algometry, thermography, kinematic gait analysis, and response to analgesia (e.g., nerve blocks). The horse may be placed on analgesics (usually NSAIDS) as a trial to see if pain is present. If the problem does not improve with this single medication, then the horse is often incorrectly declared to not be in pain. This can lead to much more severe riding or controlling techniques (e.g., double twisted wire bit) being used on a painful horse to "control" perceived bad behavior when the problem is actually a normal response to pain.

The credentialed rehabilitation veterinary technician will be assisting the CERP veterinarian in carrying out the treatment plan for alleviation of this pain. Initially, the work is all on the ground to strengthen the abdominals and core musculature, followed by introduction of a rider (Davies, 2014a, b).

Ways to treat equine pain include:

1) Analgesics
2) Acupuncture
3) Physical rehabilitation therapy
4) Local heat
5) Osteopathy
6) Veterinary spinal manipulation or "Veterinary Chiropractic"
7) Massage

Conclusion

The certified rehabilitation veterinarian, certified rehabilitation veterinary technician, physical therapist, and owner must work as a **team** to have successful management of pain and restore the patient (no matter what species) to a functional life. Each animal should have its own tailored plan. Nothing should be "cook-book" in this process. The aim should be to restore the patient to an active and pain-free lifestyle, whether this is in the context of a leisurely walk or full athletic activity (Davies, 2014a, b).

Resources

https://www.aaha.org/aaha-guidelines/2022-aaha-pain-management-guidelines-for-dogs-and-cats/home/.

https://wsava.org/Global-Guidelines/Global-Pain-Council-Guidelines/.

Bockstahler, B. and Levine, D. (2011). Physical therapy and rehabilitation. In: *The Feline Patient*, 4the (ed. G.D. Norsworthy), 687–690. Ames, IA: John Wiley & Sons, Inc.

Bockstahler, B. and Levine, D. (2012). Physical therapy and rehabilitation. In: *Nursing the Feline Patient* (ed. L.E. Schmeltzer and G.D. Norsworthy), 138–144. Ames, IA: John Wiley & Sons, Inc.

Drum, M.G., Bockstahler, B., and Levine, D. (2015). Feline rehabilitation. *Vet Clin North Am Small Anim Pract* 45: 185–201.

Medina, C. and Robertson, S. (2015). Non-pharmacological pain management in cats. *Feline Focus* 1 (6): 195–199.

Sharp, B. (2012). Feline physiotherapy and rehabilitation. 1. Principles and potential. *J Feline Med Surg* 14: 622–632.

Sharp, B. (2012). Feline physiotherapy and rehabilitation. 2. Clinical application. *J Feline Med Surg* 14: 633–645.

Langford, D.J., Bailey, A.L., Chanda, M.L., and Clarke, S.E. (2010). Coding facial expressions of pain in the laboratory mouse. *Nat Methods* 7 (6): 448.

Sotocinal, S.G., Sorge, R.E., Zaloum, A. et al. (2011). The Rat Grimace Scale: A partially automated method for quantifying pain in the laboratory rat via facial expressions. *Mol Pain* 7: 55.

Edmunson, A.M., Boynton, F.D.D., Rendahl, A.K. et al. (2021). Indicators of postoperative pain in Syrian hamsters (*mesocricetus auratus*). *Comp Med* 71 (1): 76–85. Available at: 10.30802/aalas-cm-20-990056.

Keating, S.C.J., Thomas, A.A., Flecknell, P.A., and Leach, M.C. (2012). Evaluation of EMLA cream for preventing pain during tattooing of rabbits: Changes in physiological, behavioural and facial expression responses. *PloS One* 7 (9): e44437.

Reijgwart, M.L., Schoemaker, N.J., Pascuzzo, R. et al. (2017). The composition and initial evaluation of a grimace scale in ferrets after surgical implantation of a telemetry probe. *PloS One* 12 (11): e0187986.

Dalla Costa, E., Minero, M., Lebelt, D. et al. (2014). Development of the horse grimace scale (HGS) as a pain assessment tool in horses undergoing routine castration. *PloS One* 9 (3): e92281.

Orth, E.K., Navas, G.F., Pastrana, C.I. et al. (2020). Development of a donkey grimace scale to recognize pain in donkeys (Equus asinus) post castration. *Animals* 10: 1411. https://doi.org/10.3390/ani10081411.

Tomacheuski, R.M., Monteiro, B.P., Evangelista, M.C. et al. (2021). Measurement properties of pain scoring instruments in farm animals: A systematic review protocol using the Cosmin Checklist. *PLOS One* 16 (5): e0251435. Available at: https://doi.org/10.1371/journal.pone.0251435.

Gleerupa, K.B., Andersenb, P.H., Munksgaardc, L., and Forkmanaa, B. (2015). Pain evaluation in dairy cattle. *Appl Anim Behav Sci* 171 (25): 32.

McLennan, K.M., Rebelo, C.J.B., Corke, M.J. et al. (2016). Development of a facial expression scale using footrot and mastitis as models of pain in sheep. *Appl Anim Behav Sci* 176 (19): 26.

Muri, K. and Valle, P.S. (2012). Human animal relationships in the Norwegian dairy goat industry: Assessment of pain and provision of veterinary treatment (Part II). *Anim Welfare* 21 (547): 558.

Giminiani, P.D., Brierley, V.L.M.H., Scollo, A. et al. (2016). The assessment of facial expressions in piglets undergoing tail docking and castration: Toward the development of the piglet grimace scale. *Front Vet Sci.* 3: 100. https://doi.org/10.3389/fvets.2016.00100. PMID: 27896270; PMCID: PMC5107875.

Holden, E., Calvo, G., Collins, M. et al. (2014). Evaluation of facial expression in acute pain in cats. *J Small Anim Pract* 55: 615–621.

References

Belli, M., de Oliveira, A.R., de Lima, M.T. et al. (2021). Clinical validation of the short and long UNESP-Botucatu scales for feline pain assessment. *Peer J* 9: e11225.

Braid-Lewis, D. (2002). Electrotherapy – A guide for practitioners. *UK Vet* 7 (7): 43–48.

Brondani, J.T., Mama, K.R., Luna, S.P. et al. (2013). Validation of the English version of the UNESP-Botucatu multidimensional composite pain scale for assessing postoperative pain in cats. *BMC Vet Res* 9: 143.

Brown, D.C., Boston, R.C., Coyne, J.C. et al. (2008). Ability of the canine brief pain inventory to detect response to treatment in dogs with osteoarthritis. *J Am Vet Med Assoc* 233: 1278–1283.

Bucknoff, M. (2019). Pain: The underdiscussed vital sign. *Vet Pract News* https://www.veterinarypracticenews.com/pain-management-september-2019/.

Cachon, T., Frykman, O., Innes, J.F. et al. (2018). Face validity of a proposed tool for staging canine osteoarthritis: Canine OsteoArthritis Staging Tool (COAST). *Vet J* 235: 1–8. https://doi.org/10.1016/j.tvjl.2018.02.017. Epub 2018 Feb 27. PMID: 29704933.

Davies, L. (2014a). Chapter 11: Canine rehabilitation. In: *Pain Management in Veterinary Practice* (ed. C. Egger, L. Love, and T. Doherty), 133–146. Ames, IA: John Wiley & Sons, Inc.

Davies L (2014b) Chapter 12: Equine rehabilitation. In *Pain Management in Veterinary Practice*, 1st edn (eds. CM Egger, L Love, and T Doherty). John Wiley and Sons, Inc, Ames, IA, pp. 147–154.

Enomoto, M., Lascelles, B.D.X., Robertson, J.B., and Gruen, M.E. (2022). Refinement of the Feline Musculoskeletal Pain Index (FMPI) and development of the short-form FMPI. *J Feline Med Surg* 24 (2): 142–151. https://doi.org/10.1177/1098612X211011984. Epub 2021 May 18. PMID: 34002643.

Essner, A., Zetterberg, L., Hellström, K. et al. (2017). Psychometric evaluation of the canine brief pain inventory in a Swedish sample of dogs with pain related to osteoarthritis. *Acta Vet Scand* 59 (1): 44. https://doi.org/10.1186/s13028-017-0311-2. Erratum in: *Acta Vet Scand* 2017 Jul 25;59(1):50. PMID: 28668080; PMCID: PMC5493851.

Evangelista, M.C., Watanabe, R., Leung, V.S.Y. et al. (2019). Facial expressions of pain in cats: The development and validation of a feline grimace scale. *Sci Rep* 9: 19128.

Evangelista, M.C., Benito, J., Monteiro, B.P. et al. (2020). Clinical applicability of the feline grimace scale: Real-time versus image scoring and the influence of sedation and surgery. *Peer J* 8: e8967.

Evangelista, M.C., Monteiro, B.P., and Steagall, P.V. (2021). Measurement properties of grimace scales for pain assessment in nonhuman mammals: A systematic review. *Pain* 163: e697–e714.

Firth, A.M. and Haldane, S.L. (1999). Development of a scale to evaluate postoperative pain in dogs. *J Am Vet Med Assoc* 214: 651–659.

Flaherty, M.J. (2019). Rehabilitation therapy in perioperative pain management. *Vet Clin North Am Small Anim Pract* 49 (6): 1143–1156. https://doi.org/10.1016/j.cvsm.2019.07.006. Epub 2019 Aug 28. PMID: 31473030.

Frank, L.R. and Roynard, P.F.P. (2018). Veterinary neurologic rehabilitation: The rationale for a comprehensive approach. *Top Companion Anim Med* 33 (2): 49–57. https://doi.org/10.1053/j.tcam.2018.04.002. Epub 2018 May 16. PMID: 30236409.

Gingerich DA and Strobel JD (2003) Use of client-specific outcome measures to assess treatment effects in geriatric, arthritic dogs: Controlled clinical evaluation of a nutraceutical. *Vet Ther* 4(1):56–66. 12756636.

Goldberg ME (2016) Feline Physical Rehabilitation, Today's Veterinary Nurse, November/December. 1–10 https://todaysveterinarynurse.com/rehabilitation/feline-physical-rehabilitation/.

Goldberg, M.E. (2022). An overview of feline pain management through physical rehabilitation. *Feline Pract* 1: 45–48.

Groppetti, D., Pecile, A.M., Sacerdote, P. et al. (2011). Effectiveness of electroacupuncture analgesia compared with opioid administration in a dog model: A pilot study. *Br J Anaesth* 107 (4): 612–618.

Gruen, M.E., BDX, L., Colleran, E. et al. (2022). AAHA pain management guidelines for dogs and cats. *J Am Anim Hosp Assoc* 58: 55–76. https://doi.org/10.5326/JAAHA-MS-7292.

Halkett, E.V.C. and Romano, L. (2018). Rehabilitation of the feline patient: Physiotherapy treatment as part of a multidisciplinary team approach – Part 1. *Vet Nurse* 8 (10): 548–552.

Han, J., Chen, X., Sun, S. et al. (1991). Effect of low and high frequency TENS on Met-enkephalin-Arg-Phe and dynorphin A immunoreactivity in human lumbar CSF. *Pain* 47 (3): 295–298.

Harris, J.E. and Dhupa, S. (2008). Lumbosacral intervertebral disk disease in six cats. *J Am Anim Hosp Assoc* 44 (3): 109–115.

Harris-Hayes, M., Mueller, M.J., Sahrmann, S.A. et al. (2014). Persons with chronic hip joint pain exhibit reduced hip muscle strength. *J Orthop Sports Phys Ther* 44 (11): 890–898.

von Hehn, C.A., Baron, R., and Woolf, C.J. (2012). Deconstructing the neuropathic pain phenotype to reveal neural mechanisms. *Neuron* 73 (638): 52.

Hielm-Björkman, A.K., Rita, H., and Tulamo, R.M. (2009). Psychometric testing of the Helsinki chronic pain index by completion of a questionnaire in Finnish by owners of dogs with chronic signs of pain caused by osteoarthritis. *Am J Vet Res* 70: 727–734.

Vasiliadis, H.M.I., Collet, J.P., Shapiro, S. et al. (2002). Predictive factors and correlates for pain in postpoliomyelitis syndrome patients. *Arch Phys Med Rehabil* 83 (8): 1109–1115.

Holden, E., Calvo, G., Collins, M. et al. (2014). Evaluation of facial expression in acute pain in cats. *J Small Anim Pract* 55: 615–621.

Holton, L., Reid, J., Scott, E.M. et al. (2001). Development of a behaviour-based scale to measure acute pain in dogs. *Vet Rec* 148: 525–531.

Hsieh, Y.L., Yang, S.A., Yang, C.C., and Chou, L.W. (2012). Dry needling at myofascial trigger spots of rabbit skeletal muscles modulates the biochemicals associated with pain, inflammation, and hypoxia. *Evid Based Complement Alternat Med* 2012: 342165. https://doi.org/10.1155/2012/342165. PMID: 23346198; PMCID: PMC3544533.

International Association for the Study of Pain (2023) https://www.iasp-pain.org/wp-content/uploads/2022/04/revised-definition-flysheet_R2.pdf.

Kaada, B. and Torsteinbø, O. (1989). Increase of plasma beta-endorphins in connective tissue massage. *Gen Pharmacol* 20 (4): 487–489.

Karas A (2011) Pain, anxiety, or dysphoria – How to tell? A video assessment lab. https://www.acvs.org/files/proceedings/2011/data/papers/174.pdf, *Proceedings from the American College of Veterinary Surgeons*.

Klinck, M.P., Frank, D., Guillot, M., and Troncy, E. (2012). Owner-perceived signs and veterinary diagnosis in 50 cases of Feline osteoarthritis. *Can Vet J* 53: 1181–1186.

Klinck, M.P., Gruen, M.E., del Castillo, J.R.E. et al. (2018a). Development and preliminary validity and reliability of the montreal instrument for cat arthritis testing, for use by caretaker/owner, MI-CAT(C), via a randomised clinical trial. *Appl Anim Behav Sci* 200: 96–105.2.

Klinck, M.P., Monteiro, B.P., Lussier, B. et al. (2018b). Refinement of the montreal instrument for cat arthritis testing, for use by veterinarians: Detection of naturally occurring osteoarthritis in laboratory cats. *J Feline Med Surg* 20: 728–740.

Lascelles, B.D., Hansen, B.D., Roe, S. et al. (2007). Evaluation of client-specific outcome measures and activity monitoring to measure pain relief in cats with osteoarthritis. *J Vet Intern Med* May-Jun;21(3):410–416. doi: 10.1892/0891-6640 (2007)21[410,eocoma]2.0.co;2. PMID: 17552444.

Luna, S.P.L., Trindade, P.H.E., Monteiro, B.P. et al. (2022). Multilingual validation of the short form of the UNESP-Botucatu feline pain scale (ufeps-sf). *Peer J* 10: e13134.

Maier, S.F. and Watkins, L.R. (1998). Cytokines for psychologists: Implications of bidirectional immune to brain communication for understanding behavior mood, and cognition. *Psychol Rev* 105 (83): 107.

Marks, D. (2000). Conformation and soundness. *Am Assoc Equine Practitioners' Proc* 46: 39–45.

Medline Plus 2023 National Library of Medicine https://medlineplus.gov/ency/article/003174.htm (accessed January 24, 2023).

Millis DL and Ciuperca IA (2015) Evidence for canine rehabilitation and physical therapy. *Vet Clin North Am Small Anim Pract* 45(1):1–27. https://doi.org/10.1016/j.cvsm.2014.09.001. 25432679.

Millis, D., Lewelling, A., and Hamilton, S. (2014). Range-of-motion and stretching exercises. In: *Canine Rehabilitation and Physical Therapy*, 2nde (ed. D. Millis, D. Levine, and R. Taylor), 228–243. Philadelphia: Saunders.

Monteiro, B.P., Lascelles, B.D.X., Murrell, J. et al. (2022). 2022 WSAVA guidelines for the recognition, assessment, and treatment of pain. *J Small Anim Prac* https://doi.org/10.1111/jsap.13566.

Muir, W.W. and Woolf, C.J. (2001). Mechanisms of pain and their therapeutic implications. *JAVMA* 219 (10): 1346–1356.

Murrell, J.C., Psatha, E.P., Scott, E.M. et al. (2008). Application of a modified form of the Glasgow pain scale in a veterinary teaching centre in the Netherlands. *Vet Rec* 162: 403–408.

Neal Webb, S.J., Bridges, J.P., Thiele, E. et al. (2020). The implementation and initial evaluation of a physical therapy program for captive chimpanzees (Pan troglodytes). *Am J Primatol* 82 (3): e23109. https://doi.org/10.1002/ajp.23109. Epub 2020 Feb 20. PMID: 32077522; PMCID: PMC7164683.

Paulekas, R. and Haussler, K.K. (2009). Principles, and practice of therapeutic exercises for horses. *J Equine Vet* 29: 870–893.

Petersen AM and Pedersen BK (1985) The anti-inflammatory effect of exercise. *J Appl Physiol* 98(4):1154–1162. https://doi.org/10.1152/japplphysiol.00164.2004. 15772055.

Reid, J., Nolan, A.M., Hughes, J.M.L. et al. (2007). Development of the short-form Glasgow composite measure pain scale (CMPS-SF) and derivation of an analgesic intervention score. *Animal Welfare* 16: 97–104.

Reid, J., Scott, E.M., Calvo, G. et al. (2017). Definitive Glasgow acute pain scale for cats: Validation and intervention level. *Vet Rec* 180: 449.

Rialland, P., Authier, S., Guillot, M. et al. (2012). Validation of orthopedic postoperative pain assessment methods for dogs: A prospective, blinded, randomized, placebocontrolled study. *PloS One* 7: e49480.

Richmond, M. (2016). Should pain be the fourth vital sign? *Vet Nurs J* 31 (8): 249–252. https://doi.org/10.1080/1741534 9.2016.1192966.

Riviere, S. (2007). Physiotherapy for cats and dogs applied to locomotor disorders of arthritic origin. *Vet Focus* 17 (3): 32–36.

Sharp, B. (2008). Physiotherapy in small animal practice. *In Pract* 30: 190–199.

Shearer, T.S. (2011). Managing mobility challenges in palliative and hospice care patients. *Vet Clin Small Anim* 41 (2011): 609–617.

Taylor, J. and Tangner, C.H. (2007). Acquired muscle contractures in the dog and cat. A review of the literature and case report. *Vet Comp Orthop Traumatol* 20 (2): 79–85.

Tomlinson JE (2012) Rehabilitation and pain management as aging wellness strategies. *Proceedings North American Veterinary Conference*, Orlando, Florida. 1065–1066.

Trentini, J.F., Thompson, B., and Erlichman, J.S. (2005). The antinociceptive effect of acupressure in rats. *Am J Chin Med* 33 (1): 143–150.

Valderrabano, V. and Steiger, C. (2010). Treatment and prevention of osteoarthritis through exercise and sports review article. *J Aging Res* 374653. https://doi.org/10.4061/2011/374653.

Veenman, P. and Watson, T. (2008). A physiotherapy perspective on pain management. *Vet Nurs J* 23 (4): 29–35.

Walton, M.B., Cowderoy, E., Lascelles, D., and Innes, J.F. (2013). Evaluation of construct and criterion validity for the 'Liverpool Osteoarthritis in Dogs' (LOAD) clinical metrology instrument and comparison to two other instruments. *PloS One* 8 (3): e58125. https://doi.org/10.1371/journal.pone.0058125.

Watanabe, R., Doodnaught, G.M., Evangelista, M.C. et al. (2020a). Inter-rater reliability of the Feline Grimace Scale in cats undergoing dental extractions. *Front Vet Sci* 7: 302.

Wiseman-Orr ML, Scott EM, Reid J, and Nolan AM (2006) Validation of a structured questionnaire as an instrument to measure chronic pain in dogs on the basis of effects on health-related quality of life. *Am J Vet Res* 67(11):1826–1836. https://doi.org/10.2460/ajvr.67.11.1826. 17078742.

Xie, H., Colahan, P., and Ott, E.A. (2005). Evaluation of electroacupuncture treatment of horses with signs of chronic thoracolumbar pain. *J Am Vet Med Assoc* 227 (2): 281–286.

4

Communicating the Treatment Plan

Tracy A. Darling[1], Julia E. Tomlinson[2,3], and Cynthia M. Otto[4]

[1] *Director of Canine Operations, National Disaster Search Dog Foundation, Santa Paula, CA, USA*

[2] *Twin Cities Animal Rehabilitation & Sports Medicine Clinic, Burnsville, MN, USA*

[3] *Veterinary Rehabilitation and Orthopedic Medicine Partners, San Clemente, CA, USA*

[4] *Director, Penn Vet Working Dog Center, Professor of Working Dog Sciences & Sports Medicine, University of Pennsylvania, School of Veterinary Medicine, Philadelphia, PA, USA*

CHAPTER MENU

Introduction

Veterinary patients with conditions that necessitate physical rehabilitation programs are often prescribed prolonged therapy. Sessions may be required daily or several times per week, and treatment often extends over many weeks or months. Whether the patient needs to be brought into the rehabilitation practice for therapy or is prescribed a home exercise program, it requires a serious commitment from the patient's owner/caregiver. Rehabilitation does not guarantee a complete return to function, and setbacks and/or failures are not uncommon. Thorough owner/caregiver communication regarding the treatment plan, benchmarks of progress, and expected results is essential in order to achieve a satisfactory outcome. The client/caregiver will almost always be asked to actively participate in some portion of the rehabilitation program. It is essential that the owner/caregiver has a good understanding of the basic theoretical, technical, and behavioral components of the exercises/techniques in order to safely, properly, and effectively assist with the rehabilitation plan. By understanding the basic rationale for the components of the plan, the client will have a greater investment and motivation to adhere to the prescribed plan. Incomplete or inaccurate understanding of techniques can lead to injury or failure to achieve a maximal recovery. Some owners/caregivers do not fully understand animal behavior and may misinterpret signs of stress in their pets. For the plan to be effective and fun for both the owner/caregiver and the pet, minimizing behavioral stress is critical. It is often the veterinary technician's role to provide this important client education.

Diagnosis and Progress Assessments

While clients do not always need or want a thorough understanding of the pathophysiology of the patient's disorder, at least a basic understanding of the diagnosis and dysfunction is important in order for the caregiver to be an active participant in the rehabilitation program. The veterinary technician should have a good understanding of the patient's diagnosis and the expected progression of healing (from specific tissue pathology to whole-body function) in order to answer questions that arise during rehabilitation visits.

Progress assessment markers (see Table 4.1), such as goniometry, pain scoring systems, muscle girth measurements, functional scores, and activities of daily living (ADL) are often used to document a patient's response to therapy. These assessments are an excellent way to document and demonstrate progress, especially when patient improvement may be slow or subtle. Video recording the patient initially and periodically throughout the rehabilitation process can also aid in understanding improvements. Client input is often necessary when acquiring some of the subjective assessments, such

Table 4.1 Progress assessments.

Subjective	Objective
Observations: such as sit symmetry	Girthometry
Pain assessment score	Goniometry
Lameness scores	Force plate analysis
Gait patterns	Functional scales: such as Texas Spinal Cord Injury Scale or Proposed Stifle Function Scale
Quality of Life	Time/distance to fatigue
Activities of Daily Living (ADL)	Presence of Tibial thrust/cranial drawer
Body Condition Score	Presence of conscious proprioception
Ease of position transitions (sit to stand)	

as with a pain scoring system, ADL, and quality of life (QoL) evaluation. The client should be included in the assessment and reassessment process, keeping them updated on how their pets are responding through these markers. This helps to keep the client engaged in the pet's therapy program.

Goals

Every rehabilitation program should establish a set of goals for the patient. These goals, set by the rehabilitation veterinarian, are developed in conjunction with the client's expectations for the patient's return to some level of function. These goals are customized for each patient, and in our experience are based upon a current understanding of the pathophysiology of the patient's disorder, estimated tissue healing abilities, patient's ADL, and the owner/caregiver's expectations. The goals should be communicated clearly to the owner/caregiver to ensure owner/caregiver's perception of program success. If the client and therapist have different goals in mind, they may not be satisfied with the outcome.

Goals must be reasonable and attainable. Unrealistic goals can cause clients to become discouraged and lead to abandonment of the rehabilitation effort. Setting several small goals over short periods of time, with re-assessments to confirm goals met, along with praise for reaching these small goals, can serve to keep clients motivated to continue the rehabilitation effort.

The Therapy Prescription

The discussion of the rehabilitation plan should be included in all phases of veterinary treatment planning, regardless of whether the patient has a scheduled intervention like surgery or is suffering from acute trauma or injury. The earlier the client is exposed to the idea and impact of rehabilitation, the more likely they are to become invested in the plan. Rehabilitation plans can vary in time intensity from one session per week to several sessions per day. In many cases, the plan requires a large time commitment from the individual performing the therapies. While elaborate, time-intensive therapy plans can speed recovery for the patient, it is essential to take into consideration the client's time availability and lifestyle as well as the financial commitment when developing the plan. In one study of human physical therapy patients, one of the strongest factors of noncompliance was perceived barriers by the patient (Sluijs *et al.*, 1993). These perceived barriers were often related to the time involved in completing the exercises. Clients are often busy with work, family, and other activities. If clients are asked to commit more time than they have available, there is a risk that the client will either not perform all of the therapies or become discouraged and abandon the rehabilitation effort entirely. If the client only performs a portion of the plan and neglects other segments, the program may

become unbalanced which may risk injury or failure to achieve a maximal recovery.

Many veterinary physical rehabilitation programs employ a combination of several different therapies, exercises, and modalities. Each one of these therapies offers the patient benefits, often in different ways. The veterinary technician should be well versed in the benefits and risks, if any, of each therapy so that this information can be fully communicated with the client. Clients often have questions about different modalities, especially when they may increase the cost, or result in any temporary discomfort to the patient. Clients who do not understand the benefit of a particular modality are more likely to exclude or decline these treatments even if their pets may have benefited.

Activity Restrictions

In rehabilitation practice, we often spend a large portion of time informing clients of the importance of exercise in their pet's therapy. For example, we may stress the importance of strengthening core musculature to support orthopedic incompetency, and that regular exercise is important in promoting joint health in arthritic patients. While we need to communicate the importance of exercise, we cannot overlook the critical importance of activity restriction. In most cases, restriction does not mean a complete lack of activity, it means a focus on a narrow range of acceptable activities. In fact, in most situations, a balance of both exercise and activity restrictions is required for a successful outcome. It can be challenging to communicate this need for balance with clients; there may be a feeling of depriving their pet of enjoyment if freedoms are limited. If the importance of therapeutic exercise is overemphasized, the client may push the patient too hard, resulting in injury. If activity restrictions are overemphasized, clients can become fearful of doing too much, and the pet may not improve at an acceptable rate. The trained veterinary technician can play a valuable role in educating the client on the benefits and risks of both exercise and activity restriction.

Assistive Devices

As technology and interest in animal rehabilitation increase, so does the availability of assistive devices for animals, such as orthoses, prostheses, carts, and other mobility devices. While the specific use and function of these devices are beyond the scope of this chapter (see Chapter 10), it is important for the veterinary technician to be educated on their proper use and potential adverse effects. The veterinary rehabilitation technician will often be asked to demonstrate how to properly apply and use the devices, educate the pet owner on the appropriate duration of wear of the device, and inform the client on how to monitor for discomfort and contact sores from these devices. Pictures and videos can help to communicate how to use and to jog the memory later.

Keeping It Positive

Physical rehabilitation plans often entail exercises or procedures that are performed repeatedly, or as a series of repetitions over several sessions. In addition, many of the movements or positions that we ask of our patients are not natural and may even be uncomfortable for the animal patient. Improper or uneducated application of these techniques or failure to recognize the subtle body language associated with increasing stress (Figure 4.1) can easily result in the patient developing an aversion to therapy.

This aversion can often be avoided by being alert to signs of stress and using reward-based training and low-stress handling techniques (see Chapter 9, Motivating Your Patient) to keep patients encouraged and engaged in therapy. Animals can often be trained to willingly perform exercises with very little assistance. When pets stay engaged and perform tasks willingly, it becomes a much more pleasant experience for the client, patient, and rehabilitation professional. When demonstrating rehabilitation techniques with the client, the veterinary technician can show the client how to use rewards (e.g., food, toy, or praise) to motivate the patient (see Figure 4.2). Another advantage of using training techniques to accomplish the techniques is that

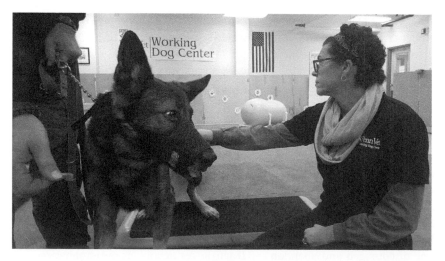

Figure 4.1 Photo of a patient showing signs of stress during a therapy session (moving away from the therapist, while ignoring a food reward). The therapist is utilizing calming body language of sitting to the side, averting the gaze, and maintaining gentle contact with the patient. *Source:* Photo by Tracy Darling (co-author).

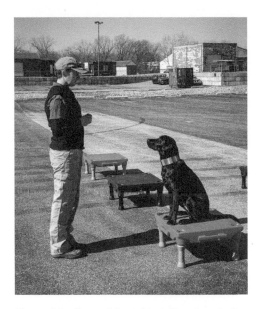

Figure 4.2 Reward-based training as part of a fitness and conditioning program. *Source:* Samantha Warner.

it provides mental exercise, which can be an effective means of releasing energy in a patient that has activity restriction. Clients should also be educated about the early signs of fatigue or aversion to therapy so sessions can be abbreviated if needed. When used successfully, most patients will show up for therapy very excited to begin each session. This engagement of the patient in turn motivates the client, and therapy is more likely to continue and be successful.

Prescriptions and Supplements

Medications and supplements are often prescribed for veterinary physical rehabilitation patients to treat infections, reduce pain and inflammation, promote joint health, and reduce anxiety, as well as many other indications. The veterinary technician is an integral part of communicating the administration and proper usage of these important pharmaceuticals. Clients often have questions or concerns about why certain drugs or supplements are prescribed, how they will help their pet, whether there are drug interactions, what side effects to look for, and how to administer medications. The veterinary technician can help increase compliance and treatment success when they have a thorough understanding of the commonly utilized medications and supplements. Sometimes medications are prescribed to be given "as needed." Clients often need specific criteria to indicate to them when these medications should be administered. For example, a dog that is being treated with a nonsteroidal anti-inflammatory drug (NSAID) to be given as needed, may become reluctant to rise or be slower climbing stairs after a therapeutic exercise session and then would benefit from receiving a dose of the NSAID. Discussions about the clinical signs of conditions like discomfort or nausea can help to reassure clients that they have the knowledge to properly use these medications. Reinforcing these discussions by providing written instructions, and/or handouts can ensure that medications are administered properly.

Adverse Events and Setbacks

When communicating with clients about physical rehabilitation treatment plans, a discussion about the possibility of setbacks or adverse events should always be included. While our goals are always to improve a patient's condition, there may be times during therapy when clinical signs worsen, or a new injury occurs. Besides being detrimental to the patient, these incidents can be devastating to clients and can strain the relationship between the client and the rehabilitation team. For these reasons, clients should always be educated about the potential for setbacks during therapy, what steps should be taken to mitigate them, how to identify signs of injury early, and how these setbacks will be addressed by the rehabilitation team. This information may be especially important when clients have elected physical rehabilitation in lieu of surgical options. Clients should be advised to discontinue activities at home and contact the therapist immediately upon the suspicion of an injury or adverse event with their pets.

Compliance

The nature of the condition may impact owner commitment and compliance. Any treatment including rehabilitation may be considered to be an optional extra (icing on the cake), or even an extreme measure because of the option of euthanasia in veterinary medicine. The presence of sudden disease versus gradual decline, the age of the pet, the general health of the pet, the relationship with the owner, as well as the outlook for return of function may influence the initial commitment to rehabilitation of a pet. Once a client commits to a course of physical rehabilitation, the next challenge is to ensure compliance with the recommended plan.

In one study of human physical therapy patients, only 35% of adult patients fully complied with their prescribed regimen (Sluijs *et al.*, 1993). Compliance becomes even more complicated when the client providing the rehabilitation is not the patient but rather the caretaker. This model of care is most similar to parents undertaking rehabilitation therapy for their children. Adherence to a recommended treatment plan has been associated with parental expectations and belief in the impact of the program. These factors are strongly influenced by the professionalism of, communication by, and trust in the health care professional (Rabino *et al.*, 2013; Dimatteo, 2004). It has also been proposed that parents are most likely to adhere to their child's recommended physiotherapy if

they perceive a severe disease threat (Rabino *et al.*, 2013); although not documented, in veterinary medicine, adherence may be impacted by the potential for return to acceptable function and QoL. Based on human data, compliance is also influenced by how the therapist fulfills the individual's preference for an active versus passive role in health care of their dependent. A report published by the American Animal Hospital Association stated "using multiple approaches to client education and communication increases compliance" (AAHA Compliance report, p. 16).

In both adults and children with chronic conditions, treatment adherence is less than 50% (Simons *et al.*, 2010). In older adults, the most common barriers to treatment adherence are time, transportation, perception of treatment efficacy, and fear of pain or injury (Austrian *et al.*, 2005). With children and adolescents suffering from chronic pain, the most common barrier was a negative attitude about the treatment recommendation; however, early success with exercise increased the future compliance for physical therapy (Simons *et al.*, 2010). These findings emphasize both communication and design of a plan that can be implemented early and have measurable success. Based on the adage that "past behavior is the best predictor of future behavior," clients who have participated in fitness and conditioning programs with their dogs prior to an injury or illness are more likely to adhere to therapist recommendations.

Communication

There are several aspects of the rehabilitation program that are essential to communicate in order to maximize patient success. Shortcomings in any of these areas may compromise patient recovery. Setbacks during a therapy program are not uncommon, and often clients require frequent coaching and encouragement to keep them motivated. The veterinary technician works very closely with the client and patient throughout the rehabilitation process and is, therefore, a vital part of the communication effort.

Communication skills are at the heart of the effective home rehabilitation plan. All communication should be based on recognition of the value of the client, attention to the client's needs and concerns, acknowledgment of the client's message, empathy with the client, and a goal of providing the best care for both the client and the pet (Dreeben, 2011) (also see Chapter 7, Supporting the Client and Patient).

The communication style of the veterinary technician needs to be adjusted to each client. Clients will respond differently to verbal and nonverbal communication. Clients will be particularly attuned to the nonverbal communication between the technician and the pet, paying attention to the veterinary technician's level of comfort, empathy, and compassion. Any discrepancy between verbal expression of empathy and nonverbal cues will undermine the trust of the client and their confidence in the treatment plan. While authentic expression of empathy, (being able to understand and share the feelings held by the client) is one of the most powerful components of effective communication, the skilled veterinary technician also needs to be sensitive to cultural diversity and beliefs of the client. Verbal communication will be the foundation of sharing information and teaching the client. Effective verbal communication includes written and oral communication. The learning style and emotional state of the client will help determine how the client will most effectively receive information. There are several recognized learning styles. Please see the following website for further instructions.

http://www.learning-styles-online.com/overview/

For people who learn by hearing (aural), the therapist will need to articulate in words the full therapy plan, whereas verbal learners or patients under emotional duress may benefit from a combination of verbal and written communication and may be more likely to return with the need to "talk through the plan," providing a conduit for additional follow-up communication, such as an email address, is extremely beneficial. When explaining and demonstrating therapeutic exercises, some clients may be able to learn from watching the therapist perform the exercise, whereas others need to have hands-on experience. Demonstration can be effective especially if the therapist describes each action and demonstrates common errors to avoid. Many individuals, however, will require the kinesthetic experience of having their hands/body move in the proper motion. This can be augmented by the therapist guiding the movements, or by feedback for the caretaker of watching themselves in a mirror or on video. The visual reminders of videos, photos, or drawings are particularly important to visual learners and provide a guide to remind all clients of the proper technique that they have learned. Some clients will learn best by understanding the theory behind the actions; for example, explaining how exercises that encourage eccentric muscle contraction, such as crouching through a tunnel, are used to strengthen muscles of the limbs and core (see Figure 4.3).

In a study of children with cystic fibrosis, parents found written and video instructions were a valuable adjunct to verbal and practical training; however, the documents must be professional, current, and credible (Tipping *et al.*, 2010). Information overload is a risk, especially for a client who is dealing with a sudden and unexpected event. Repetition and patience will be critical in the communication process (see Table 4.2).

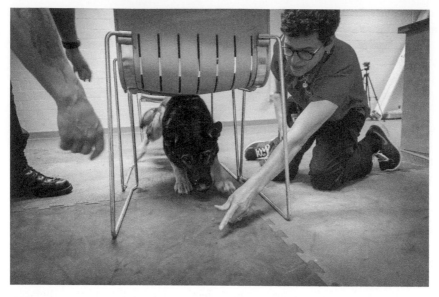

Figure 4.3 A patient performing a crawl exercise for a treat reward. *Source:* Photo by Tracy Darling (co-author).

Table 4.2 Standard learning styles: from http://www.learning-styles-online.com/overview/.

Descriptions of learning modalities*
Visual: Learn by seeing shapes, pictures, and three dimensional objects.
Tactile (kinesthetic): Learn by touch, manipulating objects or the body, and gestures.
Auditory: Learn by hearing words, sounds, tones, and rhythms.
Verbal: Learn by articulating, reading, or writing words.
Logic: Learn by deriving information from reasoning.

Learning Styles

1) Accommodator = *Concrete Experience + Active Experiment*: strong in "hands-on" practical doing (e.g., physical therapists)
2) Converger = *Abstract Conceptualization + Active Experiment*: strong in practical "hands-on" application of theories (e.g., engineers)
3) Diverger = *Concrete Experience + Reflective Observation*: strong in imaginative ability and discussion (e.g., social workers)
4) Assimilator = *Abstract Conceptualization + Reflective Observation*: strong in inductive reasoning and creation of theories (e.g., philosophers) (Kolb, 2015).

---

* Adapted from https://en.wikipedia.org/wiki/Learning_styles and http://www.learning-styles-online.com/overview/, Barbe *et al.* (1979), and Leite *et al.* (2010).

Note: it is important to emphasize the privacy of clinic-provided videos; they should not be shared online or used for therapy on other animals.

Continued advances in technology allow us the ability to communicate with clients in a variety of ways. Utilizing multiple communication modalities can help enhance client understanding and retention of what can sometimes be an overwhelming amount of information. There is so much information about clinical findings, diagnosis, treatment options, side effects, and many other aspects of a patient's condition that cannot always be communicated effectively using one form of communication alone. One of the most common ways, we communicate with clients is verbally, either over the telephone or in person during an appointment session. The use of verbal communication is an effective way to relay information, and it is also a means to build relationships with clients. Pairing verbal communication with something visual, like anatomical models or pictures can help clients' understanding of disorders and disease processes. When communicating a treatment plan with a client, hands-on instruction on how to properly perform exercises and other therapies is essential in developing client confidence in carrying out such treatments at home (Figure 4.4). Online videos demonstrating commonly used techniques are a great way to reinforce hands-on instruction, as they can be accessed on-demand by the client after they leave the clinic. Videos can be customized by the rehabilitation clinic, or there are many great online resources on physical rehabilitation-related topics that can be shared with clients. Treatment schedules can often be quite elaborate; therefore, it is helpful to provide a treatment schedule in written format. Home exercise plans can be printed and handed to the client or sent via email after each visit.

The nature of the condition and expectation for the necessary duration of home rehabilitation is variable. Lessons from parents of children with cystic fibrosis provide some insights into approaches to client education with severely affected or chronic disease patients (Tipping *et al.*, 2010). In a qualitative study evaluating factors that impair delivery and retention of physiotherapy education of parents and impact effective home physiotherapy treatment, three major themes were identified. These themes are transition from one life or disease stage or even location to another, psychological distress often associated with the learning process as well as the underlying condition and social connectedness with the health professional, and social networks. In the case of pets, no doubt the connectedness with the pet is also a major factor.

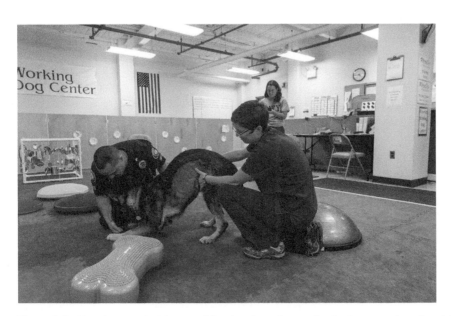

Figure 4.4 Veterinary technician providing hands-on instruction in the execution of assisted exercise. *Source:* Tracy Darling.

Telemedicine

Telemedicine represents a communication opportunity for providing care of veterinary patients. Telemedicine is the practice of medicine using electronic communications, information technology, or other means between a licensee in one location and a patient in another location, with or without an intervening health care provider. Initial evaluations should be with the patient physically present, the only exception being if the veterinarian or therapist is doing a rehabilitation consultation, with a primary care veterinarian present in the room with the client and patient. Telemedicine can be used for quick check-ins, or for full follow-ups. Remote repeat evaluations are often within the patient's home, providing the advantage of observing the animal in its home environment. Facilitating the evaluation is an important role for the rehabilitation veterinary technician. Prior to launching an appointment, the client needs to be educated to ensure that the client is comfortable using the digital platform and equipment and that there is enough space and visibility so that the patient can be observed moving. The client also needs to be comfortable handling their pet to demonstrate reactions to certain exercises, touch, or activities. The connection needs to be clear enough that you can assess progress and teach new home therapies easily. Phone calls are less than ideal, and video connections should be considered essential. In preparation for the appointment, the technician should allow time for the setup of the connection to occur; recruiting the front desk team to initiate the connection can save time. The front team can facilitate the appointment by gathering data beforehand as to the preferred communication platform for the client (e.g., Facetime, Meet, Zoom, Skype, etc.). The clinic should have high-speed internet and have several small computer tablets available to alleviate stress on the main computers, and to allow movement of the screen to follow the patient, doctor, or demonstration of equipment with a different pet in the clinic. If telemedicine is being used to augment an appointment while maintaining physical distancing with the client outside the clinic building, then the clinic Wi-Fi should extend into the parking area, which may require a repeater or an extra modem.

Telemedicine is most frequently used when the care provider is in a different location than the client and patient; however, in cases where the client is not in the same location as the patient receiving rehabilitation therapies, the technician can share short videos of treatments. This type of communication can reassure clients, reinforce the veterinarian–client–patient relationship (VCPR), and build trust in your establishment. Recordings of less than 10 seconds can generally be shared by email. Alternatively, you can post longer videos as private or unlisted links on one of the many cloud-based hosting sites (e.g., Vevo, Twitch, Vimeo, and YouTube). Clients should also be encouraged to share videos of progress or observations of their pets' movements.

Although telemedicine can be an appealing approach to communication, legal ramifications and restrictions must be clearly understood, as regulations can vary between countries. There are guidelines from the American Veterinary Medical Association in cooperation with the AAHA, but the veterinarian and technician should consult their state guidelines in defining the VCPR. The Australian Veterinary Association has produced guidelines including that the veterinarian must be registered or recognized in the location in which the *patient* (not the veterinarian) is located. The Federation of

Veterinarians of Europe has provided recommendations in the context of a VCPR by setting up standard operating procedures, codes of conduct, and proportionate regulation but states that it believes that a physical examination is necessary to make a diagnosis and issue a prescription. The Royal College of Veterinary Surgeons (the United Kingdom) provides information in their code of conduct for professionals that remote advice should only be given to the extent appropriate without a physical examination and to avoid highly specific advice if it could compromise welfare.

In the case of remote follow-ups, the question often is raised as to when the next in-person physical evaluation is needed. That will be largely governed by the condition treated, the expected timeline for recovery or a change in patient status, and veterinarian's discretion. For example, a patient with ongoing static neurologic deficits (unchanged for over a year) should be physically examined every six months to guard against contracture, check for decline, and check overall physical health (cardiovascular and pulmonary issues can be missed in patients who are minimally active). A post-operative patient who is in the later stages of recovery should still have a physical evaluation every six weeks.

In the case of patients living a large distance from the clinic, a mix of in-person and remote rechecks is suitable in order to reduce unnecessary trips – this is an option only provided that they have a valid VCPR with a primary care veterinarian in their region. Email communications with pictures and videos of any areas of concern (e.g., skin sores in a case with an orthosis) can help to define when a physical examination is needed and if the primary care provider can take over for that purpose.

Discussing Finances

When discussing treatment plans with clients, it is often necessary for the veterinary technician to discuss the estimated cost of services. Finances can be a stressful topic to discuss for some clients. In our experience, there are some ways to approach the topic without added difficulty. Focusing on the needs of the patient and explaining how the services will benefit the patient is an excellent way to increase client acceptance (AAHA Six Steps, p. 19). Clients may be more willing to accept the cost associated with a treatment when they can appreciate the value of the service. For example, a therapy visit of $150 might sound expensive to a client, especially when told that their pet will need weekly visits for 12 weeks. On the other hand, if they first learn that each 1-hour therapy visit will include massage therapy, therapeutic laser, an underwater treadmill session, and assisted exercise, they may be surprised to hear that each visit will only cost $150. Disclosing all costs and obtaining written consent before providing services are good ways to avoid financial conflict after therapy sessions are completed.

Follow-up

In a study of rehabilitation compliance in human athletes, patients with emotional support were more likely to adhere to their rehabilitation regimen (Byerly *et al.*, 1994). This concept is likely to be the case with caregivers of veterinary patients undergoing rehabilitation. Client communication should not end when the client leaves the clinic. The veterinary technician can be utilized to maintain an open line of communication with clients in between rehabilitation visits. Clients often leave an appointment excited to start rehabilitating their pets but are often overwhelmed or nervous about carrying out treatments properly. Clients also may have questions after they leave, but might not be inclined to reach out until their next visit. A follow-up phone call or email the day after an initial visit to check in will not only help answer client questions but will keep the line of communication open and reassure the client that you are behind them 100%. This support should continue throughout the treatment program. The veterinary technician can provide valuable support during follow-up therapy visits. Technicians often perform many of the functional assessments and can discuss these results with the client, providing praise for improvements and being prepared to discuss the potential causes for lack of improvements.

Special Considerations for Working Dogs

Working dogs represent a unique population with special needs for both the handlers and the dogs. Working dogs include dogs that provide service or assistance to individuals (e.g., guide, hearing, mobility support, and medical detection), single-purpose detection dogs (e.g., explosives, drugs, search, and rescue), and dual-purpose law enforcement (also referred to as police dogs) that may perform patrol/criminal apprehension work in addition to a detection task. See the AAHA practice guidelines for general definitions and considerations (Otto *et al.*, 2021). All working dogs have a unique and often life-saving relationship with their handler. In general, the handler should always accompany a working dog for the duration of the treatment. Communication should be adapted to the special needs of the handler. For example, a blind handler will benefit from clear verbal communication throughout the

visit and from written communication that can be shared electronically in a format that can be read by a screen reader. A hearing-impaired client will require written communication throughout the visit. For any working dog, the handler may be able to assist by providing appropriate commands to facilitate compliance and maximize safety for the team. When communicating with a working dog handler, it is important to understand the nature of the dog's job, the terminology associated with that job, and the impact that treatment may have on the ability to perform their necessary tasks. The goals of rehabilitation may be different for a working dog than for a companion dog. The technician will be critical in helping define the handler's goals and the impact on performance. A working dog may require a much higher level of function and fitness in order to safely return to their job. Managing expectations and communicating progress benchmarks will be important, as a prolonged recovery period may trigger the discussion of retirement or repurposing, for example, a dog that was doing patrol work and detection work may be moved to performing only detection work. Clear communication on activity restrictions as they relate to training will also be critical to clearly communicate, with an explanation of the rationale and the benchmarks for progression. Rehabilitation of working dogs can be incredibly rewarding as the dog is able to return to work, but clear and regular communication will be imperative in making that journey successful.

Conclusion

The way in which a treatment plan is presented and communicated with clients will have a powerful effect on patient outcomes and should not be overlooked. There are many ways that the rehabilitation team can use effective communication to maximize success in the veterinary rehabilitation patient. This aspect of rehabilitation practice is often tasked to the veterinary technician. The unique knowledge, and perspective of the trained veterinary technician make them well-suited for this important responsibility.

Websites

Learning Instructions http://www.learning-styles-online.com/overview (accessed January 8, 2023).

https://www.aaha.org/aaha-guidelines/telehealth-guidelines/telehealth-home/ (accessed March 4, 2022).

https://www.ava.com.au/policy-advocacy/policies/professional-practices-for-veterinarians/telemedicine-practice/ (accessed March 4, 2022).

https://fve.org/publications/fve-position-and-recommendations-on-the-use-of-telemedicine/ (accessed March 4, 2022).

https://veterinaryevidence.org/index.php/ve/article/view/349 (accessed March 4, 2022).

Further Reading

Albers, J. and Hardesty, C. (ed.) (2009). *Compliance: Taking Quality Care to the Next Level*. Lakewood, CO: American Animal Hospital Association.

Albers, J. and Hardesty, C. (ed.) (2009). *Six Steps to Higher-Quality Patient Care*. Lakewood, CO: American Animal Hospital Association.

References

Austrian, J.S., Kerns, R.D., and Reid, M.C. (2005). Perceived barriers to trying self-management approaches for chronic pain in older persons. *J Am Geriatr Soc* 53: 856–861.

Barbe, W.B., Swassing, R.H., and Milone, M.N. (1979). *Teaching through modality strengths: Concepts and practices*. Columbus, Ohio: Zaner-Bloser ISBN 0883091003. OCLC 5990906.

Byerly, P.N., Worrell, T., Gahimer, J., and Domholdt, E. (1994). Rehabilitation compliance in an athletic training environment. *J Athl Train* 29 (4): 352–355.

Dimatteo, M.R. (2004). The role of effective communication with children and their families in fostering adherence to pediatric regimes. *Patient Educ Couns* 55: 339–344.

Dreeben, O. (2011). Ch 9: Communication basics. In: *Introduction to Physical Therapy for Physical Therapist Assistants*, 2nde (ed. O. Dreeben-Irimia). Sudbury, MA: Jones and Bartlett Learning.

Kolb, D.A. (2015) [1984]). *Experiential Learning: Experience as the Source of Learning and Development*, 2nde. Upper Saddle River, NJ: Pearson Education ISBN 9780133892406. OCLC 909815841.

Leite, W.L., Svinicki, M., and Shi, Y. (2010). Attempted validation of the scores of the VARK: Learning styles inventory with multitrait–multimethod confirmatory factor analysis models. *Educ Psychol*

Measurem 70 (2): 323–339. https://doi.
org/10.1177/0013164409344507.

Otto, C.M., Cohen, J.A., Darling, T. et al.
(2021). 2021 AAHA working, assistance,
and therapy dog guidelines. *J Am Anim
Hosp Assoc* 57: 253–277. https://doi.
org/10.5326/JAAHA-MS-7250.

Rabino, S.R., Peretz, S.R., Kastel-Deutch, T.,
and Tirosh, E. (2013). Factors affecting
parental adherence to an intervention
program for congenital torticollis. *Pediatr
Phys Ther* 25 (3): 298–303.

Simons, L.E., Logan, D.E., Chastain, L., and
Cerullo, M. (2010). Engagement in
multidisciplinary interventions for
pediatric chronic pain: Parental
expectations, barriers, and child outcomes.
Clin J Pain 26 (4): 291–299.

Sluijs, E.M., Kok, G.J., and van der Zee, J.
(1993). Correlates of exercise compliance
in physical therapy. *Phys Ther* 73:
771–782.

Tipping, C.J., Scholes, R.L., and Cox,
N.S. (2010). A qualitative study of
physiotherapy education for parents of
toddlers with cystic fibrosis. *J Cyst Fibros*
9 (3): 205–211.

5

Manual Techniques in the Clinic

Amie Lamoreaux Hesbach

EmpowerPhysio, Maynard, MA, USA

CHAPTER MENU

Introduction

Manual therapy (MT) is an approach in which skilled, goal-focused, passive or assisted active movement techniques (forces) are applied with (through) the hands (or hand-held instruments, as an adjunct to the hands) in order to induce structural or functional changes within myofascial, neuromuscular, or articular connective tissues (American Physical Therapy Association, n.d.). MT incorporates a comprehensive, immediate, and continuous evaluative process, including examination and assessment, and a therapeutic intent and goal focus in the selection and application of interventions or manual techniques based on a functional diagnosis. The practitioner utilizes critical thinking, clinical problem-solving, and decision-making skills in this practice, based on current evidence and the practitioner's knowledge, skills, and experience (Hesbach, 2014). MT might be utilized in coordination with other rehabilitation interventions, leading to a symbiotic, summative result (Goff and Jull, 2007; Veterinary Manual Therapy Working Group, 2022).

Physical Rehabilitation for Veterinary Technicians and Nurses, Second Edition.
Edited by Mary Ellen Goldberg and Julia E. Tomlinson.
© 2024 John Wiley & Sons, Inc. Published 2024 by John Wiley & Sons, Inc.
Companion website: www.wiley.com/go/goldberg/physicalrehabilitationvettechsandnurses

MT approaches and manual techniques might include:

- Light touch MT (LIMT),
- Passive range of motion (PROM),
- Stretching,
- Soft tissue mobilization,
- Neuromuscular facilitation,
- NeuroDynamics,
- Peripheral joint and spinal *mobilization,*
- Peripheral joint and spinal *manipulation,*

The animal physical therapy and rehabilitation practitioner must have pre-requisite knowledge in the following areas to ensure safe and effective implementation of MT and manual techniques:

- Species-specific neuromusculoskeletal anatomy, including muscle, tendon, and ligament origins; insertions and actions; fascial system attachments; and nervous tissue course and connections.
- Species-specific biomechanics with regards to forces applied to the body from an external origin, for example, through the hands of the rehabilitation practitioner, and by the patient's body, originating internally, causing isolated or gross body movements or having an effect on the patient's external environment.
- Osteokinematics and arthrokinematics.
- Structure and function (anatomy and physiology) of the various body systems involved in and responsive to MT and manual techniques, including the musculoskeletal, integumentary, nervous, myofascial, as well as other body systems, such as the cardiovascular, gastrointestinal, and endocrine systems.

MT in animal rehabilitation might be practiced by veterinarians and veterinary technicians or nurses with proficiency in the application of manual techniques from additional post-professional education or certification training programs addressing the didactic and practical knowledge necessary (Brunke *et al.*, 2021), by physical therapists, chiropractors, osteopaths, massage therapists, or other practitioners licensed, chartered, registered, certified, or otherwise possessing the knowledge, skills, expertise, and experience with specific MT approaches in animals. It is the position of the author that practitioners limit practice based on the scope appropriate and as designated by licensing or regulatory authorities in the practitioner's country, province, or state, but with a spirit of interprofessional collaboration, always, with the veterinarian of record and the entire rehabilitation team.

Purpose

The purpose of this chapter is to provide a description of MT and manual techniques which have been adapted to and utilized in the practice of animal rehabilitation. Though it does provide a more detailed discussion of basic PROM, stretching, and massage techniques, it is understood that the practice of MT and performance of manual techniques in practice requires in-depth practical instruction, which is beyond the scope of this publication.

Manual Examination, Evaluation, and Assessment

A thorough and objective evaluation, with an MT focus, must be performed prior to selection and application of any manual technique (Sprague, 2013). This evaluation will focus on the neuromusculoskeletal systems and should include:

- Subjective history, including client-specific outcome measures, questionnaires, and medical history,
- Synthesis of diagnostic imaging results or specialist interpretation of such,
- Assessment of the patient's general health (e.g., body weight and condition score, vital signs),

- Examination of the integumentary (including skin and fur or hair coat), cardiovascular, and respiratory systems,
- Examination of neurological status, including reflexes, reactions, and sensory and proprioceptive tests,
- Observation of static postures, including conformation, weight-bearing, stance, tail and head position or carriage, and bony symmetry,
- Observation of dynamic functional mobility, gait, and other functional tasks, including coordination, balance, strength, functional active range of motion (AROM), and quality of movement or motor control,
- Observation or measurement of PROM and flexibility,
- Observation or measurement of muscle development and symmetry,
- Objective outcome scores and scales, where applicable,
- Palpation or manual evaluation, which is defined as the use of special diagnostic techniques which use the hands to assess the structure and function of soft tissues, joint lines, and bony prominences, and
- Accessory motion testing, especially with regards to quality and quantity of motion which might reveal motion limitations, joint dysfunctions, hypomobility or hypermobility, the presence of pain or sensitivity, normal or abnormal end feel, and soft tissue reaction (e.g., hypertonicity, hypotonicity, or spasm). Accessory motion testing might include the Ortolani test, cranial drawer test, and varus or valgus tests, for example.

Pathoanatomic and Functional Diagnosis

The practitioner, synthesizing subjective and objective data, will consider the potential origin of the patient's symptoms (pathoanatomic diagnosis) and impairments, functional limitations, and disability (functional diagnosis) prior to formulation of functional goals and selection of treatment strategies and tactics to address those goals, which might include an MT approach and manual techniques, in addition to other rehabilitation interventions.

Indications, precautions, contraindications, and prognosis must also be considered and integrated with the practitioner's knowledge, skill, and experience, and will vary dependent upon the pathoanatomic diagnosis, functional diagnosis, and specific goals of rehabilitation for the individual patient (and client). Knowledge of the pathoanatomic or differential diagnosis will enhance the specificity of manual techniques chosen and utilized, allowing for a more efficient and effective resolution of impairments related to that diagnosis (Basmajian and Nyberg, 1992; Lascelles *et al.*, 2012).

The pathoanatomic diagnosis specifically describes the local, regional, or systemic structural or tissue-based pathology present, based on positive or abnormal findings as identified on physical examination and through diagnostic imaging or histologic testing. Examples of pathoanatomic diagnoses include gracilis fibrotic myopathy, coxofemoral osteoarthritis, and cranial cruciate ligament rupture (CCLR).

Pathoanatomic diagnoses that might benefit from the application of manual techniques include but are not limited to, osteoarthritis, spondylosis, intervertebral disk disease, muscle strains, ligament sprains, post-orthopedic or neurologic surgery, and tendinopathies (Baltzer, 2020).

The functional diagnosis is a "movement-based" diagnosis and describes the impact or effect of an injury, disorder, or disease process on function, resulting in functional limitations or disability. Examples of functional diagnoses include: cervical spine stiffness, stifle joint instability, thoracolumbar pain exacerbated by trunk extension, etc. Successful treatment of a functional diagnosis will result in improvements in symptoms, as well as in restoration of function.

In general, MT is indicated in cases in which function is limited by the following impairments:

- Reduced ROM
- Reduced flexibility
- Swelling, effusion, edema, and lymphedema
- Pain of neuromusculoskeletal origin (Grayson *et al.*, 2012)
- Reduced sensory awareness

Effects of the Application of Manual Techniques

Before initiating any treatment and following the comprehensive evaluation, the practitioner will specify the goals of rehabilitation, which should be specific, measurable, achievable, realistic, and timely (or SMART). Utilization of an MT approach and application of manual techniques will assist in the achievement of these goals if the approach or techniques are indicated. Effects of the application of manual techniques can be generalized and multisystemic (see Table 5.1), but they also might be specific relative to the manual technique applied (Bialosky *et al.*, 2018).

Table 5.1 General systemic effects of the application of manual techniques.

Body system	Primary effects	Secondary effects	Tertiary effects
Cardiovascular	• Increased circulation • Reduced heart and respiratory rate • Reduced blood pressure	• Lubrication of joint • Reduced muscle soreness • Decreased swelling and edema	• Increased ROM • Increased flexibility • Promotion of tissue healing
Neurological	• Activation of sensory receptors	• Reduction in pain • Relaxation/sedation • Reduction in anxiety	• Facilitation of muscle contraction • Improved neuromuscular tone • Improved sensory awareness and proprioception • Promotion of neuroplasticity • Improved motor control
Musculoskeletal (incl fascia and connective tissue)	• Assisted glide and movement of tissue		• Increased ROM • Increased flexibility • Increased tissue mobility
Endocrine and immune	• Decreased arginine-vasopressin, interleukin and cortisone • Increased lymphocyte circulation		• Promotion of tissue healing • Relaxation
Gastrointestinal	• Increased peristalsis		

Source: Information from Lima *et al.* (2020), Kirkby-Shaw *et al.* (2020), Rapaport *et al.* (2010), and Banker *et al.* (2014).

Precautions, Contraindications, and Red Flags

Precautions are based on the possibility that a treatment could cause harm or damage to a patient. They are specific to an individual patient, based on synthesis of information gathered during the evaluative process, and require continuous assessment and reassessment prior to, during, and following treatment. Examples of precautions might include:

- Acute injury or surgery with integumentary involvement
- Joint hypermobility
- Recently healed fractures
- Post-operative tendon repair
- Vigorous stretch post-immobilization
- Infection
- Neoplasia

Contraindications are specific conditions in which expert recommendation or advice is to not utilize a treatment based on the significant likelihood of harm occurring with or after treatment. Contraindications to the application of manual techniques might be general, relative, or absolute, and are sometimes specific to the MT approach or manual technique chosen. Some absolute contraindications, also referred to as red flags, might require urgent referral for further medical or surgical management and should be identified through a comprehensive evaluation. In general, contraindications for the application of manual techniques include:

- Instability
- Recent fracture or dislocation
- Intractable pain
- Thromboembolic diseases, clotting disorders, or hematoma
- Acute inflammation
- Active infection
- Inability to communicate pain or discomfort (i.e., the patient is sedated or under anesthesia)

- Over open wounds, incisions, or burns and near staples or sutures (Furlan *et al.*, 2002)

Outcomes Measurement and Determining the Effectiveness of Manual Therapy

Functional goals based on objective outcome measures which have been established as standardized, valid, and reliable are essential in rehabilitation and can assist the practitioner in the identification of red flags and in determining the effectiveness of treatment, the need for alteration of the treatment plan, or whether an external referral is indicated. Outcomes might include goniometry, girth measures, infrared thermographic imaging, objective measures and markers in kinematic or kinetic assessment of postures, gait, and functional mobility, pain scales and scores, functional measures, and questionnaires and client-reported outcome measures, among others (Dutton, 2015; Jaegger *et al.*, 2002).

For more immediate feedback with regards to effectiveness of or patient responsiveness to therapy, pre-tests and post-tests can be utilized (Hendrickson *et al.*, 1993). These are functional activities or efficiently measured outcomes (e.g., goniometric measures of a single joint) that can be assessed prior to (pre-test) and immediately following (post-test) application of a manual technique or other treatment. Pre-tests and post-tests can relate directly to the functional goal of focus during a single treatment session and might include: symmetry of weight bearing in a sit-to-stand transition, tarsal flexion range of movement (ROM) in a sitting position, or frequency of weight bearing at a walk, for example.

Outcomes of the rehabilitation episode of care (i.e., the period of time from initial assessment to final discharge in rehabilitation), incorporating MT approaches and the application of manual techniques, are dependent upon multiple variables, both patient-dependent and practitioner-dependent. When setting a prognosis or client expectations, consideration must be made of such variables as the pathophysiology of the disorder or injury, the age of the patient, comorbidities which might be present, expected tissue healing timeframes, other interventions utilized (i.e., medical, surgical, complementary, or rehabilitative), home instruction compliance, and persistence of the condition, among others.

Role of Palpation in Manual Therapy

Palpation is the basis of MT, both of evaluation and of treatment, and is the use of the hands to assess the structural or functional features of superficial bony and soft tissues (e.g., muscle, ligament, tendon, and fascia). Palpation skills must be developed through practice and the acquisition of detailed knowledge and understanding of anatomy. Palpation is essential in preparation for the application of manual techniques.

Bony and soft tissues can be palpated with regards to:

- Temperature,
- Tone (i.e., normal, hypertonicity, or hypotonicity),
- Muscle development (or atrophy),
- Texture or consistency,
- Pliability (or tissue movement),
- Symmetry (or asymmetry),
- Presence or absence of effusion, edema, swelling, or pitting edema,
- Pain response (e.g., hyperalgesia and allodynia), and
- Skin integrity.

The method of palpation can vary based on the goal of the practitioner, including variation of hand or finger positions or pressures, and can be static or dynamic. Static palpation is performed with the patient in a static (preferably relaxed) position, though the practitioner might move, deform, or displace the skin and superficial tissues. Dynamic palpation is performed as the practitioner palpates a specific structure while the patient is mobile, whether actively or passively. Dynamic palpation might provide further information to the practitioner, for example:

- Integrity or stability (or instability) of a joint-associated structure (e.g., sesamoid bone, meniscus, labrum, and ligament)
- Presence (or absence) of crepitus
- Relative motion of bony or soft tissues (e.g., tendon and sesamoid bone)
- Symmetry (or asymmetry) of deviations or prominences
- Muscle activation

Palpation might also serve a value in the identification of specific red flags (e.g., subcutaneous emphysema).

Manual Technique Selection and Communication

The MT approach or manual technique is selected based on:

- The evaluation (examination and assessment)
- Patient-specific indications, contraindications, and precautions
- The functional goal of the patient and client
- The therapeutic goal of the technique

For example, if manual techniques are to be applied to address limitations in stifle flexion ROM due to reduced rectus femoris flexibility, chronic inflammation of the patellar tendon, and chronic joint effusion, resulting in asymmetry of the sitting posture in a dog after a tibial plateau leveling osteotomy (TPLO) procedure for a CCLR, then a soft tissue mobilization (STM) technique might be selected in combination with PROM and stretching techniques.

As MT approaches and manual techniques are selected specific to the individual patient as described above, they do require somewhat generic labels as the method of application of techniques is very practitioner-specific and difficult to reproduce across the rehabilitation team. Further details regarding specific variables of the treatment, including patient position, location and extent of treatment area, specific technique utilized, depth and rate of application, and patient response, should be documented in the patient record utilizing accepted and defined terminology for adequate communication within and outside of the rehabilitation team. As well, variables associated with different MT approaches and manual techniques selected require modification based on the patient's status, thus emphasizing the need for continuous evaluation and re-evaluation of the patient.

Preparation for the Application of Manual Techniques

Though there is an understanding that the practitioner is educated and skilled in the performance of the manual technique(s) to be utilized in the rehabilitation session, it is also necessary to be mindful in the preparation of the patient, the client, the environment, and the practitioner herself, prior to initiation of treatment. This preparation will ensure that the patient is trusting of the practitioner, relaxed and comfortable during treatment, and perceives the practitioner as being non-threatening, all of which contribute to the session as being more likely to be successful with regards to meeting pre-test and post-test goals and progressing towards more long-term functional outcomes.

With regards to the treatment environment, a quiet location with few sensory distractions is preferable. If possible, a location that is devoid of excessive noises, windows for visual distractions, or smells that, though they might be familiar, might elicit a stress or threat response (i.e., within an animal hospital). The practitioner should allow the patient to safely explore and familiarize himself with the environment prior to the session. Provision of a mattress, cushion, bed, or surface that is supportive, comfortable, and easy to access, might further ensure that the patient is relaxed during the session.

The patient will respond to the client's behaviors, especially in an unfamiliar environment. If the client is calm and trusting of the practitioner, the patient will more likely be so as well. The practitioner should be sure to speak calmly with the client and explain the selected manual procedures to ensure their understanding and comfort. Allowing the client to be helpful during the session, whether sitting calmly with the patient, offering treats, toys, petting, or other forms of positive feedback, or assisting with positioning of the patient, can also reassure the patient that he is safe with the practitioner and in the treatment environment.

When applying manual techniques to the patient, the practitioner should position herself in a non-threatening way and use movements and a tone of voice that are reassuring to the patient (and to the client). Avoiding direct eye contact and avoiding handling a known painful body part (at least initially during the session) will reduce the potential that the patient to feel threatened or stressed. The practitioner should begin any MT session by gently resting both hands on the patient, allowing him to settle and become accustomed to the sensation, prior to progression to the application of more specific manual techniques (Robinson and Sheets, 2015). The practitioner should maintain some manual or physical contact with the patient throughout the session. The focus should be on the patient using calm, non-threatening verbal and non-verbal communication. The practitioner might find it helpful to verbally describe the manual technique while it is being applied, so as to appropriately set client expectations (Coates, 2017).

If the patient is lying in a laterally recumbent position, the practitioner should sit near the "back" or dorsal aspect of the patient. This is potentially a safer position, both with regards to avoiding any aggressive movements on the part of the patient, as well as allowing for safe body mechanics involved in reaching movements during the session. The patient should not be forced to assume specific movements or positions and the practitioner should avoid restraint if at all possible. Observation of the patient during the session can provide non-verbal feedback with regards to level of comfort, anxiety, or stress which can be reflected in eye, tail, and ear positions or movements, alteration in heart rate or respiratory rate, or vocalizations. The practitioner should always be responsive to this feedback and alter her approach or technique appropriately (Yin, 2009).

Manual Therapy Approaches and Manual Techniques

MT and the application of manual techniques are part of a comprehensive rehabilitation approach with technique selection, dosage, and protocol based on multiple factors, including pathoanatomic or functional diagnosis, acuity and severity of the condition, tissue healing timeframes, and the stage of healing, and location of the tissues being manipulated via the manual techniques. Unfortunately, due to the number of MT approaches and manual techniques potentially applicable to animal patients,

there are few well-defined protocols or standards of practice (Haussler *et al.*, 2021). The practitioner, therefore, should make attempts to educate, communicate, and collaborate with the entire rehabilitation team, including the client, prior to administering any manual technique to an animal.

The subsequent sections will provide descriptions of the following MT approaches and manual techniques; however, it is understood that application of such techniques requires further, more in-depth, education beyond the scope of this text. Such manual techniques include:

- Light touch MT (LIMT)
- PROM
- Stretching
- Soft tissue mobilization
- Peripheral joint and spinal mobilization
- Peripheral joint and spinal manipulation
- Neuromuscular facilitation and sensory stimulation approaches, and
- NeuroDynamics (Veterinary Manual Therapy Working Group, 2022).

Light Touch Manual Therapy (LTMT)

LTMT or minimal contact MT approaches include energy work, energy healing therapies, energy manipulative therapies, and biofield therapies (Hammerschlag *et al.*, 2014), such as external qigong, healing touch, therapeutic touch, johrei, reiki, craniosacral therapy, reconnective healing, brain curriculum, and visceral manipulation, among others. These techniques utilize gentle manual contact (MC) with the patient but might require only energy manipulation, focus, or intent by the practitioner. Effects are debated but are suggested to include support of healing processes, relaxation, reduction of stress, tension, anxiety, and pain; assistance in fascial release; and promotion of health, immunity, and well-being (Davis *et al.*, 2016). These therapeutic approaches have been studied with variable levels of understanding and acceptance by the scientific and veterinary medical community. There is considerable debate as to whether LTMT should be considered an MT approach or manual technique at all (Cleveland Clinic, n.d.).

Passive Range of Motion (PROM)

Range of motion or ROM is the movement capability of a joint or body part. ROM is a combination of both osteokinematic and arthrokinematic motion. Osteokinematic motion is the movement of bones around a joint axis, resulting in an alteration of the angle of the joint, measurable by goniometry. The movement is named based on the direction of movement (i.e., flexion, extension, abduction, adduction, internal rotation, external rotation, lateral flexion, or side-bending). Arthrokinematic motion, also known as accessory or translatory motion, is the movement that occurs between joint surfaces, primarily rolls, spins, and slides or glides. This movement is predictable with regards to direction, based on the shape of the joint surfaces in the normal, non-pathologic joint. Arthrokinematic motion cannot be isolated by the patient with muscle contractions but can be reproduced manually by the skilled practitioner (Norkin and Levangie, 1992). Both osteokinematic and arthrokinematic motion influence the selection of manual techniques, specifically mobilization or manipulation, in an MT approach (Hesbach, 2014).

PROM is the movement of a joint through the desired ROM without participation or muscle contraction provided by the patient, but through an outside or external force, usually manually by the rehabilitation practitioner (though it can also be performed mechanically). Active ROM (AROM) is movement of a joint through active contractions of surrounding muscle groups, performed by the patient (Figure 5.1).

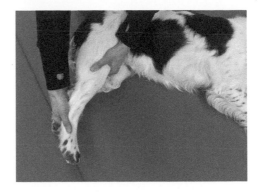

Figure 5.1 Passive range of motion of the stifle into extension. *Source:* This photo is Courtesy Dr Amie Hesbach (co-author).

When performing PROM, the practitioner will note restrictions, potentially due to passive articular structures, including the articular surface, meniscus or labrum, joint capsule, ligaments, and myofascial tissues. The end ROM, which is normally indicated by an elastic barrier, has a characteristic quality, also known as end feel, specific to each joint and each motion direction. Normal and abnormal end feels are defined (see Table 5.2) and indicate the potential pathology of the components of the joint which are being passively moved and which might restrict or otherwise alter the sensation experienced by the practitioner at the end ROM, whether at the expected position or prior to that expected position.

The normal excursion or ROM of the joint can be altered or limited in the presence of pathology or changes in tissues within the joint or surrounding the joint (e.g., inflammation or joint effusion, soft tissue tightness or thickness, pain, and articular cartilage pathology). These changes might also contribute to the patient's pain perception. There are standards with regard to ROM of the peripheral joints in many species (e.g., dog, cat, and horse), however, these standards vary depending upon the breed and other conformational characteristics of the animal.

Table 5.2 Normal and abnormal end feels (Physiopedia, n.d.).

	Descriptor	Definition
Normal (ROM is normal)	Soft (Soft Tissue Approximation)	Normal muscular bulk, tissue meets tissue, feeling of soft compression, and painless.
	Firm (Tissue Stretch)	Firm, springy movement with a slight give, normal elastic resistance, and painless.
	Hard (Bony or Bone to Bone)	Hard, unyielding, abrupt sensation, and painless.
Abnormal (ROM is greater or less than normal, painful)	Empty	No physical restriction to ROM, but considerable pain
	Bony (Bony Block)	Hard, unyielding, restriction occurs before the normal end ROM
	Spasm	Sudden and hard dramatic arrest of movement accompanied by pain, springy, rebound, reflexive/protective muscle guarding
	Springy Block (Internal Derangement)	Springy or rebound sensation in a non-capsular pattern before the end of ROM
	Capsular Stretch (Leathery)	Hard capsular: thick quality, ROM limitation is abrupt
		Soft capsular: acute, stiffness early in ROM increasing until end ROM
	Boggy (Soft)	Mushy, soft quality

Normal ROM is essential for normal function and biomechanics of associated tissues for efficient functional mobility (DiBerardino *et al.*, 2012). If joint ROM is limited, abnormal stresses can occur at the joint and in its periphery. Regardless of limited ROM, the patient might be able to maintain independence with functional activities by increasing movement at an adjacent joint or elsewhere within that limb. This compensation can result in secondary joint hypermobility or irritability or increase the likelihood of pain in or injury to joints or soft tissues in the proximity of or distant from the original injury (Weiner, 2001). Early attention to these limitations can potentially reduce the risk of secondary injury through compensation (Coates, 2017).

When performing PROM to a peripheral joint, it is necessary that the practitioner move slowly and cautiously, respecting the expected or anatomical limit of the PROM as well as the end feel, so as to not cause undue damage to joint-associated tissues or articular structures (Wise, 2015). Positioning the hands close to the point of interest, to reduce the torque applied to the patient's body, will reduce the risk of injury during application of PROM techniques. For example, when performing PROM techniques on the stifle joint of a dog, the practitioner should place her hands on the thigh and crus of the hind limb, close to the stifle joint. When flexing the stifle passively, the practitioner will bring her hands together, reducing the angle between the two segments of the limb until an end feel is noted.

When extending the stifle passively, the practitioner will move her hands apart, increasing the angle between the two segments of the limb until an end feel is noted.

Stretching

Stretching is a manual technique used to increase the extensibility or flexibility of musculotendinous tissues (Page, 2012). Reduced extensibility or flexibility can result from adaptive shortening due to chronic postures or positioning; scarring, adhesion, or fibrosis; and overuse, injury, or spasm (Weiner, 2001). It can also occur secondary to abnormal neurologic input. Chronic changes in extensibility or flexibility can result in abnormal stresses on the joint and associated tissues, which can potentially lead to further compensation by the patient (Jarvis *et al.*, 2013).

In general, a stretch can be performed by moving the involved joint(s) in the direction opposite the action of the muscle or muscle group (Wise, 2015). For example, a stretch of the biceps brachii would require that the shoulder be positioned in flexion and elbow in extension. Attention should be paid to end feel and tolerance or comfort of the patient when applying a passive static stretch.

Stretching can be applied in a static or dynamic method. Static or passive stretching requires that the practitioner hold the stretch position for a prolonged period of time, with no movement at end range. Static stretching has been found to be effective in increasing muscle flexibility through the addition of sarcomeres to the length of the muscle. In the same manner, a prolonged stretch might provide relaxation to the musculotendinous and fascial tissues through neurological input, allowing for a greater excursion of the musculotendinous unit, without active contraction of the muscle as it resists the stretch (McHugh and Cosgrave, 2012).

A dynamic or active stretching technique can be utilized prior to an athletic event, for example. In this case, the patient does not require restraint or recumbent positioning while the targeted muscle group is stretched by luring the patient into a position of stretch. Active stretches are less specific as the origin of the muscle is not stabilized, but are considered to be more functional, incorporating full body movements and active muscle contractions by the patient. For example, the hip flexor muscle group can be actively stretched by encouraging the dog to put his front legs up onto a step, bringing the hips into an extended position (Figure 5.2).

There are varying opinions regarding the variables required to ensure optimal results in gaining and maintaining flexibility when stretching. Research has demonstrated that stretching more than once each day does not have significant benefits in long-term flexibility gains. Alternatively, Brady (2013) suggested that stretching four times per week led to 82% greater improvements in flexibility when compared to stretching only twice weekly. And Taylor *et al.* (1990) suggested that there was no increase in muscle length after two to four repetitions of a stretch.

The length of time that a stretch is held has also been widely investigated. Research suggests that a 30-second sustained stretch results in effects which are maintained significantly longer than that of a 15-second

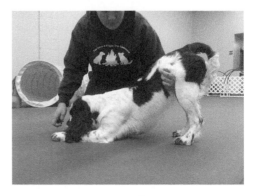

Figure 5.2 Active stretch "play bow."
Source: Courtesy Dr Amie Hesbach (co-author).

stretch. Holding a stretch for longer than 30 seconds has not been found to have an increased benefit in human subjects, however (Bandy and Irion, 1994).

As canine muscle has a different fiber type composition compared to human muscle, the response to an applied stretch may differ as well (Coville, 2016). Unfortunately, current evidence is lacking and we extrapolate from our understanding of the effects of stretching in other species (Reese and Brandy, 2010). It is recommended that practitioners continue to assess and gauge the response of the patient, both in progress towards functional therapeutic goals and tolerance of the applied treatment technique both during and following application of any manual technique.

Soft Tissue Mobilization (STM)

STM is the induced movement of superficial and deep layers of soft tissues (i.e., skin, fascia, tendon, ligament, joint capsule, and muscle) (Hesbach, 2014). STM is used in conjunction with other therapeutic techniques as part of a systematic therapeutic approach, designed to achieve functional goals. STM can include such techniques as:

- Massage
- Manual lymphatic drainage (MLD)
- Myofascial techniques
- Trigger point techniques
- Instrument assisted techniques

The effects of STM are largely based on hypothesis and clinical experience as underlying tissue changes, especially long-term, are not well researched. Short-term effects are demonstrated subjectively in human medicine; however, there are no studies to support the efficacy of STM in the long term. STM can be used in combination with or prior to the application of other interventions and should be applied with a functional goal or therapeutic intent (Formenton *et al.*, 2017).

Regardless, STM is hypothesized to have indirect (or reflexive) effects, due to stimulation of the nervous and endocrine systems, and direct (mechanical) effects, because of forces applied to the body (see Table 5.3).

Table 5.3 Proposed effects of soft tissue mobilization.

System	Effects
Circulatory and endocrine systems	- Increased local circulation (blood and lymphatic) - Reflex vasodilation - Decreased edema - Release of endorphins, neurotransmitters, and hormones (e.g., vasopressin, oxytocin)
Neurological system	- Generalized relaxation - Decreased motor unit activity, spasm (via Golgi tendon organ and muscle spindles) - Stimulation (facilitation or inhibition) of sensory receptors (e.g., cutaneous mechanoreceptors and muscle spindles) - Pain reduction
Musculoskeletal system (mechanical effects)	- Improved gliding of soft tissue layers - Increased tissue extensibility - Increased ROM

Source: Information from Billhult *et al.* (2009), Austin *et al.* (2012), Furlan *et al.* (2002), Gay *et al.* (2015), Sefton *et al.* (2011), and Wang *et al.* (2014).

Soft Tissue Mobilization: Massage

Massage is an STM technique which includes a variety of methods. Effleurage, French for "to skim" or "to touch lightly on," is often used as an introductory technique and is a rhythmic, long, broad, gliding, continuous stroke of light to moderate pressure, often performed parallel to the fibers of the muscle and on larger muscle groups, or throughout an entire limb. When applying effleurage, the practitioner's hands are open and relaxed, working in a hand-over-hand pattern (Salvo, 2012; Fritz, 2004). Petrissage, French for "to knead," includes movements such as lifting, kneading, compressing, wringing, and rolling of soft tissues, performed as the practitioner "picks up" the soft tissues between the thumb and the flat side of the index finger(s) or between the hands (DeLisa *et al.*, 2005).

In general, when performing massage, the practitioner should start with gentle, but firm MCs, progressing to light effleurage strokes moving from distal to proximal and from areas distant from a painful or edematous body part and slowly approaching the involved area. More vigorous petrissage strokes should be introduced as tolerated and as necessary to achieve therapeutic goals (Fehrs, 2010). Variables with regard to amount of pressure or force and frequency, speed, direction, and location of strokes utilized during massage are selected specific to the functional goals of the individual patient (Fritz and Grosenbach, 2009). It is not uncommon to utilize massage as an introductory technique prior to application of PROM, stretching, or other manual techniques, including joint or spinal mobilization or manipulation (Corti, 2014).

Additionally, tapotement, derived from the French word for "tap or pat," is a STM technique which involves the application of rapid, repetitive, stimulatory tapping, hacking, slapping, cupping, pinching, or plucking contact with the patient's body (Fritz, 2004). Tapotement or percussion is also utilized in respiratory or chest physical therapy approaches. The concussive force applied to the thorax with a cupped palm creates a "shock wave" which helps to loosen secretions within the lung fields for eventual movement out of the airway through coughing and expectoration. These techniques are utilized in small animal critical care medicine, especially in pets that are recumbent or restricted in mobility, whether due to the use of medical sedation or reduced active mobility due to acute pathology. These techniques, in combination with postural drainage strategies, can reduce the risk of the development of pneumonia in these cases.

Soft Tissue Mobilization: Manual Lymphatic Drainage (MLD)

MLD is a specialized manual technique, popularized by Still and Vodder, incorporating a sequence of gentle (low pressure), rhythmic, circular manual movements, stimulating lymphatic flow from the distal superficial lymphatic vessels to the more proximal lymph nodes and finally into generalized circulation. MLD results in reduction of persistent tissue swelling or edema, also known as lymphedema or lymphatic congestion, which can result in movement and ROM restrictions.

Primary lymphedema is considered an inherited condition in humans, but it also has been reported in a case study of two Whippet siblings (Schuller *et al.*, 2011) and in draft horses (Affolter, 2013). Secondary lymphedema can occur following trauma, surgery, removal of lymph vessels or nodes, or irradiation (Lee *et al.*, 2011).

Complex decongestive physiotherapy (CDP) is an approach which utilizes MLD in combination with compressive elastic bandaging, prescription of customized elastic sleeves or stockings, and therapeutic exercises

(Vairo *et al.*, 2009). CDP has demonstrated efficacy when compared to MLD alone in systematic reviews and meta-analyses and has been traditionally utilized in treatment of lymphedema in human patients undergoing surgical and oncologic treatment for breast cancer (Huang *et al.*, 2013).

Soft Tissue Mobilization: Myofascial Techniques

Fascia is a three-dimensional, web-like, continuous sheet of connective tissue composed of collagen fibers and a glycosaminoglycan matrix. It attaches to, stabilizes, encloses, and separates muscles, bones, internal organs, and neurovascular structures and is classified as superficial, deep, or visceral based on its location and composition (Salvo, 2012).

Fascial restrictions, including densification and fibrosis, are theorized to be caused primarily by inflammation, trauma, or surgical procedures but can also be secondary to repetitive movements and postures. Densification is the thickening and increased viscosity of the loose fascia between the more fibrous, deep fascial layers (Pavan *et al.*, 2014). Densification is reversible and can be altered through movement, either passively through the application of manual myofascial techniques or actively through muscle contractions. Fibrosis or adhesion is a permanent change, similar to scarring, in which there is excessive and disorganized deposition of Type III collagen over an area, leading to disruption of the fascia (Schleip and Klingler, 2019).

Myofascial techniques are STM techniques which specifically focus on mechanical manipulation of the superficial and deep layers of fascia. Effects are both mechanical and neurological, resulting in altered neuro-myofascial tone, improved circulation, increased mobility through and between fascial layers, reduction in densification, and reduced pain.

Myofascial release (MFR) is a manual technique during which the practitioner utilizes her hands to place the patient's body and superficial tissues in a position in which the fascia might stretch either into (placing tissues on slack) or out of (placing tissues on tension) a "restrictive barrier" until the sensation of a release or "unwinding" is felt by the patient or practitioner. The goal is to reduce movement restrictions through mobilization or stretching of fascia. The literature regarding the effectiveness of MFR is mixed in both quality and results. Although the quality of randomized controlled trial (RCT) studies varies greatly, the results are encouraging (Ajimsha *et al.*, 2015) (Figure 5.3).

Friction massage is a manual technique, developed by James Cyriax, a British orthopedic physician. In the application of this technique, the practitioner uses the pad of the fingertip or thumb, first applying pressure to increase the depth of the technique, usually and specifically to the level of an interface between two tissues, then creating a shear force parallel, perpendicular, or diagonally across the fibers which are to be treated (Chamberlain, 1982). The practitioner's hand moves together with the superficial tissue, while the subcutaneous tissue is static. More aggressive techniques might utilize friction massage with passive or active movement of the body in the opposite

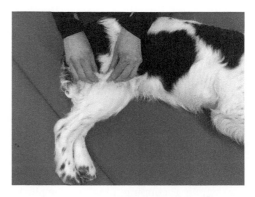

Figure 5.3 Skin rolling. *Source:* Courtesy Dr Amie Hesbach (co-author).

direction, further increasing the shear forces (DeLisa *et al.*, 2005). In physical therapy for human patients, friction massage techniques are utilized for 5–15 minutes; however, this duration might not be realistic for use in the animal patient (Goats, 1994).

Friction massage is a technique which is theorized to:

- Maintain or improve mobility within and between ligaments, tendons, and muscles (Sharma and Maffulli, 2005)
- Prevent fibrotic and adherent scar tissue from forming (Robinson and Sheets, 2015)
- Assist in re-alignment of collagen fibers (Salvo, 2012)
- Cause hyperemia (Chamberlain, 1982)

Certainly, all manual techniques have effects on the fascial system, due to their integration within the entire body; however, these myofascial techniques are specific in their focus and therapeutic goal.

Soft Tissue Mobilization: Trigger Point Techniques

A trigger point (TrP) is a hyperirritable point that is palpable within a taut band of muscle and fascia and can be active or latent. An active TrP is painful at rest, with active muscle contraction, and with manual compression. Pain results in a localized twitch response or "jump sign," tenderness, and pain referred in a predictable, distant pattern (i.e., referred pain pattern), which "frequently occurs within the same dermatome, myotome, or sclerotome as that of the TrP but does not include the entire segment" (Travell and Simons, 1983). Active TrPs prevent full lengthening of the muscle, leading to muscle weakness, and can produce referred motor and autonomic phenomena, generally within its pain reference zone. A latent TrP is painful only with compression or when palpated but may have clinical characteristics similar to an active

TrP. It always has a taut band that increases muscle tension and restricts ROM (Bron and Dommerholt, 2012).

TrPs can be managed with:

- Medications
- Injections, either wet (i.e., trigger point injection [TPI] or prolotherapy) or dry (i.e., TrP or dry needling) (Gattie *et al.*, 2017)
- Osteopathic approach
- Acupuncture or acupressure
- Modalities (i.e., phototherapy, therapeutic ultrasound, and focused shockwave)
- Manual TrP release, stress point therapy, or ischemic compression

Manual trigger point release (TPR), stress point therapy, or ischemic compression is the treatment of tender, hyperirritable foci located within the muscle belly or musculotendinous junction using sustained digital pressure. The practitioner progressively applies moderate to heavy pressure perpendicular, directly over, and into a TrP until an increase in tissue resistance is noted. The digital pressure is theorized to restrict the superficial blood supply to the underlying painful tissue so that, upon release of the pressure, there is a resurgence of blood. The pressure is maintained until there is a sense of release of the taut band, which can be repeated up to three times (Lewit, 1991), and, upon release of the manual compression, the muscle is gently stretched. This technique is theorized to increase local circulation, resulting in flushing of waste products, increased oxygenation of tissues, and promotion of healing (Jannsens, 1991; Travell and Simons, 1983; Physiopedia, n.d.).

This topic will be further discussed in Chapter 26: Myofascial Trigger Point Therapy.

Instrument-Assisted Techniques

Manual techniques might be performed mechanically, via the utilization of an instrument or tool as an adjunct or extension of the hands, in STM or peripheral joint and spinal mobilization and manipulation. Instrument-assisted techniques might incorporate the use of hand-held instrument-assisted soft tissue mobilization (IASTM) devices (e.g., Graston, ASTYM, and FASCIQ), therapy guns (e.g., TheraGun), massagers, mechanical adjusting devices or manually assisted adjusting instruments (MADs) (e.g., actuators/activators), vibrators, or other electromechanical devices and require additional training specific to the device (and often provided by the manufacturer). Though some practitioners consider instrument-assisted techniques less specific in application than using the hands alone, others suggest that the use of instruments in the application of manual techniques provides more or different information about the target tissues than the hands alone (Seffrin *et al.*, 2019).

The use of MADs in combination with an adaptor has been shown to not pose an increased risk of injury when used in manipulation on animal patients (Colloca *et al.*, 2005; Duarte *et al.*, 2014; Taylor *et al.*, 2004). Though patients may have a fear or anxiety response to the sensation or noise and so feedback of positive effects can be obscured. The current literature provides support for IASTM in improving ROM in uninjured individuals and improving pain and patient-reported function (or both) in injured patients (Seffrin *et al.*, 2019). IASTM has been shown to increase tissue perfusion in collateral ligaments of the rat knee (Loghmani and Warden, 2013). More high-quality research involving a larger variety of animal patients and products is needed to further substantiate and allow for generalization of these findings.

Peripheral Joint and Spinal Mobilization

Since 1998, the American Physical Therapy Association's (APTA) Guide to Physical Therapist Practice has defined mobilization and manipulation as "a MT technique comprised of a continuum of skilled passive movements that are applied at varying speeds and amplitudes, including small-amplitude, high-velocity therapeutic movements" (American Physical Therapy Association, n.d.). The International Federation of Orthopaedic Manipulative Physical Therapists (IFOMPT) further defines joint mobilization as "a MT technique comprising a continuum of skilled passive movements that are applied at varying speeds and amplitudes to joints, muscles or nerves with the intent to restore optimal motion, function, and/or to reduce pain" (Physiopedia, n.d.).

As previously discussed, joint ROM consists of both osteokinematic and arthrokinematic motions. Arthrokinematic motion is passive, involuntary motion that occurs between two joint surfaces during osteokinematic motion. Arthrokinematic motion, also known as accessory or translatory motion, is the movement that occurs between joint surfaces, primarily rolls, spins, and slides or glides. It cannot be isolated by the patient with muscle contractions but can be reproduced passively and manually by the skilled practitioner as both an assessment and a treatment technique (Hesbach, 2014).

"Accessory motion testing" is the method by which the practitioner can assess arthrokinematic motion and is the use of mobilization with a stretch articulation or assessment of end feel to assess or evaluate mobility of the joint-associated tissues (i.e., joint capsule, ligament, muscle, tendon, fascia, and articular cartilage). Upon performance of these tests, the practitioner will designate each joint (and direction of arthrokinematic motion) as hypermobile, hypomobile, normal, and/or painful. Additionally, the practitioner might note the presence of spinal segmental dysfunction, somatic dysfunction, or facilitated segments (Björnsdóttir and Kumar, 1997).

Assessment and reassessment of accessory motion are necessary prior to and during the application of peripheral joint and spinal mobilization techniques. When an abnormality or dysfunction is noted through accessory motion testing, the practitioner must understand when or if the dysfunction is indicative of a red flag and warrant referral or can be managed through the application of traditional and advanced MT techniques, such as peripheral joint and spinal mobilization, or other interventions (Edge-Hughes, 2013; Goff, 2009; Hesbach, 2014).

Peripheral joint or spinal mobilization techniques might include traction, approximation or compression, or gliding of one joint surface on an opposing and stabilized joint surface (Bialosky *et al.*, 2018; Reed *et al.*, 2021). Treatment variables which are prescribed based on the results of accessory motion testing include: type, grade or amplitude (see Table 5.4),

Table 5.4 Grades of peripheral joint and spinal mobilization and manipulation (Maitland).

Grade	Descriptor
I	Small-amplitude, rhythmic oscillations performed at beginning of range
II	Large-amplitude, rhythmic oscillations performed within range, below tissue resistance, not reaching anatomic limit
III	Large-amplitude, rhythmic oscillations performed to the limit of available motion and into tissue resistance
IV	Small-amplitude, rhythmic oscillations performed to the limit of available motion and to tissue resistance
V	A small-amplitude, high-velocity thrust technique is performed to stretch to the limit of available motion

Source: Adapted from Kaltenborn (1989).

direction, speed, duration, and frequency of mobilization (Zusman, 1986). Each of these variables should be documented in the animal rehabilitation record (Saunders *et al.*, 2005).

Peripheral Joint and Spinal Manipulation

Manipulation is the passive movement of a peripheral joint or axial spinal segment beyond the normal range of motion. It is characterized by the application of controlled short-lever or long-lever manual or mechanical thrusts applied within or at the end ROM to induce therapeutic responses in joint function (Bialosky *et al.*, 2018; Chaitow, 2010). Manipulation, also known as high-velocity, low-amplitude (HVLA) thrust technique, non-thrust technique, or Grade V Maitland mobilization, requires specialized training which is standard in many chiropractic and physical therapy educational programs (Haussler, 2016).

Neuromuscular Facilitation and Sensory Stimulation Approaches

Though quite specialized and requiring further education and practical instruction for safe clinical application, neuromuscular facilitation and sensory stimulation approaches utilize a variety of inputs, both manually and through the application of sensory stimuli, positional and postural changes, and assisted and resisted active movements to elicit both reflexive and functional motor responses for normalization of postures and movement (Elizabeth, 1966). Examples of such approaches include proprioceptive neuromuscular facilitation (PNF), neurodevelopmental training (NDT), and rood sensorimotor therapy (Prentice, n.d.). While these approaches were traditionally utilized with human patients with neurological disorders, they have been successfully applied in animal patients with both neurological and orthopedic diagnoses.

NeuroDynamics

Formerly called neural mobilization, NeuroDynamics is an MT approach including neural tissue mobilization and traction techniques, a consolidation of the research and clinical practice of Michael Shaklock, Geoffrey Maitland, James Cyriax, and David Butler (Shaklock, 1995). A NeuroDynamic evaluation will include examination of the patient-specific to the mechanics and physiology of the nervous system. With regards to mechanics, NeuroDynamics considers both the passive positioning (or neural tension) and the active dynamic mobility (or neural gliding, tensioning, compressing, or elongating) of the nervous tissues with regard to the influence and interface of the fascia and meninges and its effect on the adequate functioning of the nervous tissues (Bialosky *et al.*, 2018). Physiologically, NeuroDynamics is concerned with the impaired microcirculation and axonal transport that occurs as a result of injury, chronic postures (i.e., neural entrapment), or pathology. NeuroDynamic treatment might include passive movements or mobilizations (i.e., mobilization of the nervous system [MOTNS]) of the spine and extremities in specific combinations or sequences to elongate or tension components of the nervous system, which effectively could allow for restoration of pain-free postures and active functional mobility and optimization of physiologic functioning of the nervous tissues (Ellis and Hing, 2008). Practitioners have developed and successfully utilized a NeuroDynamic approach adapted for use in small and large animals.

Osteopathy, Chiropractic, and Physical Therapy

Osteopathy, chiropractic, and physical therapy are fields which include MT approaches and manual techniques within their overall approach to patient management. As it is beyond the scope of this text to describe these in detail, the field of animal physical rehabilitation is a multi-disciplinary field with collaborators from these varied backgrounds, among others.

Client Instruction, Education, and Home Exercise Programs (HEP)

To optimize functional outcomes, the client should be educated and instructed in basic manual techniques in order to ensure progression through the animal rehabilitation program. Such instruction might include basic PROM, stretching, and massage techniques.

As well, consideration of other variables under the control of the client is necessary as they will influence the eventual achievement of functional goals. The practitioner should consider such variables as:

- Biomechanical stresses due to inappropriate saddle, bit, harness, leash, or collar use and fit
- Biomechanical stresses due to the patient's physical home or work environment (e.g., flooring surfaces, bedding, variable terrain, and obstacles)
- Training or sport-specific stresses, including physical and mental stresses (e.g., overload to tissue failure, and overtraining)

The client should also be instructed in a HEP supportive of the goals of rehabilitation, encouraging active mobility to promote tissue mobility, circulation, and other gains made through the clinical practice. Home programs should be simple and sensitive to the client's ability, skill, and time limitations in order to ensure an optimal level of compliance. The program should be easy to implement and a positive experience for both client and patient.

To enhance compliance, the practitioner should educate the client with regards to the purpose and benefit of any MT approach or manual technique applied and relate it to the patient's condition and established functional goals. Understanding the expected response to the application of these techniques will better prepare the client to ensure appropriate progression of treatment and assist the practitioner in identifying red flags or a need for referral in the case of a negative or detrimental response.

When instructing in a HEP (which is essential for motor learning and neuroplasticity) and basic manual techniques, the practitioner should provide:

1) A visual and verbal demonstration with explanation of appropriate and safe positioning, handling, and other necessary variables,
2) Practice with appropriate supervision, assistance, and feedback to ensure that all prescribed activities are performed safely and effectively, and
3) Take-home instruction in hard-copy form, with written instructions and images, as well as links to online videos or other interactive technology. Instructions should be specific with regard to frequency, intensity, and duration.

Conclusion

The utilization of an MT approach and application of manual techniques in tandem with other rehabilitation strategies and tactics can support the restoration of and return to maximal function in animal patients. A multitude of approaches and techniques are available, with varied levels of skill, knowledge, expertise, and supervision necessary for safe, efficient, and effective application by the animal rehabilitation practitioner. Though only the basics of ROM, stretching, and massage techniques were described, this chapter introduces other approaches and techniques which could be beneficial for inclusion in the comprehensive, goal-focused, multi-disciplinary rehabilitation plan as an adjunct to and supportive of other interventions, including the application of therapeutic exercise, functional mobility retraining, and physical modalities.

References

Affolter, V.K. (2013). Chronic progressive lymphedema in draft horses. *Vet Clin North Am Equine Pract* 29 (3): 589–605.

Ajimsha MS, Al-Mudahka NR, and Al-Madzhar JA (2015) Effectiveness of myofascial release: Systematic review of randomized controlled trials. *J Bodyw Mov Ther* 19(1):102–112. https://doi.org/10.1016/j.jbmt.2014.06.001. Epub 2014 Jun 13. 25603749 (accessed March 20, 2022).

American Physical Therapy Association (n.d.) Available at: www.apta.org (accessed April 26, 2016).

Austin, P.J., Kim, C.F., Perera, C.J., and Moalem-Taylor, G. (2012). Regulatory T cells attenuate neuropathic pain following peripheral nerve injury and experimental autoimmune neuritis. *Pain* 153 (9): 1916–1931.

Baltzer, W.I. (2020). Rehabilitation of companion animals following orthopaedic surgery. *NZ Vet J* 68: 157–167.

Bandy, W.D. and Irion, J.M. (1994). The effect of time on static stretch on the flexibility of the hamstring muscles. *Phys Ther* 74: 845–850.

Basmajian, J.V. and Nyberg, R.E. (1992). *Rational Manual Therapies*. Philadelphia, PA: Williams and Wilkins.

Bialosky, J.E., Beneciuk, J.M., Bishop, M.D. et al. (2018). Unraveling the mechanisms of manual therapy: Modeling an approach. *J Orthop Sports Phys Ther* 48 (1): 8–18. https://doi.org/10.2519/jospt.2018.7476.

Billhult, A., Lindholm, C., Gunnarsson, R.K., and Stener-Victorin, E. (2009). The effect of massage on immune function and stress in women with breast cancer—A randomized controlled trial. *Auton Neurosci* 150 (1–2): 111–115.

Björnsdóttir SV and Kumar S (1997) Posteroanterior spinal mobilization: State of the art review and discussion. *Disabil Rehabil* 19(2):39–46. https://doi.org/10.3109/09638289709166826. 9058028.

Brady D (2013) How often and long should I stretch to improve flexibility? Available at: www.Sports Science.com. (accessed March 20, 2022).

Bron C and Dommerholt JD (2012) Etiology of myofascial trigger points. *Curr Pain Headache Rep* 16(5):439–444. https://doi.org/10.1007/s11916-012-0289-4. 22836591; PMC3440564 (accessed July 4, 2022).

Brunke, M., Broadhurst, M., Oliver, K., and Levine, D. (2021). Manual therapy in small animal rehabilitation. *Adv Small Anim Care* 2: 19–30. 10.1016/j.yasa.2021.07.008.

Chaitow, L. (2010). *Modern Neuromuscular Techniques: Advanced Soft Tissue Techniques*, 3e. Wellingborough, Northamptonshire: Churchill Livingstone.

Chamberlain GJ (1982) Cyriax's friction massage: A review. *J Orthop Sports Phys Ther* 4(1):16–22. https://doi.org/10.2519/jospt.1982.4.1.16. 18810110.

Cleveland Clinic (n.d.). Available at: https://my.clevelandclinic.org/health/treatments/17677-craniosacral-therapy (accessed January 24, 2022).

Coates, J. (2017). *Manual Therapy Treatment. Physical Rehabilitation for Veterinary Technicians and Nurses*, 59–78. Ames, IA: John Wiley and Sons, Inc. https://doi.org/10.1002/9781119389668.ch5.

Colloca CJ, Keller TS, Black P, *et al.* (2005) Comparison of mechanical force of manually assisted chiropractic adjusting instruments. *J Manipulative Physiol Ther* 28(6):414–422. https://doi.org/10.1016/j.jmpt.2005.06.004. 16096041.

Corti, L. (2014). Massage therapy for dogs and cats. *Top Companion Anim Med* 29: 54–57.

Coville, J. (2016). *Muscular System. Clinical Anatomy and Physiology for Veterinary Technicians*, 3rde, 210–225. St. Louis, MO: Elsevier.

Davis, L., Hanson, B., and Gilliam, S. (2016). Pilot study of the effects of mixed light touch manual therapies on active duty soldiers with chronic post-traumatic stress disorder and injury to the head. *J Bodywork Movement Ther* 20: 42–51. https://doi.org/10.1016/j.jbmt.2015.03.006.

DeLisa, J.A., Gans, B.M., and Walsh, N.E. (2005). *Physical Medicine and Rehabilitation: Principles and Practice*, vol. 1. Philadelphia: Lippincott Williams and Williams.

DiBerardino, L.A., Ragetly, C.A., Hong, S. et al. (2012). Improving regions of deviation gait symmetry analysis with pointwise T tests. *J Appl Biomech* 28 (2): 210–214.

Duarte FC, Kolberg C, Barros RR, *et al.* (2014) Evaluation of peak force of a manually operated chiropractic adjusting instrument with an adapter for use in animals. *J Manipulative Physiol Ther* 37(4):236–241. https://doi.org/10.1016/j.jmpt.2014.02.004. Epub 2014 May 2. 24793371.

Dutton, M. (2015). *Goniometry in Orthopaedic Examination, Evaluation, and Intervention*, 2nde. http://highered.mheducation.com/sites/0071474013/student_view0/chapter8/goniometry.html.

Edge-Hughes L (2013) Manual therapy and the canine thoracic spine. Available at: https://www.orthopt.org/uploads/content_files/CSM_2014/ManualTherapy_CanineThoracicSpine.pdf.

Elizabeth, R. (1966). Sensory stimulation techniques. *Am J Nurs* 66 (2): 281–286.

Ellis, R.F. and Hing, W.A. (2008). Neural mobilization: A systematic review of randomized controlled trials with an analysis of therapeutic efficacy. *J Man Manip Ther* 16 (1): 8–22. https://doi.org/10.1179/106698108790818594.

Fehrs L (2010) Massage stroke review. Institute for Integrative Health Care.

Formenton, M.R., Pereira, M.A.A., and Fantoni, D.T. (2017). Small animal massage therapy: A brief review and relevant observations. *Top Companion Anim Med* 32: 139–145.

Fritz, S. (2004). *Fundamentals of Therapeutic Massage*. St. Louis: Mosby.

Fritz, S. and Grosenbach, M.J. (2009). *Essential Sciences for Therapeutic Massage*. St. Louis: Mosby.

Furlan, A.D., Brosseau, L., Imamura, M., and Irvin, E. (2002). Massage for low-back pain: A systematic review within the framework of the Cochrane Collaboration Back Review Group. *Spine* 27 (17): 1896–1910.

Gattie, E., Cleland, J.A., and Snodgrass, S. (2017). The effectiveness of trigger point dry needling for musculoskeletal conditions by physical therapists: A systematic review and meta-analysis. *J Orthop Sports Phys Ther* 47 (3): 133–149. Available at: doi: 10.2519/jospt.2017.7096. Epub 2017 Feb 3. PMID: 28158962.

Gay, A., Aimonetti, J.-M., Roll, J.-P., and Ribot-Ciscar, E. (2015). Kinesthetic illusions attenuate experimental muscle pain, as do muscle and cutaneous stimulation. *Brain Res* 1615: 148–156.

Goats, G.C. (1994). Massage: The scientific basis of an ancient art. Part 1: The techniques. *Br J Sports Med* 28 (3): 149–152.

Goff, L.M. (2009). Manual therapy for the horse: A contemporary perspective. *J Equine Vet* 29 (11): 799–808.

Goff, L. and Jull, G. (2007). Manual therapy in animal physiotherapy. In: *Assessment, treatment, and rehabilitation of animals* (ed. C. McGowan, L. Goff, and N. Stubbs), 164–176. Ames, IA: Blackwell.

Grayson, J.E., Barton, T., Cabot, P.J., and Souvlis, T. (2012). Spinal manual therapy produces rapid onset analgesia in a rodent model. *Manual Ther* 17 (4): 292–297.

Hammerschlag R, Marx BL, and Aickin M (2014) Nontouch biofield therapy: A systematic review of human randomized controlled trials reporting use of only nonphysical contact treatment. *J Altern Complement Med* 20(12):881–892. https://doi.org/10.1089/acm.2014.0017. 25181286.

Haussler, K.K. (2016). Joint mobilization and manipulation for the equine athlete. *Vet Clin North Am Equine Pract* 32: 87–101.

Haussler, K.K., Hesbach, A., Romano, L., and Goff, L. (2021). A systematic review of musculoskeletal mobilization and manipulation techniques used in veterinary medicine. *Animals* 11: 2787. Available at: https://doi.org/10.3390/ani11102787.

Hendrickson, A.R., Massey, P.D., and Cronan, T.P. (1993). On the test-retest reliability of perceived usefulness and perceived ease of use scales. *MIS Q* 1993: 227–230.

Hesbach, A.L. (2014). Manual therapy in veterinary rehabilitation. *Topics in Comp An Med* 29 (1): 20–23. Available at: ISSN 1938-9736. https://doi.org/10.1053/j.tcam.2014.02.002.

Huang, T.W., Tseng, S.-H., Lin, C.-C. et al. (2013). Effects of manual lymphatic drainage on breast cancer-related lymphedema: A systematic review and meta-analysis of randomized controlled trials. *World J Surg Oncol* 11 (15): Available at: https://doi.org/10.1186/1477-7819-11-15.

Jaegger, G.H., Marcellin-Little, D.J., and Levine, D. (2002). Reliability of goniometry in Labrador retrievers. *Am J Vet Res* 63 (7): 979–986.

Jannsens LA (1991) Trigger points in 48 dogs with myofascial pain syndromes. *Vet Surg* 20(4):274–278. Available at: https://doi.org/10.1111/j.1532-950x.1991.tb01263.x.1949567.

Jarvis, S.L., Worley, D.R., Hogy, S.M. et al. (2013). Kinematic and kinetic analysis of dogs during trotting after amputation of a thoracic limb. *Am J Vet Res* 74 (9): 1155–1163.

Kaltenborn, F.M. (1989). *Manual Mobilization of the Extremity Joints, Basic Examination and Treatment Techniques*, 4the. Minneapolis: Orthopedic Physical Therapy Products.

Kirkby-Shaw, K., Alvarez, L., Foster, S.A., and Tomlinson, J. (2020). Fundamental principles of rehabilitation and musculoskeletal tissue healing. *Vet Surg* 49: 22–32.

Lascelles, B.D., Hansen, B.D., Roe, S. et al. (2012). Relationship of orthopedic examination, goniometric measurements, and radiographic signs of degenerative joint disease in cats. *BMC Vet Res* 8: 10.

Lee, B.B., Bergan, J., and Rockson, S.G. (2011). *Lymphedema: A Concise Compendium of Theory and Practice*. New York City: Springer.

Lewit, K. (1991). *Manipulative Therapy in Rehabilitation of the Locomotor System*. Woburn, MA: Butterworth-Heinemann.

Lima, C.R., Martins, D.F., and Reed, W.R. (2020). Physiological responses induced by manual therapy in animal models: A scoping review. *Front Neurosci* 14: 430.

Loghmani, M.T. and Warden, S.J. (2013). Instrument-assisted cross fiber massage increases tissue perfusion and alters microvascular morphology in the vicinity of healing knee ligaments. *BMC Complement Altern Med* 13: 240.

McHugh, M.P. and Cosgrave, C.H. (2012). To stretch or not to stretch: The role of stretching in injury prevention and performance. *Scand J Med Sci Sports* 20 (2): 169–181.

Norkin, C.C. and Levangie, P.K. (1992). *Joint Structure and Function: A Comprehensive Analysis*. Philadelphia: F.A. Davis Company.

Page, P. (2012). Current concepts in muscle stretching for exercise and rehabilitation. *Int J Sports Phys Ther* 7 (1): 109–119.

Pavan, P.G., Stecco, A., Stem, R., and Stecco, C. (2014). Painful connections: Densification versus fibrosis of fascia. *Curr Pain Headache Rep* 18: 441.

Physiopedia (n.d.). Available at: https://www.physio-pedia.com/Trigger_Points. Accessed 31 January 2022. https://www.physio-pedia.com/End-Feel (Accessed 17 March 2022).

Prentice WE (n.d.) Proprioceptive neuromuscular facilitation techniques in rehabilitation. Available at: https://musculoskeletalkey.com/proprioceptive-neuromuscular-facilitation-techniques-in-rehabilitation/ (Accessed 31 January 2022).

Rapaport, M.H., Schettler, P., and Breese, C. (2010). A preliminary study of the effects of a single session of Swedish massage on hypothalamic-pituitary-adrenal and immune function in normal individuals. *J Altern Complement Med* 16 (10): 1079–1088. Available at: doi: 10.1089/acm.2009.0634. PMID: 20809811; PMCID: PMC3107905.

Reed, W., Gudavalli, M., Lima, C., and Singh, H. (2021). In vivo measurement of intradiscal pressure changes related to spinal manual therapy in an animal model: A feasibility study. *Arch Phys Med Rehabil* 102 (10): e94–e95. Available at: ISSN 0003-9993. https://doi.org/10.1016/j.apmr.2021.07.757. https://www.sciencedirect.com/science/article/pii/S0003999321012818.

Reese, N.B. and Brandy, W.D. (2010). *Joint Range of Motion and Muscle Length Testing*, 2nde. St. Louis: Saunders.

Robinson, N.G. and Sheets, S. (2015). *Treatment Techniques: Canine Medical Massage Techniques and Clinical Applications*. Lakewood, CO: American Animal Hospital Association Press.

Salvo, S.G. (2012). *Massage Therapy: Principles and Practice*, 4the. St. Louis: Saunders.

Saunders, D.G., Walker, J.R., and Levine, D. (2005). Joint mobilization. *Vet Clin North Am Small Anim Pract* 35: 1287–1316, vii–viii.

Schleip, R. and Klingler, W. (2019). Active contractile properties of fascia. *Clin Anat* 32: 891–895.

Schuller, S., Le Garrérès, A., Remy, I., and Peeters, D. (2011). Idiopathic chylothorax and lymphedema in 2 whippet littermates. *Can Vet J* 52 (11): 1243–1245.

Seffrin, C.B., Cattano, N.M., Reed, M.A., and Gardiner-Shires, A.M. (2019). Instrument-assisted soft tissue mobilization: A systematic review and effect-size analysis. *J Athl Train* 54 (7): 808–821. Available at: doi: 10.4085/1062-6050-481-17. Epub. PMID: 31322903; PMCID: PMC6709755.

Sefton, J.M., Yarar, C., Berry, J.W. et al. (2011). Physiological and clinical changes after therapeutic massage of the neck and shoulders. *Man Ther* 16 (5): 487–494.

Shaklock, M. (1995). Neurodynamics. *Physiotherapy* 81 (1): 9–16.

Sharma, P. and Maffulli, N. (2005). Tendon injury and tendinopathy: Healing and repair. *J Bone Joint Surg Am* 87 (1): 187–202.

Sprague, S. (2013). Introduction to canine rehabilitation. In: *Canine Sports Medicine and Rehabilitation*, 1ste (ed. M.C. Zink and J.B. VanDyke). Ames, IA: John Wiley and Sons, Inc.

Taylor, D.C., Dalton, J.D., Saeber, A.V., and Garrett, W.E. (1990). Viscoelastic properties of muscle-tendon units: The biomechanical effects of stretching. *Am J Sports Med* 18 (3): 300–309.

Taylor, S.H., Arnold, N.D., Biggs, L., and Colloca, C.J. (2004). A review of the literature pertaining to the efficacy, safety, educational requirements, uses and usage of mechanical adjusting devices. *J Can Chiropr Assoc* 48 (1): 74–108. Available at: PMID: 17549220; PMCID: PMC1840033.

Travell, J.G. and Simons, D.G. (1983). *Myofascial Pain and Dysfunction: The Trigger Point Manual*. Baltimore: Williams and Wilkins.

Vairo, G.L., Miller, S.J., NM, M.B. et al. (2009). Systematic review of efficacy for manual lymphatic drainage techniques in sports medicine and rehabilitation: An evidence-based practice approach. *J Man Manip Ther* 17 (3): e80-9. https://doi.org/10.1179/jmt.2009.17.3.80E. PMID: 20046617; PMCID: PMC2755111.

Veterinary Manual Therapy Working Group (2022). *Definition of Veterinary Manual Therapy*. Unpublished.

Wang, Q., Zeng, H., Best, T.M. et al. (2014). A mechatronic system for quantitative application and assessment of massage-like actions in small animals. *Ann Biomed Eng* 36–49.

Weiner, R.S. (2001). *Pain Management: A Practical Guide for Clinicians*, 6the. Boca Raton: CRC Press.

Wise, C.H. (2015). *Orthopaedic Manual Physical Therapy from Art to Evidence*. Philadelphia: F.A. Davis Company.

Yin, S. (2009). *Low Stress Handling, Restraint and Behavior Modification of Dogs and Cats: Techniques for Developing Pets Who Love Their Visits*. Davis, CA: Cattle Dog Publishing.

Zusman M (1986) Spinal manipulative therapy: Review of some proposed mechanisms, and a new hypothesis. *Aust J Physiother* 32(2):89–99. Available at: https://doi.org/10.1016/S0004-9514(14)60645-0. 25026443.

6

Home Exercises: Teaching the Client to be an Extension of You

Jacqueline R. Davidson and Sherri Jerzyk

Small Animal Clinical Sciences, College of Veterinary Medicine & Biomedical Sciences, Texas A&M University, College Station, TX, USA

Introduction

Client involvement in a rehabilitation program may be minimal, or the therapy may be performed entirely by the client in the home environment. To design the ideal program, the client, the patient, and the environment must first be assessed. The client must be committed to the plan, and have the mental, emotional, and physical capability to work with the patient. The patient should be assessed for motivation and cooperation. And the home environment should be assessed to take obstacles into consideration as well as using resources in the home environment such as inclines or exercise equipment. The rehabilitation team must work with the client to create a program that is effective and fits with the client's capabilities and resources. The therapist must ensure that the client can correctly perform the therapies, and the patient should be assessed regularly until the therapeutic goals are reached.

Assessing the Client

Level of Commitment

Several factors can affect a client's level of commitment to a rehabilitation program. It is important to understand some of the factors that may impede the client from participating in the therapy. Once the rehabilitation team is aware of potential factors that may reduce client compliance, they may be able to adjust the program to improve the client's ability to commit.

Physical Rehabilitation for Veterinary Technicians and Nurses, Second Edition.
Edited by Mary Ellen Goldberg and Julia E. Tomlinson.
© 2024 John Wiley & Sons, Inc. Published 2024 by John Wiley & Sons, Inc.
Companion website: www.wiley.com/go/goldberg/physicalrehabilitationvettechsandnurses

One of the key factors in client compliance is how they perceive the value of rehabilitation as a treatment. The client's personal experience with exercise or physical therapy may have a positive or negative effect on their attitude toward rehabilitation for the patient. The client's cultural background may also affect their beliefs in the value of therapy. A basic understanding of the patient's health condition and how rehabilitation can help is also important. Client education by the rehabilitation team can make a significant difference in the clients' understanding of the value and purpose of rehabilitation. This may help motivate them to follow a program.

Financial considerations may also affect client compliance. Clients must be willing and able to pay for a rehabilitation program. Financial considerations will affect the type of program the client chooses for their pet. If clients have minimal financial constraints, they may be able to take advantage of extensive in-house therapy. For many patients and clients, it is appropriate to consider some in-house therapy along with home exercises. However, if funds are limited, the client may request a program that is strictly carried out at home with minimal intervention on the part of the rehabilitation team. A frank discussion of the cost of rehabilitation enables the rehabilitation team to develop a program that is affordable for the client to perform and maintain. In some cases, the less expensive option may be less ideal for the patient. However, this may be preferable to the client electing to pursue no therapy because it is unaffordable.

Time constraints may also affect the degree to which the client adheres to a program. If the rehabilitation program recommended is too time-intensive, the client may become overwhelmed and entirely abandon it in frustration. It is important to have a nonjudgmental discussion to establish how much time the client can realistically commit to the program each day. Once this has been established, a program can be designed to maximize the available time.

The clients' understanding of the value of rehabilitation, along with any financial or time constraints should all be discussed prior to creating the rehabilitation program. Any factors that may be barriers to commitment must be considered when designing the program. The "ideal" program will not be effective if the client is unable to remain committed to it.

Physical Abilities

Rehabilitation can be very physically and mentally demanding for the client or the animal handler. The client's general physical abilities should be assessed during the initial discussion about the rehabilitation program. It is a good idea to simply ask the client or handler if they have any physical limitations that need to be considered when designing the home exercise program. You do not need to ask for any specific details of their condition. Explain how the program may be designed to adapt to these conditions. If the client does not wish to share any information, the therapist should create a home exercise plan they feel is appropriate. Most clients are willing to give you the information needed to properly care for their pet if approached with sincerity.

The therapist should carefully observe the client during any training sessions where the client is demonstrating proficiency in handling the patient. The client may be required to get down on the ground with the patient for some exercises and may transition from squatting to a standing position frequently. In some cases, the client may need to lift and support the patient. Additionally, some exercises may require a certain level of agility or speed on the part of the client, to have the patient perform correctly. Exercises that are complex or require precise timing may be too difficult for some clients to understand and perform well. If the therapist suspects that the client may have physical or mental difficulty with certain exercises, they may need to be modified or dropped from the home program.

There are situations where multiple handlers are required to have the patient perform the treatments correctly. This most commonly occurs in large dogs that are non-ambulatory or have severe physical impairments. In these situations, the client must be able to identify other individuals in the home environment who will be able to participate in the patient's care.

It is particularly important for the client to be physically fit for them to perform rehabilitation on their pet. Many home exercise programs include a lot of walking or stair climbing. If clients have been sedentary or have any potential risk associated with an increase in activity, it should be recommended that they consult their physician before beginning the rehabilitation program for their pet. The goal is to improve the patient's physical ability, not decrease the client's! However, sometimes the patient's need for exercise is helpful motivation for the clients to improve their own physical fitness.

Animal Handling Skills

The animal handling skills of the client can affect the design of the rehabilitation home program. Knowledge of basic obedience commands is nice but not necessary. However, the client must be able to control or redirect the patient's behavior. If the client is unable to control the patient's movements they may be performed ineffectively, or even worse, could result in further injury to the patient.

As clients understand more about animal training, they are better able to motivate or alter the patient's behaviors. While this is not essential for passive types of therapy, it becomes more important for active exercises, particularly if the movements become more complex. For example, controlled leash walking can be performed with minimal handling skills (although this can vary with the patient's personality and level of training). However, having a patient perform sit-to-stand exercises requires a higher level of control that can be made easier if the client can shape the patient's behavior.

The client should also have a basic understanding of animal behavior. Some clients may need guidance to understand body language. This is particularly important if the patient may be inclined to bite or scratch, so the client can avoid becoming injured during a therapy session. The client should also be instructed to interpret signs that the patient may be in pain. This is helpful because additional therapies may be indicated if the patient is in pain. In addition, clients are fearful of creating pain and become reluctant to perform the therapy. If they can more accurately assess the patient's pain, they are more likely to perform appropriate therapy.

Clients may benefit from some instruction to improve their animal handling skills. It is important to not only explain handling skills to the client but to also show them physically, and then have them demonstrate proficiency. In this way, the therapist can identify potential problems in the animal handling techniques. An instruction appointment can be made with a technician therapist to help troubleshoot with the client and to teach luring behaviors (see Chapter 9) for each therapeutic exercise.

Client–Patient Bond

The relationship between the client and the patient plays a crucial role in successful rehabilitation. The client's emotional bond often provides significant motivation for the client to persist in helping with the recovery and rehabilitation process. Clients may understand what toys or treats best motivate their pets, as well as which activities they particularly enjoy. A more intimate knowledge of the patient's personality may give clients an advantage because they may be able to "think outside the box" to motivate the patient to perform an exercise or movement.

In some cases, the client relationship may hinder the rehabilitation program. Some clients may be reluctant to push the patient to do any activity when they encounter resistance. In addition, some clients may be concerned that they are going to create pain or further injury. These clients should be educated so they understand what needs to be done, and gain confidence that their efforts are necessary and beneficial.

Clients need to be able to notice any subtle changes in the patient. They need to be instructed to take note of any physical changes that are either seen or felt by physical palpation and take note of any behavior change that arises during their in-home treatments. As previously mentioned, the clients must also be able to watch for signs of pain and distinguish it from fatigue or stress. Some clients are very skilled at understanding their pet's personality and behaviors, while others may need some guidance and education related to typical animal behaviors. Having clients fill out regular brief pain indexes is a way to track pain progression.

Rehabilitation Goals

Rehabilitation goals should be discussed early in the assessment process. The rehabilitation team can help establish realistic end goals, based on their knowledge of the condition and prognosis. It is helpful for many clients to not only establish an end goal but to break it down into baby steps. For example, a post-operative disc dog may have an end goal of walking. If we give a first goal of motor function while ambulating with support, or positioning the rear feet in an appropriate position to stand, the client can see the progress easier and does not feel like they are never getting to their goal. The team can also suggest whether the goals are likely to be achievable with the patient receiving home care only. In many cases, a combination of in-house therapy and home care, or extensive in-house therapy may be more appropriate.

Client expectations should also be explored during this discussion. It is important for the therapy team to know what the client anticipates and desires as the outcome. Do they want their pet to return to full working duty or do they just want it to be able to climb up on the couch again? If there is a disparity between what the client expects and the probable outcome, this should be recognized before beginning the therapy program. While it is beneficial to be optimistic, a realistic outcome needs to be discussed.

Assessing the Patient

Concurrent Medical Issues

When assessing a patient for rehabilitation, it is important to take the patient's history into account. If the patient has concurrent medical issues, the exercises you choose must not aggravate any underlying condition. For example, if a patient has had an FHO but also has a partial cruciate tear on the other leg, or has a history of intervertebral disc disease (IVDD), the exercises would not be the same as for a dog that is otherwise healthy. In trauma cases or senior pets, concurrent medical problems are common and should be monitored closely.

Motivation

Motivating patients to work can be one of the most difficult aspects of rehabilitation. There are several factors that can affect individual motivation. Patients that are painful, fatigued, or stressed may be distracted or reluctant to be active. Very young patients may have a brief attention span, while geriatric patients may have cognitive impairments that reduce their ability to follow directions (Salvin *et al.*, 2010). See Chapter 9 for more details.

Training

It is important to consider the patient's level of training. If patients do not already know basic obedience commands like "sit," then it may be more difficult to have them perform sit-to-stands. The therapist may be able to train basic skills as the therapy progresses. However, if the client is performing home therapy, they may be unwilling or unable to train the patient. The complexity of the exercises must be chosen with the patient's level of training in mind. If the patient is not trained to do a certain command, it is still possible to lead them through the movement or shape the behavior, with the right type of motivation. Bear in mind that the client must possess or learn training skills if the therapy program is being done at home.

Some patients already have a high level of training. This can make it easier to design a varied therapy program. However, this type of patient may lose focus if the therapeutic activities are overly simplistic and repetitive. This type of patient may also anticipate what you are going to ask them to do and make it more challenging to get them to slow down and focus. For this type of patient, it may be necessary to challenge them not only physically but mentally as well.

Goal of Exercise Program

The goal is to return the patient to the highest level of function possible. To do this, the therapist must understand which exercises are beneficial and which are contraindicated. To meet the goal sometimes it is best to focus on accomplishing short-term goals or individual exercises. It is important to remember that the patient must be evaluated at regular intervals throughout the rehabilitation program. When checking in with the client to see how the home exercises are going, ask which exercises are going well and which ones are a struggle.

If the client is asked a closed-ended question (one that can be answered with one word) about how they are doing with the home program, they often give a generic "good" or "bad" response without details. This makes it difficult to assess and modify their exercises. It may be necessary to adjust goals or the expected time the goals are reached as the patient progresses through the program.

Assessing the Resources

Environment

Factors in the home environment will influence the development of the therapeutic exercise program. As the activity level is increased, walking up the stairs or hills may be recommended, if available. A pond, lake, hot tub, or swimming pool may be recommended for water therapies such as walking in water or swimming. However, these may not be appropriate to include in the therapeutic plan if the client has limited access to these resources or is unable to use them safely.

The patient's environment may also need to be controlled to prevent further injury. Most patients need to be housed indoors and often need to be confined to a small area when they are unsupervised. This is typically best accomplished by the use of a kennel or a small room. Early in the rehabilitation program, it may be undesirable for patients to traverse flights of stairs, and this can present a challenge if they are in the habit of sleeping in an upstairs bedroom. In addition, patients who are recumbent need a padded area to rest. If the home has hardwood or tile floors, weak patients may need nonskid boots or assistance to prevent slipping. Also, dog doors may need to be temporarily inactivated due to limited unsupervised access to the yard. Appropriate activity levels should be discussed to ensure the patient is prohibited from doing too much too soon.

Equipment

Knowledge of the client's available equipment is just as important as understanding the home environment. The equipment that the client has or that they can make will heavily impact the structure of the home exercise program. Most therapeutic exercise equipment can be purchased inexpensively at a local department store, but clients who are crafty and willing can make some of the equipment. For some exercises, common household items may be used. For example, broomsticks and drink containers make nice cavaletti. Two cans can make endpoints for marking a figure-of-eight pattern. Another option may be for the rehabilitation business to loan, rent, or sell equipment to clients.

A basic rehabilitation home program can often be created with minimal to no equipment. If the patient needs to reach an elevated level of function, particularly if they need to return to sports-specific or work-specific activity; some specific exercise equipment may be needed. However, for this type of patient, clients usually have access to necessary training equipment.

Training the Client

Initial Instruction of Exercises

The initial instruction with the client must be detailed. This begins with a handout that explains the home program. A home exercise program should not only list the exercises but also give detailed descriptions and photos of the exercises and explain how to perform them. The client is given so much information during the discharge that it is easy for them to forget what was said or lose a piece of paper. Providing a video of the exercises is also extremely helpful. Sometimes, taking a video of their pet doing the exercise is helpful. The correct form can more easily be conveyed by video as compared to written instructions. Clients may be overwhelmed by all the instructions, so it is helpful for them to have information that they can refer to once they get home.

Providing verbal and written instructions is essential, but these alone are not sufficient. The therapist should demonstrate the correct techniques to the patient. The client should then practice the techniques with the therapist's guidance. This allows the therapist to ensure that the client understands the exercises and can perform them correctly with the patient. This session also gives the client the opportunity to ask questions, and the practice activities improve their self-confidence. A client who has demonstrated appropriate technique, and who is confident that they can perform the therapy is more likely to adhere to the program.

Finally, if any assistive devices are sent home, the therapist should ensure that the client is completely comfortable with how they work and how to correctly apply them. Slings, harnesses, carts, and braces should be evaluated by the therapist or veterinary team to ensure they fit the patient properly. It is best to have the client practice applying and removing the device several times until the client and therapist are confident that the client can use it correctly. In most cases, it is recommended to avoid leaving any assistive devices on the patient while not supervised. This includes any time the client leaves home and at bedtime. Even if the client insists the patient will not chew it, other considerations include the risk of Velcro or metal rings getting caught on objects in the home environment. The client must also be advised to watch for complications. Specific regions of the body where an apparatus may pinch or rub should be pointed out, and specifics of when to act should be given "any issue more than hair loss needs to be addressed." In general, the client should be instructed to call immediately if they notice any potential problems and to avoid the use of the device if possible until examination can be performed.

Education Regarding the Patient's Condition

It is particularly important for the client to be aware of the patient's condition. Client education on pain assessment is key in ensuring that the patient's comfort level is adequately addressed. In educating clients about pain, they must be told the signs to watch for during exercises that may indicate a problem. Signs of pain can include vocalizing, excessive panting, dilated pupils, limping, restlessness, and changes in behavior or personality (Gaynor and Muir, 2015).

Clients also need to know what complications may occur from any of the recommended treatments, physical or pharmaceutical. The potential complications will vary depending on the initial problem and the patient's condition, and must be identified by the rehabilitation team. The potential complications should be explained to the clients, and they should also be given a written description of potential signs. Clients should also be given guidelines that outline when an exercise should be stopped and when to seek additional help. In addition, the clients should be given an idea of the rate of progress to expect as they progress through the program.

In some cases, the discussion may include quality of life or end of life issues. In senior pets or cases such as degenerative myelopathy, rehabilitation may be used to improve function or quality of life but will not change the prognosis. These clients often want to do everything and search online for magic cures. They also tend to worry so much about helping their pet that they forget to enjoy their time together. Having honest, and frank discussions about what to expect, the science behind what they find online, and how to maintain and assess quality of life is helpful.

Follow-Up

The follow-up evaluations are as important as the initial exam. These evaluations are used to determine whether the patient is improving as expected or new problems are noted. If the patient is not improving as expected, the reasons should be evaluated. It is possible that the initial goals were overly optimistic. It is also possible that the client is having difficulty following the rehabilitation program, or the patient may be experiencing complications. Regardless, the rehabilitation program may need to be modified to address any problems. In some cases, rehabilitation may need to be halted and the patient referred back to the surgeon or veterinarian managing the patient.

A phone call or email are excellent way to see how the client is coping with the exercises at home. Weekly check-ins allow the therapist to assess whether the client is comfortable with the prescribed exercises and to obtain an update on the patient's progress. Bear in mind that the client's self-report of patient progress may be inaccurate. In addition, a client may be unaware that they are performing therapy incorrectly. Therefore, it is important to have the client repeat the exercises after they are shown how to perform them during the initial assessment. The therapist may also help motivate the client by phone or email if they are having difficulty performing the exercises or becoming frustrated with lack of progress. If a client struggles with the exercises at home, making a video of their pet doing the exercises for you is sometimes helpful for them. Maintaining contact and open discussion with the client makes rehabilitation more successful.

Ideally, the patient should be re-evaluated roughly every four weeks depending on the problem. Some will need to be seen sooner and some later. If the patient is also receiving in-house therapy, a re-evaluation can be scheduled during one of these visits. The patient should not be released to full activity until a final evaluation is performed.

Home Exercises

Thermotherapy

Application of cold packs is beneficial after any surgery because it helps reduce inflammation and aids in pain control (Cameron, 2003). Cold packs may also be applied after exercise to reduce inflammation. This may be especially beneficial for patients with arthritis because the cold can reduce the pain and inflammation of arthritic joints. A cold pack can also be applied to an area that has been traumatized, to reduce hemorrhage and inflammation (Cameron, 2003).

Several different forms of cold packs are available for use. Commercially available gel packs are nice because they remain pliable even when frozen, can be easily disinfected and usually can double as a hot pack (Figure 6.1). Crushed ice can be placed in a sealable plastic bag to create an ice pack. A small amount of water may be added to help eliminate the dead space. Ice can be placed in a pillowcase or moist towel, although this can be messy. Using a bag of frozen vegetables has been recommended for emergency situations. This is a less effective method because of the dead space between the vegetables, so it is not recommended for use during therapy sessions. An ice slush can be made by mixing four parts of water with one part rubbing alcohol in a sealed bag and placing it in a freezer. Note that this alcohol–water mixture performs at

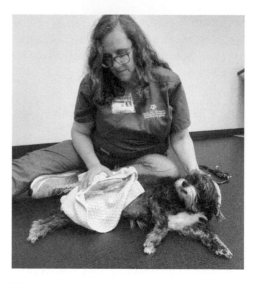

Figure 6.1 Application of a cold pack. *Source:* Sherri Jerzyk (chapter author).

a lower temperature than crushed ice. Therefore, this type of cold pack should never be applied directly to the skin because it carries an increased potential for causing cold-induced injuries (Cameron, 2003).

Before applying a cold pack, it may be wrapped in a cloth or thin towel to protect the skin and keep the cold pack clean. For maximal cooling effect of a cold pack, the towel may be moist. However, when using a true ice pack or alcohol slush pack, the cooling is more intense, so the towel should be dry. The cold pack may be held firmly in place or secured with an elastic bandage to ensure good skin contact. The application time should be at least 10 minutes to effectively reduce pain and swelling and may be repeated every 1–2 hours (Cameron, 2003). It may not be necessary to treat that often and may be impractical for the clients. A typical recommendation is to apply the cold pack for 10–20 minutes (Dragone *et al.*, 2014), 2–4 times daily, or after each therapy session.

Heat therapy can also be used in a home program. Some of the effects of heat are peripheral vasodilation, increase in metabolic rate, relax muscle spasms, improve soft tissue elasticity, and reduce pain. Indications to use heat would be to help reduce pain and muscles spasm, to enhance stretching, or to warm the tissues before activity. Use of local heat therapy is contraindicated in the presence of active bleeding, acute inflammation or infection, swelling or edema, neoplasia, or impaired sensation in the area (Cameron, 2003). This means that heat should not be applied near a surgical incision during the first few postoperative days when there is inflammation associated with the surgical procedure! A hot pack encourages dilation of blood vessels, resulting in increased blood flow and metabolic activity to the area (Cameron, 2003); this is undesirable in the face of postoperative inflammation.

The most commonly used hot packs are sacks or bags filled with beans, rice, cracked corn, bentonite (a hydrophilic silicate gel), or other inert materials. As mentioned above, the same gel packs can be used as either cold packs or hot packs. A hot pack can also be created by heating a damp towel or bag of water in the microwave; however, these methods may result in less effective heating. Although hot packs can be beneficial, bear in mind that heat from a hot pack only penetrates a few centimeters beneath the tissue surface.

The hot pack should be checked against a person's skin to ensure that it does not feel too warm for the patient, encourage a prolonged test of at least one minute as the sensation may build. A towel or cloth may be placed between the hot pack and skin if there are any concerns about overheating the skin. In addition, the skin should be observed intermittently for signs of excessive redness. In addition, animals with normal sensation should be monitored for evidence of discomfort. Hot packs are generally applied to an area for 15–30 minutes. This may be done two or three times daily and may be done as a warm up prior to exercise or stretching.

Passive Range of Motion

Passive range of motion (PROM) is performed by moving a joint within its available range of motion, using an external force. The benefits of PROM include: maintain range of motion, help prevent joint contracture, reduce pain, and improve synovial fluid production and diffusion (Millis and Levine, 2014). It is important to remember that PROM does not prevent muscle atrophy, nor does it improve strength or endurance. PROM can enhance blood and lymphatic flow, but not as effectively as active range of motion (ROM) does (Kisner and Colby, 2007). ROM exercises are contraindicated if the movement could cause further injury or instability. For example, a tenuous fracture repair could be compromised by excessive movement, so it is important to discuss the therapeutic plan with the surgeon before beginning therapy. In most cases, PROM is beneficial if performed at a slow, controlled speed and within a comfortable ROM for the patient.

It is best to perform PROM in a quiet room with as few distractions as possible, so the patient can relax. The patient should be in lateral recumbency with the affected leg up. If the patient is aggressive, it may need to be muzzled. If the patient is painful, the pain management protocol may need to be modified prior to performing PROM. In some cases, two people are needed to perform PROM; one person to restrain or calm the patient and one person to do the exercises.

When performing PROM on a postoperative orthopedic patient, it may be most efficient to focus on the affected joint; however, it is important to maintain normal ROM in all joints of the affected limb. When performing PROM on a neurologic patient with a spinal cord injury, PROM should be performed on all major joints. For example, if the patient is paraplegic, PROM should be performed on the joints of both hind limbs; and if the patient is tetraparetic PROM should be performed on the joints of all four limbs.

It may be necessary to spend a few minutes gently massaging the affected limb to promote further relaxation, and gradually move toward the affected joint. Some patients do not like their feet being touched so it may be better to start proximally and move slowly, rather than grabbing hold of the patient's foot. Motions should be slow and controlled. This is not a race! One hand should be positioned to support the limb proximal to the joint, while the other hand supports the limb distal to the joint. To avoid grabbing or pulling on the limb, using an open-handed approach to guide the limb may be beneficial. The entire limb should be supported with the joints in neutral positions to prevent any excessive joint stresses. The two hands are slowly moved to gently flex the affected joint, while the other joints are allowed to maintain neutral positions. The joint is flexed as completely as possible until some resistance is met or until the patient displays signs of discomfort. Discomfort may be displayed by muscle tension, pulling the limb away, or turning the head towards the affected area. With hands in the same supportive positions, the joint is extended fully, stopping before the patient displays signs of discomfort. An alternative method is to support the entire limb and flex and extend all the joints by moving the limb in a way that mimics an exaggerated walking step, or "bicycling" movement. This method of PROM is more appropriate when the patient is nearly using the leg actively. Remember that the stifle and hock positions are related, so maximum flexion of one of these joints requires simultaneous flexion of the other. When done correctly, PROM should not be a painful experience, nor should it cause any signs to worsen.

The most appropriate treatment prescription will vary with the condition. However, for most postoperative conditions, 15–20 repetitions (for each joint), 2–4 times daily is adequate (Millis and Levine, 2014). PROM is typically discontinued when the patient can use the leg, and flex and extend the affected joint voluntarily. Although the patient may not be completely normal at this point, the focus of therapy changes to promote active ROM exercises.

It is important to show the clients how to correctly perform PROM so that it can be done correctly and safely at home (Figures 6.2 and 6.3). If the client struggles to master the technique or the patient is

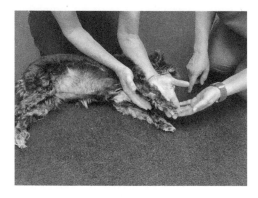

Figure 6.2 Teaching passive range of motion. *Source:* Sherri Jerzyk (chapter author).

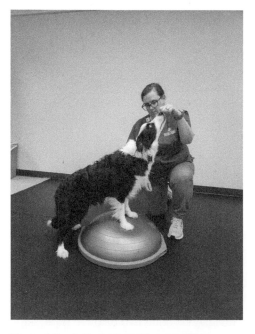

Figure 6.3 Actively stretching on a Bosu. *Source:* Sherri Jerzyk (chapter author).

uncooperative, the therapy team must decide whether the client should persist in attempting to do the PROM. It is possible that the potential risk of injury (to the patient or the client) outweighs the anticipated benefit of PROM. However, most clients can learn how to perform effective PROM. In these cases, it is still recommended that they demonstrate their technique during patient re-evaluations because they may not realize when their technique is suboptimal. Most clients enjoy learning this skill, and it can be empowering for them to feel that they are contributing to the successful recovery of their pet.

Stretching

Various stretching techniques may be used to improve joint ROM and extensibility of periarticular tissues, muscles, and tendons. Passive stretching is not the same as PROM. Passive range of motion activities occurs within the unrestricted ROM of the joint, while stretching moves a restricted joint beyond the available ROM to elongate the soft tissues (Kisner and Colby, 2007).

A static stretch is performed using a similar technique as PROM and the patient is still not actively involved in the movement. The patient should be as relaxed as possible, and the limb should be held and supported on either side of the affected joint. The joint is then moved to the end of its available range. This may be flexion or extension, depending on where the joint restriction is located. There is limited evidence to determine the most effective stretching protocol. In healthy adults, stretching for 30 or 60 seconds was more effective than 15 seconds or less (Bandy *et al.*, 1997). There is reportedly no increase in muscle elongation beyond two to four repetitions of static stretching (Page, 2012). The optimal frequency and duration for static stretches are still being researched. Static stretching is typically a little uncomfortable for the patient and can

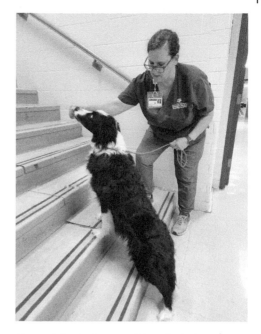

Figure 6.4 Active stretching of a large dog using some stairs. *Source:* Sherri Jerzyk (chapter author).

be more challenging to perform than PROM. In addition, there is a higher risk of causing injury to the patient. For these reasons, static stretching may not be the best choice for a home program.

Active stretches can be performed by coaxing or luring the patient to move into positions that accentuate joint flexion or extension, which stretches the associated soft tissues. Stretching exercises may be facilitated with the use of a disc or Bosu (Figure 6.4). Since the patient is controlling the motion, the risk of overstretching is relatively low. These stretches are often performed by use of a toy or treat to lure the patient into various positions, hence they may be termed "cookie stretches." One example of an active stretch is to coax a dog to stand with the hind legs on the floor and the front legs on a stair step (which step depends on the size of the patient and degree of stretch desired). These elevated positions could be used to encourage hind limb extension, promoting stretch of the hip and stifle flexors (Figure 6.5).

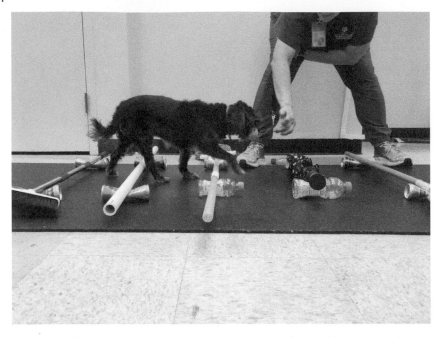

Figure 6.5 Dog can be encouraged to step over various linear objects, such as broom sticks or PVC pipes, to encourage joint flexion. *Source:* Sherri Jerzyk (chapter author).

"Cookie" or treat-lured stretches can be used to promote stretching of the cervical and thoracic spine. They also encourage weight-shifting that may simultaneously help improve balance, and limb and back strength. This is performed by having the patient stand on a surface with good traction. The cookie is used to slowly lure the patient's head to one side, and then the other. Luring the patient's nose to the shoulder will focus on stretching the neck while luring to the hip or hock will focus on stretching the trunk. The nose may also be lured up and down to stretch the ventral and dorsal aspects of the neck. The patient can be enticed to hold the stretch by delaying delivery of the treatment, while the patient is maintaining the end range position. Although this is a straightforward exercise, it can be challenging for some clients to master the luring techniques, so the patient remains in a standing position without moving their feet. The therapist must decide on an individual basis whether this type of stretch is indicated, and if so, whether the client will be able to perform it correctly.

Massage

Massage is the manipulation of soft tissues, and several different styles have been developed. The basic concept is to apply pressure and friction to the patient's skin. Massage can improve lymphatic flow, and one of the indications is to reduce limb edema. Massage helps reduce anxiety and pain, but there is limited scientific evidence to support other potential benefits (Sutton and Whitlock, 2014).

Clients often enjoy giving massages to their pets. The pet may become more relaxed as a direct result of the massage, and it often appears to improve the bond between the client and the patient. Massage may be performed prior to a therapy session to calm the patient. Massage may also be performed following exercise, particularly to reduce muscle spasms and pain.

The type and extent of massage may depend partly on the client's level of comfort and skill. The first step in performing a massage is to have the patient lie in lateral recumbency in a quiet room. The client may be instructed in basic stroking, effleurage, and petrissage techniques (*see Chapter 5; Manual Therapies for details on massage*). The massage may be general (for general relaxation and pain reduction) or focused on tissues of the affected area. The initial massage may be supervised by the therapist to ensure that the client is using appropriate techniques. The massage should not cause pain or discomfort.

Weight Shifting

Weight shifting exercises are relatively simple activities that most clients can easily learn to perform. This type of activity can be done for patients who can stand but need to work on improving balance and fine motor control. Shifting of the body increases mechanoreceptor firing in the joints and soft tissues, which increases feedback to the central nervous system regarding body position. This feedback results in increased muscle recruitment to stabilize the body (Deliagina *et al.*, 2014). Weight shifting may also be performed to encourage weight bearing on a limb. The simplest type of weight shifting is done with the patient standing (with assistance if needed), while someone gently pushes the patient from side to side or front to back in a rhythmic fashion.

For example, the client may place one hand on each shoulder or hip and gently sway the patient from side to side. Making the movements larger or more rapid will increase the difficulty of the exercise. Another method of weight shifting is to use the "cookie stretches" as previously described. Weight-shifting activities can be made even more challenging by having the patient perform them while standing on an air mattress or couch cushion. There are many other types of weight-shifting exercises, but they require equipment that most clients do not have at home. In addition, these are more complex and require more skill to do correctly, so may not be appropriate for many clients.

For more details about weight shifting, see Chapter 19: *Therapeutic Exercises Part 1: Land Exercises.*

Assisted Walking

Patients that are weak or non-ambulatory may need assistance to stand and to walk. The patient should be fitted with the most appropriate sling or harness to be used by the client at home. It is important to instruct the clients on proper techniques for lifting and assisting patients, to preserve client health. In some cases, the patient may be fitted for a cart, particularly if the dysfunction is anticipated to be prolonged or permanent.

Clients with patients that spend most of their time recumbent must be instructed on basic nursing care to prevent urine scalds and decubital ulcers. *For more information, see Chapter* 11: *The Disabled Patient Part 2: The Neurologic Patient.* The clients must also be alerted to watch for foot abrasions in patients that have neurologic deficits or abnormal postures. They should seek veterinary care as soon as they notice any reddened skin beginning to develop. Foot abrasions can often be prevented by boots.

Controlled Leash Walking

Slow leash walks are typically a key component of most rehabilitation programs, particularly early in the rehabilitation process. Slow leash walking is indicated for patients who have lameness, weakness, or proprioceptive deficits. The authors have observed that the patient is more likely to use each leg in the proper gait sequence and more likely to bear weight on a lame leg when encouraged to walk slowly. It may help to praise lame patients whenever they touch the affected foot to the ground.

Instructions for the clients must be clear and detailed. For maximum control, the leash must be a short (four to six feet long) lead and not a retractable leash. Some patients may be better controlled with the use of a harness. Ideally, the patient should be walked in a normal "heel" position. If the client–patient team lacks obedience training, the patient may walk a few steps ahead or to the side of the client, but it must be as controlled as possible. Retractable leashes are strongly discouraged because the tendency is for the client to relinquish control of the patient, allowing activity that is inappropriate or too vigorous.

The appropriate duration and frequency of the walks vary with the patient's condition. A typical postoperative program might start with five-minute walks, two to four times daily. Over time the duration of the walks may gradually increase. In general, the duration or frequency of the walking sessions should only be increased after being instructed to do so by the rehabilitation team. A guideline that can be used to increase cardiorespiratory conditioning is to increase the duration of the walks by 10–15% each week (Millis *et al.*, 2014a). However, this guideline may not be appropriate for patients recovering from orthopedic or neurologic injuries or surgeries.

Balance, strength, and active ROM exercises may be incorporated into the patients' walking program. During each walking session, the patient may spend a portion of the time walking on uneven or unstable surfaces, such as grass, sand, or snow, if available. Walking over different terrain may challenge the patient's balance, and it can also encourage flexion of the limb joints. Joint flexion may also be enhanced by exercises in which the patient steps over objects, such as a garden hose, broomstick, PVC pipe, or rungs of a ladder placed on the ground. Clients who have working or sporting dogs may have agility equipment, such as cavaletti rails that they can use. Inclines, declines, or stairs may also be integrated into the walking program, depending on what is accessible to the client. Walking downstairs is particularly beneficial for increasing ROM of the stifles and hocks (Millard *et al.*, 2010), while walking up ramps promotes ROM of the forelimb joints (Carr *et al.*, 2013).

Strength Exercises

A walking program will improve the strength of the limbs. Walking up hills or stairs may be used to focus on strengthening the hind limbs. The client must understand the importance of moving slowly to discourage the patient from hopping or skipping up the steps. The client must also be able to recognize signs of fatigue and avoid pushing the patient too quickly. Hills or stairs can be challenging for the cardiorespiratory endurance and muscular strength, so these exercises should be gradually introduced into the program, particularly if the patient is deconditioned.

Sit-to-stand exercises can also be incorporated into a home program to improve strength and ROM of hind limbs (Millis *et al.*, 2014a). It is best to have the client include some sit-to-stand exercises after five minutes of walking to warm up the muscles. Although sit-to-stand exercises look simple, they can be difficult to perform correctly. The patient must sit and stand symmetrically, without leaning to one side or favoring one leg. In the authors' experiences, patients often tend to abduct the affected limb to avoid fully flexing it during the sit or fully bearing weight during the transitions. The client must be instructed to watch for this method of "cheating." It may be prevented by positioning the patient with the affected leg next to a wall or other object that prevents lateral movement of the leg during the exercise. It may be most efficient to start by including 5–10 sit-to-stand exercises once or twice daily, during the walking sessions (Millis *et al.*, 2014b). The number of daily sessions and repetitions can be increased over time as the patient's strength improves.

Crouched walking is another relatively simple exercise to improve limb strength and ROM. One technique is to have the patient walk through a child's play tunnel or dog agility tunnel. However, the tunnel must be small enough that the patient cannot stand up inside it. This type of equipment may not be available to the client; however, other objects may have the same effect. For example, the client may have a chair or table that the patient could walk under. Another convenient and inexpensive option is a telescoping shower rod. It can be placed in a doorway or hallway at an appropriate height to force the patient to flex the limbs to walk under it.

Sport Specific Exercises

The end goal of the rehabilitation program is that the patient returns to full function. In many cases, this does not involve a high degree of athleticism. However, the goal for some patients is to return to a competitive sporting activity or to return to strenuous work. For these patients, the clients typically have a good understanding of the type of strength, endurance, and agility that is required. These clients also tend to have

more experience with animal training and access to specific training equipment.

The final portion of the rehabilitation program for these patients should focus on building the specific skills and endurance needed for that individual. The rehabilitation team can work with the client to design a program that is gradual, yet progressively improves patient function. Although this type of client tends to be very observant, it is still important to reassess the patient at regular intervals to ensure they are meeting retraining goals and not sustaining any injuries or setbacks.

Conclusion

The therapist must assess the client, patient, and home environment carefully before creating a home exercise program. The therapist and the client must establish realistic outcome goals. Clients must be committed to the therapeutic plan. The therapist must determine which therapies are realistic for the clients to perform at home, considering their available resources and their animal handling skills. Under the therapist's guidance, most clients can learn basic skills to provide effective therapy for their pets. Clients with working dogs or high-level athletes may carry out more complex home exercises to refine specific skills. Recheck evaluations are needed to ensure that the client is performing the therapies correctly and the patient is progressing toward the therapeutic goals.

References

Bandy, W.D., Irion, J.M., and Briggler, M. (1997). The effect of time and frequency of static stretching on flexibility of the hamstring muscles. *Phys Ther* 77 (10): 1090–1096.

Cameron, M.H. (2003). *Physical Agents in Rehabilitation: From Research to Practice*, 2nde. St. Louis: Saunders.

Carr, J.G., Millis, D.L., and Weng, H.Y. (2013). Exercises in canine physical rehabilitation:

Range of motion of the forelimb during stair and ramp ascent. *J Small Anim Pract* 54 (8): 409–413.

Deliagina, T.G., Beloozerova, I.N., Orlovsky, G.N., and Zelenin, P.V. (2014). Contribution of supraspinal systems to generation of automatic postural responses. *Front Integr Neurosci* 8: 1–20. https://doi.org/10.3389/fnint.2014.00076.

Dragone, L., Heinrichs, K., Levine, D. et al. (2014). Superficial thermal modalities. In: *Canine Rehabilitation and Physical Therapy*, 2nde (ed. D.L. Millis and D. Levine), 312–327. Philadelphia: Elsevier Saunders.

Gaynor, J.S. and Muir, W.W. (2015). *Handbook of Veterinary Pain Management*, 3rde. St Louis: Elsevier.

Kisner, C. and Colby, L.A. (2007). *Therapeutic Exercise*, 5the. Philadelphia: F.A. Davis Company.

Millard, R.P., Headrick, J.F., and Millis, D.L. (2010). Kinematic analysis of the pelvic limbs of healthy dogs during stair and decline slope walking. *J Small Anim Pract* 51 (8): 419–422.

Millis, D.L. and Levine, D. (2014). Range-of-motion and stretching exercises. In: *Canine Rehabilitation and Physical Therapy*, 2nde (ed. D.L. Millis and D. Levine), 431–446. Philadelphia: Elsevier Saunders.

Millis, D.L., Drum, M., and Levine, D. (2014a). Therapeutic exercises: Early limb use exercises. In: *Canine Rehabilitation and Physical Therapy*, 2nde (ed. D.L. Millis and D. Levine), 495–505. Philadelphia: Elsevier Saunders.

Millis, D.L., Drum, M., and Levine, D. (2014b). Therapeutic exercises: Joint motion, strengthening, endurance, and speed exercises. In: *Canine Rehabilitation and Physical Therapy*, 2nde (ed. D.L. Millis and D. Levine), 506–525. Philadelphia: Elsevier Saunders.

Page, P. (2012). Current concepts in muscle stretching for exercise and rehabilitation. *Int J Sports Phys Ther* 7 (1): 109–119.

Salvin, H.E., McGreevy, P.D., Sachdev, P.S., and Valenzuela, M.J. (2010). Under diagnosis of canine cognitive dysfunction: A cross-sectional survey of older companion dogs. *Vet J* 184 (3): 277–281.

Sutton, A. and Whitlock, D. (2014). Massage. In: *Canine Rehabilitation and Physical Therapy*, 2nde (ed. D.L. Millis and D. Levine), 464–483. Philadelphia: Elsevier Saunders.

7

Supporting the Client and Patient

Megan Ridley and Renée Yacoub

Integrative Pet Care, Chicago, IL, USA

CHAPTER MENU

Introduction

Rehabilitation is a rapidly growing field in veterinary medicine that combines services in high demand with exceptional patient care and significant client participation. As pets live longer and clients demand that their pets receive the same standard of care as humans, the number of veterinary professionals in the field has grown significantly. The first two certification programs in canine physical rehabilitation started in 1999 (University of Tennessee) and 2002 (Canine Rehabilitation Institute), and there are now several other programs in the United States that also provide certification. The American Association of Rehabilitation Veterinarians (AARV), whose members include veterinary students, veterinarians, physical therapists, and veterinary technicians and nurses, was started in 2008 with about 50 members (Nolen, 2009). In 2010, the American Veterinary Medical Association's (AVMA) American Board of Veterinary Specialists (ABVS) approved the formation of the American College of Veterinary Sports Medicine and Rehabilitation (ACVSMR) as a Recognized Veterinary Specialty Organization (RVSO). In 2017, the Academy of Physical Rehabilitation Veterinary Technicians (APRVT) was granted provisional accreditation by the National Association of Veterinary Technicians in America (NAVTA) Committee on veterinary technician specialties (VTS), and the first certifying exam was administered in 2018. As of 2022, there are 18 VTS in Physical Rehabilitation. In 2022, AARV's membership reached nearly 500 members.

Veterinary medicine overall is growing as well. Research showed that US pet healthcare spending will increase by 33% between

Physical Rehabilitation for Veterinary Technicians and Nurses, Second Edition.
Edited by Mary Ellen Goldberg and Julia E. Tomlinson.
© 2024 John Wiley & Sons, Inc. Published 2024 by John Wiley & Sons, Inc.
Companion website: www.wiley.com/go/goldberg/physicalrehabilitationvettechsandnurses

2019 and 2029 (Lloyd, 2021a). The US Bureau of Labor Statistics (BLS) reports that the employment outlook for animal care professionals is generally strong. BLS predicts a 16% growth in the number of veterinarian jobs between 2019 and 2029 with an identical growth rate for veterinary technician jobs in that same time frame (Best Accredited Colleges, 2022; BLS, 2022).

However, not all prospects in the field are rosy since there is concern that we may be heading into a critical shortage of veterinary professionals. While there is speculation that a "pandemic pet" adoption boom is responsible, data from the AVMA indicate a more serious explanation for this looming workforce crisis is a decrease in practice productivity coupled with employee turnover and attrition. Productivity has decreased for various reasons over the past few years. Safety protocols that were instituted during the COVID-19 pandemic such as curbside care, increased sanitizing in between appointments, and splitting staff members into rotating teams have led to a 25% decline in productivity in 2020 compared to 2019. Practices have also struggled with losses of staff members due to illness, quarantining, and a shortage of childcare. While the number of appointments grew in 2021, practices were still playing catch-up with patients that had not been seen for over a year (Salois and Golab, 2021). High turnover also impacts productivity. In the American Animal Hospital Association's (AAHA) 2020 compensation and benefits survey, the average veterinary employee turnover was 23% (VBA, 2021). While this rate is concerning, recent research performed by Mars Veterinary Health (MVH) is even more unsettling. Findings indicate that 2,000 baby boomer veterinarians are retiring each year and that the number of US veterinarians is increasing by just 2.7% annually. MVH projects that more than 40,000 additional veterinarians will be needed to meet the needs of companion animal healthcare by 2030 and that over 75 million pets in the United States may not have access to veterinary care by 2030 if no actions are taken to mitigate current trends (MVH, 2022).

The industry needs to tackle the professional shortage by investing in equity and diversity initiatives, building a larger talent pipeline, offering student debt relief, and decreasing attrition rates through improved mental health and well-being resources (MVH, 2022). These changes need to be made not only to increase productivity but to sustain the industry as a whole. Much of this focus will be on veterinary technicians and nurses. Research indicates that the positive contribution to practice productivity and revenue of one additional veterinary technician/nurse is approximately 18.3% and by some estimates, technicians and nurses may be using only about 30% of the skills for which they have been educated (Lloyd, 2021b). Using veterinary technicians and nurses to their full capacity will help resolve retention issues. As a result, career satisfaction, which among veterinary technicians and nurses is largely tied to the application of skills and support in caring for patients (Davidow, 2019; AVMA, 2022c) will improve. There will also be more opportunities for career advancement. Additionally, as technicians and nurses are utilized to their full potential, veterinarians' time will be freed up such that they, in turn, can use their skills more appropriately, and the whole practice will operate more efficiently (Salois and Golab, 2021) and be able to accommodate more patients and clients.

It is commonly understood that veterinarian–client interactions are already brief (Shaw *et al.*, 2010; Pun, 2020). As this trend continues with a rise in cases, reliance on veterinary technicians and nurses to provide much of the communication with clients will increase. The discipline of veterinary rehabilitation requires significant interaction and communication with clients, and client cooperation and participation are paramount. In order for the veterinary technicians/nurses in this field to provide appropriate support for the clients and patients, they need to be trained in rehabilitation and communication skills, be empowered to advocate for patients, and to be given organizational support that promotes their well-being and career satisfaction.

Training

For the technician/nurse to be able to support the rehabilitation patient fully, training beyond the two-year veterinary technician associate degree is necessary. Completing a certification program in animal rehabilitation and complementing it with additional formal instruction and on-the-job training will enable the technician to become a highly qualified patient advocate.

Certification in Rehabilitation

As detailed in Chapter 1, several animal rehabilitation certification programs are available to the veterinary technician/nurse. These courses provide training in anatomy, biomechanics, diagnoses and conditions referred for rehabilitation, therapeutic modalities, and patient assessment. By gaining clinical competency in these areas, technicians and nurses can gain autonomy over their practice, leading to the improvement of patient experiences and clinical outcomes.

Advanced Techniques

Advanced training is also available and can further benefit the support of the patient. Massage therapy, manual trigger point therapy, and kinesiology taping are a few advanced certifications that can be obtained by the technician/nurse.

Lastly, as previously stated, qualified technicians/nurses can pursue a VTS in physical rehabilitation, which can enhance both efficiency and effectiveness (Lloyd, 2021b). More information can be obtained at: https://www.aprvt.com.

Knowledge of Orthopedic and Neurologic Conditions

To provide medically appropriate care to rehabilitation patients, it is imperative that the veterinary technician/nurse have knowledge of the diagnoses determined by the rehabilitation veterinarian. Familiarity with orthopedic and neurologic conditions, clinical signs, prognoses, and treatments will enable the technician/nurse to communicate clearly with both the supervising veterinarian and the client.

Knowledge of Equipment and Modalities

Because many physical modalities and equipment are prescribed in animal rehabilitation treatment plans, the technician/nurse needs to understand both why they are being recommended for a patient and how to use them appropriately and effectively (see Figure 7.1). If a patient is not responding as desired, the technician/nurse needs to discuss a possible change in modalities or modality parameters with the supervising veterinarian.

Knowledge of Medications, Supplements, and Other Products

Medications, supplements, assistive devices, and home treatment equipment are often prescribed in veterinary rehabilitation. As is discussed in Chapter 4, the veterinary technician/nurse is an integral part of communicating the administration and proper use of these products with the client. Proficiency in how the products work, how to administer them, and what side effects to watch for will improve client compliance.

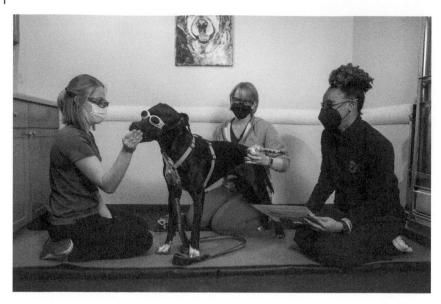

Figure 7.1 An in-house training session on photobiomodulation with new staff members. Regularly scheduled in-house training improves staff communication and patient care. *Source:* Courtesy of Dr Megan Ridley/Renee Yacoub (co-author).

Patient Assessment

Because of the frequency and duration of therapeutic visits that occur in the rehabilitation setting, the technician/nurse will have ample opportunity to observe the patients they work with, thus becoming skilled at recognizing changes in body condition, gait, lameness, discomfort, and even a patient's quality of life (QoL). The resulting observations can be communicated directly to the supervising veterinarian who can then intervene as needed.

Body Condition Scoring

A body condition score or BCS is a method of determining if a patient is a healthy weight. BCS can range from 1 to 9 or 1 to 5 depending on what scale is being used. The World Small Animal Veterinary Association (WSAVA) body condition score is based on visual body morphology and palpable body fat around the ribs, lumbar vertebrae, and pelvic bones. WSAVA also has a muscle condition score chart that can be used to assess muscle mass in a dog. Assessment

is by visualization and palpation of the spine, scapula, skull, and wings of the ilia (WSAVA, 2011).

Gaiting Evaluation

Rehabilitation technicians and nurses should be well-versed in gait analysis and, with training, will not only be able to determine what constitutes a normal versus abnormal gait but also which limb or limbs are affected and to what degree (Davies, 2021). This will help the technician/nurse communicate progress or setbacks more objectively to the supervising veterinarian. Gaiting analysis includes visual observation of the patient from a number of angles, both walking and trotting on a flat surface (Carr and Dycus, 2016; see Figure 7.2).

Lameness Scales

Many lameness scales exist, and the entire rehabilitation team should be using the same scale for consistency. Most scales are numeric, while some are more descriptive in nature, quantifying lameness as mild,

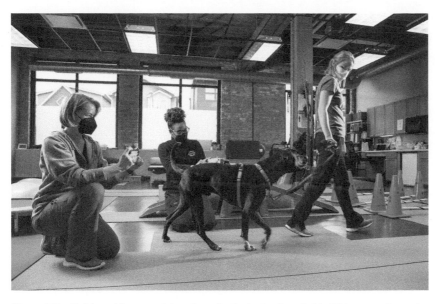

Figure 7.2 Gaiting videos are taken from both the back and side. Videos can be reviewed later to further analyze gaiting abnormalities and to help evaluate patient progress. *Source:* Courtesy of Dr Megan Ridley/Renee Yacoub (co-author).

moderate, or severe. An example of a numeric lameness scale is listed here (DeCamp, 1991):

- Grade 0 – Normal, no lameness
- Grade 1 – Off weight bearing at a stance, no lameness noted at a walk/trot
- Grade 2 – Mild lameness at a walk/trot
- Grade 3 – Moderate lameness at a walk/trot
- Grade 4 – Places foot when standing, intermittently carries limb when trotting
- Grade 5 – Non-weight bearing lameness

Pain Scales

As discussed in Chapter 3, recognition and assessment of pain are essential for its effective management. Because technicians/nurses have the most contact with patients, they are uniquely positioned to evaluate patient discomfort and to advocate for pharmacologic intervention when needed (Tabor, 2016; Clapham, 2012; Shaffran, 2008). Although technicians/nurses do not have the freedom to prescribe or initiate therapy, when the supervising veterinarian trusts the judgment and experience of the technician/nurse, the patient

benefits (Shaffran, 2008). Along with their general observations, the technicians/nurses can use an objective, validated pain scale to evaluate the patient and then work with the prescribing veterinarian to determine a pain management protocol and adjust it as needed (Nugent-Deal, 2017; see Figures 7.3 and 7.4).

Quality of Life Scales

The rehabilitation team can also support the clients with making difficult, end-of-life decisions for their pets. A QoL scale, called the HHHHHMM scale, was developed by Dr. Alice Villalobos (Villalobos, 2004). Each letter stands for a category and each category is rated on a 1–10 scale, with 10 being the best. Categories include:

- Hurt
- Hunger
- Hydration
- Hygiene
- Happiness
- Mobility
- More good days than bad

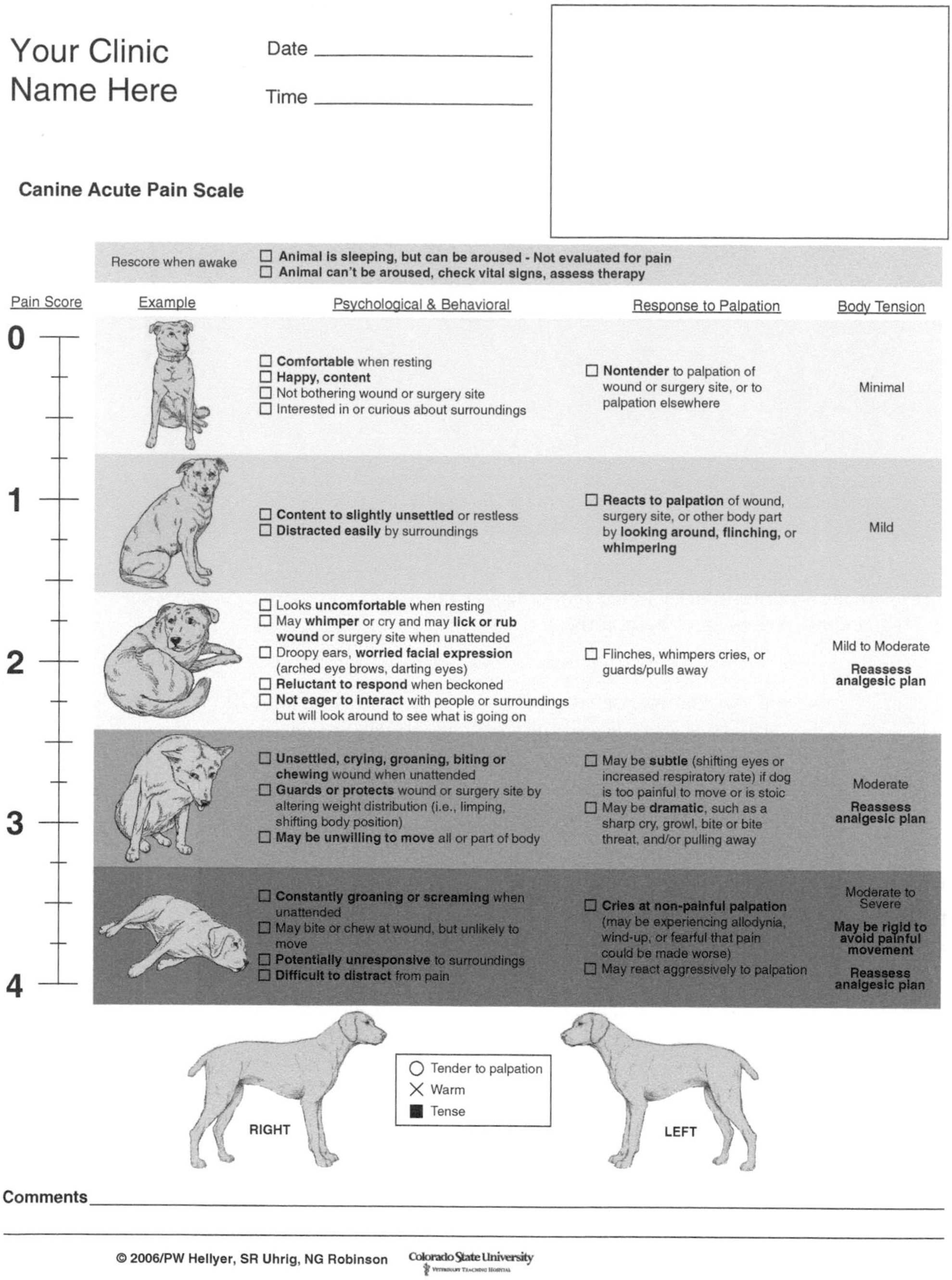

Your Clinic Name Here

Date _____

Time _____

Canine Acute Pain Scale

Rescore when awake	☐ **Animal is sleeping, but can be aroused - Not evaluated for pain** ☐ **Animal can't be aroused, check vital signs, assess therapy**

Pain Score	Example	Psychological & Behavioral	Response to Palpation	Body Tension
0		☐ **Comfortable** when resting ☐ **Happy, content** ☐ Not bothering wound or surgery site ☐ Interested in or curious about surroundings	☐ **Nontender** to palpation of wound or surgery site, or to palpation elsewhere	Minimal
1		☐ **Content to slightly unsettled** or restless ☐ **Distracted easily** by surroundings	☐ **Reacts to palpation** of wound, surgery site, or other body part by **looking around, flinching,** or **whimpering**	Mild
2		☐ Looks **uncomfortable** when resting ☐ May **whimper** or cry and may **lick or rub wound** or surgery site when unattended ☐ Droopy ears, **worried facial expression** (arched eye brows, darting eyes) ☐ **Reluctant to respond** when beckoned ☐ **Not eager to interact** with people or surroundings but will look around to see what is going on	☐ Flinches, whimpers cries, or guards/pulls away	Mild to Moderate **Reassess analgesic plan**
3		☐ **Unsettled, crying, groaning, biting or chewing** wound when unattended ☐ **Guards or protects** wound or surgery site by altering weight distribution (i.e., limping, shifting body position) ☐ **May be unwilling to move** all or part of body	☐ May be **subtle** (shifting eyes or increased respiratory rate) if dog is too painful to move or is stoic ☐ May be **dramatic**, such as a sharp cry, growl, bite or bite threat, and/or pulling away	Moderate **Reassess analgesic plan**
4		☐ **Constantly groaning or screaming** when unattended ☐ May bite or chew at wound, but unlikely to move ☐ **Potentially unresponsive** to surroundings ☐ **Difficult to distract** from pain	☐ **Cries at non-painful palpation** (may be experiencing allodynia, wind-up, or fearful that pain could be made worse) ☐ May react aggressively to palpation	Moderate to Severe **May be rigid to avoid painful movement** **Reassess analgesic plan**

○ Tender to palpation
✕ Warm
■ Tense

RIGHT   LEFT

Comments _____

© 2006/PW Hellyer, SR Uhrig, NG Robinson   Colorado State University
Veterinary Teaching Hospital

Figure 7.3 Therapists can use a pain scale such as The Colorado State Acute Pain Scale to assess pain at each session. The therapist will then communicate with the case veterinarian if additional pain interventions are needed. Canine SCU Acute Pain Scale. *Source:* Adapted from Colorado State University.

Your Clinic Name Here

Date _____

Time _____

Feline Acute Pain Scale

Rescore when awake	☐ **Animal is sleeping, but can be aroused** - Not evaluated for pain ☐ **Animal can't be aroused, check vital signs, assess therapy**

Pain Score	Example	Psychological & Behavioral	Response to Palpation	Body Tension
0	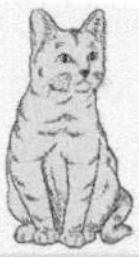	☐ **Content and quiet** when unattended ☐ **Comfortable** when resting ☐ Interested in or **curious** about surroundings	☐ **Not bothered** by palpation of wound or surgery site, or to palpation elsewhere	Minimal
1	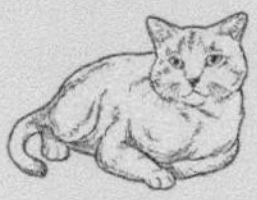	☐ **Signs are often subtle and not easily detected in the hospital setting**; more likely to be detected by the owner(s) at home ☐ Earliest signs at home may be **withdrawal from surroundings or change in normal routine** ☐ In the hospital, may be content or slightly unsettled ☐ **Less interested** in surroundings but will look around to see what is going on	☐ May or may not react to palpation of wound or surgery site	Mild
2	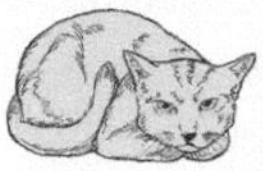	☐ Decreased responsiveness, **seeks solitude** ☐ **Quiet**, loss of brightness in eyes ☐ **Lays curled up or sits tucked up** (all four feet under body, shoulders hunched, head held slightly lower than shoulders, tail curled tightly around body) with eyes partially or mostly closed ☐ **Hair coat appears rough** or fluffed up ☐ May intensively groom an area that is painful or irritating ☐ Decreased appetite, **not interested in food**	☐ **Responds aggressively or tries to escape** if painful area is palpated or approached ☐ Tolerates attention, may even perk up when petted as long as painful area is avoided	Mild to Moderate **Reassess analgesic plan**
3	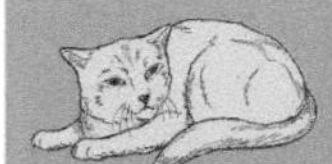	☐ Constantly **yowling, growling, or hissing** when unattended ☐ May bite or chew at wound, but **unlikely to move** if left alone	☐ **Growls or hisses at non-painful palpation** (may be experiencing allodynia, wind-up, or fearful that pain could be made worse) ☐ **Reacts aggressively** to palpation, **adamantly pulls away** to avoid any contact	Moderate **Reassess analgesic plan**
4	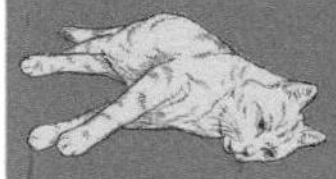	☐ Prostrate ☐ Potentially **unresponsive** to or unaware of surroundings, difficult to distract from pain ☐ Receptive to care (even aggressive or feral cats will be more tolerant of contact)	☐ **May not respond** to palpation ☐ **May be rigid to avoid painful movement**	Moderate to Severe **May be rigid to avoid painful movement** **Reassess analgesic plan**

○ Tender to palpation
✕ Warm
■ Tense

RIGHT   LEFT

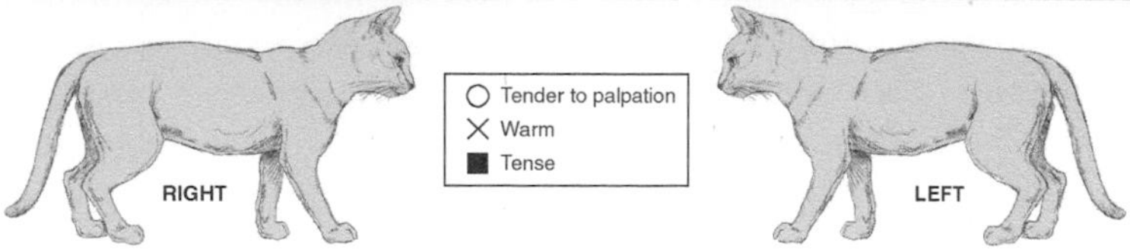

Comments _____

© 2006/PW Hellyer, SR Uhrig, NG Robinson   Colorado State University
Veterinary Teaching Hospital

Figure 7.4 CSU Acute Pain Scale Feline. *Source:* Adapted from Colorado State University.

A score of 35 or more out of 70 reflects an acceptable QoL. The client can be directed by the rehabilitation team to score their pet's QoL at a certain frequency (such as daily, weekly, or monthly) and the team can then provide support to the client in terms of making end-of-life decisions based on those scores. The Villalobos QoL scale can be obtained here: https://www.merckvet-manual.com/multimedia/table/the-hhhhhmm-scale.

Communication

Team Communication

Effective and clear communication among members of the rehabilitation team is essential. Research has shown that team communication in the veterinary practice is challenging (Ruby and DeBowes, 2007), and while some training on team communication is included in the veterinary curriculum, key elements are missing. Displaying transparent governance, setting clear expectations, and avoiding unwarranted assumptions are fundamentals of successful leadership in veterinary practice. The team leader also needs to maintain a supportive and positive working environment (Pun, 2020; Ruby and DeBowes, 2007).

In such an environment, the technician/nurse is empowered to work collaboratively with the prescribing veterinarian. Patient updates including setbacks, progress, changes in pain status, and concomitant medical issues can be relayed to the case manager who can then adjust patient treatment accordingly (see Figure 7.5). The technician/nurse and veterinarian must have consistent messaging regarding diagnoses, prognoses, treatment parameters, medication and supplement recommendations, activity instructions, and client home care programs. If more than one technician/nurse is working with a patient, all involved need to have consistent messaging with one another so that the patient receives proper care, and the client receives proper instruction.

The necessity for strong team communication extends to other staff as well. Assistants to the veterinarians and technicians/nurses need to be apprised of patient temperament, dietary restrictions, and mobility limitations. Last, but perhaps most important, the patient/client service representatives need to be updated by veterinary team members so that they are aware of any changes in treatment recommendations, medications/supplements, and patient status. These front-line communicators are imperative to the success of the veterinary rehabilitation practice. They are the first and last team members to interact with clients. Including them in the exchange of information in the hospital setting will ensure smooth clinic flow and client satisfaction.

To maximize connectivity and communication among staff members, many types of media may be used including in-person meetings, email, practice software memos, group chats, and messaging platforms. Hospital meetings such as case rounds and all-staff meetings can keep the entire team informed about workflow and patient status. Documented and effective means of communication can also include email exchanges between staff members. The practice's software may have note or memo functions for team members to provide updates to each other. A group text or chat can also be a useful means of giving in-the-moment information to the entire team. Lastly, there are now many messaging platforms such as Microsoft Teams, Slack, and others that may streamline messaging within a practice. All these channels of communication can boost employee engagement, morale, productivity, and satisfaction and will ultimately benefit both the client and the patient.

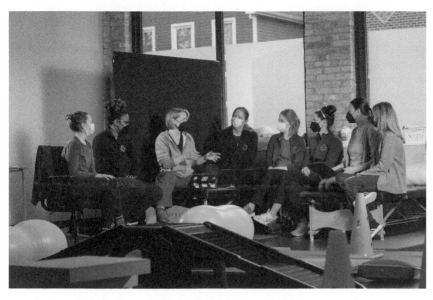

Figure 7.5 Weekly case meetings give the patient care team an opportunity to communicate on case progression. *Source:* Courtesy of Dr Megan Ridley/Renee Yacoub (co-author).

Communication with Clients

Exemplary communication with veterinary clients is an essential skill for the technician/nurse, perhaps especially in the rehabilitation practice due to the amount of time that is spent with clients and the level of client participation that is required for successful patient outcomes. In fact, the client experience is often the basis for how a veterinary rehabilitation practice will be judged (Kelly, 2019). The rehabilitation technician/nurse needs to be adept at non-verbal and verbal communication, client interviewing, listening, managing expectations, providing frequent patient updates, and encouraging client participation.

Non-verbal cues while communicating with clients can include eye contact, facial expression, level of body tension, touch, and movement (Pun, 2020; Baker, 2008). Pitch, tone, volume, and speaking rate are also important voice-related components that can help convey empathy to the client (Pun, 2020; AAHA, 2022). Emotions, a key component of effective communication, are more often communicated non-verbally than verbally (Garrett, 2021).

Verbal techniques that can help the technician/nurse gain client trust include clearly introducing oneself and using both the client's and patient's names while conversing (Baker, 2008). Speaking clearly, being relaxed, and conveying confidence are imperative. Verbalizing acceptance of clients' emotions can also enhance communication. Non-judgmental, normalizing, and self-disclosing comments can make a client feel heard and understood. Examples of these comments were supplied by Dr. Laura D. Garrett at the 2021 ACVIM Virtual Forum (Garrett, 2021):

- Non-judgmental comment: "You were in a very difficult situation."
- Normalizing comment: "It is so common for people to miss these masses until they get very large."
- Self-disclosing comment: "My cat has behavioral issues too."

Proper client interviewing techniques are also crucial. Research has shown that when veterinarians did not actively solicit clients' concerns at the beginning of an interaction, clients were four times more likely to raise concerns at the end of the appointment (Dysart *et al.*, 2011). Open-ended inquiries at patient drop-off can allow the technician/nurse to obtain an accurate patient history and have a fruitful discussion with the client (AAHA, 2022). Questions such as "How is Rex doing?" and "Do you have any concerns today?" leave room for the client to expand. Motivational interviewing, a practice first described by William R. Miller and Stephen Rollnick in the 1980s, consists of four processes: engaging, focusing, evoking, and planning. This practice is defined by an underpinning philosophy of compassion, acceptance, partnership, and evoking which helps the interviewer elicit client ideas rather than imposing ideas on them (Bard *et al.*, 2017).

Once the open-ended questions have been posed, the technician/nurse should remain silent in order to give the client time to speak and to reassure the client that they are being heard (Shadle, 2016). Reflective listening techniques such as parroting and paraphrasing can then be used to ensure that the client's viewpoint is understood and to allow the client to correct any misconceptions (AAHA, 2022; see Figures 7.6–7.8).

Technology for Client Communication

Technology innovations are transforming veterinary medicine, perhaps at an even more rapid pace due to the COVID-19 pandemic. Practices have had to adapt rapidly to provide telemedicine as well as improve and diversify how they communicate with clients. Due to that crisis, communication with clients now extends well beyond in-person interactions and includes telemedicine, text messaging, e-mail, and alerts through social media. In rehabilitation, where clients are encouraged to participate in home care programs for their pets, there is the additional need to transmit demonstration videos and pictures to clients. These can include the demonstration of passive

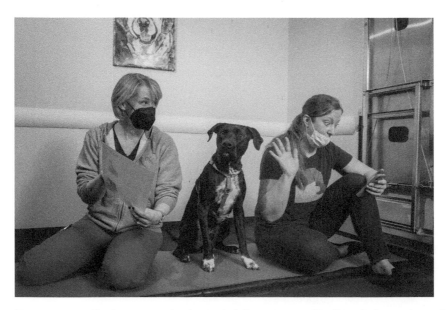

Figure 7.6 Ineffective communication style fails to engage the client during, and exercise demonstration. *Source:* Courtesy of Dr Megan Ridley/Renee Yacoub (co-author).

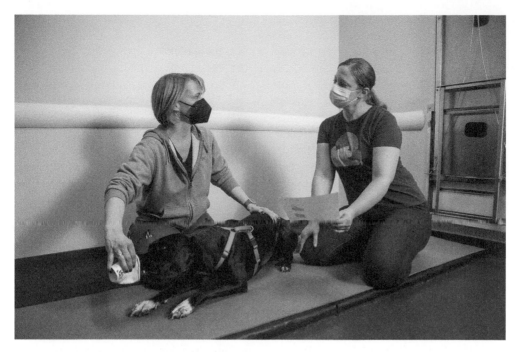

Figure 7.7 The therapist uses several communication styles to engage the client during an exercise demonstration. Following the demonstration, the therapist will follow up with an email summary including videos of the exercise and massage techniques discussed. *Source:* Photo courtesy of Dr. Megan Ridley and Renee Yacoub.

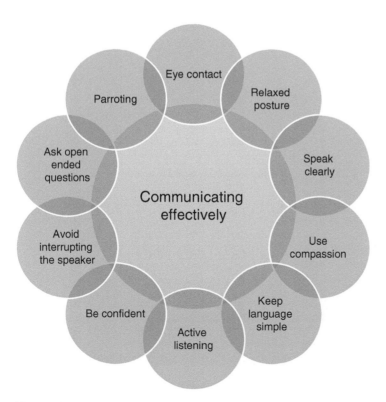

Figure 7.8 A combination of verbal and non-verbal communication skills is essential for good communication.

range of motion, stretching, therapeutic exercises, and massage techniques. It is important for each practice to find the most efficient way possible to transmit media to clients depending on the technology available. The information needs to be digital, updatable, and easily accessible to clients.

Veterinary practice management systems have evolved, and many are now highly customizable. Diagnostics and images can now often be directly integrated into a patient record (Covetrus, 2022). Depending on functionality, these attachments can then be e-mailed directly to the client through the management system. An alternative is to have cloud-based storage such as Dropbox where media can be stored. A link to the desired videos or pictures, easily accessed and clicked, can be e-mailed to the client. If documentation of the e-mails is not automatically posted in the patient record or if the practice management software does not have the ability to e-mail the client directly, the cloud-based link and e-mail communication to the client should be cut and pasted into the patient record so that team members can identify what media has been sent.

Video conferencing platforms such as Zoom and Skype were widely used during the COVID-19 pandemic for both personal and professional purposes. Veterinary-specific telemedicine platforms (e.g., AirVet, Anipanion, Medici, and PetsApp) have also become popular. These platforms are generally inexpensive and have both web browser and app capabilities. This technology can be used for the demonstration of rehabilitation home care techniques when clients cannot be present for sessions (see Figure 7.9). Lastly, client engagement platforms, also known as veterinary client communications software (e.g., PetDesk, Rapport, and Vet2Pet), have multiple capabilities for distributing information to clients, such as push notifications, e-mail, and chat/video. Although these platforms are generally more expensive than telemedicine-only apps, they encompass more features and eliminate the need for multiple apps, which can be confusing to clients (Wallis, 2021).

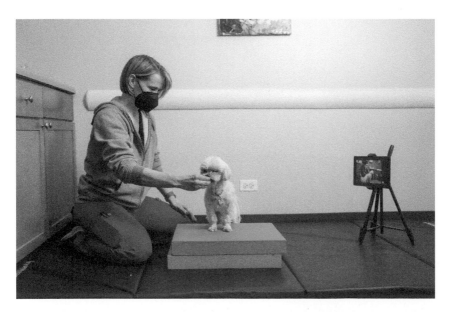

Figure 7.9 A therapist demonstrates home exercises via Zoom. The client then has an opportunity to practice the technique virtually while the therapist troubleshoots with the client to ensure proper technique. *Source:* Courtesy of Dr. Megan Ridley and Renee Yacoub.

Managing Expectations

The veterinarian should discuss goals for each patient at the initial consultation when client expectations should be discussed and adjusted if needed. The technician/nurse will be seeing the client and patient on a frequent basis, so the messaging regarding expectations needs to be unambiguous and consistent with that defined by the veterinarian. Being open and clear about what can be delivered and what the plan is can instill confidence and cooperation in the client (RCVS, 2016). It has also been found that clients who have realistic expectations tend to be more satisfied, less litigious, and more eager to give positive feedback on hospital satisfaction surveys. They are also more likely to follow through on agreed-upon treatment plans and to refer other clients to the hospital (Baker, 2008). If setbacks occur during a patient's treatment program, goals should be re-evaluated, and the veterinarian should explain adjustments in expectations to the client. The technician/nurse should then also be updated so that the team is again on the same page.

Setting Boundaries

Working in veterinary medicine requires a combination of compassion, patience, and positivity when dealing with patients, clients, and coworkers alike. In rehabilitation, due to the frequency with which we see our patients, the extent of communication with clients, and the requisite high level of interaction between coworkers, healthy boundaries need to be set to perform our duties effectively without becoming depleted.

Setting boundaries does not come easily but is rather a skill that requires practice. Normalize the setting of boundaries by discussing them openly with clients and coworkers. Communicate your boundaries in advance and proactively to avoid conflict (Tricarico, 2021). Examples of boundary setting can include:

- Set an out-of-office (OOO) message or an autoresponder email message that defines when you check your messages and when people can expect a response from you.
- Establish the set hours you work.
- Use your paid time off (PTO).
- Discuss upfront with clients the length of appointment times and the importance of being on time for appointments.

Once boundaries have been identified and communicated, they need to be upheld. If a boundary is infringed upon, determine how to assert that boundary better going forward (Tricarico, 2021). Standing by boundaries will promote resilience by preserving the time and energy to engage in coping strategies for well-being (Holowaychuk, 2018). This self-care will in turn help maintain effectiveness in caring for patients and clients (Squires, 2016).

Well-Being and Workplace Wellness

The well-being of veterinary professionals is one of the most important issues facing the profession (Salois and Golab, 2021). The effects of helping others who are experiencing suffering and trauma, coupled with the often overwhelming needs of patients and clients, can take a toll on the healthcare provider. Over time, burnout and/or compassion fatigue can develop, which can affect emotional and physical health, job satisfaction, job performance, productivity in the workplace, and turnover (ProQOL, 2021b). Compassion fatigue and burnout of employees can also affect revenue. A study by Neill *et al.* suggested that the economic cost of burnout is large and the cost of turnover per veterinary technician is as high as $59,000. The study considers the loss of potential income given absenteeism ($35,000) as well as replacement costs ($24,000) (Neill *et al.*, 2022). Given both the personal and economic effects of these workplace stresses, an understanding of their definitions and signs as well as their quantification is important. Hospital management can then develop prevention and intervention programs to help employees maintain fulfillment and satisfaction in the workplace, leading to a successful practice and the ability of employees to continue fully supporting their patients and clients.

Key Definitions

Compassion – The willingness to relieve the suffering of another.

Sympathy – Being able to understand what a person is feeling.

Empathy – Experiencing what a person is feeling.

Understanding the difference between compassion, sympathy, and empathy is important for people who work in the veterinary field. Although the necessity of being empathetic towards clients is commonly discussed in the training of veterinary professionals, experts have recently begun to assert that it may not be healthy to experience empathy on a routine basis (Harrison, 2021; Singer and Klimecki, 2014). In fact, excessive empathy can lead to internalizing another person's feelings and dwelling on their sadness. If that person's pain cannot be alleviated, the caregiver can experience frustration, disappointment, and depression. In place of empathy, Dr. Paul Bloom recommends rational compassion, which is a feeling of goodwill, caring for people, and wanting them to thrive (Paul, 2017). Singer *et al.* also discuss the important distinction between empathy and compassion, both on a psychological and neurological level. They describe how empathic distress can give rise to negative health outcomes, while compassionate responses are based on positive,

other-oriented feelings and the activation of prosocial motivation and behavior (Singer and Klimecki, 2014).

Compassion satisfaction – The pleasure, fulfillment, and sense of purpose derived from assisting others and being a care provider (AVMA, 2022a).

Compassion stress – The unavoidable stress experienced when helping others in distress. Compassion stress is derived from a sense of responsibility and a desire to alleviate suffering. If not addressed, it can lead to compassion fatigue (AVMA, 2022a).

Compassion fatigue – A state of exhaustion and biological, physiologic, and emotional dysfunction resulting from prolonged compassion stress (AVMA, 2022a), which can occur due to repeated exposure to traumatic events such as illness and euthanasia (AVMA, 2022d). Compassion fatigue can lead to a reduced capacity for empathy toward suffering in the future (Scheidegger, 2015). Signs of compassion fatigue in an individual can include:

- Sadness and apathy
- Isolation
- Feeling mentally and physically tired
- Chronic physical ailments
- Lack of self-care, including poor hygiene
- Difficulty concentrating
- Inability to get pleasure from activities that previously were enjoyable
- Substance abuse or other compulsive behaviors (AVMA, 2022d)

Compassion fatigue can also lead to organizational symptoms that affect not just the individual but permeate throughout the practice. These symptoms can include:

- High rate of employee absenteeism and/or excessive workers' compensation claims
- Changes in co-workers' relationships
- Inability of teams to work well together
- The breaking or challenging of company rules by staff members

- Outbreaks of aggressive behavior among staff
- Inability of staff to complete assignments and tasks, or to respect and meet deadlines
- Inflexibility regarding change among staff members
- Negativity toward management
- Inability of staff to believe that improvement is possible
- Lack of a vision for the future (AVMA, 2022b)

Burnout – Studies show that both technicians/nurses and veterinarians are experiencing high levels of burnout (Kogan *et al.*, 2020; Ouedraogo *et al.*, 2021). The World Health Organization includes burnout in the International Classification of Diseases (ICD-11) and defines it as a syndrome resulting from chronic workplace stress that has not been successfully managed (WHO, 2022). It is characterized by emotional exhaustion, cynicism, personal inefficiency, and ineffectiveness in the work environment (AVMA, 2022a). Compassion fatigue and burnout are similar, but according to Dr. Jennifer Brandt, burnout results from the stresses in the work environment, whereas compassion fatigue is associated with the type of work performed (Scheidegger, 2015).

Assessment Tools

The AVMA recommends using the professional quality of life (ProQOL) assessment to measure compassion satisfaction, compassion stress, and compassion fatigue. The ProQOL was developed for use among human health care providers so some modifications in wording are needed such as replacing "people" with "patients" or "clients." The ProQOL, a widely validated, self-administered tool that can be used as a guide to assess one's balance of positive and negative personal and work-related experiences, can be a starting point for change.

The ProQOL assessment is available through the AVMA website at https://www.avma.org/resources-tools/wellbeing/assess-your-wellbeing and at https://proqol.org/proqol-measure (ProQOL, 2021a).

Other assessment resources can potentially be used by veterinary professionals. The Maslach Burnout Inventory (MBI), first developed by Christina Maslach and Susan E. Jackson in 1981, measures several dimensions of burnout (Mind Garden, Inc, 2022; Kogan *et al.*, 2020). New versions have since been developed that apply to different groups such as students, educators, and medical personnel. The MBI was used in a study to measure burnout among veterinary technicians, with participants reporting high levels of burnout across all three dimensions of the inventory, with high emotional exhaustion, high cynicism, and low professional efficacy (Kogan *et al.*, 2020). Another assessment tool, the Professional Fulfillment Index (PFI), designed to measure professional fulfillment and burnout in human physicians (Trockel *et al.*, 2018), can potentially also be adapted to the veterinary profession. Several other assessment tools exist that can help determine an individual's resiliency if compassion fatigue develops (Monaghan *et al.*, 2020; Vaglio *et al.*, 2004; Ogińska-Bulik, 2005). These tools are all meant to help determine if a caregiver is at risk for burnout and/or compassion fatigue so that appropriate interventions can be taken.

Intervention and Well-being Initiatives

Compassion fatigue and burnout affect not just the individual professional but also impact overall patient care, potentially leading to medical errors, workplace toxicity, reduced productivity and profitability, and decreased client satisfaction (Stoewen, 2020). Therefore, interventions are imperative with an emphasis not just on individual self-care but on the resiliency of the entire practice and organization.

Developing a self-care plan will help to build resiliency to prevent burnout and compassion fatigue and promote compassion satisfaction. Start by getting a baseline reading of your own current health by taking an assessment such as the ProQOL and then developing a prevention plan. Such a plan might include proper sleep and exercise, healthy eating, adequate vacation time, the setting of professional boundaries, and access to mental health services (see Figure 7.10). Both the AVMA and NAVTA have valuable resources available on their websites. NAVTA has a Well-Being Task Force to help members with physical, mental, and professional well-being. Also consider taking workshops and continuing education courses about compassion and empathy and asking your employer to help find the resources and finance the training (Singer and Klimecki, 2014; Harrison, 2021).

Prepare a professional growth plan and ask practice management to discuss your plan.

In a study of burnout among physicians in human medicine, Panagioti *et al.* found that organization-directed approaches to burnout intervention such as changes in schedule, and reductions in workload were associated with more significant reductions in burnout compared with individual-directed interventions such as mindfulness techniques and cognitive behavioral therapy (Panagioti *et al.*, 2017). Similar strategies can also be adopted at the veterinary practice level. Optimal workflows should be developed that set realistic productivity measures, adequate administrative time to support the clinical volume and realistic documentation requirements (Bohman *et al.*, 2017). Through investigating burnout among veterinary technicians in specialty teaching hospitals, Hayes *et al.* determined that burnout could be reduced by maintaining an appropriate patient-to-caregiver

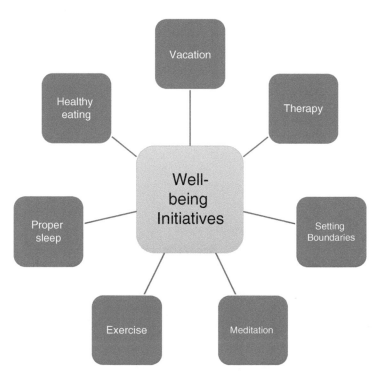

Figure 7.10 A self-care plan can help mitigate burnout and compassion fatigue.

ratio, giving technicians/nurses control of their schedules, allowing them to use their skills fully, providing them with opportunities for learning and growth, and showing them respect (Hayes *et al.*, 2020; Holowaychuk, 2022). Many of these recommendations are paralleled by Kogan *et al.* who further describe the importance of mitigating emotional exhaustion and cynicism through professional development and career mobility for technicians/nurses (Kogan *et al.*, 2020).

Leadership within practices and larger organizations also plays a critical role in shaping a culture of self-care and well-being. Shanafelt *et al.* surveyed physicians in human medicine for burnout and had them rate the leadership qualities of their immediate supervisors. Supervisor scores strongly correlated with the burnout and satisfaction scores of individual physicians. The findings have implications for the selection and training of physician leaders (Shanafelt *et al.*, 2015). Similarly, leadership is also key in veterinary medicine. To develop a framework that promotes well-being, veterinary leaders need to foster a sense of community and transparency and promote an inclusive, healthy workplace that nurtures both individual and workplace well-being (Salois and Golab, 2021).

Conclusion

Veterinary medicine is in a time of critical stress and needs to be bolstered and reformed to accommodate client and patient needs. The role of veterinary technicians/nurses in the industry will be a key part of that change. Their role in veterinary rehabilitation, where frequent patient visits, active client participation, and a high level of team collaboration are standard, cannot be overestimated. Providing technicians/nurses with proper training, respect, the potential for career growth, and resources for well-being will lead to a practice environment that ensures that clients and patients are fully supported.

References

AAHA (American Animal Hospital Association) (2022) *Client support and communication*. https://www.aaha.org/aaha-guidelines/oncology-configuration/client-support-and-communication/ (accessed July 11, 2022).

AVMA (American Veterinary Medical Association) (2022a) *Assess your wellbeing*. https://www.avma.org/resources-tools/wellbeing/assess-your-wellbeing (accessed August 10, 2022).

AVMA (American Veterinary Medical Association) (2022b) *Organizational symptoms of compassion fatigue*. https://www.avma.org/resources-tools/wellbeing/organizational-symptoms-compassion-fatigue (accessed August 10, 2022).

AVMA (American Veterinary Medical Association) (2022c) *Utilizing veterinary technicians to improve practice success*. https://www.avma.org/resources-tools/how-empowering-veterinary-technicians-supports-practice-success (accessed July 3, 2022).

AVMA (American Veterinary Medical Association) (2022d) *Work and compassion fatigue*. https://www.avma.org/resources-tools/wellbeing/work-and-compassion-fatigue (accessed August 10, 2022).

Baker, S.K. (2008). Managing expectations: The art of finding and keeping loyal clients. *J Vet Med Educ* 35 (1): 1–5.

Bard, A.M., Main, D.C., Haase, A.M. et al. (2017). The future of veterinary communication: Partnership or persuasion? A qualitative investigation of veterinary communication in the pursuit of client behaviour change. *PloS One* 12 (3): e0171380.

Best Accredited Colleges (2022) *Careers in Domestic Animal Rehabilitation: Education and Job Info.* https://bestaccreditedcolleges. org/articles/careers-in-domestic-animal-rehabilitation-education-and-job-info.html (accessed August 5, 2022).

BLS (Bureau of Labor Statistics) (2022) *Occupational Outlook Handbook.* https:// www.bls.gov/ooh/healthcare/ veterinarians.htm (accessed August 8, 2022).

Bohman B, Dyrbye L, Sinsky CA, *et al.* (2017) Physician well-being: The reciprocity of practice efficiency, culture of wellness, and personal resilience. *NEJM Catalyst.* https:// www.schulich.uwo.ca/oncology/about_us/ strategic_planning/Physician-Well-Being-NEJM.pdf (accessed August 12, 2022).

Carr, B.J. and Dycus, D. (2016). Recovery and rehab; canine gait analysis. *Today's Vet Pract* 6 (2): 93–100.

Clapham, L. (2012). The VN's role in pain management. *Vet Nursing J* 27 (12): 446–448.

Covetrus (2022) *The Growing Role of Technology in a Veterinary Practice.* https:// northamerica.covetrus.com/resource-center/education/case-studies/growing-role-of-technology-in-a-veterinary-practice (accessed September 24, 2022).

Davidow B (2019) Veterinary nurses – The heart of quality veterinary care. *The Veterinary Idealist.* https://vetidealist.com/ veterinary-nurses-heart-of-quality-veterinary-care/ (accessed August 10, 2022).

Davies W (2021) Key Components of Canine Gait Analysis in the Rehabilitation Exam. *Today's Veterinary Nurse.* https:// todaysveterinarynurse.com/rehabilitation/ key-components-of-canine-gait-analysis-in-the-rehabilitation-exam/ (accessed August 16, 2022).

DeCamp, C.E. (1991). Kinetics and kinematic gait analysis and the assessment of lameness in the dog. *Vet Clin North Am Small Anim Pract* 27 (1): 825–840.

Dysart, L.M., Coe, J.B., and Adams, C.L. (2011). Analysis of solicitation of client concerns in companion animal practice. *J Am Vet Med Assoc* 238 (12): 1609–1615.

Garrett L (2021) Communication Tools for Clients and Coworkers. *2021 ACVIM Virtual Forum.* https://www.vin.com (accessed July 14, 2022).

Harrison, K. (2021). Compassion fatigue: Understanding empathy. *Vet Clin North Am Small Anim Pract* 51 (5): 1041–1051.

Hayes, G.M., LaLonde-Paul, D.F., Perret, J.L. et al. (2020). Investigation of burnout syndrome and job-related risk factors in veterinary technicians in specialty teaching hospitals: A multicenter cross-sectional study. *J Vet Emerg Crit Care (San Antonio)* 30 (1): 18–27.

Holowaychuk MK (2018) Setting Boundaries to Foster Personal and Professional Wellbeing. *Conference Proceedings: New York Vet Show.* www.vin.com (accessed August 5, 2022).

Holowaychuk MK (2022) *What You Can Do to Reduce Veterinary Technician Burnout.* https://marieholowaychuk.com/2021/ 10/05/what-you-can-do-to-reduce-veterinary-technician-burnout/ (accessed August 12, 2022).

Kelly M (2019) Managing Clients' Expectations. *Onlinepethealth.* https:// onlinepethealth.com/managing-clients-expectations/ (accessed August 20, 2022).

Kogan, L.R., Wallace, J.E., Schoenfeld-Tacher, R. et al. (2020). Veterinary technicians and occupational burnout. *Front Vet Sci* 7: 328.

Lloyd JW (2021a) Pet Healthcare in the US: Are There Enough Veterinarians? *Animal Health Economics, LLC.* https://www. marsveterinary.com/wp-content/ uploads/2022/03/Characterizing%20 the%20Need%20-%20DVM%20-%20 FINAL_2.24.pdf (accessed August 9, 2022).

Lloyd JW (2021b) Pet Healthcare in the US: Are There Enough Veterinary Nurses/Technicians? Is There Adequate Training Capacity? *Animal Health Economics, LLC.* https://www.marsveterinary.com/wp-content/uploads/2022/03/Characterizing%20the%20Need%20-%20VN%20-%20FINAL_2.24.pdf (accessed August 5, 2022).

Mind Garden, Inc (2022) *Maslach Burnout Inventory (MBI).* https://www.mindgarden.com/117-maslach-burnout-inventory-mbi (accessed August 12, 2022).

Monaghan H, Rohlf V, Scotney R, and Bennett P (2020) Compassion fatigue in people who care for animals: An investigation of risk and protective factors. *Traumatology* Advance online publication (accessed August 10, 2022).

MVH (MARS Veterinary Health) (2022) *Tackling the Veterinary Professional Shortage.* https://www.marsveterinary.com/tackling-the-veterinary-professional-shortage/ (accessed August 9, 2022).

Neil, C.L., Hansen, C.R., and Salois, M. (2022). The economic cost of burnout in veterinary medicine. *Front Vet Sci* 9: 814104.

Nolen S (2009) *Pet Rehab Becoming Mainstream Practice.* https://www.avma.org/javma-news/2009-10-01/pet-rehab-becoming-mainstream-practice (accessed August 5, 2022).

Nugent-Deal J (2017) Pain management and becoming a patient advocate. *Today's Veterinary Nurse.* https://todaysveterinarynurse.com/articles/pain-management-and-becoming-a-patient-advocate (accessed August 10, 2022).

Ogińska-Bulik, N. (2005). Emotional intelligence in the workplace: Exploring its effects on occupational stress and health outcomes in human service workers. *Int J Occup Med Environ Health* 18 (2): 167–175.

Ouedraogo, F.B., Lefebvre, S.L., Hansen, C.R., and Brorsen, B.W. (2021). Compassion satisfaction, burnout, and secondary traumatic stress among full-time veterinarians in the United States (2016–2018). *J Am Vet Med Assoc* 258: 1259–1270.

Panagioti, M., Panagopoulou, E., Bower, P. et al. (2017). Controlled interventions to reduce burnout in physicians: A systematic review and meta-analysis. *JAMA Intern Med* 177 (2): 195–205.

Paul M (2017) Empathy: An unhealthy path for veterinarians. *dvm360.* https://www.dvm360.com/view/empathy-unhealthy-path-veterinarians (accessed October 3, 2022).

ProQOL (2021a) *Professional Quality of Life.* https://proqol.org/proqol-measure (accessed October 8, 2022).

ProQOL (2021b) *ProQOL Health Manual.* https://proqol.org/proqol-health-manual (accessed August 10, 2022).

Pun, J. (2020). An integrated review of the role of communication in veterinary clinical practice. *BMC Vet Res* 16 (1): 394.

RCVS (Royal College of Veterinary Surgeons) (2016) *Managing expectations: A vastly underutilised skill.* https://www.rcvs.org.uk/news-and-views/features/managing-expectations-a-vastly-underutilised-skill/ (accessed July 3, 2022).

Ruby, K.L. and DeBowes, R.M. (2007). The veterinary health care team: Going from good to great. *Vet Clin North Am Small Anim Pract* 37 (1): 19–35.

Salois M and Golab G (2021) *Are We in a Veterinary Workforce Crisis? Understanding Our Reality Can Guide Us to a Solution.* https://www.avma.org/javma-news/2021-09-15/are-we-veterinary-workforce-crisis (accessed August 8, 2022).

Scheidegger J (2015) Burnout, compassion fatigue, depression what's the difference? *dvm360* https://www.dvm360.com/view/burnout-compassion-fatigue-depression-what-s-difference (accessed August 9, 2022).

Shadle C (2016) Why listening is an important skill: How taking the time to listen to your veterinary clients and your staff can lead to better understanding and communication. *Vet Practice News*. https://www.veterinarypracticenews.com/why-listening-is-an-important-skill/ (accessed July 11, 2022).

Shaffran, N. (2008). Pain management: The veterinary technician's perspective. *Vet Clin Small Anim* 38: 1415–1428.

Shanafelt, T.D., Gorringe, G., Menaker, R. et al. (2015). Impact of organizational leadership on physician burnout and satisfaction. *Mayo Clin Proc* 90 (4): 432–440.

Shaw, J., Barley, G., Hill, A. et al. (2010). Communication skills education onsite in a veterinary practice. *Patient Educ Couns* 80 (3): 337–344.

Singer, T. and Klimecki, O.M. (2014). Empathy and compassion. *Curr Biol* 24 (18): R875–R878.

Squires J (2016) The Space Between Us. *Today's Veterinary Nurse*. https://todaysveterinarynurse.com/personal-wellbeing/the-space-between-us/ (accessed July 3, 2022).

Stoewen, D.L. (2020). Moving from compassion fatigue to compassion resilience Part 4: Signs and consequences of compassion fatigue. *Can Vet J* 61 (11): 1207–1209.

Tabor B (2016) Pain Recognition and Management in Critical Care Patients. *Today's Veterinary Nurse*. https://todaysveterinarynurse.com/emergency-medicine-critical-care/pain-recognition-and-management-in-critical-care-patients/ (accessed July 5, 2022).

Tricarico E (2021) Self-care: Why Boundaries Matter, Plus How to Assert Them at Your Veterinary Clinic. *dvm360*. https://www.dvm360.com/view/self-care-why-boundaries-matter-plus-how-to-assert-them-at-your-veterinary-clinic (accessed July 3, 2022).

Trockel, M., Bohman, B., Lesure, E. et al. (2018). A brief instrument to assess both burnout and professional fulfillment in physicians: Reliability and validity, including correlation with self-reported medical errors, in a sample of resident and practicing physicians. *Acad Psych* 42: 11–24.

Vaglio, J. Jr., Conard, M., Poston, W.S. et al. (2004). Testing the performance of the ENRICHD social support instrument in cardiac patients. *Health Qual Life Outcomes* 2: 24.

VBA (Veterinary Business Advisors, Inc) (2021) *Compensation Best Practices in 2021*. https://veterinarybusinessadvisors.com/compensation-best-practices-in-2021/ (accessed August 21, 2022).

Villalobos A (2004) Quality of Life Scale Helps Make Final Call. *Veterinary Practice News*. https://www.veterinarypracticenews.com/quality-of-life-scale-helps-make-final-call/ (accessed August 12, 2022).

Wallis C (2021) How to Navigate the Virtual Care Platforms without Suffering from Information Overload. *Atlantic Coast Veterinary Conference 2021*. https://www.vin.com/members/cms/project/defaultadv1.aspx?id=10485691&pid=27741& (accessed September 24, 2022).

WHO (World Health Organization) (2022) *Burn-out an "Occupational Phenomenon": International Classification of Diseases*. https://www.who.int/news/item/28-05-2019-burn-out-an-occupational-phenomenon-international-classification-of-diseases (accessed August 12, 2022).

WSAVA (World Small Animal Veterinary Association) (2011) *Global Nutrition Guidelines*. https://wsava.org/Global-Guidelines/Global-Nutrition-Guidelines/ (accessed August 27, 2022).

8

Nutritional Counseling

Kara M. Burns

Academy of Veterinary Nutrition Technicians, Independent Nutritional Consultant Lafayette, IN, USA

Introduction

Nutrition plays a vital role in the prevention and management of many conditions seen by veterinary healthcare team members. This can especially be seen in the rehabilitation of certain disease conditions and should be considered an integral component of the physical rehabilitation protocol. This chapter will look at how nutrition supports the goals of veterinary rehabilitation as well as the technician's role in counseling clients on the importance of nutrition.

Nutritional Assessment

Proper nutrition is a critical component for maintaining the health of pets. Every patient,

healthy or ill, that enters the veterinary hospital should have an evaluation of their nutritional status, and healthcare team members should make a nutritional recommendation based on this evaluation. The goal of patient assessment is to establish the key nutritional factors and their target levels in light of the patient's physiologic or disease condition. This assessment is vital and is in fact the fifth vital assessment to be performed by the healthcare team.

The nutritional assessment considers several factors, including the animal, the diet, feeding management, and environmental factors. The nutritional assessment is an iterative process in which each factor affecting the animal's nutritional status is assessed and reassessed as often as required (Cline *et al.*, 2021).

Although the impact of nutrition on health is a complicated area of study, the American Animal Hospital Association (AAHA) and the World Small Animal Veterinary Association (WSAVA) nutritional guidelines can be abridged into three steps:

1) Incorporate a nutritional assessment and specific dietary recommendation in the physical exam for every pet, every visit.
2) Perform a screening evaluation (nutritional history/activity level, body weight, and body/muscle condition score) – every pet, every visit
3) Perform an extended evaluation for a patient with abnormal physical exam findings or nutritional risk factors such as life-stage considerations, abnormal body condition score or muscle condition score, poor skin or hair coat, systemic or dental disease, diet history of snacks or table food that is greater than 10% of total calories, unconventional diet, gastrointestinal (GI) upset or inadequate or inappropriate housing.

Obesity

Pet obesity has reached epidemic proportions in the United States and other industrialized countries. In 2018, the Association for Pet Obesity Prevention estimated that 56% of dogs and 60% of cats in the United States were overweight or obese (Association for Pet Obesity Prevention, 2019). **It is estimated that 35% of adult pets and 50% of pets over age 7 are overweight or obese** (German et al., 2006). Additionally, a long-term study has documented that the prevalence of osteoarthritis (OA) is greater in overweight/obese dogs compared with ideal-weight dogs (83% versus. 50%) (Burns, 2011, 2020; Kealy *et al.*, 2000). Given these data, it is reasonable to assume that a significant portion of arthritic dogs will be overweight/obese and vice versa.

Obesity can be defined as an increase in fat tissue mass sufficient to contribute to disease. Dogs and cats weighing 10–19% more than the optimal weight for their breed are considered overweight; those weighing 20% or more above the optimum weight are considered obese. Obesity has been associated with a number of diseases as well as with a reduced lifespan. A combination of excessive caloric intake, decreased physical activity, and genetic susceptibility are associated with most cases of obesity and the primary treatment for obesity is reduced caloric intake and increased physical activity. Obesity is one of the leading preventable causes of illness/death and with the dramatic rise in pet obesity over the past several decades, weight management and obesity prevention should be among the top health issues healthcare team members discuss with every client.

Causes of Obesity

Obesity is an imbalance of energy intake and energy expenditure. It is a simple equation – too much in, too little out! There are a number of risk factors that affect energy balance. Indoor pets in North America are typically neutered. There are many positive health benefits associated with neutering: however, it is important that metabolic impacts of neutering are addressed as well. Studies have demonstrated that neutering may result in decreased metabolic rate and increased food intake, and if energy intake is not adjusted, body weight, body condition score, and amount of body fat will increase resulting in an overweight or obese pet. Other recognized risk factors for obesity include breed, age, decreased physical activity, type of food and feeding method, and consumption of "other" foods such as treats or table scraps (Verbrugghe, 2019; Burkholder and Toll, 2000).

Health Risks Associated with Obesity

There are many health conditions associated with obesity in pets, including arthritis, diabetes mellitus, cancer, skin diseases, lower urinary tract problems, hepatic lipidosis, and heart disease. Obese pets are also more difficult to manage in terms of sample collection (blood and urine) and catheter placement and may be more prone to treatment complications, including difficulty intubating, respiratory distress, slower recovery time, and delayed wound healing. It is widely believed that obesity affects quality of life and leads to reduced life expectancy. The dramatic impact of excess body weight in dogs and cats has been demonstrated. In cats, it is estimated that 31% of degenerative myelopathy (DM) and 34% of lameness cases could be eliminated if cats were at optimum body weight. In dogs, lifespan was increased by nearly two years in dogs that were maintained at an optimal body condition (Kealy *et al.*, 2000). It is important to recognize and communicate to our clients that fat tissue is not inert. Obesity is not an aesthetic condition that only affects our pet's ability to interact with us on a physical activity level. Fat tissue is metabolically active and, in fact, is the largest endocrine organ in the body and has an unlimited growth potential (Ahima, 2006). Fat tissue is an active producer of hormones and inflammatory cytokines and the chronic low-grade inflammation secondary to obesity contributes to obesity related diseases (Laflamme, 2006; Witzell Rollins and Shepherd, 2019).

Evaluating Weight and Nutrition

Most pet owners do not recognize or admit that their pet is overweight. The entire healthcare team needs to commit to understanding and communicating the role of weight management in pet health and disease prevention. In particular, the veterinary technician is the primary source for client education; the interface between the client, the doctor and the rest of the hospital team, and is the key advocate for the patient.

Again, every patient needs an assessment to establish nutritional needs and feeding goals. These goals will vary depending on the pet's physiology, obesity risk factors, and current health status. Designing and implementing a weight management protocol supports the team, the client, and most importantly the patient (Wortinger and Burns, 2015b).

A comprehensive history, including a detailed nutritional profile, and a thorough physical examination, including a complete blood count, serum chemistry, and urinalysis, are the first steps in patient evaluation. Signalment data should include species, breed, age, gender, neuter status, weight, activity level, and environment. The nutritional history should determine the type of food (all food) fed, the feeding method (how much and how often), who is responsible for feeding the pet, and any other sources of energy intake (no matter how small or seemingly insignificant) (see Box 8.1).

Obtaining a complete nutritional history supports consistency and accuracy of patient information, helps to pinpoint potential barriers to client compliance, guides client discussion, and supports the optimal weight management program for the pet.

Be sure to weigh the pet and obtain a body condition score at every visit and record the information in the patient's medical record. It is helpful to use the same scale and chart the findings for the client. Body condition scoring (BCS) is important to assess a patient's fat stores and muscle mass. A healthy and successful weight management program results in loss of fat tissue while maintaining lean body mass and consistent and accurate assessment of weight and BCS are important tools to track progress. The use

---

Box 8.1   The following questions should be part of every nutritional assessment

- What brand of food do you feed your pet (try to get specific name)?
- Tell me what your pet eats in a day?
- Do you feed moist or dry or both?
- How do you feed your pet – feeding method (how much, how often)?
- What types of snacks and/or treats do your pets receive? What and how often?
- What if any supplements do you give pets?
- What medications, including chewable medication, does your pet receive? Obtain name and dosage.
- What types of chew toys does your pet play with?
- What foods and/or treats not specifically designated for pets (such as human foods) does your pet receive? What and how often?
- Who is responsible for feeding your pet?
- Does your pet have ANY access to other sources of food (neighbor, trash, family member, etc.)

---

of body condition charts and breed charts are helpful tools in discussing the importance of weight management with clients and help them visualize what an optimal weight would look like on their pet.

Although subjective, BCS is a tool to evaluate body fat. The goal for most patients is a body condition of 2.5–3.0 out of 5 or a 4–5 out of 9, which is ideal (see Figures 8.1 and 8.2).

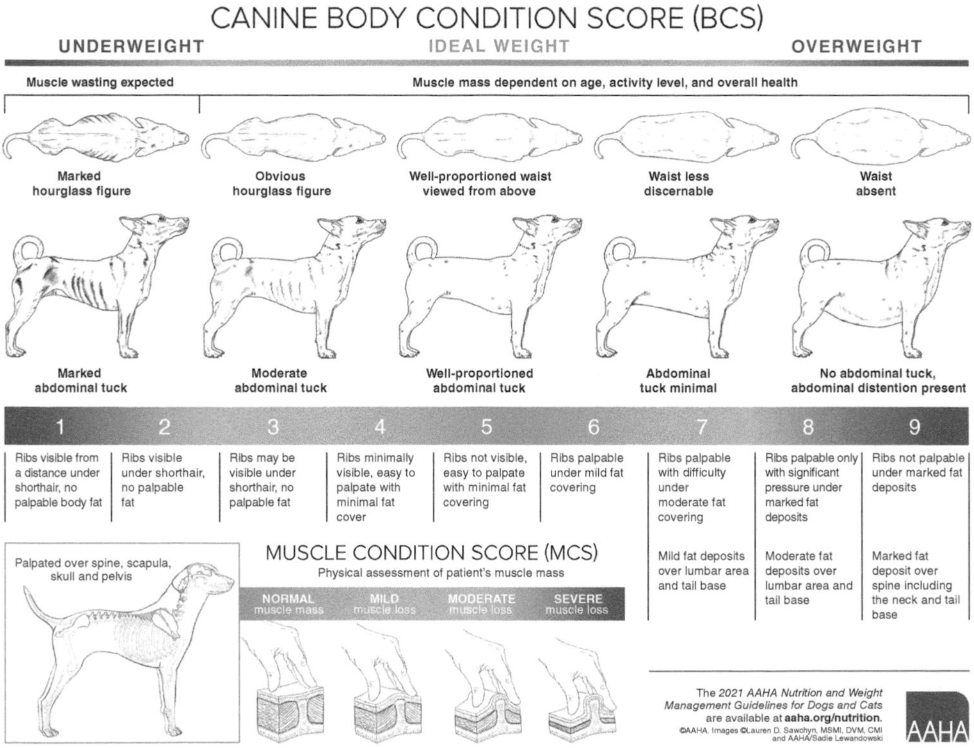

Figure 8.1   AAHA Canine Body Condition Score. *Source:* The 2021 AAHA Nutrition and Weight Management Guidelines for Dogs and Cats, aaha.org/nutrition. ©AAHA. Images ©Lauren D.Sawchyn, MSMI, DVM, CMI and AAHA/Sadie Lewandowski.

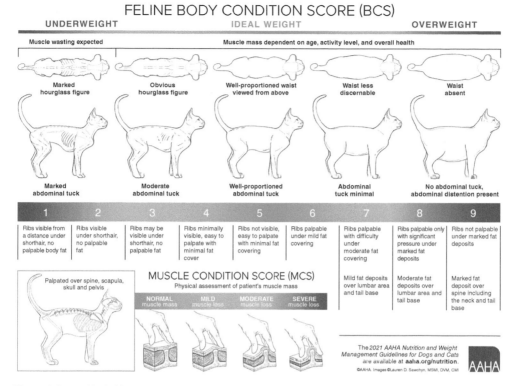

FELINE BODY CONDITION SCORE (BCS)

| UNDERWEIGHT | IDEAL WEIGHT | OVERWEIGHT |

Muscle wasting expected — Muscle mass dependent on age, activity level, and overall health

| Marked hourglass figure | Obvious hourglass figure | Well-proportioned waist viewed from above | Waist less discernable | Waist absent |

| Marked abdominal tuck | Moderate abdominal tuck | Well-proportioned abdominal tuck | Abdominal tuck minimal | No abdominal tuck, abdominal distention present |

1	2	3	4	5	6	7	8	9
Ribs visible from a distance under shorthair, no palpable body fat	Ribs visible under shorthair, no palpable fat	Ribs may be visible under shorthair, no palpable fat	Ribs minimally visible, easy to palpate with minimal fat cover	Ribs not visible, easy to palpate with minimal fat covering	Ribs palpable under mild fat covering	Ribs palpable with difficulty under moderate fat covering	Ribs palpable only with significant pressure under marked fat deposits	Ribs not palpable under marked fat deposits
						Mild fat deposits over lumbar area and tail base	Moderate fat deposits over lumbar area and tail base	Marked fat deposit over spine including the neck and tail base

MUSCLE CONDITION SCORE (MCS)
Physical assessment of patient's muscle mass

Palpated over spine, scapula, skull and pelvis

| NORMAL muscle mass | MILD muscle loss | MODERATE muscle loss | SEVERE muscle loss |

The *2021 AAHA Nutrition and Weight Management Guidelines for Dogs and Cats* are available at **aaha.org/nutrition**.
©AAHA. Images ©Lauren D. Sawchyn, MSMI, DVM, CMI

Figure 8.2   AAHA Feline Body Condition Score. *Source:* The 2021 AAHA Nutrition and Weight Management Guidelines for Dogs and Cats, aaha.org/nutrition. ©AAHA. Images ©Lauren D.Sawchyn, MSMI, DVM, CMI and AAHA/Sadie Lewandowski.

An ideal BCS is believed to help decrease health problems, including musculoskeletal conditions. The evaluation of muscle mass independent from body fat content assessed by body condition score, is known as muscle condition scoring. Muscle condition scoring includes visual examination and palpation over temporal bones, scapulae, lumbar vertebrae, and pelvic bones. The loss of muscle unfavorably affects the strength, immune function, and wound healing of pets. After all information is collected and analyzed in the assessment phase a treatment plan is implemented. This is followed by repeated assessment and adjustment of the plan.

A newer tool for obtaining an accurate fat percentage on the pet's body is body fat indexing (BFI) – especially for overweight and obese pets (Witzel *et al.*, 2014a, b; Burns, 2011, 2014, 2020, 2021; Wortinger and Burns, 2015a–d). This method of obtaining a more accurate body fat percentage has been utilized and confirmed by veterinary nutritionists and provides a better method for pinpointing the amount of fat on a specific pet. Thus, aiding in accurately calculating an amount to feed for an overweight pet, better identifying the pet's ideal body weight, ensuring proper and safe weight loss, and increasing the overall success of the weight management program.

Weight Management Program

As with many aspects of healthcare, designing a successful weight management program is not a "one program fits all" for our patients. The components of a successful weight management program include consistent and accurate weight measurement/patient monitoring, effective client communication, identification of compliance gaps and utilization of tools to reinforce compliance, client and patient support, and program re-structure as needed.

Setting a goal for weight loss and calculating the appropriate energy intake starts with determination of the pet's ideal body weight. Ideal body weight is a starting goal that is adjusted for appropriate body condition as the pet loses weight. It is important to determine the number of daily calories that will result in weight loss while providing adequate protein, vitamins, and minerals to meet the pet's daily energy requirement (DER). The DER reflects the pet's activity level and is a calculation based on the pet's resting energy requirement (RER).

There are a couple of basic formulas that all veterinary healthcare team members should memorize or have on laminated note cards in every exam room (along with a calculator)! The most accurate formula to determine the RER for a cat or a dog is:

$$RER \, kcal / day = 70$$

$$\left(\text{ideal body weight in kg} \right)^{0.75}$$

or

$$RER \, kcal / day = \left(kg \times kg \times kg, \sqrt{}, \sqrt{} \right) \times 70$$

RER is determined initially followed by the DER. DER may be calculated by multiplying RER by "standard" factors related to energy needs. The calculations used to determine energy needs for obese prone pets or for pets needing to lose weight are (Wortinger and Burns, 2015a):

Obese prone dogs	$DER = 1.4 \times RER$
Weight loss / dogs	$DER = 1.0 \times RER$
Obese prone cats	$DER = 1.0 \times RER$
Weight loss / cats	$DER = 0.8 \times RER$

Gathering the above information is crucial and takes only a few minutes. This information provides the foundation for developing a weight loss program that includes:

1) Target weight or weight loss goal
2) Maximum daily caloric intake
3) Specific food, amount of food, and method of feeding.

The program should also include specific protocols for monitoring the pet's weight (schedule these before the client leaves and send reminder cards/e-mails/texts). Also prior to leaving the healthcare team should adjust the pet's energy intake accordingly and exercise guidelines/suggestions (see Box 8.2).

Successful weight management begins with recognition of the importance of weight control in our pets. It is essential that the healthcare team, specifically the

---

Box 8.2 There are specific recommendations that support a successful weight loss program including:

1) Feeding consistency, including feeding the pet designated dish only
2) Ensure the use of an eight ounce measuring cup
3) Recommend the appropriate weight loss food and calculate the initial amount to feed
4) Discuss the importance of total energy intake (do not feed anything other than the recommended food at the designated amount)
5) Make appropriate recommendations for treats and adjust the caloric intake of the base food accordingly
6) Encourage clients to feed their pets separately if possible
7) Recommend appropriate exercise for the pet
8) Offer suggestions on ways other than food to reward or bond with their pet
9) Evaluate, adjust, communicate, and encourage on a consistent basis.

veterinary technician, communicate the serious effects that even a few excess pounds can have on the health and longevity of their pet's life. Weight management should be a cornerstone wellness program in every clinic and the veterinary technician the champion of the program and advocate for the patient.

Osteoarthritis

As in humans, OA is the most common form of arthritis recognized in all veterinary species. A slowly progressive condition, OA is characterized by two main pathologic processes: degeneration of articular cartilage with a loss of both proteoglycan and collagen; and proliferation of new bone. Furthermore, there is a variable, low-grade inflammatory response within the synovial membrane (Anandacoomarasamy *et al.*, 2008). Current estimates of the prevalence of arthritis range from 20% in dogs older than one year up to 80% in dogs older than eight years (Johnston, 1997; Autefage and Gossellin, 2007). The prevalence of OA in adult cats is 33% with the prevalence in senior cats rising to 90% (Lascelles and Robertson, 2010). The objectives of treatment for OA are multifaceted; reduce pain and discomfort, decrease clinical signs, slow the progression of the disease, promote the repair of damaged tissue, and improve the quality of life. A multimodal approach to OA provides the best results for dogs with chronic pain due to OA and includes a combination of anti-inflammatory and analgesic medications, disease-modifying osteoarthritis agents (DMOAs), nutraceuticals, weight reduction, exercise programs, physical therapy, and therapeutic foods. Applying an individualized combination of these management options to each patient will enhance quality of life which is the ultimate goal of therapy.

Weight Reduction

We have discussed the fact that obesity is epidemic in companion animals. Reportedly, 56% of dogs and 60% of cats in the United States are overweight or obese. Similar to the center for disease control and prevention (CDC) estimates that approximately 33% of all adults suffer from arthritis, an estimated 20% of the adult canine population suffers from OA. One long-term study has documented that the prevalence of OA is greater in overweight/obese dogs compared to ideal-weight dogs (83% versus 50%) (Kealy *et al.*, 2000; Burns, 2011). Consequently, it is reasonable to assume a significant portion of arthritic dogs will be overweight/obese and vice versa. Managing these concurrent conditions presents many challenges.

Before a disease can be treated it must first be diagnosed. As disease entities, OA and overweight/obesity present diagnostic challenges for very different reasons. Clinical signs of OA are often not obvious on examination, particularly early in the disease process. Signs of overweight/obesity may be readily apparent, but often they are overlooked or dismissed as inconsequential. Diagnosis of OA requires a combination of history, physical examination findings, and radiographic evidence of degenerative joint disease. Although this may seem straightforward, historical clues crucial to diagnosis may not be readily apparent on routine veterinary examination. Owners often believe many signs of OA are a part of "normal" aging and consequently fail to report them unless prompted by the healthcare team.

Clinical signs of arthritis include difficulty rising from rest, stiffness, or lameness. A thorough, disease-specific history should be taken and may reveal evidence of subtle changes early in the course of OA such as reluctance to walk, run, climb stairs, jump, or play. Signs may be as discreet as lagging behind on walks. Owners are often unaware of the correlation between behavior changes and arthritis.

Yelping or whimpering and even personality changes (i.e., withdrawal, aggressive behavior) may be indicative of the chronic pain of OA. It is recommended to use an owner questionnaire with every potential OA patient to assist with early detection of OA.

Recognizing signs of OA in cats is much more difficult. Cats often suffer in silence and the veterinary healthcare team must rely upon the owner's evaluation and a thorough history to discover potential signs and symptoms of OA in cats. The changes often noted by owners can be categorized into four groups: mobility, activity level, grooming, and temperament. Mobility changes include reluctance to jump; not jumping as high; and changes in toileting behavior due to inability to climb into the litter box. Activity level changes manifest in decreased playing and hunting and a change in sleep patterns. Grooming changes may be noticed when the cat is more matted or unable to groom certain areas, and the claws may be overgrown because they cannot stretch out to "scratch/sharpen" claws. Changes in temperament are demonstrated by the cat hiding from owners or other pets in the house and seeming "grumpy" (Bennett and Morton, 2009; Paster *et al.*, 2005). Many of these signs are again attributed to "old age" in the cat by the owner. Thus it is important for the technician to take a thorough history and ask open-ended questions that may help uncover otherwise overlooked signs of OA in cats.

Diagnosing overweight/obesity is of the utmost importance and leads to diagnostic, curative, and preventive strategies that may be lost in the absence of a diagnosis. The first step to diagnosing overweight/obesity is consistent recording of both a body weight and body condition score.

Prevention

In dogs, risk factors for developing OA include age, large or giant breeds, genetics, developmental orthopedic disease, trauma, and obesity. Risk factors for overweight/ obesity in dogs include age, certain breeds, being neutered, consuming a semi-moist, homemade, or canned food as their major diet source, and consumption of "other" foods (meat or other food products, commercial treats, or table scraps). The radiographic prevalence of canine hip dysplasia, a leading cause of OA in dogs, has been reported to be as high as 70% in Golden Retrievers and Rottweilers (Eby and Colditz, 2008). Golden Retrievers, Rottweilers, and Labrador Retrievers are overrepresented in the population of overweight/ obese dogs.

Dogs found to be overweight at nine to 12 months of age were 1.5 times more likely to become overweight adults (Eby and Colditz, 2008; Kienzle *et al.*, 1998; Anandacoomarasamy *et al.*, 2009; Christensen *et al.*, 2007). Owners of dogs at risk for obesity and OA must be educated on the importance of lifelong weight management. The incidence and severity of OA secondary to canine hip dysplasia (CHD) can be significantly influenced by environmental factors such as nutrition and lifestyle (Anderson *et al.*, 2020; Kealy *et al.*, 2000; Impellizeri *et al.*, 2000). A long-term study has acknowledged that the prevalence and severity of OA is greater in dogs with BCS above normal compared to dogs maintained at an ideal body condition throughout life. Over the lifespan of these same dogs, the mean age at which 50% of the dogs required treatment for pain attributable to OA was significantly earlier (10.3 years, $P < 0.01$) in the overweight dogs as compared to the dogs with normal BCS (13.3 years). Obesity is also a risk factor for the most common traumatic cause of OA in dogs, ruptured cruciate ligaments. Overweight/obese dogs have a two–three times greater prevalence of ruptured cruciate ligaments compared to normal weight dogs. Understanding the correlation between maintaining their dog at a healthy weight and decreasing the risk of disease may be a powerful motivator for many owners.

In humans, the epidemic of obesity is largely attributed to changes in the availability, quantity, and composition of food and the decrease in the amount of physical activity needed for daily living. Physical activity levels of dogs often mirror those of their human companions. Owners should be encouraged to respond with play activities or praise rather than food rewards.

Nutritional Management

Historically, the stress of excess weight on the skeletal system has been thought to be the primary offender of the pathophysiology and progression of OA. Yet, adipose tissue is no longer considered simply a storage site for energy; rather it is now recognized as a multifunctional organ. Adipose tissue plays an active role in a variety of homeostatic and pathologic processes. Recent studies have documented that adipocytes secrete several hormones, including leptin and adiponectin, and produce a diverse range of proteins termed adipokines. Among the currently recognized adipokines is a growing list of mediators of inflammation: tumor necrosis factor-α, interleukin-6, interleukin-8, and interleukin-10 (Towell and Burns, 2011; Ahima, 2006). These adipokines are found in human and canine adipocytes. Production of these proteins is increased in obesity, suggesting that obesity is a state of chronic low-grade inflammation. Low-grade inflammation may add to the pathophysiology of several diseases commonly associated with obesity, including OA. This also explains why somewhat small reductions in body weight can result in significant improvement in clinical signs.

Nutrigenomics and Osteoarthritis

Nutritional supplementation of omega-3 fatty acids is recommended in the management of dogs with OA. Recent studies provide high-quality data has shown that a food with high levels of total omega-3 fatty

acids and eicosapentaenoic acid (EPA), can improve the clinical signs of canine OA. The use of a therapeutic canine food with higher levels of omega-3 fatty acids (specifically EPA) for the management of OA has been supported by four randomized, double-blinded, controlled clinical trials using client-owned dogs (Roush *et al.*, 2010a, b; Fritsch *et al.*, 2010a, b). One 6-month study and two 3-month studies were conducted in US veterinary hospitals. Additionally, a three-month prospective study was carried out in two veterinary teaching hospitals. Overall, 500+ dogs with OA were studied. Participating dogs were diagnosed with OA based on history, clinical signs, and radiographic evidence. Dogs were fed either a typical commercial dog food or a test mobility food, which has higher concentrations of total omega-3 fatty acids and EPA and lower omega-6: omega-3 fatty acid ratios. At baseline and throughout the studies, subjective and objective veterinary evaluations were executed. Owners were also asked to subjectively evaluate their dogs throughout the studies.

These studies provide high-quality evidence that illustrates the benefits of incorporating a food with high levels of omega-3 fatty acids, into the management of the pain of OA in dogs. In normal canine cartilage, there is a balance between synthesis and degradation of cartilage matrix. In arthritic joints, damage to chondrocytes incites a vicious circle which culminates in the destruction of cartilage, inflammation, and pain. The mechanisms responsible for the demonstrated clinical benefits of omega-3 fatty acids include controlling inflammation and reducing the expression and activity of cartilage degrading enzymes.

Cartilage degradation begins with loss of cartilage aggrecan and is followed by loss of cartilage collagens. This results in the loss of ability to resist compressive forces during movement of the joint. EPA is the only omega-3 fatty acid able to considerably decrease the loss of aggrecan in canine cartilage. EPA inhibits the upregulation of aggrecanases by blocking the signal at the level of messenger RNA (Caterson *et al.*, 2000; Caterson, 2004).

Inflammation is not only a vital reaction, but it also plays an essential role in the pathophysiology of OA. The polyunsaturated fatty acids are critical components in the initiation and mediation of inflammation. Arachidonic acid (AA, 20:4n-6) and EPA (20:5n-3) act as precursors for the synthesis of eicosanoids, a significant group of immunoregulatory molecules that function as local hormones and mediators of inflammation. The amounts and types of eicosanoids synthesized are determined by the availability of the fatty acid precursor and by the activities of the enzyme systems that synthesize them. In most conditions, the principal precursor for these compounds is AA, although EPA competes with AA for the same enzyme systems. The eicosanoids produced from AA are proinflammatory and when produced in excess amounts may result in pathologic conditions. In contrast, eicosanoids derived from EPA promote minimal to no inflammatory activity (Wander *et al.*, 1997).

Eating foods which contain omega-3 fatty acids results in a decrease in membrane AA levels as omega-3 fatty acids replace AA in the substrate pool. This yields an accompanying decrease in the capacity to synthesize eicosanoids from AA. Studies have documented that inflammatory eicosanoids produced from AA are depressed when dogs consume foods with high levels of omega-3 fatty acids. In addition to their role in modulating the production of inflammatory eicosanoids, omega-3 fatty acids have a direct role in the resolution of inflammation. Resolution of inflammation is a progressive, active process involving a switch in the production of lipid-derived mediators over time. Proinflammatory products of omega-6 fatty acids metabolism (PGE2, PGE12, and LTB4) are thought to initiate this sequence. Arachidonic acid-derived mediators foster the extravasation of inflammatory cells. With time and in the presence of sufficient levels of omega-3 fatty acids, a class shift occurs toward production of pro-resolving omega-3-derived mediators (resolvins, protectins). These mediators serve as endogenous stop signals by preventing inflammatory cell recruitment, stopping "cell entry" and promoting resolution by removing inflammatory cells from the site. The identification of these two new families of omega-3-derived chemical mediators (resolvins and protectins) may clarify the mechanisms that underlie the many reported benefits of dietary omega-3 PUFAs. Absence of sufficient dietary levels of omega-3 fatty acids may contribute to "resolution failure" and perpetuation of chronic inflammation.

Nutritional supplementation of omega-3 fatty acids should also be part of overall management of cats with OA. As with dogs, high levels of omega-3 fatty acids control inflammation in cats; however, in cats, docosahexaenoic acid (DHA) is the inhibitor of the enzymes responsible for cartilage degradation (Innes *et al.*, 2008; Burns, 2020). The efficacy of therapeutic nutrition for cats with OA is also supported by research (Sparkes *et al.*, 2010; Fritsch *et al.*, 2010c; Frantz *et al.*, 2010). One study looking at therapeutic nutrition containing high levels of DHA, natural sources of glucosamine and chondroitin, methionine, and manganese found that veterinarian-assessed arthritis scores improved in 70% (33/47) of cats and owner-evaluated mobility scores improved in 96% (45/47) of cats after 1 month of therapy (Sparkes *et al.*, 2010). Another randomized, controlled clinical trial looked at this same therapeutic nutritional profile in cats with moderate to severe arthritis (Fritsch *et al.*, 2010c). Alterations in both the ability to jump and the height of jump were the most frequent signs of disease. After 1 month of therapy, 61% of owners noted marked improvement in their cat's clinical signs. Activity monitors worn by the cats documented significant increases in activity in the cats on the OA diet. This study also evaluated a variety of biomarkers. Cats on the OA diet had decreased biomarkers and metabolomic markers of inflammation and cartilage degradation.

Research suggest therapeutic nutrition provides an effective and safe way to manage both dogs and cats with OA. Foods with high levels of n-3 fatty acids have the dual value of controlling inflammation and pain while slowing progression of the disease by reducing cartilage degradation. Efficacy of therapeutic nutrition for OA is supported by multiple clinical trials in arthritic pets.

Developmental Orthopedic Disease

The goal of a feeding plan for pediatric pets is simple – to create a healthy adult. The specific objectives of a good feeding plan are to achieve healthy growth, optimize trainability and immune function, and minimize obesity and developmental orthopedic disease. Growth is a complex process involving interactions between genetics, nutrition, and other environmental influences. Nutrition plays a role in the health and development of growing pets and directly affects the immune system body composition, growth rate, and skeletal development.

Developmental orthopedic diseases (DOD) are a diverse group of musculoskeletal disorders that occur in growing puppies and may be related to nutrition. CHD and osteochondrosis are the most common musculoskeletal problems with a nutrition related etiology. Specific nutritional factors that are thought to increase the risk of DOD in young dogs include:

1) free choice feeding (excess energy consumption)
2) feeding high-energy foods (rapid growth)
3) excessive intake of calcium from food, treats, or supplements (dietary imbalance) (Burns, 2014; Richardson *et al.*, 2010; Wortinger and Burns, 2015b).

OA secondary to DOD can be minimized by educating young dog owners to offer appropriate nutrition during the critical growth phase. All puppies whose adult weight is estimated to be ≥50 lbs should be fed a growth food specifically formulated for large breed dogs. As discussed earlier, maintaining an ideal body condition score throughout life will decrease trauma to joints and the development of OA.

Patient Assessment

Pediatric patients should be assessed for risk factors before weaning to allow implementation of recommendations for appropriate nutrition. A thorough history and physical evaluation are necessary. Special attention should be paid to large- and giant-breed puppies, breeds, and genders (including intact and neutered) at risk for obesity. Furthermore, growth rates and BCS provide valuable information about nutritional risks. Growth rates of young dogs are affected by the nutrient density of the food and the amount of food fed. It is important that puppies be fed to grow at an optimal rate for bone development and body condition rather than at a maximal rate. Growing animals reach a similar adult weight and size whether growth rate is rapid or slow. Feeding for maximum growth puts puppies at increased risk for skeletal deformities and has been found to decrease longevity in another species (Burns, 2014). In Labrador Retrievers, even moderate overfeeding resulted in overweight adults and decreased longevity. The most practical indicator of whether or not a puppy's and kitten's growth rate is healthy is its BCS. Healthcare team members should be comfortable BCS all patients; and with growing patients should reassess at least every two weeks to allow for adjustments in amounts fed and, thus, growth rates. Owners can and should be taught to assess body condition and are likely to become more aware of the appearance of a healthy growing puppy and kitten. Regularly assessing body condition provides immediate feedback about optimal nutrition.

Key Nutritional Factors

The requirements for all nutrients are increased during growth compared with requirements for adult dogs. Most nutrients supplied in excess of that needed for growth cause little to no harm. However, excess energy and calcium are of special concern; these concerns include energy for puppies of small and medium breeds (for obesity prevention) and energy and calcium for puppies of large and giant breeds (for skeletal health). Also, essential fatty acids can affect neural development and trainability of puppies.

Energy

Energy requirements for growing puppies consist of energy needed for maintenance and growth. During the first weeks after weaning body weight is relatively small and the growth rate is high; puppies use about 50% of their total energy intake for maintenance and 50% for growth. Gradually, the growth curves reach a plateau, as puppies become young adults. The proportion of energy needed for maintenance increases progressively, whereas the part for growth decreases. Energy needed for growth decreases to about 8–10% of the total energy requirement when puppies reach 80% or more of adult body weight. A puppy's DER should be about three times its RER until it reaches about 50% of its adult body weight (Wander *et al.*, 1997). Thereafter, energy intake should be about 2.5 × RER and can be reduced progressively to 2 × RER. When approximately 80% of adult size is reached, 1.8–2 × RER is usually sufficient.

- RER (kcal/day) = $70 \times BW(kg)^{0.75}$
- RER (kcal/day) = $(BW_{kg} \times BW_{kg} \times BW_{kg}, \sqrt{}, \sqrt{}) \times 70$

These factors are general recommendations or starting points to estimate energy needs. BCS should be used to adjust these energy estimates to individual puppies.

Prevention of obesity is essential and should start at weaning. After puppies and kittens become overweight, it is challenging to return to, and maintain normal weight. Too much food intake during growth may contribute to skeletal disorders in large- and giant-breed puppies. If the pet is overweight and/or obese and this is carried into adulthood, the risk for several important diseases is increased. These include hypertension, heart disease, diabetes mellitus, dyslipidemias, OA, heat exercise intolerance, and decreased immune function. Studies show that moderate energy and food restriction during the postweaning growth period reduces the prevalence of hip dysplasia in large-breed (Labrador Retriever) puppies and increases longevity in rats without hindering adult size (Burns, 2014; Richardson *et al.*, 2010; Wortinger and Burns, 2015b). Nonetheless, the pet may not receive enough energy and nutrients to support optimal growth if fed a food with a very low energy density and low digestibility. This may result in consumption of large quantities of the food, which can overload the GI tract resulting in vomiting and diarrhea. Healthcare team members should initiate monitoring of energy and food intake and body condition at an early age to help keep the pet at a healthy weight throughout life.

Protein

Protein requirements of growing dogs differ from the requirements of adult dogs. During puppyhood, protein requirements are highest at weaning and decrease progressively until adulthood. Puppies

14 weeks and older, should receive at least the minimum recommended allowance for crude protein which is 17.5% DM. The recommended protein range in foods intended for growth in all puppies (small, medium, and large breeds) is 22–32% DM. Most dry commercial foods marketed for puppy growth provide protein levels within this range (Burns, 2014; Wortinger and Burns, 2015c).

Protein levels above the upper end of this range have not been shown to be detrimental but are well above the level in bitch's milk. Protein requirements of growing dogs differ from those of adults. An important difference is that arginine is an essential amino acid for puppies, whereas it is only conditionally essential for adult dogs. Foods formulated for adult dogs should not be fed to puppies (Burns, 2014). Although protein levels may be adequate, energy levels and other nutrients may not be balanced for growth.

Fat

Growing dogs have an estimated daily requirement for essential fatty acids (linoleic acid) of about 250 mg/kg body weight, which can be provided by a food containing between 5–10% DM fat. Research has shown that DHA is essential for normal neural, retinal, and auditory development in puppies. Inclusion of fish oil as a source of DHA in puppy foods improves trainability and should be considered essential for growth. The minimum recommended allowance for DHA plus EPA is 0.05% DM; EPA should not exceed 60% of the total. Thus, DHA needs to be at least 40% of the total DHA plus EPA or 0.02% DM (Richardson *et al.*, 2010) (see Box 8.3).

When feeding young pets, we must remember that fat contributes greatly to the energy density of a food and excessive energy intake can cause overweight/obesity and developmental orthopedic disease. The

---

> ### Box 8.3 Dietary fat serves three principal functions:
>
> 1) Source of essential fatty acids
> 2) Carrier for fat-soluble vitamins
> 3) Concentrated source of energy

---

minimum recommended allowance of dietary fat for growth (8.5% DM) is much less than that needed for nursing but more than is needed for adult maintenance (5.5% DM). In order to deliver a DM energy density between 3.5–4.5 kcal/g; 10–25% DM fat is necessary. This range of dietary fat is recommended from post-weaning to adulthood (Richardson *et al.*, 2010).

Calcium and Phosphorus

Although growing dogs need more calcium and phosphorus than adult dogs, the health-care team must remember and educate owners that the minimum requirements are relatively low. Puppies have been successfully raised when fed foods containing 0.37–0.6% DM calcium and 0.33% DM phosphorus (Richardson *et al.*, 2010).

Large- and giant-breed puppy foods should contain 0.7–1.2% DM calcium (0.6–1.1% phosphorus). Foods with a calcium content of 1.1% DM provide more calcium to puppies just after weaning than if bitch's milk is fed exclusively. Small- to medium-sized breeds are less sensitive to slightly overfeeding or underfeeding calcium; thus the level of calcium in foods for these puppies can range from 0.71.7% DM, (0.6–1.3% phosphorus) without risk. The phosphorus intake is less critical than the calcium intake, provided the minimum requirements of 0.35% DM are met and the calcium–phosphorus ratio is between 1:1 and 1.8:1. For large- and giant-breed dogs, the calcium/phosphorus ratio should be between 1:1 and 1.5:1 (Richardson *et al.*, 2010).

Digestibility

Puppies that are fed foods with decreased energy density and decreased digestibility will need to eat larger amounts of food to achieve growth. Consequently, this increases the risk of flatulence, vomiting, diarrhea, and the potential development of a "pot-bellied" appearance. As a result, foods recommended for puppies should be more digestible than typical adult foods. An indirect indicator of digestibility is energy density. Foods with a higher energy density are likely to be more digestible (Burns, 2014; Richardson *et al.*, 2010).

Carbohydrates

While no specific level of digestible (soluble) carbohydrates exists for growing puppies, it is recommended that the level of digestible (soluble) carbohydrates around 20% (DM) may optimize health.

Successful treatment and prevention of musculoskeletal disease conditions require a comprehensive approach which includes preventive measures and a multimodal management program. Clinical signs of musculoskeletal diseases are often not obvious on examination, especially early in the disease process. Although signs of overweight/obesity are readily apparent they are often overlooked or dismissed as inconsequential. Documenting a diagnosis of overweight/obesity is critical to the management of these disease conditions. Diagnosing overweight/obesity requires consistent recording of both a body weight and body condition score. Early diagnosis of OA and DOD enables early intervention which in turn often improves the long-term outcome for the patient. Consistent use of a thorough, disease specific history may raise awareness of subtle changes early in the course of OA and DOD. Successful management of OA/DOD and obesity requires nutritional intervention.

Conclusion

Rehabilitation programs are designed to be part of a multimodal approach. One important part of the rehabilitation of veterinary patients is nutrition. Healthcare teams should have knowledge of nutrition and specific nutrients which play a role in certain disease conditions. Rehabilitation incorporates a number of treatment modalities. A nutritional plan should be part of each patients' rehabilitation therapy and should continue following successful completion of the rehabilitation program. Reassessment is required until nutritional and rehabilitative goals are met.

References

Ahima, R.S. (2006). Adipose tissue as an endocrine organ. *Obesity* 14 (Suppl 5): 242S–249S.

Anandacoomarasamy, A., Fransen, M., and March, L. (2009). Obesity and the musculoskeletal system. *Curr Opin Rheumatol* 21: 71–77.

Anandacoomarasamy, A., Caterson, I., Sambrook, P. et al. (2008). The impact of obesity on the musculoskeletal system. *Int J Obes (London)* 32: 211–222.

Anderson, K.L., Zulch, H., O'Neill, D.G. et al. (2020). Risk factors for canine osteoarthritis and its predisposing arthropathies: A systematic review. *Front Vet Sci* 7: 220. https://doi.org/10.3389/fvets.2020.00220. PMID: 32411739; PMCID: PMC7198754.

Autefage, A. and Gosselin, J. (2007). Efficacy and safety of the long-term oral administration of carprofen in the treatment of osteoarthritis in dogs. *Rev Méd Vét* 1: 119–127.

Bennett, D. and Morton, C. (2009). A study of owner observed behavioural and lifestyle changes in cats with musculoskeletal disease before and after analgesic therapy. *J Feline Med Surg* 11 (12): 997–1004.

Burkholder, W.J. and Toll, P.W. (2000). *Obesity, Small Animal Clinical Nutrition*, 4the, 402–426. Missouri: Walsworth Publishing Company.

Burns, K.M. (2011). Are your patients suffering in silence? Managing osteoarthritis in pets. *NAVTA J* 16–22.

Burns KM (2014) Pediatric Nutrition: Optimal Care for Life! *NAVC Proceedings*. Orlando, FL January 18–22.

Burns KM (2020) Mobility matters: Nutritional management of canine joint disease. *Vetted*. July pp. 8–11.

Burns KM (2021) Osteoarthritis: Getting Patients Moving Through Nutrition. *Today's Veterinary Nurse*. Winter edition. pp. 34–43.

Caterson, B., Flannery, C.R., Hughes, C.E. et al. (2000). Mechanisms involved in cartilage proteoglycan catabolism. *Matrix Biol* 19: 333–344.

Caterson G (2004) Omega-3 Fatty Acids-Incorporation in Canine Chondrocyte Membranes. *Unpublished data*. Cardiff university, Wales, UK.

Christensen, R., Bartels, E.M., Astrup, A., and Bliddal, H. (2007). Effect of weight reduction in obese patients diagnosed with knee osteoarthritis: A systematic review and meta-analysis. *Ann Rheum Dis* 66: 433–439.

Cline, M., Burns, K.M., Coe, J.B. et al. (2021). 2021 AAHA nutrition and weight management guidelines for dogs and cats. *J Am Anim Hosp Assoc* 57: 153–178.

Eby, J. and Colditz, G. (2008). Obesity/overweight: Prevention and weight management. In: *International Encyclopedia of Public Health* (ed. S. Quah and K. Heggenhougen), 602–609. St. Louis: Elsevier.

Frantz, N.Z., Hahn, K., MacLeay, J. et al. (2010). Effect of a test food on whole blood gene expression in cats with appendicular degenerative joint disease. *J Vet Intern Med* 24: 771.

Fritsch, D., Allen, T.A., Dodd, C.E. et al. (2010a). Dose-titration effects of fish oil in osteoarthritic dogs. *J Vet Intern Med* 24: 1020–1026.

Fritsch, D.A., Allen, T.A., Dodd, C.E. et al. (2010b). A Multi-Center Study of the effect of dietary supplementation with fish oil omega-3 fatty acids on carprofen dosage in dogs with osteoarthritis. *JAVMA* 236: 535–539.

Fritsch, D., Allen, T.A., Sparkes, A. et al. (2010c). Improvement of clinical signs of osteoarthritis in cats by dietary intervention. *J Vet Intern Med* 24: 771–772.

German, A.J., Holden, S.L., Moxham, G.L. et al. (2006). A simple, reliable tool for owners to assess the body condition of their dog or cat. *J Nutr* 136: 2031S–2033S.

Impellizeri, J.A., Tetrick, M.A., and Muir, P. (2000). Effect of weight reduction on clinical signs of lameness in dogs with hip osteoarthritis. *JAVMA* 216: 1089–1091.

Innes et al. (2008). *Proceedings Hill's Global Mobility Symposium*, 22–26.

Johnston, S.A. (1997). Osteoarthritis – Joint anatomy, physiology, and pathobiology. *Vet Clin North Am Small Anim Pract* 27: 699–723.

Kealy, R.D., Lawler, D.F., Ballam, J.M. et al. (2000). Evaluation of the effect of limited food consumption on radiographic evidence of osteoarthritis in dogs. *JAVMA* 217: 1678–1680.

Kienzle, E., Bergler, R., and Mandernach, A. (1998). A comparison of the feeding behavior and the human-animal relationship in owners of normal and obese dogs. *J Nutr* 128: 2779S–2782S.

Laflamme, D.P. (2006). Understanding and managing obesity in dogs and cats. *Vet Clin Small An Pract* 36: 1283–1295.

Lascelles, B.D. and Robertson, S.A. (2010). DJD-associated pain in cats: What can we do to promote patient comfort? *J Feline Med Surg* 12: 200–212.

Paster, E.R., LaFond, E., Biery, D.N. et al. (2005). Estimates of prevalence of hip dysplasia in Golden Retrievers and Rottweilers and the influence of bias on published prevalence figures. *JAVMA* 226 (3): 387–392.

Richardson, D.C., Zentek, J., Hazewinkel, H.A.W. et al. (2010). Developmental orthopedic disease in dogs. In: *Small Animal Clinical Nutrition*, 5the (ed. M. Hand, C.D. Thatcher, R. Remillard, et al.). Topeka, KS: Mark Morris Institue.

Roush, J.K., Dodd, C.E., Fritsch, D.A. et al. (2010a). Multicenter practice assessment of the effects of omega-3 fatty acids on osteoarthritis in dogs. *JAVMA* 236 (1): 59–66.

Roush, J.K., Cross, A.R., Renberg, W.C. et al. (2010b). Evaluation of the effects of dietary supplementation with fish oil omega-3 fatty acids on weight bearing in dogs with osteoarthritis, 3-month feeding study. *JAVMA* 236 (1): 67–73.

Sparkes, A., Debraekeleer, J., and Hahn, K.A. (2010). An open-label, prospective study evaluating the response to feeding a veterinary therapeutic diet in cats with degenerative joint disease. *J Vet Intern Med* 24: 771.

Towell TL and Burns KM (2011) Multimodal Management of Osteoarthritis. *NAVC Proceedings* Orlando, FL, NAVC Conference 2011, January 15–19.

Verbrugghe, A. (2019). Epidemiology of small animal obesity. In: *Obesity in the Dog and Cat* (ed. M.G. Cline and M. Murphy), 1–15. Boca Raton: CRC Press.

Wander, R.C., Hall, J.A., Gradin, J.L. et al. (1997). The ratio of dietary (n-6) to (n-3) fatty acids influences immune system function, eicosanoid metabolism, lipid peroxidation and vitamin E status in aged dogs. *J Nutr* 127: 1198–1205.

Witzell Rollins, A. and Shepherd, M. (2019). Pathophysiology of obesity: Metabolic effects and inflammation mediators. In: *Obesity in the Dog and Cat* (ed. M.G. Cline and M. Murphy), 17–37. CRC Press.

Witzel AL, Kirk CA, Henry GA, *et al.* (2014a) Use of a novel morphometric method and body fat index system for estimation of body composition in overweight and obese dogs. *J Am Vet Med Assoc* 244(11):1279–1284. https://doi.org/10.2460/javma.244.11.1279. 24846427.

Witzel AL, Kirk CA, Henry GA, *et al.* (2014b) Use of a morphometric method and body fat index system for estimation of body composition in overweight and obese cats. *J Am Vet Med Assoc* 244(11):1285–1290. https://doi.org/10.2460/javma.244.11.1285. 24846428.

Wortinger, A. and Burns, K. (2015a). *Nutritional management of Disease for Veterinary Technicians and Nurses*. Ames, IA: Wiley Blackwell.

Wortinger, A. and Burns, K.M. (2015b). *Weight Management. Nutrition for Veterinary Technicians and Nurses*, 159–167. Ames, IA: Blackwell.

Wortinger, A. and Burns, K.M. (2015c). *Pediatric Nutrition. Nutrition for Veterinary Technicians and Nurses*, 159–167. Ames, IA: Blackwell.

Wortinger, A. and Burns, K.M. (2015d). *Musculoskeletal. Nutrition for Veterinary Technicians and Nurses*, 159–167. Ames, IA: Blackwell.

Association for Pet Obesity Prevention (2019) 2018 Pet obesity survey results: U.S. pet obesity rates plateau and nutritional confusion grows. Association for Pet Obesity Prevention website: https://petobesityprevention.org/2018. Published March 12, 2019. Accessed January 8, 2023.

9

Motivating Your Patient

Megan Nelson[1] and Julia E. Tomlinson[1,2]

[1] *Twin Cities Animal Rehabilitation & Sports Medicine Clinic, Burnsville, MN, USA*
[2] *Veterinary Rehabilitation and Orthopedic Medicine Partners, San Clemente, CA, USA*

CHAPTER MENU

Introduction: Why We Need to Motivate the Rehabilitation Patient

Patients that need rehabilitation are often in pain. It is also likely that the patient has undergone multiple previous examinations for the issue that the patient is presenting before the rehabilitation examination and treatment even occur. This means that the painful area has been palpated repeatedly for the purpose of diagnosis and monitoring response to any prior therapy instituted. The natural guarding of an injured body part, which is part of protecting an injury while it heals, can be compounded and amplified by the repeated experiences of physical examination. In veterinary medicine, we expect this from many of our patients, often without giving them coping mechanisms. Training a dog rarely includes teaching the dog what to expect or how to tolerate veterinary exams. The exam during a

Physical Rehabilitation for Veterinary Technicians and Nurses, Second Edition.
Edited by Mary Ellen Goldberg and Julia E. Tomlinson.
© 2024 John Wiley & Sons, Inc. Published 2024 by John Wiley & Sons, Inc.
Companion website: www.wiley.com/go/goldberg/physicalrehabilitationvettechsandnurses

rehabilitation visit is often a foreign concept with the amount of patient handling necessary, and that can cause undue stress for the patient, the client, and the team.

A relaxed patient is more compliant, easier to examine, and affords the doctor more hands-on time to gather information for a diagnosis. Muscle tension is reduced, and pain signs are easier to discern when the overall stress level of a patient is lowered. It is mutually beneficial for the patient and for the veterinary team to have the examination and subsequent therapies in a low-stress, high-reward environment for the patient.

After examination and diagnosis, a prescription for rehabilitation and a plan are made. This plan can involve both in-clinic therapies and daily in-home therapies. By creating a relaxed environment for the initial evaluation process, we set the expectation of a calm patient; this also helps the client to fully participate in learning about the pet's condition and the at-home and in-clinic therapy plan without distractions of stress and concern for the pet. Both active and passive exercises may be prescribed for the patient. A motivated patient will comply with the plan, whereas forcing an exercise by using restraint without motivation often leads to increasing reluctance from the patient. Reluctance reduces both patient and client compliance for at-home and in-clinic therapy. The rehabilitation team should aim a happy patient engagement, if possible, to achieve the best results. Building and maintaining a good relationship with each patient is important for the rehabilitation team working with the patient in the clinic, but vital for success with at-home exercises.

Understanding Animal Psychology

It is important to understand that reinforcement and punishment are defined by their effect, not by the intent of anyone who may be delivering them. When discussing positive and negative aspects of a handling or motivation technique, we need to be aware of how the patient handles the information given. It is common to assume that since no harm is meant, the procedures are not perpetuating fear in the patient. Teaching this approach to the client starts with understanding and explaining the situation from the animal's point of view. There are many resources that make understanding canine body language easier. For example, in Doggie Drawings (www.doggiedrawings.net, www.doggielanguagebook.com), drawings starring a Boston Terrier named Boogie illustrate important information such as "How Not to Greet a Dog" and "Doggie Language" in an informal and entertaining way. The American Association of Feline Practitioners has created an online resource for cat behavior that covers many topics (www.catvets.com). "Teaching staff and clients how to improve experiences for the cat at the veterinary clinic also improves patient behavior. Fewer staff, less time, and fewer resources are needed to work with well-behaved patients" (American Association of Feline Practitioners, 2004).

Helping clients understand how to better read their pet's body language leads to being able to apply that knowledge and then change their approach to their pet during an exercise as needed to improve comfort and compliance. This will foster a successful relationship long term. It is important for us, as professionals, to use correct terminology when discussing and teaching behavior modification and training. For a glossary of terms, see Box 9.2.

Classical Conditioning Versus Operant Conditioning

Reinforcing Behaviors

The most well-known example of classical conditioning is Ivan Pavlov's experiments with salivating dogs (Pavlov, 1928). Present food, and the dog salivates. Ring a bell, and the dog does not salivate. Ring a bell, then present food, and the dog salivates. Ring the bell, and the dog now salivates. Pavlov effectively used classical conditioning to associate a ringing bell with food (Overall, 2013). We often use this to our advantage when working with our patients in the clinic. Many of the patients that we treat are fearful of new surroundings, strangers, and new activities. When we pair a primary reinforcer – something innately reinforcing to the dog or cat (typically food) – with a neutral (uninteresting) or stressful experience, we can create a positive association and change how the patient perceives the situation in the present, and how he or she will perceive the same situation in the future. It is important to note that we should make every effort to create positive experiences, not just neutral experiences. At our clinic, Twin Cities Animal Rehabilitation and Sports Medicine, a few treats utilized are freeze-dried meat (which is also popular with our feline patients), peanut butter, and frozen peanut butter yogurt cups, along with soft food in a tube or on a lick mat (Figure 9.1). For the increasing number of dogs with food intolerances, hydrolyzed (hypoallergenic) treats are available as well.

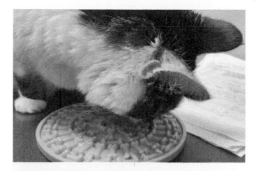

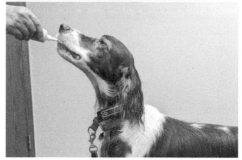

Figure 9.1 Soft food takes time to consume when dispensed on a lick mat (above) or in a squeezable container (below), allowing the animal to work at the reward.

Real Life Example

A client was unwilling to use food rewards in the clinic.

Client – "Sparky doesn't need treats to behave."

Technician – "We want to build the best association with us, the building, and the equipment we can. Using food helps us to reinforce calm, cooperative behavior."

Client – "He needs to listen because I said so."

Technician – "We use food to see how willing Sparky is to do exercises for us. If we know Sparky likes food and knows how to earn food but will not sit, I will ask for other behaviors (down, stand) first. Then ask for a sit; if he will make the other movements, but still shows hesitation to sit, this can help us to identify pain and understand where it hurts so that we can help Sparky to recover."

Emotional Response – Creating Associations with the Environment

Where Pavlov is known for his work with the bell, B.F. Skinner is known for the four quadrants of operant conditioning (Skinner, 1938). Skinner's principles were that desired behaviors should be reinforced; behaviors can be built in incremental steps; and that immediate reinforcement generally provides a better learning experience than delayed reinforcement. These principles have been used extensively in training. Operant conditioning breaks learning down into four areas, or subsets. In each area, we evaluate our training/motivation based on whether we have successfully increased or

Box 9.1	Positive reinforcements	
	Positive (add)	**Negative (remove)**
Reinforcement (desirable)	Add something desirable to increase the frequency of a behavior	Remove something aversive to increase the frequency of a behavior
Punishment (undesirable)	Add something undesirable to decrease the frequency of a behavior	Remove something desirable to decrease the frequency of a behavior

Source: Adapted from Martin and Martin (2009).

decreased the frequency of a behavior (Martin and Martin, 2009) (see Box 9.1).

Positive reinforcement is often used, and usually without thinking too much about it. Successful influence on behavior using this technique generally occurs, but we can always try to do a better job of communicating with our patients more clearly. A key piece, often missing when motivating a patient, is looking closely at what exact behavior or action is being reinforced. This requires precise attention to detail. Dogs are uniquely attuned to small motions; for example, the handler may be rewarding a "behavior chain" of brief contact of one foot on a balance disc with a step back off again when the goal is to reinforce standing still with both front feet on a balance disc.

Improving the timing of rewards, typically by adding in a "secondary reinforcer," will shorten the amount of training time. The most common secondary reinforcer is a "marker" (a unique way to mark a behavior), such as a clicker, verbal tongue clicks, verbal yes, or other less commonly heard words such as "good" or "yes" (avoid "okay"). The purpose of the secondary reinforcer is to give the handler more time between desired behavior and getting around to giving the primary reinforcer (reward). A secondary reinforcer helps to give the animal clarity about the exact behavior (e.g., limb placement) that is desired and so being reinforced. The animal knows that a reward will follow the secondary reinforcer. The patients typically learn about a secondary reinforcer without too much dedicated training if there is consistency with the type of marker used. Mark the behavior, then deliver the reward. Practice mark, followed by reward, for multiple new behaviors to build value for the marker. Since both hands are usually needed for restraint and carrying out exercises, using a secondary reinforcer that is a verbal marker will help an animal to identify the behavior being rewarded, and this will give the handler time to access and then deliver the treat reward.

In cases where a verbal marker is utilized, remember that inflection (the tone and pitch of your voice as it says the word) can impact the effect. For this reason, a tongue click may be preferred over a verbal "yes." One of the rules of good training is to always pair the secondary reinforcer with food, or it will quickly lose value. Using these techniques while the client is in clinic with the patient allows time for observation and learning techniques to apply at home and time for answering questions if needed (see Box 9.2).

Working to make positive or neutral associations with the environment in the clinic can include more than just the use of reinforcers. Maintaining a quiet environment is extremely important for some patients. Patients who are reactive to noise can react to something as small as a beep from an ultrasound machine. It is possible to get the sounds turned off on some ultrasound and e-stim machines. Shockwave units can make a lot of sound. The use of ear mufflers can help patients that are not

Box 9.2   Key terms used for reinforcement

Reinforcer – Any consequence that causes the preceding behavior to increase (e.g., treats)

Behavior chain – Specific sequence of discrete responses, each associated with a stimulus

Primary reinforcer – Primary reinforcers are biological (e.q., food, pleasure from a toy)

Secondary reinforcer – A conditioned reinforcer; the dog knows something good is coming

Marker – A unique way to mark behavior (e.g., "yes!")

Luring – Using a reward to increase attention and interest (e.g., to initiate motion)

Conditioning – Associations between stimuli and response

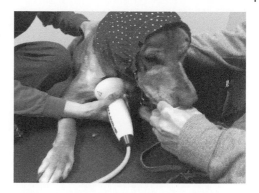

Figure 9.2   Patient undergoing shockwave therapy. He is wearing ear muffs and licking a frozen treat.

Understanding Body Language

Evaluating stress while in the clinic can be challenging. A stress level scale developed by Dr. Karen Overall is a helpful tool to accurately assess the current stress level of a dog while in clinic (Overall, 2013). There is a fear, anxiety, and stress scale for cats (https://fearfreepets.com/resources/fear-free-store/fear-anxiety-and-stress-spectrum-cat/). Knowing how to properly evaluate the behavior of a patient is going to help foster the best relationship so that we can meet our goals. We can also provide some assignments for the client to work on these handling situations in a positive way at home.

sedated for therapy and can also help lightly sedated patients (Figure 9.2). Sometimes a white noise machine can help reduce sounds outside the treatment room. The white noise of some underwater treadmill units can dull general clinic noise in some cases. All staff members should be cognizant of raising their voices, even in laughter. Calming music can help some patients relax, and there are specific tempos of music made to calm dogs (e.g., Through A Dog's Ear™). It is recommended to have individual stereos/speakers in each room to allow for volume control rather than having music playing at the same level throughout the clinic. The importance of comfortable, traction flooring should not be underestimated; a patient will feel more relaxed if they are better able to grip the floor. Examination tables, if used, should have traction; low-matted tables are recommended (Figure 9.3).

The most basic signs of stress are yawning, lip-licking, or blinking. The most severe is biting for carnivores (biting and kicking for equids and ungulates). Most patients fall somewhere in the middle of this spectrum; they are not completely comfortable with what is going to happen but are not predisposed to bite. Dr. Overall suggests taking note of body posture, tail posture, ear posture, gaze, pupils, respirations, lips, activity, and vocalization. If we take the time to learn about what patient behaviors mean, we can make decisions about how thorough

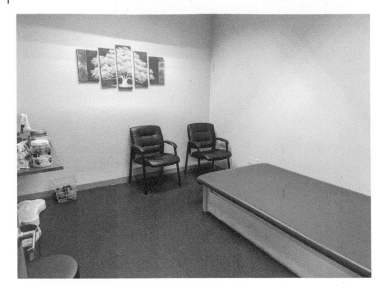

Figure 9.3 A low-matted table for examination and therapy in a quiet room with matted floor, the table is 40 cm high.

and lengthy the hands-on portion of each visit is (see Figures 9.4 and 9.5). We can quickly discern when a patient needs a break so that stress (cortisol) levels can drop back to a more neutral state. In cases of rising stress with danger signs, we can evaluate whether we need to postpone the examination or restrain the patient for safety of personnel; the best option for all concerned is to postpone the examination/therapy when patient stress is reaching concerning levels.

Building Motivation and Value Through Food Rewards

As discussed previously, food is a powerful primary reinforcer for our patients. Utilizing this effectively includes gathering information about diet and feeding rituals in the home. Two of the most common reasons for lack of food motivation are free feeding at home and weight control issues. Free feeding is when food is left out always for the pet. This can be a measured amount or filled at will. The measured amount still

often means no portion control. Free feeding makes our primary reinforcer (food) far less rewarding as it is always available; there is no drive to eat from a human hand. Many free-fed animals are also overweight, so by addressing one problem, we address both. Food is such a powerfully useful tool, and it is often overlooked. Help the client to set up a feeding schedule that works for everyone. For dogs with a necessity for low caloric intake, a common recommendation is to use meals as treats. By teaching the dog to work for meals, a lot is accomplished; when appetite is high, so is drive and attention to the reward. Using the normal diet as reinforcement in familiar environments allows for a wider variety of high-value reinforcement in more stimulating (usually also more stressful) environments. Reserving a variety of treats specifically for therapy appointments can help the whole process proceed more smoothly. For cats, very high-value foods with strong odors (freeze-dried meat and baby food) can help to stimulate a cat to eat; for example, move to eat while stretching front legs up onto a raised surface, elongating the spine and extending the

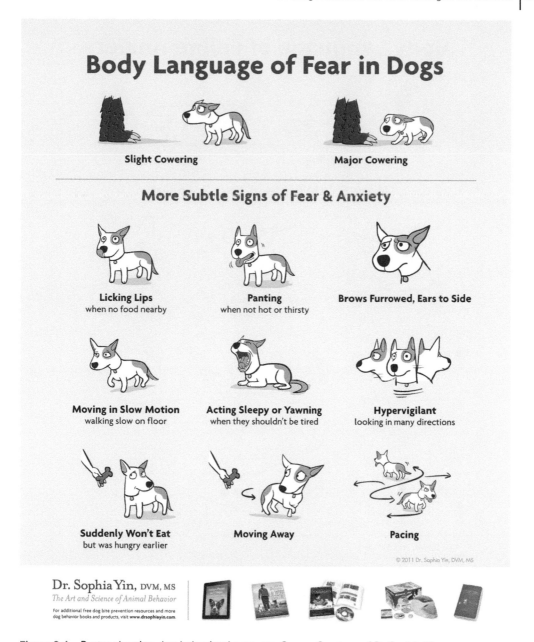

Figure 9.4 Poster showing dog behavioral postures. *Source:* Courtesy of Dr. Sophia Yin.

hips (see Figure 9.6). Many horse clients and trainers use treats. For both cats and horses, it is even more important than it is for dogs to have a treat that takes multiple bites or licks to consume, as these patients tend to gain less reinforcement from interaction with people.

A positive relationship is fostered if the goal of motivation and training is cooperation. Prescribed rehabilitation exercises provide an opportunity for training, thereby providing the patient with mental stimulation and the client with strengthening of the human–animal bond. Patients who are

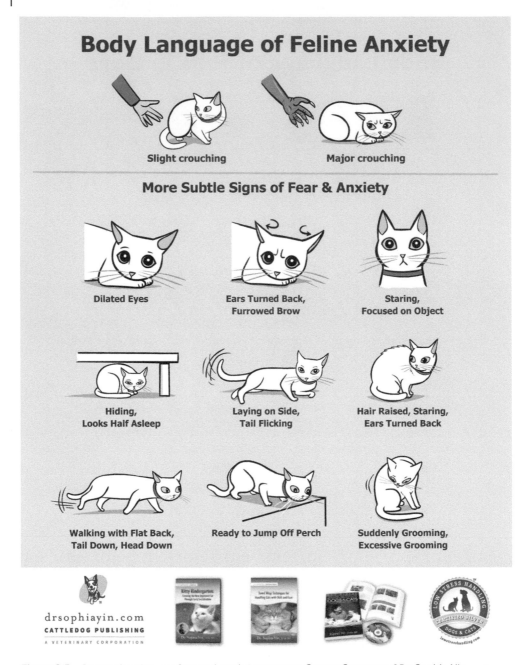

Figure 9.5 Poster showing cat fear and anxiety postures. *Source:* Courtesy of Dr. Sophia Yin.

undergoing rehabilitation are usually exercise-restricted. This can lead to unwanted behaviors due to boredom and excess energy. Training requires concentration from the animal (as well as the handler); this mental activity and stimulation cause some fatigue and decreases boredom.

Replacing the normal food bowl with a work-to-eat toy (also known as a food toy) is another great way to encourage mental stimulation and avoid boredom. For horses, work-to-eat toys such as the Amazing Graze™ treat toy (www.HorsemensPride.com) can help alleviate the boredom of stall

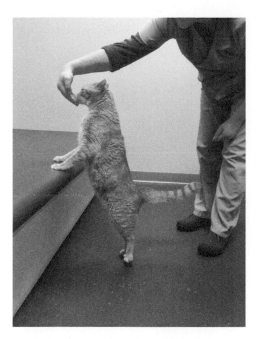

Figure 9.6   A feline patient being lured into a stretch using freeze-dried meat. Note his left rear extends less. The patient has had a left femoral head excision.

confinement. The rehabilitation team needs to be cognizant of the type of toy and the effort and motions required to release food from the toy. Choosing an appropriate work-to-eat toy needs to be taken into consideration. A toy that requires a lot of movement, with the patient concentrating on rolling the toy instead of on their gait compensations, may result in relative overload of an injury. The disabilities of the patient need to be considered, and the team should be sure to counsel the client about providing the work-to-eat toy in a confined area.

Luring, Shaping, and Marking Behaviors

Luring is the motivating technique that is used most often, as most patients can be motivated by food. Having an assortment of high-value reinforcers (treats and fun toys) as well as instructing clients to bring known

favorite treats from home can help. Even the most outgoing and typically social dogs can be unsettled by new experiences. The rehabilitation team should be creative with the treats, but as mentioned previously, reserve the exciting stuff for situations where it will be harder to motivate due to distraction and stress (for example, a treatment such as dry needling of myofascial trigger points, which causes some discomfort). A helpful recommendation is to make a bag of goodies to be kept in the refrigerator or freezer that combines a few tasty snacks and some regular food. An example snack "grab bag" ready to go with everything cut up into small pieces would contain cubes of cheese, strips of boiled chicken, regular dry food, and a commercially available soft treat.

Although it may seem to be a skill that most dogs are born with, teaching an animal to "lure" is invaluable. Luring is when the animal follows the treat (Martin, 2009b) to perform a desired behavior. Most clients are familiar with luring without realizing it, but may not be maximally successful. It is important to feed often during the luring process to keep the patient focused more on the food than on the goal behavior (a desired motion or simply remaining still during therapy). For this reason, treats that can be nibbled on or something that can be licked at, providing a slow, continuous reward, are great options. When teaching a dog to lure, start with small steps. Do not have the complete behavior as the goal; instead, reward small behaviors. Many dogs tend to sink to the ground instead of standing still when manipulated. When we need a dog to stand for examination, luring him into that position would be a multistep process. First, let the dog nibble from their current, undesired position. Next, bring the treat up and forward just a little so the dog continues to be engaged. Finally, reward the full stand with a rapid succession of treats in a short "burst" (see Figure 9.7). The posture is maintained by continued, intermittent rewards.

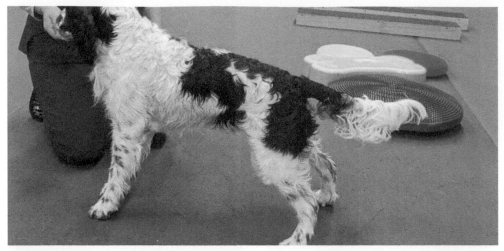

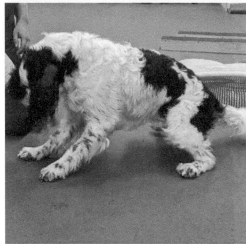

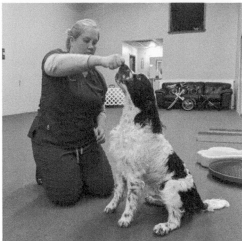

Figure 9.7 Luring a patient from a sit into a standing position for examination.

Teaching a horse or a cat to lure is a very similar process, but motivation may differ between individuals.

Luring requires focus on the part of the animal. Overly exuberant dogs are approached in a similar manner to shy dogs so that stress/unfocused energy does not distract from the food-luring process. Present the food to the patient without eye contact, and with your body turned to the side; if the dog acknowledges you but does not take it from your hand, then gently toss a treat across the floor. Aim to toss the treat behind the dog, not in their face. Once the patient recognizes you as the source

of the treatment, they are more likely to accept a treatment given by your hand. These non-assertive behaviors by rehabilitation team members will keep the dog focused on the treats and avoid stressors, overexcitement, and other distractions.

Simple Games: Set Up for Success

As mentioned previously, a patient that can be lured into different positions is much easier to work with. Starting with behaviors that are easily lured helps keep patient and client motivated with success being the reinforcer for both individuals. Having the patient follow a food luring head up, head down, body in a circle, into a sit, or into a stand are some basic behaviors that most dogs do on a regular basis. Cats will stretch and move their bodies in response to luring, too. Breaking the final behavior down into smaller, incremental steps helps set up both client and patient for success. If the end goal is to have the patient lie in lateral or sternal recumbency, it is necessary to think of the behaviors that build up to that. Clients who get involved in the whole process of making the prescribed rehabilitation therapies into a game tend to be more successful in maintaining, or in many cases, strengthening, their human–animal bond and in completing the rehabilitation goals.

Having Intent and Understanding Trust

Leading by example is a powerful way to teach clients about building and maintaining trust with their animals and their animal's trust in the rehabilitation team. During an initial consultation, while the veterinarian is learning about the patient's history, the technician can build a relationship with the patient. The luring process can initially be time-consuming (e.g., tossing treats to a shy or fearful patient and slowly building trust), so beginning the process during the time taken to record patient history and during the time taken to make initial observations about the patient before handling (postures, gait, and transitions, etc.) is efficient. This approach means that by the time the patient needs to be handled, they have had some exposure to the luring/reward process.

Home Exercises – Knowing When to Stop

Many clients who bring a pet in for rehabilitation are unaware of subtle signs of pain. Vocalizing is typically the only sign recognized by clients, so education about pain-related behaviors and understanding pain levels at home is an important part of the initial evaluation process. Every exercise prescribed by the veterinarian must be performed with comfort in mind. Improper application of technique, changes in patient status/function, or fatigue can be the difference between an exercise going smoothly without pain and one being met with resistance due to pain and stress. Pain and fatigue levels can vary day to day depending on other activity levels and additional compounding factors. Counseling clients with typical pain and stress-related body language will help set the stage for knowing when to stop (see Figure 9.8). A patient who is averting their eyes, shifting away, lip-licking, or pulling ears back is showing signs of pain and discomfort; these signs occur at relatively mild levels of discomfort, and long before vocalizing will happen. Proceeding with more caution and modifying the exercise to decrease physical pressure (e.g., limiting end-range joint motions) will not only keep the patient more comfortable physically, but it will also help to preserve the relationship between patient and client. If in doubt, the client should stop the exercise, and it should be re-evaluated with the client in the rehabilitation clinic. Video footage of the exercise (see Videos 9.1 and 9.2) and associated behaviors at home may also be helpful. Hesitation is often the first sign of fatigue, but it can also be the first sign of discomfort. Be sure to counsel about rest and about not pushing through an exercise if the patient's willingness decreases.

Rehabilitation therapy can cause mild transient discomfort but should not be an

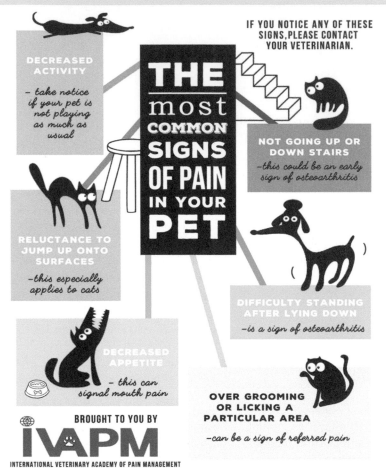

Figure 9.8 International Veterinary Academy of Pain Management (IVAPM) pet pain awareness poster for client education, 2016. *Source:* Courtesy of IVAPM.

uncomfortable process beyond this. In the veterinary world, we rely on patient compliance, and a breakdown of this compliance can mean an end to therapy; we cannot force our way through a patient's pain by reasoning with the patient about long-term gains being worth the discomfort. We aim to avoid philosophies espoused in human therapy and sports training such as "no pain, no gain." Instead, we focus on teaching cooperation and compliance to develop a willing partnership between patient, client, and the rehabilitation team.

Problem Solving and Dealing with Challenging Patients

Case Examples

Case No. 1: Human Reactive and Handler Aggressive

Arlo, a three-year-old intact male Doberman Pinscher bred for bite sports, is a powerful dog with significant specialized training that does not include tolerance of a comprehensive examination. He will alarm bark and growl when uncomfortable in a situation.

He does not want interaction with strangers. The client brought high-value soft food (meatballs) and had previously brought a dog to the clinic, so was familiar with handling techniques. During initial evaluation, after settling from alarm barking, Arlo would eat food from the client. After a few minutes to acclimate, he would take food from the rehabilitation technician; however, he was not motivated enough for him to eat while the doctor examined him. Some bite sport dogs respond best to their handler; however, the client was nervous and uncomfortable restraining and feeding him for examination, and the rehabilitation technician quietly voiced concern about adequate restraint. Having the client leave the room caused an increase in anxiety-related behavior (turning to watch the door, trembling). The team, a collaboration between technician and veterinarian, learned through trial and error that having the client in the room but not handling him made examinations the smoothest. A basket muzzle was used at initial examination so feeding could continue whenever he was comfortable enough to eat. Therapy visits (therapeutic ultrasound for a shoulder injury) involved the client in the room and two technicians, one to handle and feed, and the second to perform the therapy. Once Arlo became familiar with his therapy visits, the client suggested a head halter, and Arlo was calmer in this than in the basket muzzle. The halter was used for light restraint, and Arlo was given a target to put his front feet on during therapy and examination (with patient behavioral goal of understanding his job was to stay still). Arlo went on to have many successful visits handled this way, including follow-up on general physical health after resolution of the shoulder tendinopathy.

Case No. 2: Fearful Patient

A five-year-old medium-sized mixed-breed dog presented for back pain. The dog was not very treat-motivated at home, and even less so when stressed. The client brought multiple types of treats to the consultation and used massage techniques to aid compliance. Chewy strips of sweet potato and peanut butter in a very thin consistency were readily consumed. He received laser treatments for three weeks, where he learned to relax.

When hydrotherapy was initiated, the patient had higher stress levels than he had demonstrated before, even at his consultation. He would not take food. The underwater treadmill was a change in environment and expectation, and changes were stressful for him. He also had the added stressor of movement (whereas for laser therapy he had been relatively still, in a quiet room), along with being in a higher-traffic, open-plan area. For three appointments, the technician and the client tried the same approach as was used in the consultation. The same treats, essential oils, and predictable massage were used while the patient walked on the underwater treadmill. Despite this, the patient demonstrated higher levels of stress than at the initial consult. Social pressure, in the form of paying direct attention, added stress for the patient; the client repeatedly offered peanut butter for the patient to lick without expecting him to do so. The client and technicians continued to try offering a variety of treats but stopped interacting with the patient purposefully while in the water. When the client and technician had a conversation without paying attention to the patient, he was calmer. This was repeatable with future appointments. By the fourth underwater therapy appointment, the patient could walk calmly and take treats, provided attention was not obviously focused on him. The use of non-assertive body language and avoiding eye contact worked well for this patient.

Case No. 3: Food Allergy and Anxiety

A 10-year-old Australian Shepherd with food allergies presented with biceps muscle pain and elbow osteoarthritis. The patient was already taking the medication fluoxetine for anxiety at initial presentation. During visits, she would shake and retreat into the corners of the room. Even light handling would result in a struggle to escape touch. Attempts were made to allow acclimatization; she visited just briefly for treats and then left. During these acclimatization visits, she was very nervous, but when she took food, she relaxed. Treats used were dry kibble from home, supplemented with hypoallergenic treats in the clinic. After several desensitization visits, examinations were possible using this approach, but treatment procedures (even the low stimulus of a modality) resulted in an escalation of her stress response. After several therapy sessions, she began to reach her threshold more quickly with each follow-up visit. Premedication was elected, using trazodone at home two hours before the car ride, but unfortunately had minimal effect. After communication with her primary care veterinarian, alprazolam was prescribed for situational use. This raised her threshold for stressors and enabled the team to complete rehabilitation.

The patient has some long-term issues; therefore, her visits for follow-up at the clinic are very ordered with the aim of minimizing stress. She enters the room at least 10 minutes before the appointment time and listens to her favorite music from home (country and western from her client's phone). With each visit, time is consciously allocated to talk about her progress at the start of the visit with no hands-on for at least five minutes. The hypoallergenic treats given in clinic are not the same as her everyday home treats; therefore, they provide higher motivation for luring and reward. Therapy decisions always take into consideration the stress of each plan and modality and handling needed (e.g., contact needed along with beeping sounds of the laser versus soundless, no-contact pulsed electromagnetic field therapy).

Case No. 4: Home Environment Issues

A six-year-old straight-line racing Whippet presented with a deltoid muscle strain. It was an acute injury that had occurred at an event. His client had mobility problems and usually exercised her dogs to maintain fitness by letting them run in her large yard every day, chasing a Frisbee™. Practice on a lure line was once weekly but only in racing season. Visits for in-clinic therapy were not a problem; however, the patient had to be exercise-restricted at home, in a multi-dog household. A dog walker was utilized. In the clinic, appropriate modalities and manual therapies were used. Daily stretching was prescribed for home with consideration for the client's disabilities. The patient was not making adequate progress in the rehabilitation plan; shoulder extension continued to be restricted, and some intermittent lameness was seen at a trot. After some discussion, it was determined that the client had not been utilizing the dog walker daily and was tired of restricting her dog, so had allowed some yard time for a mental break. The client reported that the dog was much more relaxed, having been able to freely run, and was holding his front leg up only a little, a lot less than he had initially. She suggested she allow more activity and use an anti-inflammatory to help the pain. The pros and cons of this approach were discussed at great length, and a compromise was achieved. The patient could have off-leash yard time alone, not with the other dogs, and no Frisbee.

The client agreed to make the long drive to the clinic twice weekly for exercise therapy for another month to bridge the gap between limited home exercise and full home exercise. The situation was not ideal, but the yard time alone progressed to Frisbee retrieves as the patient progressed, and then on to yard time with other dogs.

An issue of lack of conditioning remains, and straight-line racing fitness has not been achieved.

Case No. 5: Too Much Fun/Equipment Cues

A seven-year-old Rottweiler presented for strengthening and gait retraining. Previously, he had been exercised on a land treadmill at home, but it was overstimulating for him so had to be managed carefully. At his first underwater therapy session, he was put in a non-restrictive harness and then led into the empty underwater treadmill. Since he seemed to be comfortable, although very excited, the treadmill started to fill with water. The patient began to thrash happily in the water. Attempting to hold him back with the harness only escalated his behavior more. His handler then remembered that a harness had only been used previously when doing bite sport work (a high-adrenaline and very reinforcing activity). He bit at it, splashed, and tried to spin in circles in the water. He had never been exposed to water outside of a kiddy pool in the yard, to which his response had been similar. At this appointment, he was barely responsive to cues from his handler. He would not take food, and he could not be distracted by toys.

We developed a training plan to desensitize him to water. He had to perform obedience to earn access to the water. The sound of water splashing made it very difficult for him to perform the behaviors he was asked for. He had to demonstrate calmness to be able to stay in the water. We used a martingale lead to be able to prevent him from biting at the water if he was unresponsive to cues and a calming cap (http://www.thundershirt.com/thundercap.html) to help him tune out external stimuli. His handler worked on his responses to his obedience position cues (sit, down, stand, and walk forward specifically). Initially, he vocalized when not allowed to be in the water. After only two sessions in clinic, he could walk into and out of the underwater treadmill without trying to dig at or bite the low-level water sitting in there. He was responsive to cues from his handler. Homework included walking in and out of the edge of the water at a boat-loading dock. By the fourth session, the patient could walk on the moving treadmill in the water, although continued use of a calming cap was needed.

Case No. 6: Curbside Issues

An eight-year-old Mini Aussie presented for left hind lameness. The client informed us that Leni has been getting more anxious at the vet since curbside service had started. The client was allowed to be present in the room for the consultation, and while Leni was worried, she was compliant for the comprehensive examination. Team members were masked, as well as the client, and Leni did not appear concerned about masks. The client held Leni's collar and fed her treats. Under clinic pandemic protocols, Leni was brought in for her first photobiomodulation (laser) therapy treatment without the client. Leni was nervous but allowed the handling and treatment to happen. Leni would take treats tentatively but would not eat while the technician or laser probe was touching her (there was no difference in behavior with the treatment probe on or off). At the second treatment appointment, the technician began feeding Leni treats. Leni ate the treats but stopped eating as soon as there was *intent* to touch her. Leni's behavior escalated significantly during this appointment. She vocalized and then lunged toward the technician about halfway through the treatment, even with the active laser probe touching her and switched off. When the client was brought into the clinic to handle and restrain Leni, she relaxed immediately. Trying to abide by clinic pandemic protocols, the third treatment was attempted without the client, but the technician could not even touch Leni. The client was brought into the room, and the therapy was completed without issue. Leni did not vocalize or try to bite when the client restrained her. It was determined that we needed to make an exception for this client and Leni, in the best interest of everyone. The client was allowed to be present for all future visits.

Case No. 7: Motivating the Feline Patient

Peanut, a 15-year-old cat with bilateral quadriceps contracture, following therapeutic ultrasound to improve stifle flexion, had been prescribed exercise in clinic on the treadmill. She had remaining limitations on active range of motion and stifle flexion but could now stand and walk.

Peanut was a very agreeable cat and tolerated a lot of handling but was not motivated to do any kind of physical activity. She could be bribed to walk short distances at home but not move for any set amount of time. The veterinarian's goal was to get Peanut to walk for minutes at a time to keep her quadriceps as functional as possible. Underwater treadmill therapy was attempted briefly, but it caused too much stress for Peanut. The plan was changed to see how she would tolerate the land treadmill. When we first tried having her walk on the land treadmill, she was not too afraid of it but she had no motivation to walk on the moving track. While she would accept treats in other situations, Peanut was not motivated by food enough to walk forward on the treadmill. Placing her carrier at the height of the treadmill in the direction she was walking with the door open got her moving very quickly! She was very motivated to walk toward her career. Initially, she got to dive into her carrier as her reward during each walking break. The more she got used to this routine, she only got to enter into the carrier at the end of the last walking interval. She needed a higher rate of reinforcement (diving into her crate between each interval) initially, but once she learned the expectation, she would continue to walk after each break when her rest was either lying in a lap or on the treadmill. This was successful for years.

Motivating the Client

Motivating the patient is always the most necessary step for in-clinic rehabilitation. For home rehabilitation, we have two factors – we must motivate the client to motivate the patient. Daily home exercises (often several times a day) can become difficult to fit into a busy schedule, and therefore knowing the importance of the prescribed exercises along with the reasoning for each exercise can help to motivate the client (and every person involved in home care of the patient). Some clients want to know exactly why the prescribed exercises will help; others just want to know that the exercise will help. Explaining the exercise verbally when first introducing it and explaining in written handouts and videos helps to aid motivation (see Videos 9.1 and 9.2). Demonstrating the exercise with the patient shows the client that the patient is willing to perform the exercise. Sometimes, when compliance is poor, we will rank the home exercise prescription – those exercises that should be done even if you have a super busy day versus those that must be done at least three times a week. It is a fine balance between giving a pragmatic recommendation and giving the client an excuse to skip some exercises.

The next hurdle is to use the client to motivate the patient. This can be a significant challenge. It helps to meet all members of the family, as there may be one member who is particularly adept at motivating and working with the pet. This may not be the primary caregiver. Sometimes, the client's compassion for the patient may present a roadblock in that the caregiver does not want to hurt their pet. Explaining how the exercise should feel and the relative "cost" (slight initial discomfort during a stretch, for example) versus benefit can help motivate the client to perform the exercise. As stated earlier, no exercise should be truly painful; in the veterinary world, we rely on patient compliance, and a breakdown of this compliance can mean an end to therapy. Motivating your patient and client in a low-stress way can achieve great goals.

Conclusions

A behavior-centered rehabilitation clinic will be a successful clinic. Motivating a patient with positive (usually food) rewards in a calm environment aids in a low-stress visit for examination and subsequently for therapy. As the number of visits increases, the stress level of the patient should ideally decrease, or at least not escalate. Minimizing handling and other stressors is vital where possible. A compliant, relaxed patient will greatly benefit from rehabilitation therapy. Home compliance for exercises is an important part of therapy, and motivating both the patient and the client leads to a successful outcome and a rewarding experience with rehabilitation. The trust gained from a low-stress therapeutic course for a patient and client will stand the practice in good stead for reaching therapeutic goals and for future referrals.

Video 9.1 Intermittent versus continuous feeding for reward.
Video 9.2 Luring to shape a simple handshake.

Resources

Through A Dog's Ear. www.throughadogsear.com
Understanding canine body language. http://www.doggiedrawings.net

Interactive feeding toys for dogs

Busy Buddy Toys. http://www.petsafe.net/busybuddy
Green slow feeder. http://northmate.com/category/products/green/
Kong. www.kongcompany.com
Orka. https://outwardhound.com/brands/petstages/

Interactive feeding toys for cats

Slimcat.http://store.petsafe.net/slimcat-interactive-feeder

Trixie Fun Board. https://www.trixie.de/heimtierbedarf/en/shop/Cat/

Interactive feeding toys for horses

Amazing Graze. www.horsemenspride.com/products/#tour-5

Posters

Dr. Sophia Yin Dog Postures. https://store.lowstresshandling.com/product/body-language-of-fear-in-dogs/
Dr. Sophia Yin Cat Postures. https://store.lowstresshandling.com/product/body-language-of-feline-anxiety-free-download-or-donation/

References

American Association of Feline Practitioners (2004) Pleasant veterinary visits for cats. In *Feline Behavior Guidelines*. www.catvets. com/public/PDFs/PracticeGuidelines/FelineBehaviorGLS.pdf, p. 20 (accessed March 9, 2016).

Martin, K.M. and Martin, D. (2009).
How dogs learn. In: *Puppy Start Right:
Foundation Training for the Companion
Dog* (ed. K.M. Martin and D. Martin),
28. Waltham, MA: Sunshine
Books Inc.

Overall, K.L. (2013). Changing behavior, roles
for learning, negotiated settlements and
individualized treatment plans. In: *Manual
of Clinical Behavioral Medicine for Dogs
and Cats* (ed. K.L. Overall), 76. St. Louis,
MO: Elsevier Mosby Publishing.

Pavlov, I.P. (1928). *Lectures on Conditioned
Reflexes (transl WH Gantt)*. London: Allen
and Unwin.

Skinner, B.F. (1938). *The Behavior of
Organisms: An Experimental Analysis*.
New York: Appleton-Century.

10

Fitness Conditioning for the Veterinary Technician and Owner

Dawn Rector and Darryl Millis

The College of Veterinary Medicine, University of Tennessee, Knoxville, TN, USA

CHAPTER MENU

Introduction

What Is Fitness and Conditioning?

Exercise and conditioning give the dog and owner the tools to maintain good health and quality of life (QOL), potentially reduce injury and recovery time, and hasten the return to work or competition. Conditioning is the augmentation of body systems to create and maintain peak fitness. Each system (cardiovascular, respiratory, musculoskeletal, and nervous) must work together and function equivalently and efficiently to improve exercise capacity (Zink and Schlehr, 1997). Fitness is a state of health and well-being that enhances the ability to play sports, retain occupations, and perform activities of daily living. Fitness is obtained with proper nutrition, exercise, rest, and recovery. Fitness also helps create confidence and body awareness by strengthening both mind and body as well as maintaining a strong human–animal bond between owner and pet.

Why Fitness and Conditioning?

Many family pets do not get enough exercise or mental stimulation which may lead to loss of QOL due to boredom, obesity, and

---

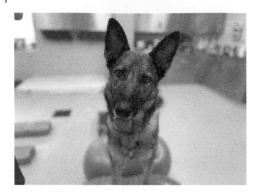

Figure 10.1 Happy dog. *Source:* Courtesy of Dawn Hickey Rector.

a deterioration of the human–animal bond for owner and pet. With exercise, the brain releases endorphins which cause a feeling of pleasure and well-being in humans. It is easy to extrapolate that this may also happen in animals. The happiness in a dog's expression can be witnessed when they are doing an activity they enjoy (see Figure 10.1)! Mental and physical activity can be used to avoid or decrease a pet's obsessive or destructive behavior, improving the well-being of the pet and the owner.

As in humans, proper conditioning may help to prevent injury, especially in sporting and working dogs, as well as to facilitate quicker recovery and return to function should an injury occur.

Attaining fitness requires optimizing function of the musculoskeletal, nervous, respiratory, and cardiovascular systems. The bones must be strong enough to bear the weight of activity. The nervous system tells the muscles when to contract to move bones efficiently, as well as communicating where the body is in space (proprioception) for body awareness, which is crucial for proper form and to help prevent injury. For efficient muscle contraction, muscles must receive an adequate amount of oxygen and nutrients circulated and delivered by the heart and lungs. If there is a breakdown in any of these systems, fatigue and injuries can occur.

Healthy dogs may enjoy a slower onset of physical and cognitive deterioration associated with aging. From decreased body weight and fat stores (resulting from faster metabolism with increased muscle mass and activity), to greater muscle strength, improved organ function, less stress, and improved mental health, the benefits of an active lifestyle are hard to dispute. According to the 2016 National Pet Obesity Awareness Day Survey, 53.9% of US dogs are estimated to be overweight or obese. That amounts to over 41.9 million overweight dogs that may benefit from increased physical exercise (http://petobesityprevention.org/2016-u-s-pet-obesity-statistics/). Accelerated aging, chronic diseases, and increased behavior challenges may also occur because of limited exercise and conditioning (Bellows *et al.*, 2015). For the working, sporting, and performance dogs, more injuries may occur if dogs are not properly conditioned leading up to job performance and competition.

Who Needs Fitness and Conditioning?

Dogs in a fitness program benefit from increased mobility and decreased boredom. Even athletic dogs like greyhounds, bulldog breed type dogs, and other well-muscled dogs need to refine movement patterns, build confidence, and perform enough mental and physical activity to help them rest well and not destroy property. Just because they "look fit" to the eye does not mean there is no room for improvement and enrichment. Puppies need environmental socialization, balance, and body awareness to build confidence and life-long healthy patterns. Conditioning programs for performance dogs can improve their skills, prevent injury, and have quicker return to function should an injury occur. Aging dogs can also benefit from exercise and conditioning. Senior dogs tend to slow down (and owners allow this because they think it is part of the natural aging process), but maintaining muscle strength prevents obesity and helps manage osteoarthritis, thereby providing higher quality, longer life.

Poor movement patterns cause dogs to work harder (Campa *et al.*, 2019). To compensate, they become more susceptible to injury by overstressing other areas of the body. Therapeutic exercise and conditioning are beneficial for dogs recovering from injury or surgery. It is also likely that exercise and conditioning after recovery can help to prevent injury from happening again (Steib *et al.*, 2017). To stay healthy, dogs must be taught to move better and more efficiently.

How to Create Individual Conditioning Programs

Conditioning programs should include cardiovascular and endurance exercise, strength training, proprioceptive and body awareness exercises, flexibility exercises, and mental challenges. Each individual program should include a variety of exercises, incorporating groundwork and balance and conditioning equipment. The program should be fluid and constantly evolve and involve all planes of motion since dogs function and move in all planes. The program must account for the capabilities of the patient, considering limitations of any injury, age, and beginning fitness levels. A successful program involves a combination of behavior principles, anatomy, exercise biomechanical and physiology knowledge, and most importantly, PLAY! It must be fun for both the owner and dog.

Principles of Conditioning

There are important principles that are involved in creating a conditioning program. A crucial one to understand is the Overload Principle (Millard, 2014). This is the need to exercise the cardiovascular system and musculoskeletal system to a level beyond what it is accustomed to for effective training progress. For cells to replicate and build strength or muscle mass, they must be challenged. If a dog is going to run an endurance race, a daily 1-mile training run is not sufficient – they must be pushed beyond what the normal resting cells are accustomed to for them to adapt and grow. Athletes must work beyond normal levels to progress, either by increasing the length of exercise, speed of exercise, or working against higher-than-normal loads. Chemically, fatigue is an imbalance between the muscles' need for adenosine triphosphate (ATP) and the cell's ability to make more. Depleting ATP indicates to the cell that it must create more which ramps up the metabolism for future workouts. The body makes physiologic changes to resist or adapt to the increased demands placed on it. During this phase, the body increases its capacity to handle the stress by making changes in structure, enzyme levels, and increased motor unit recruitment. The result is better cardiovascular fitness, coordination, and strength, which is the desired response to fitness training. The factors that most influence overload are intensity, duration, and frequency of specific exercises. Increases in these factors should occur slowly and contact with the client must be maintained to determine whether the changes are adequate or too much.

Equally important is the specific adaptation to imposed demands principle (SAID) (Sevier *et al.*, 2000; Millard, 2014). SAID relates to what the dog is expected to do. It is important to determine if the dog is a sporting or working dog with greater physical demands or if is it a pet that needs to be able to move around better, climb stairs, etc.? If it is a sporting dog, is endurance, strength, or both required? Which specific movements must be performed well to be successful? Working dogs may perform search and rescue (SAR), apprehension (bite), tracking, or detection. Dogs performing nose work (tracking/detection/SAR) must have excellent endurance and cardiovascular fitness because when they are panting, they may not sniff effectively, and they may work in dry arid environments where temperatures remain high for long periods (Niedermeyer *et al.*, 2020). Apprehension dogs need a strong core, neck, and shoulders to hit and bring down suspects. Conditioning for pulling a sled is more effective when dogs trot or run against resistance rather than simply trotting on a treadmill. Dogs that perform in agility need to be conditioned differently than dogs that perform skijoring. Knowing the demands that a patient will undergo as well as what the client requires will result in a greater likelihood of success in all areas.

Box 10.1   Steps to break down a movement and gradually progress it

1) Always teach new behaviors off of equipment – on the floor
2) Start basic and/or simple then move to advanced and/or complex – break down the movements to their simplest form as much as possible
3) Start slow and gradually increase speed
4) Low force to high force – low jump height/low exercise height to higher height
5) Short distance to long distance – less reps to gradually more reps or duration
6) Gradually use the Overload Principle

Anatomy and Exercise Physiology

Progression of Exercises

As individuals, dogs will progress at variable rates. Exercise should be significantly progressed every four weeks. Smaller increases of 5–10% can be made weekly. Exercise can be progressed by changing one or more variables including number of repetitions, number of sets, frequency, duration, tempo, equipment choice, and rest interval. It is best to increase only one variable at a time based on the needs and lifestyle of the dog. In general, shorter, more frequent bouts of exercise form the initial conditioning program. As fitness improves, the length of the sessions should increase to form a firm cardiovascular foundation. Speed and/or strength conditioning may proceed after basic cardiovascular fitness is achieved. Core strengthening and flexibility exercises are incorporated throughout all phases of conditioning including all planes of motion in the exercises (sagittal, dorsal, and transverse). Use the fitness variables (reps/sets/duration/volume/frequency) to create the correct intensity for each dog. Intensity is the degree of effort (both mental and physical) involved in an exercise. Be sure the amount and intensity of exercise are attainable both for the dog and the owner's lifestyle and time constraints (see Box 10.1).

An exercise program should be SMART – specific/measurable/attainable/relevant/timebound (Bovend'Eerdt *et al.*, 2009). Be sure to include all components in the evaluation (cardiovascular, strength/endurance, proprioception/balance, flexibility, and mental). Set specific time points for reassessment to measure progress, such as every two weeks or monthly.

Signs of Fatigue

The ability to interpret body language – canine and human – is essential when working with dogs and their owners. One of the most important skills to develop is recognizing fatigue. Although every dog is different, signs of fatigue can include appeasement behaviors such as yawning, licking lips, disengagement from the activity after a period of intense engagement, scratching, shaking off (such as when they are wet but dry), or simply stopping the exercise. Signs of fatigue while exercising on a treadmill include wide eyes, looking around for a way out/off, and drifting back on the belt. When any of these are seen, exercise/training should be stopped. It is recommended to have the dog end with something he/she can do well, have a short treat/play session, and put the dog in a kennel or crate to decompress (once he/she has cooled down). Fatigue from excessive exercise can increase micromotion of joints due to loss of muscle strength and reaction time, which may increase the chance of injury (Rozzi *et al.*, 1999). Therefore, it is crucial to not exceed the dog's fatigue level.

Cardiovascular Conditioning

Skeletal muscle has the greatest oxygen demand of all organs of the body. At rest, skeletal muscles receive approximately 15–20% of cardiac output. This may increase to up to 80–85% during exercise (Levine, 2008; Millard, 2014). Heart and lung function are critical to fitness, especially in performance dogs, primarily to deliver oxygen and nutrients to body tissues, to remove wastes, and to aid in temperature regulation. Vasoconstriction of inactive tissues and organs as well as splenic contraction increases oxygen delivery to muscles during exercise by increasing blood delivery to active skeletal muscle (see Box 10.2).

Type of Exercise

The initial type of exercise depends on what the dog and owner can do. An older, arthritic, poorly conditioned dog may only

---

Box 10.2 To maximize overload, cardiorespiratory training should include these four training variables
1) Be the correct type 2) Be of sufficient duration 3) Occur with adequate frequency 4) Performed at the proper intensity

---

be capable of short, frequent walks. However, a healthy dog or performance athlete may be able to sustain a 2-hour hike in the woods or a 30-minute trot on a land treadmill. Owner goals, intended activity of the dog, and dog life stage should also be considered when selecting exercise type.

Duration

Duration refers to the number of minutes of aerobic exercise during the conditioning phase of a session. For cardiovascular benefit, duration is related to exercise intensity. With more intense exercise, the duration should be shorter (Gillette and Dale, 2014). It is helpful to ask the owner about the exercise program that the dog is currently performing. Begin with that level of activity. Very deconditioned dogs may be better suited for multiple sessions of short duration. It is often difficult to set a time limit when creating a fitness program for the dog as they cannot "tell" you how they are feeling. **Body language must be evaluated to determine when to end the session based on recognizing signs of fatigue.** The duration must be sufficiently intense to increase heart rate for an amount of time, typically more than 15 minutes. Playing fetch is not a cardiovascular exercise unless the dog does not stop in between each throw. For swimming to be cardiovascular exercise, the dog must stay in the water and not get out or rest for a prolonged period. The amount of time differs for each dog, but the goal is to increase the duration by 5–10% each week.

Frequency

Frequency refers to the number of exercise sessions per day or week. The frequency depends on the duration and intensity of each session. For example, if the exercise is of lower intensity for a short duration, more frequent sessions may be performed each day or week. For dogs starting a fitness program, it is recommended to begin with a frequency of at least three times per week with at least one day of rest between sessions. This allows the body time to recover between sessions. Healthy dogs and canine athletes can participate in cardiorespiratory sessions more frequently. Again, one must also consider the variables of intensity and duration.

Intensity

The degree of exercise intensity depends on the speed, work, and power of the exercise and will be limited by the condition of each individual dog. Depending on the capability of the dog, the intensity of an exercise can be varied by changing the speed, surface (adding incline, moving from a smooth surface to taller grass, sand, water, etc.), or duration. Interval training is utilized in conditioning programs and uses several repetitions of intense activity with short periods of rest between episodes of activity. If interval training is performed, changing variables such as repetitions, sets, and rest intervals can increase the intensity for the dog (Gillette and Dale, 2014; Laursen and Jenkins, 2002).

Intensity can be difficult to measure in the dog, especially for cardiorespiratory exercise. In humans, a percentage of VO_2 max is often used in laboratories for stress tests. VO_2 max is the maximum (max) rate (V) of oxygen (O_2) the body uses during exercise. Personal trainers often use the "talk test" to determine if the subject has gone past their anaerobic threshold which causes them to rapidly ventilate and be unable to have a conversation. Another test that is used in human fitness is the target heart rate test (THR). Evidence-based studies that have evaluated THRs are limited to dogs. Heart monitoring devices have been used to monitor heart rate during exercise (Moïse *et al.*, 2021). Heart rate monitoring may also be performed manually but requires the dog to discontinue exercise for a brief period.

The University of Tennessee performed a study (Camp *et al.*, 2016) of adult dogs exercising on a land treadmill. The following measurements were taken in a quiet room while standing and then again immediately after exercise: resting heart rate (HR); systolic blood pressure (SBP), diastolic blood pressure (DBP), and mean blood pressure (MBP); rectal temperature; and respiratory rate (RR). The dogs were exercised to mild fatigue (unwilling to exercise beyond verbal or treatment encouragement). The results showed there were no significant changes in SBP, DBP, MBP, or temperature to indicate fatigue. However, a mild increase in HR of 10 beats per minute above steady state HR or a 5-fold increase in the RR resulted in fatigue within 10 minutes. These findings may help to direct cardiovascular conditioning programs without causing end-exercise fatigue and possible injury as a result.

Strength Training

Strength fitness refers to the ability of the muscles to produce force, work, and power and overcome resistance. Muscle strength is the maximal force that a muscle or group of muscles can generate during one repetition. Muscle strength is gained by an increase in muscle fiber size. There are two main types of muscle fibers characterized by the metabolism with which they burn energy. Type I fibers (aerobic muscle fibers) use oxygen to metabolize energy, are the main muscle fibers in postural stability muscles, and are resistant to fatigue. Type II muscle fibers (anaerobic muscle fibers) use the energy that has been stored in the muscle, comprise large muscle groups that provide power to jump and run, and fatigue more quickly due to limited amounts of immediate energy sources that are available. Type II fibers can develop more force per cross-sectional area and contract at a higher velocity than Type I fibers due to the increase of proteins, which may be increased by high-intensity training. Type II fibers are related to strength (needed to pull or carry loads) and speed (sprinting). Genetics plays a part in the percentage of muscle fiber types that each dog (and human) is born with. For example, greyhounds have more Type II muscle fibers than beagles or foxhounds for sprinting speed (Dolan *et al.*, 2019; Williams *et al.*, 1997). Because of this, similar breeds participate in certain sports or work because they excel at performing tasks based on their genetic disposition. In racing greyhounds, studies have found that spinal muscles are the first set of muscles to fatigue (Zebas *et al.*, 1991). The paraspinal, specifically the longissimus muscles, must remain strong for limb muscles to work at capacity for sprinting activity. This is understandable when considering the gait of a sprinting dog. In the suspensory phase, all limbs are off the ground tucked under the body and the longissimus muscle is stretched with the spine in flexion. The fore and hind limbs provide forward movement through propulsion at the end of ground contact, and the spinal muscles that connect the forelimbs and hindlimbs forcefully contract to help with extension and provide a "spring effect that stores and returns internal kinetic energy" (Zebas *et al.*, 1991). As the dog fatigues, the hind limb strides shorten, the forelimb strides lengthen, and overall speed declines.

Types of Muscle Contractions

When referring to the muscular system the term "contraction" refers to the generation of tension within a muscle fiber. Muscle contractions are defined by the changes in the length of the muscle during contraction. There are several types of muscle contractions:

a) ***Isotonic contractions*** maintain constant tension in the muscle as the muscle changes length. There are two types of isotonic contractions: concentric and eccentric.

  i) **Concentric muscle contractions** shorten the muscle while maintaining constant tension. During a concentric contraction, sufficient force is generated under load and two bones are moved around a joint. A concentric contraction can be used to accelerate or increase the rate of speed for a movement. They are common in activities where power and explosive force must be generated (i.e., dock diving and flyball). An example of a concentric contraction in people is a biceps curl. In dogs, some examples are running uphill and climbing stairs (concentric contraction of the quadriceps muscles).

  ii) **Eccentric contractions** occur when a muscle opposes a stronger force which causes the muscle to lengthen as it contracts. Eccentric contractions are often referred to as deceleration, braking, or negative contractions. Examples of eccentric contractions are walking downstairs or hills and the downward motion of squats and pushups. During an eccentric muscle contraction, the muscle is activated and is trying to contract but it cannot shorten because an opposing greater force (the weight of the body going downhill or stairs) acts on the muscle, resulting in net lengthening of the muscle. As a result, surrounding muscles and tendons are called upon to control and help slow down the action, but not to reverse the force. Eccentric exercise can help to build muscle, speed, and power. However, they can also produce injury, resulting in post-exercise soreness. Most muscle strains occur under eccentric contraction.

b) ***Isometric contractions*** produce an active force on the muscle fibers while maintaining a constant length. No visible joint movement occurs during an isometric contraction but the muscle fibers still fire. The benefit of isometric exercises is that they do not place stress on the joints. Isometric contractions happen while the dog is bearing weight in a standing position either on the flat ground or on an unstable piece of equipment. The forelimb, hind limb, and core muscles must all engage for the dog to maintain balance and form.

Strength training can be accomplished by several means. The goal is to cause the muscles to adapt to the stress of exercise by getting stronger (being able to generate more force.) The SAID principle (Barfield and Oliver, 2019) tells us that if stronger muscles are necessary, then they must be targeted in a specific mechanical, neuromuscular, and metabolic manner through specific movements including resistance, tempo, and energy demands placed on the body. The Overload Principle (Plotkin *et al.*, 2022) suggests that the trainer must safely and progressively ask more of the dog's muscles than they are accustomed to. For example, the dog must overcome more resistance than it has experienced before. The stress must not be excessive or prolonged without allowing the muscles time to recover. Strengthening initially occurs through increased neural demand and recruitment of more muscle fibers to participate in the new "stressful" activity. For those dogs new to exercise, this typically occurs within two weeks of starting a fitness program. For enlargement of the muscle fibers, to occur, resistance training must be regular and consistent over time (usually several months or longer), but with appropriate rest periods to allow the body time for appropriate cellular responses to increase muscle fiber size (McArdle *et al.*, 2010).

In dogs, most strength training programs initially use the dog's own body weight as resistance. To understand how to use body weight as resistance it is necessary to understand that dogs, in general, bear approximately 60% of their body weight on their front legs and 40% in the pelvic limbs. By shifting body weight to the front end or the back end, resistance can be increased (or decreased) to stress-specific muscle groups. This is done by positioning the dog with one end elevated higher than the other, always maintaining proper form and positioning. The more weight that is shifted to the targeted muscle groups, the more force is needed to overcome the resistance (see Figures 10.2 and 10.3). To incrementally increase resistance, the height should be gradually increased during the strength training phase of the dog's fitness program. Although static weight shifting is beneficial when starting a strengthening program, the stress applied to the muscles is relatively small, necessitating dynamic strengthening exercises.

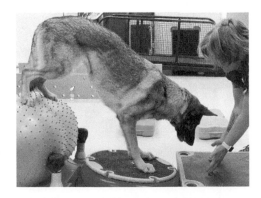

Figure 10.2 Forelimb weight shifting placement. *Source:* Courtesy of Dawn Hickey Rector.

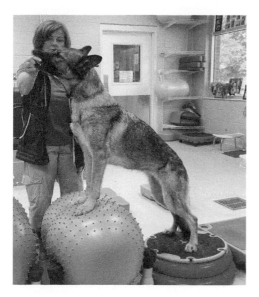

Figure 10.3 Hindlimb weight shifting placement. *Source:* Courtesy of Dawn Hickey Rector.

The next phase of strength training can be accomplished using external weights and resistance bands that are commonly used in people. External weights in dogs are primarily limited to weighted vests, leg weights, and pulling weights. The use of resistance bands or elastic ropes can be used to increase resistance by applying tension in the direction opposite the muscle group being targeted while ambulating. Weighted vests are used to strengthen the postural muscles, primarily the extensors. The use of limb weights is normally limited to strengthening the flexor muscles. Pulling a weighted sled is useful for dogs undergoing activities such as sled dog racing.

Exercises for additional strengthening of the extensors and speed development are running uphill, running, or trotting upstairs or on an inclined treadmill, swimming against jets, and pulling or carrying resistance loads.

These methods of strengthening should be done cautiously as incorrect placement and distribution of the weights or incorrect use of resistance bands have the potential to cause injury. These techniques are best used under the supervision of a certified canine rehabilitation practitioner/therapist.

Endurance Training

Endurance refers to the ability of a muscle or group of muscles to undergo many repetitions of contraction under low load. Running long distances at submaximal heart rate to increase capillaries and mitochondria in muscle fibers, especially Type 1 fibers (slow twitch, postural muscles), allows aerobic metabolism to provide continuous energy to the muscles. It should be noted that Type II or fast twitch is more aerobic in dogs compared to other species, including humans. The increase in capillary density and muscle vascularity enhances the delivery of oxygen and nutrients to the muscles. In studies, it has been shown that type II muscle fibers within a muscle can change to type I, increasing aerobic capacity in humans doing endurance training (Parsons *et al.*, 1985). These exercises benefit sporting, herding, and long-distance racing dogs, SAR dogs, and tracking or man-trailing dogs. Examples of exercises for endurance training include trotting, running, swimming, and low-load weight pulling (see Figures 10.4–10.6). The exercise should target the specific muscle groups involved in the specific action and last longer than 15 minutes.

Repetitions

Repetitions indicate how many times the exercise is repeated during each set. For strength training, low to moderate number of repetitions should be performed (with moderate to high resistance). For endurance training, a high number of repetitions should be performed (with low resistance).

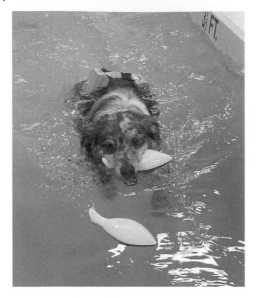

Figure 10.4 Swimming dog. *Source:* Courtesy of Dawn Hickey Rector.

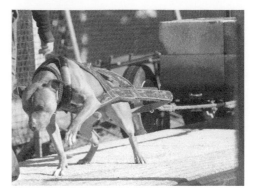

Figure 10.5 Weight pulling dog. *Source:* Courtesy of Dawn Hickey Rector.

increases in strength. Sets are not as critical with endurance training, but rest periods may be necessary for dogs that are starting endurance training.

Sets

A set is a group of consecutive repetitions of an exercise done without resting. For those new to strength training, 2–3 sets are beneficial in developing strength. More advanced dogs will need multiple sets to see

Frequency

Typically, strength training is recommended 3–5 times per week, depending on the dog's current fitness level. Since dogs are quadrupeds, it is difficult to alternate training of different muscle groups (forelimb versus

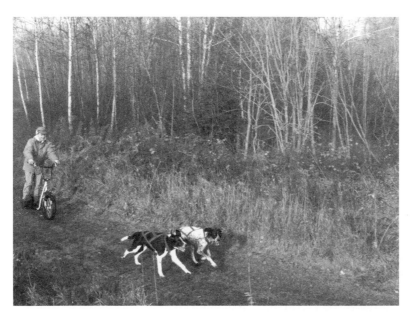

Figure 10.6 Dogs in harness pulling. *Source:* Courtesy of Dr Julia Tomlinson.

pelvic limb days) to allow one group of muscles to rest while training others. Beginning-level dogs that are new to strength training should begin only three times per week with at least one rest day in between sessions so that the muscles have time to adapt and heal.

Type

Each exercise should be selected to support the specific fitness goals of the dog. To develop greater strength in the limb muscles, exercises should be performed under more stable surface conditions (if using equipment, use stable platforms) with heavier loads or resistance. This places more emphasis on the target muscles. Unstable equipment, such as inflatable disks or wobble boards should be introduced for core muscle strengthening and body awareness.

Repetition Tempo

Tempo is the rate of performing an exercise. Slow tempos that focus on eccentric contractions are thought to increase strength and help develop muscle hypertrophy. Exercises that are done quickly, but with control, help develop power, or the rate of work. Proper technique and form must be used to be effective.

Rest Interval

Longer rest intervals allow recovery of muscle energy stores to be available for the next repetition or exercise, and heavier resistance can often be used.

Volume

Volume is the amount of physical training in each time-period. The time-period can be one day, a specific number of days, one week, etc. Add up the amount of time plus duration that specific exercises are performed per that time-period to calculate your volume. Research in people suggests that high-volume training programs promote cellular adaptations including muscle hypertrophy, while low-volume training programs promote neurological adaptations (which include strengthening by recruiting more muscle fiber involvement) (Haun *et al.*, 2019).

Balance/Proprioception/ Body Awareness

Balance fitness refers to the dog's ability to maintain its equilibrium without losing control. The ability to balance depends on both internal and external forces that help the dog's body to maintain its center of gravity over its base of support. The vestibular system works with the visual system to establish and maintain balance (Day and Fitzpatrick, 2005; Hupfeld *et al.*, 2022). Balance is learned through repetitive exposure to a variety of multisensory conditions. Conscious movement is achieved by electrical impulses sent from the brain, down the spinal cord to the limbs involved in each movement (Zink and Schlehr, 1997). In contrast, balance, and proprioception are near-automatic reactions to changes of the limb or body in space. Balance and proprioceptive conditioning are very important to create body awareness. Sensory fibers are found in all tissues throughout the body. The brain's perception of an exercise changes if the dog's hind limb is placed on a platform by a handler, as opposed to learning and initiating the motion itself. When the brain encodes an action, each specific part of the exercise is "imprinted" on the brain. If the handler places a limb on a piece of equipment the touch of the handler's hand is part of the action. Ideally, having the dog perform the exercise by luring (you would eventually fade the lure) or operant conditioning creates better neural encoding without extraneous information sent to the brain. Training proprioceptive abilities improve balance, coordination, posture, and the dog's ability to quickly adapt to changes in body position and surroundings without having to think about which movement is most appropriate in each situation. In addition, incorporating movements throughout the different planes of motion and through all muscle actions further enhances the level of neuromuscular communication throughout the body. This likely results in enhanced body awareness and reaction time that enables the body to increase its ability to stabilize and balance itself in all situations. Balance can be either static or dynamic. Static balance refers to the ability to maintain equilibrium while remaining stationary. Dynamic balance refers to being able to maintain equilibrium while moving. This must be done in a progressive, yet controlled manner for the dog's body to adapt and increase neuromuscular efficiency. Balance should progress from static to dynamic. Only after a dog has demonstrated it can safely balance in a static position should dynamic stability be challenged (see Box 10.3).

Tempo

Stability exercises should always start slowly. Balance is usually easier to maintain when an exercise is done very quickly. For example, when riding a bicycle, it is easier to keep the bicycle upright and avoid falling with the benefit of speed and momentum. Maintaining balance is much harder at a slow speed. Very slow movements require a large degree of neuromuscular control. Introducing dynamic balance exercises to challenge dynamic stability should also proceed slowly and only when the dog is able to maintain balance during static exercises. If progression is attempted too soon, the balance threshold will be exceeded, and the dog may fall or become scared and unwilling to try again.

> **Box 10.3 Balance recommendations progression**
>
> 1) **Beginner-balance recommendations:**
>   a) Unassisted weight-shifts; Assisted balance exercises – leg lifts
>   b) Foundation movements – sit to stand, tuck sit
>   c) Unassisted dynamic movement on low-level unstable surfaces – walking over a variety of multi-sensory equipment options
> 2) **Intermediate-balance recommendations:**
>   d) Unassisted dynamic movements on a variety of unstable surfaces – spins, lateral stepping, targeting, walking backward, four feet on, weight shifting off handler movement
> 3) **Advanced-balance recommendations:**
>   e) Unassisted dynamic movements on variety of unstable surfaces – hop with stabilization, crawling, leg lifts

Exercise Selection

Exercises that affect the dog's base of support can be selected to challenge balance. The dog's natural base of support is distributed over all four limbs that are evenly spaced to provide a broad base of support. When this is altered by raising one or two legs, the dog's balance threshold is challenged. Stability may also be challenged by placing the limbs in different standing positions to alter the base of support. Changing the stability of the base also challenges balance and strength.

Frequency

Balance training focuses on the Type I muscle fibers and the muscles involved in maintaining posture, including the core muscles. These muscle fibers are built for endurance and are resistant to fatigue. When they are fatigued, they tend to recover quickly. As such, balance training can be done more frequently than strength training, and rest intervals between reps and/or sets can be shorter.

Volume

Balance training requires a high degree of learning and development of neuromuscular connections (Mihara *et al.*, 2021). This typically happens quickly and is one of the rewards of balance training- improvements are obvious. Even after two weeks of consistent balance training, many dogs have better overall balance. Training volume is less with this type of training than in strength training.

Equipment

Balance should progress from the most stable to the most unstable equipment. Movements used in dynamic stability exercises should be initially performed with proper technique on the most stable surface, solid ground.

Flexibility

One of the most neglected foundation pieces of conditioning programs is flexibility. Flexible muscles and joints make everyday movements easier and can decrease the risk of certain injuries (Micheo *et al.*, 2012). As in humans, a dog's flexibility deteriorates with age and substantially decreases if the dog leads a sedentary lifestyle. With aging, collagen solubility decreases, resulting in decreased tensile strength, and increased tendon rigidity. Keeping the dog active (which includes stretching regularly) can help to prevent mobility loss. Poor flexibility can also lead to altered movement patterns as the dog becomes stiffer. A dog that does not properly

flex and extend its hind limbs during a normal walking gait will compensate and may develop an abnormal gait because of the inhibited range of motion (ROM) caused by tight muscles or joints. Tight muscles or reduced joint motion result in restricted movement, decreased joint ROM and reduced power production for peak performance (Torres *et al.*, 2017).

Flexibility requires proper joint movement to allow muscles to elongate to their optimal length. At optimal length muscles can contract with optimal force and move through full ROM if the joints are not compromised. Therefore, a flexible muscle has the potential to be a stronger muscle. Flexible muscles help to reduce the risk of injury and help improve performance in many activities.

Flexibility is especially key in warm up and cool down. As the muscle groups warm up, the blood vessels in the tissues dilate to deliver more oxygen and nutrients and remove waste products. The resulting elasticity of tissues helps to prevent strains or sprains while joint movement helps distribute synovial fluid over the surface of the joints. After extensive exercise, blood tends to pool in the extremities and the heart slows down, so blood and lymphatic fluid is not removed as quickly. The cool down ensures a gradual decrease in blood flow by slowly decreasing the heart rate. This allows the blood to replenish the area as well as remove the waste products created during exercise (see Box 10.4).

Box 10.4   Flexibility training should include the following training variables

1) Be the correct type
2) Be of sufficient duration
3) Repetitions
4) Sets
5) Tempo
6) Occur with adequate frequency
7) Performed at the proper intensity

Type

Active flexibility exercises can be incorporated into any dog's program design. Static stretching exercises can be considered post-workout depending on the dog's need, the tolerance of the dog to stretching, and the ability and knowledge of the trainer.

Duration

Duration refers to the length of the flexibility training session. It is recommended that each flexibility session should last 5–10 minutes. It is very common for this part of the training session to be eliminated or shortened when time is of the essence. Remind the client how important flexibility is to their dog's overall health and well-being and allow adequate time for stretching.

Repetitions

A repetition is one complete movement of a particular stretching exercise. Form is crucial!

1) Beginner – 1–3 reps: 5–10 seconds hold
2) Intermediate – 2–3 reps: 10–15 seconds hold
3) Advanced – 3 reps: 15–30 seconds hold

Sets

A group of consecutive repetitions performed without resting. There is an inverse relationship between sets and repetitions (i.e., fewer sets, more repetitions, more sets, and lower repetitions). Intensity is greater with more sets and fewer repetitions.

Tempo

The speed at which each repetition of a stretching exercise is performed. Flexibility exercises should be performed in a slow and easy manner. There should be no bouncing.

The idea is to have the muscle tissue relax, then stretch and elongate so that it becomes more elastic.

Rest Intervals

A rest interval is the amount of time it takes to recover between a set or exercise. The rest time between flexibility exercises need not be long as the exercises themselves are not strenuous.

Frequency

Frequency refers to the number of flexibility training sessions per week. Recovery time is generally not necessary with flexibility training as it is with strength training, so active stretching exercises can be performed in every exercise session if indicated.

Intensity

Intensity is a product of the outcome of the variables chosen and the dog itself. Stretching should NEVER be painful. Stretching should be performed slowly and deliberately and the stretch held at the point of tension working up to at least 20 seconds to derive the most benefit.

Mental Fitness

For a dog that has never exercised before, every exercise has a mental component because they are learning. Stimulating the brain in the correct way to teach and maintain correct form can be very taxing but is crucial to success in conditioning. Behavior to build neural pathways for proper form and development of body awareness is also known as "muscle memory" (Voss *et al.*, 2013; Liu and Jorgensen, 2011). If proper form is not taught from the beginning, the trainer must correct the action and teach the exercise properly. Proper and persistent training creates new neural pathways that the dog keeps for the length of its training, allowing the dog to return to form if training is stopped for an injury or other reason.

The nervous system consists of sensory and motor nerves. Sensory nerves provide information regarding the environment and location of limbs. These sensory (proprioceptive) receptors are found throughout skin, connective tissue, muscles, and joint capsules (Proske and Gandevia, 2012). These tissues send information to the brain. If a dog has an injury or surgery, the receptors may be damaged and require retraining through proper execution of exercises. The motor nerves relay the signals needed for contraction and relaxation of muscles. The motor nerves are integrated with sensory nerves. The dog must have keen body awareness to efficiently move all parts. As a conscious movement is made, the electrical impulse is sent from the brain, down the spinal cord, and to the muscles of the limbs involved in that movement. Fitness and exercise in dogs rely on the ability to respond independently to cued behaviors to complete a desired movement or position, without being manually placed or physically manipulated into position. After being certain that the dog truly understands what is being asked of them (or that learning has occurred), we then are able to use these cued behaviors to determine, and ultimately increase, exercise challenges and level of fitness. Determining whether the dog can or cannot do an exercise due to a lack of fitness, or simply because of a lack of understanding is crucial. Does the dog know what it is being asked to do, or is it not strong enough to do what is asked of it? There are many ways to teach a dog to do something and different techniques may be used. It is important to remember that a single method may not be the best for every dog. To excel at conditioning dogs, it is necessary to adjust each technique for each individual dog.

It is important to first establish a rapport with the dog. This may require using impulse control and focus exercises to engage the dog. Find out what motivates each dog to accomplish the task at hand, such as food, toys, affection/petting/praise. Every dog decides its own reward, and the trainer must be perceptive to determine what it is.

Teaching foundation behaviors helps the dog to concentrate and slow down when performing exercise. Controlled movement is key. Dogs that use momentum during exercise are basically "cheating" because the muscles do not fully activate to continue moving throughout the exercise in a controlled, deliberate fashion. By allowing momentum to take over, the dog is not using its body weight as resistance and therefore the exercise is less effective. Be sure to encourage slow, purposeful movement to help the dog concentrate on proper form and effective strengthening.

Warm Up and Cool Down

Warm Up

Never underestimate the importance of a warmup routine. In studies of human athletes, this is important to avoid injuries, especially in young non-elite athletes.

Warmup will (Woods *et al.*, 2007; Behm *et al.*, 2016):

- Dilate the blood vessels, increasing the supply of oxygen and nutrients to the muscles and nerves
- Help actively stretch the tissues
- Activate enzyme systems for energy use
- Enhance muscle contraction/reaction time and force of muscle contraction, which improves muscle strength, power, and flexibility

- Facilitate neural transmission for motor unit recruitment
- Move joints and distribute synovial fluid over the surfaces of the joints
- Prepare the muscles, tendons, and ligaments for the activity to be performed
- Provide time to strengthen the bond with your dog, increase mental focus, and create more body awareness

It takes the body a minimum of 10–15 minutes to warm up. If it is cold (building or outside temperature), that time could be longer. The warm up should gradually raise the dog's heart rate, blood pressure, respiration, oxygen delivery, and muscle temperature. Active exercises are those in which the dog performs movements that stretch the limbs and spine in ways that mimic the actions that will be performed in competition or everyday activity. The active exercises performed in a warm up should be done in multiple planes to ensure that all the major muscle groups are addressed. Warming up in this manner allows the dog to simulate actions in a slow manner in preparation for more rapid or powerful activities to prepare for performance. The warm up should continue until the dog begins an exercise, practice session, or competition. Otherwise, the dog may undergo a cool down phase and the benefits of the warm up may be lost (see Box 10.5).

Cool Down

Immediately following an exercise, practice session, or competition a proper cooldown should be performed. The cool down brings the dog's entire physiological system back to normal, including gradual reduction in heart rate, blood pressure, and respiratory rate (Van Hooren and Peake, 2018). Without a cool down, blood may pool in the extremities causing weakness. Like the warm up, the cool down promotes circulation which aids in the effective removal of metabolic

---

Box 10.5   Some examples of warmup exercises

- Weaving thru legs (neck, spine, and tail)
- Spins/circles (left and right) (spine, hind limbs, adductors, and abductors)
- Tugging – at the level of the dog's neck (gracilis and hamstring, neck)
- Front paws on a chair (paraspinals, quadriceps, and iliopsoas)
- Play bow (shoulder, triceps, and hamstrings)
- Cookie at the hip (paraspinals)
- Cookie stretches up and down (neck)
- Lateral stepping (left and right – shoulder, hips, adductors, and abductors of each limb, core)
- Wave/high 5 (shoulders and elbows)
- Squats – Front feet elevated, dog in square sit position, dog pushes into a stand w/o kicking back
- hind limbs (quadriceps, hamstrings, hips, iliopsoas, and core)
- Backup (hamstrings, core, and improves hind limb awareness)
- Sit-to-stand and down-to-stand (major joints and core)
- Passive range of motion (PROM) of Toes and Carpi-toe injuries are common in performance dogs. Be sure to gently flex/extend and spread the toes on each paw as part of your warmup and cool down routine. To warm up the carpus joints you can flex/extend the joint and then gently rotate it in both directions 2–3 times.

waste and replenishment of oxygen and energy stores in the muscle cells and liver. When performing a cool down, it is recommended to start with a trot and ease the dog into a walk over a 5–10-minute period followed by 5–10 minutes of low-intensity active exercises. The idea is to begin with quicker movements and gradually slow down, allowing the body to return to a normal state. Performing the warm up routine at a slower pace is a good way to cool down the dog. Weather indications may dictate a longer cool down period. In hot weather, it may be necessary to apply water to the dog's paws, ears, inguinal and axillary areas or have a shallow pool of water to immerse them in.

Where to Start?

For fitness conditioning, the dog should always be free of injury and if it has prior injury, there should be medical clearance from the veterinarian who treated the injury.

1) *Obtain a history* – current activities, owner goals, limitations, etc.
2) *Forms to maintain* – history/consent form/veterinary release
3) Tools for success also include obtaining photos and videos before, during, and after conditioning has been undertaken.

Functional Evaluation

Knowledge of anatomy and exercise physiology is imperative in designing an appropriate conditioning program. Bones have several main functions. The ability to bear weight and provide a location for muscles to attach are the functions most important in conditioning. It is very important to know the origin, insertion, and action of the main ambulatory and core muscles in dogs to choose proper exercises to attain and maintain fitness. Muscles work by creating actions about joints to pull bones together (flexion) and apart (extension). Dogs with normal ROM have less concussion of their joints during weight bearing and the power and force of muscles are greatest because of maximum leverage of muscles. These benefits are not seen in dogs with compromised ROM. Comfortable ROM as well as strength can be improved with exercise and rehabilitation.

There are Several Areas to Focus on in the Evaluation

Posture – How does the dog sit/stand/rise/lie down? The dog should be observed in static positions as well as in dynamic movement. Incorporate equipment into the assessment to identify limitations in dog's mental or physical ability, such as unstable surfaces, cavaletti rails, and stairs. Every dog is a beginner until proven otherwise.

Structure – Identify anomalies. Structure affects movement. Poor angulation of the joints correlates to less power because of less leverage. Dogs are also less flexible during play, landing jumps, etc. which leads to more concussion of joints and degenerative joint disease, resulting in osteoarthritis. If a dog has poor angulation of the shoulder in relation to the humerus it will have decreased reach with the forelimbs and may be more susceptible to injuries from jumping and landing. If the rear limbs are straight or "post-legged" the dog does not have as much rear-end propulsion or extension. Good forelimb reach coupled with good rear limb extension means less energy is spent covering the same amount of ground.

Too much angulation of the joints may result in unstable limbs, predisposing them to ligament damage (stretch or tear) because of abnormal amounts of stress. The damaged fibers then become scar tissue that is not as strong as the original ligament.

Increased angulation of joints leads to increased strides and should be balanced between the front and rear limbs. Often the rear limbs are more angulated than the forelimbs and the dog walks and trots sideways or paces to avoid hitting the hind limbs on the front limbs. Should fitness and conditioning be limited to dogs with perfect conformation? No! Any dog will benefit from conditioning, but the exercise program should be tailored to the dogs' needs with consideration of any structural deficiencies. The dog should not be required to perform activities that will worsen existing problems.

Gait – When assessing gait, observe the dog from the rear as it walks and trots away, and from the front while walking and trotting back. Concentrate on the hind limbs when the dog is going away, and the forelimbs when the dog is coming back. Observe it from the side as it walks and trots. Lameness is typically easier to see at a trot. If lameness is suspected but questionable, turning the dog in circles will sometimes exaggerate the lameness. From the front, the dog should have a straight line from the shoulder to the foot. When viewing from behind, there should be a straight line from the point of the ischium to the foot. Some dogs will circumduct the hind limbs or have a mildly toed-out appearance in the hind limbs to avoid interfering with the forelimbs during gait. Certain breeds have structural differences depending on their function. Border collies are typically cow-hocked which may increase maneuverability in the field. Dachshunds were bred to go underground in holes for their prey, so their limbs are bred to be shorter and have deviation from a straight line. The dog should transition from a walk to an amble to a trot: all of which are normal gaits depending on the speed of the dog. A phone or camera is useful to capture videos and pictures of the dog sitting, standing, and gaiting. Slow motion mode is especially helpful.

Body condition score (BCS) – Body condition scores are available (1–5 or 1–9) from nutrition sources and help to determine if a dog is overweight when beginning a conditioning program. Having a visual guide to show the client is very beneficial. The pictures and descriptions help neutralize what can be a difficult conversation with an unrealistic owner (see Chapter 8 Nutritional Counseling).

Muscle condition score (MCS) – Evaluation of muscle mass combines visual observation and palpation over the temporal bones, scapula ribs, lumbar vertebra, and pelvic bones (see Chapter 8 Nutritional Counseling).

Program design and implementation – Biomechanical and exercise physiology knowledge is essential to a successful program. It is important to know which exercises achieve the individual goals for each individual dog. Knowing the correct exercises, muscle anatomy, and function must be firmly ingrained in the fitness trainer's brain!

Which muscles are engaged? Quadriceps? Biceps brachii? Forelimb flexors? Core? Hindlimb extensors? Where does the muscle originate? Where does it insert? What action does the muscle contraction cause? Muscles ORIGINATE from one area of a bone and INSERT at a site more distally on a bone. Understanding the origins and insertions of the muscles helps in understanding which body parts will be moved. With this knowledge, exercises can be tailored to individual dogs.

Exercise kinematics – Certain exercises cause greater active ROM than others. Be sure to tailor the exercises in a fitness program to each individual dog, relative to conformation, fitness condition, and sport or work needs (see Box 10.6).

Box 10.6   When assessing proper exercise form consider the following as it relates to the breed
1) Neutral spine position 2) Neutral head position 3) *Limb alignment* – front feet under the shoulders and stifles under the hips (natural stance)

Equipment

The most crucial piece of equipment is a creative brain! There are so many combinations and ways to achieve complete fitness. There is a myriad of exercises to accomplish each goal. Equipment used should be based on the current fitness level of the dog, the current knowledge of foundational behaviors to achieve the desired effect, and what the owner can access. It can be purchased or created. Use stable equipment to build strength and power with isotonic contractions. Use unstable equipment for core strengthening, flexibility, strengthening with isometric contractions, and warm up and cool down. Always teach new exercises on a flat non-slip surface or minimal height platform (see Tables 10.1 and 10.2).

The basics to know are which area of conditioning does the dog need? Does it need focus and confidence? Start with an easy stable exercise and progress from there. Does it need strengthening of a particular limb after surgery? Perform repetitions on a stable surface of an exercise that stresses the muscle in that precise limb. Does it have a weak core? Use unstable equipment at the level of the dog's understanding and ability. Sometimes the ability of the dog dictates the exercise even if not planned (see Table 10.3). Many exercises have been developed that the dog created while doing a different assigned exercise! If it is working the correct part of the body with good form, it accomplishes the purpose intended.

Technology Tips

Use technology to assess the animal. Take a slow-motion video, and create a skeleton overlay on a picture of the dog at different angles to familiarize yourself with the movement of joints. Create an assessment video and teach clients how to take video; this will help when they have questions and cannot get an appointment right away. Take the video at the level of the dog – not looking up or down at the dog for adequate visuals of the ROMs of all the joints. Be certain that the camera is perpendicular to the limb being assessed. Take the video in slow motion of the dog walking away from the camera and walking toward the camera, keeping the dog in the center of the frame (at the level of the dog); video at a walk from both sides of the dog; video of the dog coming toward the camera and away at a trot, then video of the dog from both sides at a trot and lastly a video of the dog from both sides at an extended trot in order to see reach, propulsion and flexion and extension of the limbs. This may require inexpensive software such as Google Slides, iMovie, or Power Director. Apps like Coaches Eye also allow measurements of ROM angles.

In canine fitness and conditioning, this chapter is only the tip of the iceberg. There are many resources in print and online to learn from. Be selective in your choices because there is a great deal of misinformation to be found. Behavior courses should be taken from the Association of Professional Dog Trainers (APDT) certified instructors. Fitness advice should only be taken from a certified fitness professional such as a Certified Canine Fitness Trainer (CCFT) or a Certified Professional Canine Fitness Trainer (CPCFT).

Table 10.1 Hindlimb kinematics by joint.

	Increased hip flexion	Increased hip extension	Increased stifle flexion	Increased stifle extension	Increased tarsal flexion	Increased tarsal extension	Increased stance time (hindlimb)	Increased swing phase (hindlimb)	Increased stride length (hindlimb)
Trotting			X						X
LTM							X		
Incline LTM (10%)	X								
Incline ramp		X							
Decline ramp									
Stair ascent		X	X		X	X			
Stair descent			X		X	X			
Wheelbarrowing									
Dancing forward		X	X						
Dancing backward		X	X						
Cavalettis	X		X		X				
STS	X		X		X				
Swim	X		X		X				
UWTM (increased work and ROM when H2O at or above joint)	X		X		X				

Table 10.2 Forelimb kinematics by joint (as compared to walking).

	Increased shoulder flexion	Increased shoulder extension	Increased elbow flexion	Increased elbow extension	Increased carpal flexion	Increased carpal extension	Increased stance time (forelimb)	Increased stride length (forelimb)
Trotting			X		X			
LTM							X	X
Incline LTM							X	X
Incline ramp		X	X	X	X			
Decline ramp								
Stair ascent	X		X	X	X	X		
Wheelbarrowing		X	X			X		
Cavalettis			X		X			
Swim	X		X		X			
UWTM (increased work and ROM when H2O at or above joint)	X		X		X			

Table 10.3 Targeted exercises by Dr. Julia Tomlinson.

Neck muscles	Shoulder flexors	Shoulder extensors	Biceps	Triceps
• Nose through balls in container to find reward.	• Pivot with front legs	• Wheelbarrowing	• Tuck sit to stand	• Tuck sit to stand
• Resistance band while reaching for toy	• Lateral stepping	• Downstairs walking	• Stand to down	• Stand to down
• Tug	• One front foot up	• Down to stand	• Pivot with front legs	• Pivot with front legs
• Dumbbell in mouth with stride work	• Ascend stairs	• Give me 10	• Cavaletti	• Walk backwards (triceps)
• Look up, down, circle left, right while holding PVC pipe in mouth	• Swimming	• Wave, high 5	• Lateral stepping	• Lateral stepping
			• Play bow	• Play bow
			• Push up	• Push up
			• Crawl	• Crawl
			• Up stairs	• Ascend stairs
			• Descend stairs	• Weight pulling
			• Downhill walk	• Wheelbarrow
			• Wheelbarrow	• Down to stand

Forelimb add/abductor	Fore/hindlimb flexor/extensor	Abdominal muscles	Hip flexors	Hip extensors
• Lateral stepping	• Two or 3-legged stand on balance	• Tuck sit to stand	• Side leg lifts	• Rock back sit to stand
• Pivot with front limbs	• Two or 3-legged stand on paw pods	• Crawl	• Lateral step	• Down to stand
• Lift one front foot up (out to side)	• Walk in sand	• Hop forward	• Pivot with hind legs	• Hind limb targets
• Front paw targeting (out to side)	• Walk on uneven surface	• Roll over	• Uphill walking	• Ascend stairs
	• Walk backwards on uneven surface	• Crunches		• Dancing forward
	• Stand and lift leg on unstable surface	• Oblique crunches		• Dancing backward
	• Cavaletti over unstable surface	• Front limbs on rolling cart		

Quadriceps	Hamstrings	Hind limb add/abductor	Jumps/propulsion	Body control/balance/core
• Rock back sit to stand • Stand to down • Pivot with hind legs • Cavaletti • Lateral stepping • Lift one hind foot • Crawl • Ascend stairs	• Rock back sit to stand • Stand to down • Pivot with hind legs • Walk backwards • Lateral stepping • Crawl,	• Lateral stepping • Pivot with hindlimbs • Lift one hind foot out to side • Hind paw targeting to side	• Hop up to stable surface • Hop up on balance equipment • Sit to jump hurdle • Front limb elevated sit to stand • Weight pulling	• Pivot with hind legs • Pivot with front legs • 4 feet on 2 • Sit pretty • Cavaletti (for stride length & timing) • Weight shifting • Crawl • Balance work • Walk backward

Proprioception	Stride work	Flexibility	Speed	Endurance
• Pivot with hind legs • Pivot with front legs • Lateral stepping, • Cavaletti • Uneven surface walking • Weave poles	• Cavaletti (for stride length & timing • Trotting over poles 2 inches height - increase distance between poles to progress	• Cookie stretches • Weaves • Circle right/left • Crawl • Figure 8 • Play bow • Crunches standing	• Fetch • Uphill fetch • Interval training on land treadmill • Sustained trotting • Mat to mat sprints	• Uphill sprints • Swimming • Trotting on land treadmill • Underwater treadmill

References

Barfield, J.W. and Oliver, G.D. (2019). Sport specialization and single-legged-squat performance among youth baseball and softball athletes. *J Athl Train* 54 (10): 1067–1073. https://doi.org/10.4085/1062-6050-356-18. PMID: 31633412; PMCID: PMC6805059.

Behm DG, Blazevich AJ, Kay AD, and McHugh M (2016) Acute effects of muscle stretching on physical performance, range of motion, and injury incidence in healthy active individuals: A systematic review. *Appl Physiol Nutr Metab* 41(1):1–11. https://doi.org/10.1139/apnm-2015-0235. Epub 2015 Dec 8. 26642915.

Bellows J, Colitz CM, Daristotle L, *et al.* (2015) Defining healthy aging in older dogs and differentiating healthy aging from disease. *J Am Vet Med Assoc* 246(1):77–89. https://doi.org/10.2460/javma.246.1.77. 25517329.

Bovend'Eerdt, T.J., Botell, R.E., and Wade, D.T. (2009). Writing SMART rehabilitation goals and achieving goal attainment scaling: A practical guide. *Clin Rehabil* 23 (4): 352–361. 10.1177/0269215508101741. Epub 2009 Feb 23. Erratum in: Clin Rehabil. 2010 Apr;24(4):382. PMID: 19237435.

Camp, E., Dickson, R., Guevara, J. et al. (2016). CARES Center, University of Tennessee College of Veterinary Medicine, Knoxville, TN, USA, "Cardiovascular, Parameters of Exercising Pet Dogs" A44. In: (ed. E. Nemery, A. Gabriel, D. Cassart, et al.). Proceedings of the 9th international symposium on veterinary rehabilitation and physical therapy. *Acta Vet Scand* 58 (Suppl 2), 85 (2016). https://doi.org/10.1186/s13028-016-0259-7.

Campa, F., Spiga, F., and Toselli, S. (2019). The effect of a 20-week corrective exercise program on functional movement patterns in youth elite male soccer players. *J Sport Rehabil* 28 (7): 746.

Day BL and Fitzpatrick RC (2005) The vestibular system. *Curr Biol* 15(15):R583–R586. https://doi.org/10.1016/j.cub.2005.07.053. 16085475.

Dolan E, Saunders B, Harris RC, *et al.* (2019) Comparative physiology investigations support a role for histidine-containing dipeptides in intracellular acid-base regulation of skeletal muscle. *Comp Biochem Physiol A Mol Integr Physiol* 234:77–86. https://doi.org/10.1016/j.cbpa.2019.04.017. Epub 2019 Apr 25. 31029715.

Gillette, R. and Dale, R.B. (2014). Chapter 8: Basics of exercise physiology. In: *Canine Rehabilitation and Physical Therapy* (ed. D.L. Millis and D. Levine), 158. Philadelphia, PA: Elsevier.

Haun, C.T., Vann, C.G., Osburn, S.C. et al. (2019). Muscle fiber hypertrophy in response to 6 weeks of high-volume resistance training in trained young men is largely attributed to sarcoplasmic hypertrophy. *PLoS One* 14 (6): e0215267. doi: 10.1371/journal.pone.0215267. PMID: 31166954; PMCID: PMC6550381.

Hupfeld, K.E., McGregor, H.R., Hass, C.J. et al. (2022). Sensory system-specific associations between brain structure and balance. *Neurobiol Aging* 119: 102–116. doi: 10.1016/j.neurobiolaging.2022.07.013. Epub 2022 Aug 6. PMID: 36030560; PMCID: PMC9728121.

Laursen, P.B. and Jenkins, D.G. (2002). The scientific basis for high-intensity interval training: Maximizing training programmes and Maximizing performance in highly trained endurance athletes. *Sports Med* 32 (1): 53–73. https://doi.org/10.2165/00007256-200232010-00003. PMID: 11772161.

Levine, B.D. (2008). VO2max: What do we know, and what do we still need to know? *J Physiol* 586 (1): 25–34. doi: 10.1113/jphysiol.2007.147629. Epub 2007 Nov 15. PMID: 18006574; PMCID: PMC2375567.

Liu, Q. and Jorgensen, E. (2011). Muscle memory. *J Physiol* 589 (Pt 4): 775–776. https://doi.org/10.1113/jphysiol.2011. 205088. PMID: 21486844; PMCID: PMC3060353.

McArdle, W.D., Katch, F.I., and Katch, V.L. (2010). *Exercise Physiology: Nutrition, Energy, and Human Performance*, 7the, 502. Baltimore, MD: Lippincott Williams & Wilkins.

Micheo W, Baerga L, and Miranda G (2012) Basic principles regarding strength, flexibility, and stability exercises. *Phys Med Rehabil PMR* 4(11):805–811. https://doi. org/10.1016/j.pmrj.2012.09.583. 23174542.

Mihara, M., Fujimoto, H., Hattori, N. et al. (2021). Effect of neurofeedback facilitation on poststroke gait and balance recovery: A randomized controlled trial. *Neurology* 96 (21): e2587–e2598. 10.1212/ WNL.0000000000011989. Epub 2021 Apr 20. PMID: 33879597; PMCID: PMC8205450.

Millard, R. (2014). Chapter 9: Exercise physiology of the canine athlete. In: *Canine Rehabilitation and Physical Therapy*, 2nde (ed. D.L. Millis and D. Levine), 164. Philadelphia, PA: Elsevier.

Moïse NS, Flanders NH, and Gunzel ER (2021) Instantaneous and averaged heart rate profiles: Developing strategies for programming pacing rates in dogs. *Vet J* 270:105624. https://doi.org/10.1016/j. tvjl.2021.105624. Epub 2021 Jan 27. 33641808.

Niedermeyer, G.M., Hare, E., Brunker, L.K. et al. (2020). A randomized cross-over field study of pre-hydration strategies in dogs tracking in hot environments. *Front Vet Sci* 7: 292. https://doi.org/10.3389/ fvets.2020.00292.

Parsons D, Musch TI, Moore RL, *et al.* (1985) Dynamic exercise training in foxhounds. II. Analysis of skeletal muscle. *J Appl Physiol* 59(1):190–197. https://doi. org/10.1152/jappl.1985.59.1.190. 3161858.

Plotkin, D., Coleman, M., Van Every, D. et al. (2022). Progressive overload without progressing load? The effects of load or repetition progression on muscular adaptations. *Peer J* 10: e14142. doi: 10.7717/peerj.14142. PMID: 36199287; PMCID: PMC9528903.

Proske U and Gandevia SC (2012) The proprioceptive senses: Their roles in signaling body shape, body position and movement, and muscle force. *Physiol Rev* 92(4):1651–1697. https://doi.org/10.1152/ physrev.00048.2011. 23073629.

Rozzi, S.L., Lephart, S.M., and Fu, F.H. (1999). Effects of muscular fatigue on knee joint laxity and neuromuscular characteristics of male and female athletes. *J Athletic Train* 34 (2): 106–114.

Sevier, T.L., Wilson, J.K., and Helfst, B. (2000). The industrial athlete? *Work* 15 (3): 203–207. PMID: 12441489.

Steib, S., Rahlf, A.L., Pfeifer, K., and Zech, A. (2017). Dose-response relationship of neuromuscular training for injury prevention in youth athletes: A meta-analysis. *Front Physiol* 8: 920.

Torres BT, Fu YC, Sandberg GS, and Budsberg SC. (2017) Pelvic limb kinematics in the dog with and without a stifle orthosis *Vet Surg* 46(5):642–652. https://doi. org/10.1111/vsu.12634. Epub 2017 Feb 15. 28198549.

Van Hooren, B. and Peake, J.M. (2018). Do we need a cool-down after exercise? A narrative review of the psychophysiological effects and the effects on performance, injuries and the long-term adaptive response. *Sports Med* 48 (7): 1575–1595. 10.1007/s40279-018-0916-2. PMID: 29663142; PMCID: PMC5999142.

Voss, M.W., Vivar, C., Kramer, A.F., and van Praag, H. (2013). Bridging animal and human models of exercise-induced brain plasticity. *Trends Cogn Sci* 17 (10): 525–544. ISSN 1364-6613.

Williams TM, Dobson GP, Mathieu-Costello O, *et al.* (1997) Skeletal muscle histology and biochemistry of an elite sprinter, the African cheetah. *J Comp Physiol B*

167(8):527–535. https://doi.org/10.1007/s003600050105. 9404014.

Woods, K., Bishop, P., and Jones, E. (2007). Warm-up and stretching in the prevention of muscular injury. *Sports Med* 37: 1089–1099.https://doi.org/10.2165/00007256-200737120-00006.

Zebas CJ, Gillette RL, Hailey R, *et al*. (1991) Selected kinematic differences in the running gait of the greyhound athlete during the beginning and end of the race. https://ojs.ub.uni-konstanz.de/cpa/article/view/2619.

Zink, M.C. and Schlehr, M.R. (1997). Chapter 5: Conditioning the performance dog. In: *Peak Performance: Coaching the Canine Athlete*, 2nde, 109. Lutherville, MD: Canine Sports Productions.

11

The Disabled Patient Part 1: Assistive Devices and Technology

Sam Warren[1] and Julia E. Tomlinson[1,2]

[1] *Twin Cities Animal Rehabilitation & Sports Medicine Clinic, Burnsville, MN, USA*
[2] *Veterinary Rehabilitation and Orthopedic Medicine Partners, San Clemente, CA, USA*

CHAPTER MENU

Introduction

Assistive technology is an umbrella term that includes assistive, adaptive, and rehabilitative devices for individuals with disabilities and also includes the process used in selecting, locating, and using them. Assistive technology (for this chapter called devices) can be defined as "any item, piece of equipment, or product system, whether acquired commercially off the shelf, modified, or customized, that is used to increase, maintain, or improve functional capabilities of individuals with disabilities" (Nicolson *et al.*, 2012). The use of assistive devices in veterinary rehabilitation has several specific aims:

- To increase animal independence, and therefore, decrease family caregiver burden.
- To decrease effort and energy expenditure for family caregivers during the animal's activities of daily living.

Rehabilitation veterinarians and their technicians/nurses need to educate and guide family caregivers on the use of assistive devices for their pets in order to improve the chances of correct use along with patient acceptance. When we optimize movement and mobility for our patients, we can significantly affect their physical and mental health.

Physical Rehabilitation for Veterinary Technicians and Nurses, Second Edition.
Edited by Mary Ellen Goldberg and Julia E. Tomlinson.
© 2024 John Wiley & Sons, Inc. Published 2024 by John Wiley & Sons, Inc.
Companion website: www.wiley.com/go/goldberg/physicalrehabilitationvettechsandnurses

History

Canine "wheelchairs" have been on the US market for around 55 years. Dr. Lincoln Parkes, a veterinarian, designed carts in 1961 for his surgical patients, usually small-breed dogs but some German Shepherds. By the late 1970s, he had formed a company making carts for veterinarians all over the country, using specific measurements for each patient – K9 Carts (Glenn Parkes, personal communication). In 2008, a mass-market dog wheelchair was produced (Walkin' Wheels, http://walkinwheels.com/). This device fit a range of dog shapes and sizes and made dog wheelchairs easier for veterinarians to stock and have ready for future use (Bluebird Care, 2015).

The profession of bracing predates surgery when bone setters and appliance makers were the skilled artisans making braces (Mich, 2014). The development of surgical fixation caused bracing to become secondary to surgery. The correct term for braces is orthoses. Orthoses are defined as any medical device attached to the body to support, align position, prevent correct deformity, assist weak muscles, or improve function (Mich, 2014).

Originally, blacksmiths (farriers) and armor makers made prostheses for people. During the US Civil War, the number of amputations rose astronomically, forcing Americans to enter the field of prosthetics. James Hanger, one of the first amputees of the Civil War, developed what he later patented as the "Hanger Limb" from whittled barrel staves (Norton, 2007). The American Orthotic and Prosthetic Association was founded following World War I. Today's devices are much lighter and made of plastic, aluminum, and composite materials to provide amputees with the most functional devices.

Organizations such as the American Association of Rehabilitation Veterinarians (AARV), the American College of Veterinary Sports Medicine and Rehabilitation (ACVSMR), and the Academy of Physical Rehabilitation Veterinary Technicians (APRVT) are educating veterinarians on the use of assistive devices, orthoses, and prostheses to improve the mobility and functionality of the veterinary patient.

Which Patients Need Assistive Devices?

Patients who have had a physical injury, are recovering from surgery, or have a medical orthopedic or neurological issue (chronic or temporary) may need assistance. It is necessary to assist postoperative patients in getting into and out of cages and to help them up from a recumbent position, as well as assisting them while ambulating to prevent slips, excess weight bearing on a new repair, or further pain and injury. The patient must be allowed to become accustomed to any assistive device and the procedures involved in placement and assisting ambulation (Drum *et al.*, 2014). Patients with spinal cord injuries may have reduced body sensation and awareness (proprioception) but be ambulatory, or they may be nonambulatory paretic or fully paralyzed. It is important for the therapist to recognize the need for assisted standing even in a paralyzed patient. The cardiovascular system and the respiratory system benefit from being upright, in addition to the beneficial effects on muscle circulation (Olby, 2010). In patients who have some motor function, assisting motion is necessary in order to prevent falls as well as to provide the benefits of gait repatterning and strengthening (McDonald and Sadowsky, 2002).

Types of Assistive Devices

Devices Used for Assisted Standing

Standing exercises focus on strengthening shoulder, elbow, hip, and stifle extensors and reeducating muscles needed for balance and proprioception. They can also aid in lung and cardiovascular function. Several approaches can be used to facilitate standing. Particularly when a patient is large, assistive devices such as slings, physio rolls, mobility carts, wheelchairs, or lifts may be used to maintain a patient in a standing position (Drum *et al.*, 2014). Smaller patients can be supported manually to maintain a standing position, or a rolled towel can be placed under the chest and belly instead of a physio roll.

Devices that can be used include:

- Slings (see Figure 11.1)
- Therapy balls (see Figure 11.2)
- Hoyer lift (see Figure 11.3)

Devices Used for Assisted Ambulation

Devices for assisted ambulation can be used to help weak or paretic patients (see Figure 11.4). The devices used to assist companion animals may support or protect weak, unstable joints or feet (orthoses and boots), replace a missing portion of a limb (prostheses), or facilitate locomotion (slings, carts, ramps, and steps) (Marcellin-Little and Levine, 2014). Assistive devices may also decrease the complications present in recumbent patients, including decubitus ulcers (Adamson *et al.*, 2005).

Several sessions may be needed to establish acclimation. Low-stress handling techniques and positive reinforcement should be observed. In general, hair removal should be avoided as hair provides skin protection, but some devices may require that hair be clipped. Devices should be inspected for wear and damage and cleaned daily. The skin should be inspected twice daily. Cleaning is especially important if there are any incisions, wounds, or open sores in contact with the assistive device.

Pets wearing assistive devices should not be left unsupervised in nearly all cases, destructive chewing and loss of integrity can quickly occur, the device can move and result in hindering the patient rather than helping, and prolonged wear without supervision can cause any skin abrasions to become full wounds.

Boots

Boots can be used to protect paws from environmental hazards, for example, to protect working animals from ice and snow, rocky terrain, or hot surfaces. They can even provide cushion to painful arthritic feet. Patients with proprioceptive deficits may wear boots to provide more traction, protect skin, or stop them from wearing their nails down to the quick (Prydie and Hewitt, 2015). Wearing boots at home can provide traction on slippery floors, and breathable boots can be left on during the day. Boots can also be modified to provide a small "lift" in the case of a limb length discrepancy, in this case, a raised boot is only used if the length discrepancy is causing a pelvic tilt with lower back discomfort or reduced limb use.

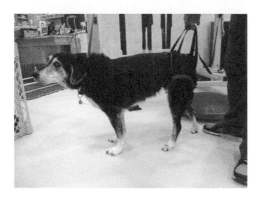

Figure 11.1   Sling for geriatric dog.

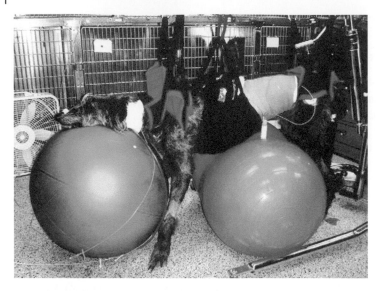

Figure 11.2 Therapy ball and sling-assisting standing.

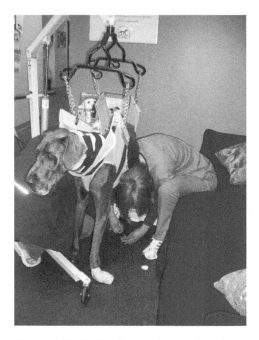

Figure 11.3 Dr. Tomlinson with a patient in a Hoyer lift.

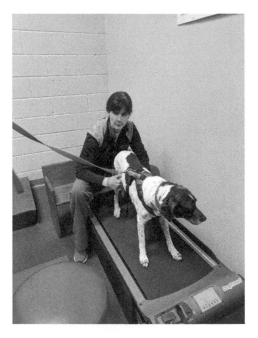

Figure 11.4 A patient in an assistive harness on a treadmill for gait patterning.

Boots act as sock-like coverings and are securely fastened by Velcro straps at the top. Most have a rubber sole to prevent slipping and are machine washable. The boots should be removed several times daily to assess the skin condition, especially in neurologically impaired patients, and, if possible, when performing therapeutic exercise to increase weight bearing and proprioception through the bottom of the pads (Adamson *et al.*, 2005). A proper fit is essential, and appropriate education instructions for skin care and rehabilitative exercises must be communicated to the owner.

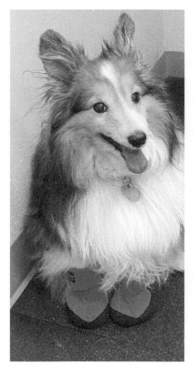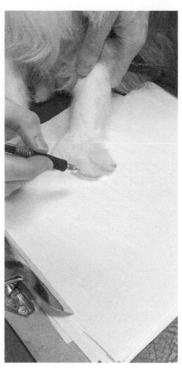

Figure 11.5 A patient with malformed, painful feet being sized for, and wearing custom cushioned slippers.

Customized grip socks are also available. These have rubber treads under the paw surface or over the whole foot, including dorsally. Old socks may also be used to help provide padding; however, if the top is secured with tape, care should be taken to avoid cutting off circulation (Marcellin-Little and Levine, 2014) (see Figure 11.5).

One study that evaluated a custom orthotic boot found that the boot was effective at immobilizing the distal extremity and reducing contact between a wound and the boot, which allowed for complete healing by contraction and epithelialization (Hardie and Lewallen, 2013).

Where Do I Get Boots?

- *Pawz*™ (http://pawzdogboots.com/boots/) are thin rubber boots without padding, so the dog is able to feel the ground. Tip: the animal's feet can get hot, so use foot powder to prevent moisture buildup or put a few small holes in the boot with a pin to create airflow around the foot (Prydie and Hewitt, 2015). The author recommends not to leave the boot on for more than three hours at a time.
- *Cushy-Paw Slippers*™ (www.therapaw.com/) are padded, grippy slippers for indoor comfort and protection. They can really help arthritic feet.
- *Ruffwear boots – Grip trex*™ (http://www.ruffwear.com/Barkn-Boots-Grip-Trex_3) are all-terrain boots and are a little thicker soled with a canvas upper. They can be adapted for sore feet by lining them with foam and can be used for multiple applications of indoor and outdoor foot protection.
- *Lewis Brand Vented Rubber Dog Boots*™ (http://www.gundogsupply.com/-950.html) protect the dog's feet from sand burrs, rocks, and brush and can also protect an injured foot or sore pad. Because they are molded to foot shape they can

help to keep the toes in proper extension for gait in animals that have mild proprioceptive issues. The boots are made of tire tread rubber with a tread on the sole to increase the life of the boot and for non-slip traction.

- *Foufoudog*™ (www.foufoubrands.com) are rubber-dipped socks with an antislip silicone sole that claim to keep paws dry, clean, and warm! The stretchy sock design makes it easy to put on, and the hook and loop allow you to wrap the sock securely so they do not fall off. The strap can be detached for quick walks or use around the house. The innovative rubber dip protects paws from outdoor elements such as water, snow, dirt, salt, and hot pavement.
- The purpose of the *Medipaw*® *X* boot (various suppliers) is to protect various appliances, such as leg bandages, splints, and casts. It can be used over incisions and is good for patients trying to bite or disturb a wound as in lick granulomas. The boots or suits are available for dogs and cats.

Nail Covers

- *Dr. Buzby's ToeGrips*™ (www.toegrips.com/) provide traction on slippery floors. These are rubber rings that fit around the dog's nail to provide grip through friction just below the nail tip. Care must be taken to pull the grips down from the cuticle as the nail grows. Dogs tolerate these well but note that some breeds, such as Dobermans, who do not have nail contact with the ground, and some individuals who do not engage the toenails when slipping, will not benefit from toe grips (Prydie and Hewitt, 2015). The grips can dislodge easily in pets with low ground clearance during ambulation.
- *Soft Claws*™ *Nail Caps* (www.mysoftclaws.com/) are glue-on caps that go over a newly trimmed nail. They stay in place

for several weeks and provide traction. They seem to be a better option for dogs with low ground clearance in gaiting. The covers are also made for cats, originally to prevent furniture damage.

Slings and Harnesses

Slings may be strapped around the belly or fitted for the forelimbs, hindlimbs, or both. They should have long, hand-held straps attached to allow proper body mechanics, avoiding personal injury to the handler when supporting the pet. Slings aid in transitioning a recumbent animal, especially larger dogs, to a standing position (Adamson *et al.*, 2005). They can also assist with ambulation and prevent falls on slippery floors, especially after surgery, to avoid further injury to the animal. Support slings are available for forelimb assistance and for patients with amputations. Patients who cross their pelvic limbs may benefit from the placement of a rolled cotton towel within a pelvic limb sling that has leg holes (Marcellin-Little and Levine, 2014). Slings used for the forelimbs should not obstruct respiration, and urine flow should not be compromised with hindlimb slings in male dogs. Slings should have a soft lining against the animal's skin to avoid irritation and sores, and they should be washable. Slings may be used for supported standing for therapeutic exercises such as repeated sit-to-stands. When documenting patient progress, the amount of assistance given through sling support can be rated as minimum, moderate, or maximal. Slings do tend to slide around in use and slide to the narrowest part of the trunk if they do not have holes for the limbs.

Harnesses are a more useful aid to mobility. They can be worn for several hours a day and provide easy access to a "handle" to lift the dog up (Prydie and Hewitt, 2015). This is particularly important if it is a larger dog to help the owners avoid injuring themselves. Animals with cervical injuries, especially following neurosurgery, will require chest harnesses to support their mobility without interfering with the injury site. There are also harnesses available with extra-long straps. These are useful for small dogs where the owners are likely to damage their back by reaching down to hold the harness.

Where Do I Get Slings and Harnesses?

- *GingerLead Sling*™ (www.gingerlead. com/) is a sling with handles and an extension leash to the collar for control of patient speed and motion. It allows the patient to feel supported while providing controlled mobility.
- *FourFlags Quick Lift*™ (http://www.four-flags.com/s.nl/sc.11/category.6990/.f) is a sling made of nylon pack cloth, available with or without fleece lining.
- *Hartmans Hip Helper*™ (www.hartman-harness.com/) is a harness, which is designed to be worn for hours at a time. It provides a handle over the rump for easy lifting assistance.
- *Help 'Em Up Dog Harness*™ (http://helpemup.com) is a padded harness designed for daily wear. Handles sit over the whithers and over the rump. The front harness and rear harness can work together or separately. This is our favorite harness because it offers the most control.
- A variety of slings and harnesses are available online (https://www.handi-cappedpets.com/walkin-lift-harnesses-slings/)

Ramps and Stairs

Ramps for dogs are useful for getting in and out of a vehicle, getting into the owner's bed, or going up and down steps. They are especially useful in geriatric patients. Ramps offer a solution that helps to protect the dog's joints when jumping and the owner's back when lifting the dog in and out of a vehicle. It is also advisable to have a ramp for getting out of a vehicle if the dog has had front-leg surgery, is prone to carpal hyperextension injuries, or has a tendency to hyperextend its carpus, as jumping out of a car will aggravate this (Prydie and Hewitt, 2015). Telescoping ramps are available. Measure the height of the bed or vehicle to calculate how steep a ramp will be based on its length.

A stool can be used for getting pets into the vehicle as an alternative to steps or a ramp in the case of a vehicle that is relatively low to the ground. The stool or single step should be solid enough to have inertia, wide enough for the caregiver to put a foot on to brace it, and have traction on the surface for the pet (see Figure 11.6).

Stairs are helpful for pets wanting to get to a higher elevation such as owner's beds, sofas, or window access. Cats particularly like using carpeted stairs. Be sure to use stairs that are strong enough for the weight of the pet and to look at pitch and overall width of the unit.

Where Do I Get Ramps and Stairs?

- *Discount Ramps*™ (www.discountramps. com) has a wide variety of ramps.
- *Pet Classics Indoor Pet Ramps*™ and *Pet Classics Outdoor Pet Ramps*™ (www.pet-classics.com/) are wooden ramps made for cats and dogs and covered with carpet.
- *Wayfair*™ (https://www.wayfair.com/keyword.php?keyword=pet) offers a variety of pet ramps and stairs for both indoor and outdoor use.

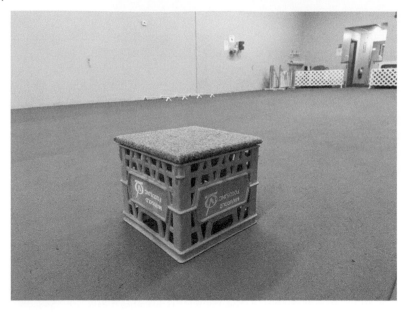

Figure 11.6 An old milk crate can be modified to create a step using a wooden block to make a flat surface, the block can be covered with traction material such as carpet.

Carts and Wheelchairs

Carts can allow functional independence for impaired animals. They aid in ambulation and can be used to provide therapeutic exercise. They are normally suggested for paretic or paralyzed patients, patients with severe osteoarthritis, and obese patients, and may be used with other devices such as boots (Borghese *et al.*, 2013). Carts have also been used for patients with long-term balance (vestibular and cerebellar) issues (Pazzaglia and Molinari, 2016).

When determining the most appropriate cart, consider the size and weight of the dog or cat, the amount of support needed, the patient's residual strength and mobility, and the caretaker's physical abilities. Getting a patient into and out of a cart can be very difficult and may require a lot of lifting, especially for larger or less mobile patients. The inertia of a cart may be too much to overcome for some patients with disabilities. Sometimes attaching a leash and using it to initiate movement of the cart will help patients move, but the leash may also be needed for braking forces.

Fitting – Cart fitting can be challenging, and rehabilitation veterinarians and their technicians or nurses should plan on spending at least 45 minutes adjusting aimed at getting the best ground clearance, allowing motion of ambulatory limbs with minimal restrictions, and balancing the weight of the cart (Pancotto, 2015). Clients should practice getting the pet into and out of the cart during the fitting. Most cart manufacturers will assist with adjustments if send a picture of the patient in the cart. Important positional factors include a straight topline (not bowed or curved), the patient should have good ground contact in the normal ambulatory limbs and toe-touch in weak or paretic limbs, and the strap on the front harness should clip just behind the scapula. Overweight dogs or those with low abdominal tone may need added belly bands.

Where Do I Get Carts?

- *Dewey's Wheelchairs for Dogs*™ (https://www.wheelchairsfordogs.com/home.html) are custom-made to a pet's measurements.
- *Doggon' Wheels USA*™ (www.doggon.com/) are custom-made to the pet's measurements, weight, and activity level. Dog and cat carts are available. The patient can be backed into the cart and the rear limb sling then snaps into straps on the cart.
- *Eddie's Wheels for Pets*™ (http://eddieswheels.com/) are custom-built for dogs and cats. The welded padded saddle gives solid support but the pet does have to be lifted into the cart. For cat patients, they send out a cat harness for the cat to get used to wearing while the wheelchair is built. The cat harness should be put on the cat to wear at all times so that he or she gets used to wearing something, and once the cart arrives, a piece of double-sided Velcro is used to attach the cat harness to the yoke of the cart.
- *K9 Carts*™ (www.k9carts.com/) are adjustable and available for dogs and cats.
- *Walkin' Wheels* (www.handicappedpets.com) comes in standard sizes that are adjustable. Different-sized wheels and bar lengths make a kit so that the cart can be modified for a patient. For larger dogs, steel reinforcement bars are added. These carts are better for rear limb issues only; a belly band can help patients with abdominal weakness.

Beds and Bedding

Orthopedic dog beds provide the necessary and supportive firmness a geriatric pet needs to sleep comfortably. These beds give a pet the support and comfort of orthopedic foam, making them the best pet beds for older, ailing, and postoperative dogs, or those with arthritis. A pet bed provides a sense of security. Advise the client to locate a comfortable place in their home for the pet bed and keep the bed in the same location so the pet learns that he or she has a special resting spot. Pet beds are comfy, and most pets would prefer to sleep somewhere soft that provides cushioning and insulation instead of on the cold, hard floor.

Important Factors to Consider Before Choosing a Pet Bed

- *Sleeping style* – Some pets like to sleep curled up in a cozy ball, but others like to sprawl out. Have the owner observe the pet's sleeping style to help determine the right bed for him or her. Does the pet like the security of leaning against something? Or does the pet like to have enough room to stretch? These are important questions to consider before choosing.
- *Pet type, size, and activity level* – Is this for a dog or a cat? Big dogs will need a larger, sturdier bed with a thick, more durable cover than a smaller dog would need. Cats prefer window perches to satisfy their curiosity. Older pets would benefit from heated pads or orthopedic beds for relief from arthritis.
- *Style and budget* – Nowadays, pet beds come in a wide range of styles, colors, materials, and prices, so there is something for every taste and budget.

Popular Types of Pet Beds

- *Orthopedic pet beds* provide extra cushioning for bones, helping to soothe painful pressure points. The large size of an orthopedic pet bed is great for pets that like to sprawl out while sleeping. The mattress type of pet bed is recommended for large dogs, while orthopedic window perches are recommended for cats. Some of the smaller orthopedic pet beds may be used for either dogs or cats.

- *Donut (bolster) beds* – If the pet likes to curl up or sleep with his or her head resting on a pillow, a donut or bolster bed is a good choice. This style of pet bed usually has a cushioned bottom and a raised side. It is cozy for smaller pets since the round shape of the pet bed helps retain body heat.
- *Pillow or cushion beds* – This pet bed is basically a large pillow or cushion. It comes in many different sizes and is a great choice for pets that like to stretch out while sleeping.
- *Heated pet beds* are recommended for older pets that may have joint pain or stiffness. The gentle heat soothes and reduces stiffness, keeping the pet warm and cozy while sleeping. Even smaller pets, such as cats, can benefit from a heated pet bed since they lose body heat easily. Consider using a heated pet bed if the client lives in a colder climate.
- *A pet cot* should be considered if the dog or cat likes to rest outdoors. Pet cots protect the pet from the rough ground, especially asphalt that may get too hot in the summer or too cold in the fall or winter. Many pet cots are made of a waterproof fabric which helps make cleaning easier. The sturdy frame makes it ideal for larger dogs.

Where Do I Get Pet Beds?

- *The PetCot™ Company* (www.petcot.com/) makes beds for homes, boarding kennels, and veterinarians. They can be vinyl, making them easy to clean, or have a fleece cover. Cage inserts are available for the veterinarian's hospital, and a raised pet bed for dogs with incontinence. Replacement parts, fleece covers, and orthopedic inserts are available as well.
- *The SleePee Time Bed*® (http://www.handicappedpets.com/sleepee-time-bed-for-incontinent-pets) is a new product specifically designed to help dogs with incontinence and older dogs get a good night's sleep. It can also be used simply as a cool, comfortable sleeping surface for any pet.
- *Care-A-Lot Pet Supply* (https://www.care-alotpets.com/Departments/Cat-Supplies/Beds-and-Cuddlers/Cuddlers-and-Bolsters.aspx) offers cat beds and cuddlers, including heated beds, plush beds, round beds, and one hanging cat condo.
- *Wayfair*® *Dog Beds* (http://www.wayfair.com/Dog-Beds-C409475.html) offer orthopedic beds, bolster beds, fleece beds, pet cots, and pet sofas.

Hydraulic Patient Lifts

Hydraulic lifts are either manual or electric. They can be found at medical supply stores and purchased new, used, or rented. A few are being made specifically for dogs. It is important to purchase a sling attachment used specifically for dogs even if you buy a human version lift. A lift can be used to manage a large tetraparetic or tetraplegic cervical patient. A patient lift (patient hoist, jack hoist, and hydraulic lift) (Figure 11.4) is usually a sling lift, allowing the patient to assume a standing position. The patient may need to be supported by therapy balls.

- The *Equa-Lift Hoist™* (http://eddieswheels.com/p/19/Hospital-Equipment) is used in conjunction with a Hoyer™ lift or overhead track system and a Help 'Em Up Harness™. The hoist provides a safe, balanced way to move disabled animals in and out of the therapy stand, clinic quad cart, or hydrotherapy unit.

Splints and Braces

A splint is a device applied to any body part to help stabilize a structure, promote healing, protect against injury/reinjury, prevent/correct deformity, and/or assist with function. A splint is lightweight, easy to apply and remove, and adaptable. It can be static or dynamic, rigid or flexible, and can be used as a coaptation device or solely for therapeutic purposes (Borghese *et al.*, 2013).

A brace is defined as a durable device used for immobilizing a body part. It renders the body part static, rigid, and fixed (Borghese *et al.*, 2013).

Splints – The primary functions of a coaptation device include protection, absorption, compression, and stabilization.

- *Air splints* can be used to help a dog to stand while the veterinarian works on them, acting as an extra set of hands to stabilize a joint or limb. Air splints are waterproof and reusable, easy to apply, inflate, deflate, remove, and clean, making them ideal for in-home use by savvy clients. When inflated, they conform to the animal's limb and are not associated with pressure sores. They are transparent and can be half filled with water, refrigerated, and then used as cold packs over an entire limb. https://www.airsplints.com/

- *Thermoplastic splints* are made of heat-sensitive plastic material heated in hot water or a low-temperature oven until it becomes soft. Once soft, the material can be cut and molded into a custom shape for the patient's needs. After the splint is made, it needs to be cooled to become solid. This process can be speeded up by running cold tap water on it or by wrapping a cold, wet crepe bandage over the splint. Hook and loop (Velcro) straps hold the splint in place, and padding/liner materials increase patient comfort. The problem with hook and loop is that it needs to be applied correctly to ensure fixation. If it is too loose, the splint will cause friction and abrasions may occur (Prydie and Hewitt, 2015). Thermoplastic sheets are widely used with human patients to make custom splints and braces that partially or totally immobilize a body part. They have now been adapted for use with animal patients (see Figure 11.7).

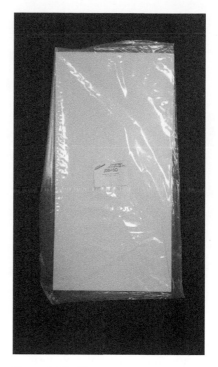

Figure 11.7 Thermoplastic sheet for devices.

- *Customizable preformed splints* are more recently available. The UPETS splint (www.dassietstore.com) is a heat moldable device with a foot part that comes in several sizes. The reusable wrap is also utilized to anchor the device (see Videos 11.1 and 11.2).

Padding materials are used with splints to protect bony prominences, areas of fragile skin, and less-protected areas of the body. Padding should only be used in the middle part of the splint and not end to end as this will significantly alter the fit of the splint, particularly with a large amount of padding. The other consideration when using padding is that it can become wet and trap distasteful smells.

Braces – Bracing is used to support and stabilize a body part. Some wraps and braces are not custom-made. These could be termed generic braces. Rigid braces that are not customized can cause pressure or

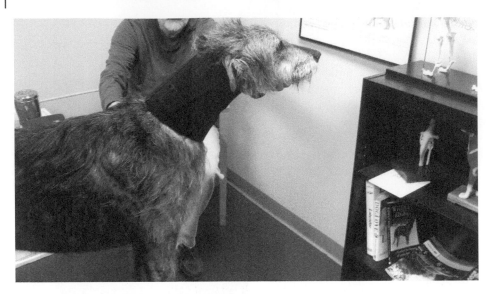

Figure 11.8 Neck brace for an Irish Wolfhound.

friction wounds and care should be taken that they are padded well and conform to the limb adequately.

Cervical neurologic patients (Drum *et al.*, 2014) may need bracing made from thermoplastic or fiberglass-cast material that extends from mid-sternum cranially to the chin. The brace prevents ventral flexion of the neck (see Figure 11.8). It should be closely monitored for excessive tightness, areas of irritation, and wetness. Many patients will have difficulty eating, so syringe feedings with water and pureed food may be required. For more severely affected cases, surgery is often required to stabilize the joint between C1 and C2. After surgical stabilization, a brace is required for 4–6 weeks postoperatively.

- *DogLeggs Therapeutic and Rehabilitative Products* (http://www.dogleggs.com/index.cfm) offer various braces. *DogLeggs' Carpal Support* is indicated for carpal hyperextension, carpal instability/sprain or strain injury, carpal osteoarthritis, immune-mediated joint disease, angular limb deformity, chondrodystrophic dogs in need of carpal support, post-op

management of carpal arthrodesis or avulsion fractures. It is made from closed-cell foam with synthetic rubber material and is laminated with a nylon jersey fabric. It is lightweight yet durable and has incredible tensile strength. The product is machine washable. *DogLeggs' Tarsal Support* is indicated for mild to moderate Achilles tendon disruption, tarsal instability/sprain or strain injury, tarsal osteoarthritis, immune-mediated joint disease, angular limb deformity, and chondrodystrophic dogs in need of tarsal support. It is constructed from a three-dimensional fleece-faced, highly breathable, and four-way stretch textile with wicking properties. It allows air to circulate while keeping the joint warm. It contains padding to protect the bony prominences of the hock. Hook and loop fastening is used to secure the product. The product is machine washable. *DogLeggs' Shoulder Stabilization System*™ is indicated for conservative management of medial shoulder instability, postoperative management of medial shoulder instability or shoulder reconstructions, conservative or postoperative management of certain scapular fractures, postoperative management of certain shoulder luxation repairs, and swimmer puppy syndrome. The system prevents abduction (moving away from the body) of the forelimbs and limits shoulder extension and flexion. The limited extension results in a mildly shortened forelimb gait when walking. The shoulder stabilization orthosis is made from breathable neoprene that can be worn continuously.

- *Thera-Paw Assistive and Rehabilitative Pet Products* (www.therapaw.com/) offer a variety of products. *Custom Carpal Wraps* are designed to provide customized support, stability, or immobilization. They come in three thicknesses. The same is true of the *Custom Tarsal Wrap. The Dorsi-Flex Assist*™ (Prydie and Hewitt, 2015) can be used to good effect in dogs and cats that knuckle over on their back legs because of reduced neural input from degenerative myelopathy, peripheral nerve injury, or proprioceptive deficits. It can be used in dogs with weakness; however, care needs to be taken to ensure that the dog has enough strength to lift the foot with the boot on and that the dog has enough stability around the hip to control the movement of the leg. The elastic straps are placed under tension and as the animal brings the leg forward, the elastic aids the foot being moved up into dorsiflexion.
- *Biko*™ *Progressive Resistance Bands* (www.animotionproducts.com/) (Prydie and Hewitt, 2015) can aid gait where there is bilateral back leg weakness such as degenerative myelopathy, wobblers, or degenerative disc disease with mild to moderate ataxia. They consist of two leg cuffs that have elastic straps clipped onto them. These elastic straps attach onto a chest harness. There are different colors of elastic relating to progressive strengths of elastic, and the device works by pulling

the foot forward as the elastic recoils after being stretched by extending the hips. Caution is needed when selecting clients to use this system, as it does not prevent knuckling and is not appropriate for acute painful conditions. It is also not suitable for patients with unilateral problems as it can increase ataxia, or those with paralysis and no motor function in one or more legs.

Custom Orthoses

Custom orthoses are made from casts of the patient's limb or are fabricated directly on the patient using a moldable thermoplastic polymer (Marcellin-Little *et al.*, 2015). These can be designed for aquatic therapy or to be worn for playing in water. The most common orthoses are used to restrict the excessive joint motion present in patients with ligamentous or tendinous problems, including patients with ruptures of their palmar fibrocartilage or common calcaneal tendon (Marcellin-Little and Levine, 2014). Custom fabrication becomes essential when a standard or semi-custom product (Borghese *et al.*, 2013):

- is not available in the correct size,
- does not meet the specific needs of the patient,
- cannot be altered to meet the patient's needs,
- incorporates a joint or joints not affected by the condition, or
- simply does not exist.

Orthoses may be hinged to enhance their functionality (Levine and Fitch, 2003). Orthoses with passive hinges may enhance limb function because part or all of the motion of the tarsus (or carpus) may be maintained. Orthoses may have dynamic hinges that can be used to enhance the support of weak joints or to stretch contracted joints. Hinges are made dynamic by using

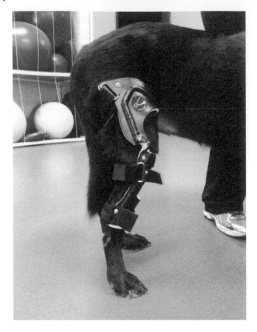

Figure 11.9 A stifle orthosis.

springs embedded in the hinges or elastic bands (Marcellin-Little and Levine, 2014) (see Figure 11.9).

A custom carpal orthosis would basically eliminate the need for cage rest while tissues are healing, but, in contrast, complete immobilization of the carpus allows some amount of tissue loading and can be removed by an owner to enable provision of passive therapeutic joint motion and daily inspection of the skin for abrasions (Tomlinson and Manfredi, 2014).

Custom orthoses have been used in conjunction with autologous mesenchymal stem cell treatment, as in the case of a four-year-old Border Collie where the owner elected conservative treatment over surgery. The owner was thoroughly informed about the experimental nature of this method of treatment (Case *et al.*, 2013).

Where Do I Go?

A professional company such as OrthoPets™ (www.orthopets.com/) needs to be employed to make custom orthotics. Examination of the patient, measuring, and continued communication between the rehabilitation veterinarian and the orthotics company help ensure custom fit of the device. Courses are available to enable the veterinarian and their rehabilitation veterinary technician to learn how to create a fiberglass mold and send the required materials to the company (http://www.caninerehabinstitute.com/Orthotics_Prosthetics.lasso).

Other companies are:

- *Animal Ortho Care, LLC (*www.animalorthocare.com/)
- *K-9 Orthotics and Prosthetics Inc.* (www.k-9orthotics.com/)
- *Handicapped Pets.com* (http://www.handicappedpets.com/k9-dog-orthoticsprosthetics)
- *My Pet's Brace* (www.mypetsbrace.com/)

Types of Custom Orthoses

- Shoulder orthoses
- Elbow orthoses
- Antebrachial and carpal orthoses
- Hip orthoses
- Stifle orthoses
- Hock orthoses
- Distal limb orthoses (distal to carpus or tarsus)
- Spinal orthoses.

Custom Prostheses

Not long ago, amputation of a limb for a small animal patient was quite normal when a salvage procedure was needed for trauma or disease. It is now being understood that the consequences of that missing limb or limb segment are not good (Goldner *et al.*, 2015). Organizations advocating pain management such as the American College of Veterinary Anesthesia and Analgesia, the International Veterinary Academy of Pain Management (IVAPM), the ACVSMR, and the AARV are understanding the importance of biomechanics in normal quadruped locomotion. If a total or partial limb is missing then there can arise limited mobility and endurance, increased metabolic demand, weight gain, support limb breakdown, chronic neck and back pain, and premature euthanasia (Mich, 2014). The reestablishment of quadruped function and structure has been made possible now in veterinary medicine. The end goal is to provide a limb that allows as close to normal ambulation as possible.

Types of Prosthesis

There are two types of prosthetic limbs available: the socket design and the intraosseous transcutaneous amputation prosthesis (ITAP). Socket-based prostheses provide a socket for the residual limb to reside in. Usually, an extension (in the form of a foot or paw) is provided for the limb to contact the ground (see Figure 11.10). The socket prosthesis requires owner care and must be put on or removed from the patient.

Contraindications for socket prostheses may be linked to the owner, the patient, or the medical condition (Marcellin-Little *et al.*, 2015). Owner-related contraindications include a potential lack of interest, motivation, supervision, or financial ability to get involved. Patient-related contraindications include being difficult to handle because of an aggressive personality (see Box 11.1).

ITAP provides an implanted endoprosthesis (into the bone) to which an exoprosthesis (external prosthesis) is attached (Mich, 2014). The clear advantage of an ITAP is direct skeletal integration of the exoprosthesis (Fitzpatrick *et al.*, 2011), and it has been shown that biological integration of osseous and dermal tissues with ITAP is

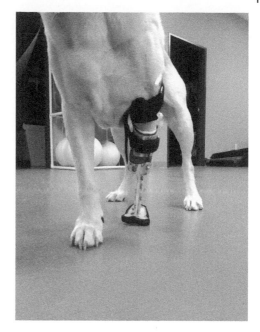

Figure 11.10 A forelimb prosthesis. *Source:* Courtesy of Dr. Douglas Stramel.

Box 11.1 Contraindications for prosthetic devices in cats and dogs

Owner
- Lack of interest
- Motivation
- Supervision
- Financial ability to get involved

Patient
- Difficult to handle because of an aggressive personality
- Medical condition
- Highly mobile skin in relation to underlying tissues
- Neurologic deficits
- Compromised joint mobility
- Local neoplasia
- Infection
- Stump pain

Adapted from Marcellin-Little et al. (2015).

Box 11.2   Orthopedic conditions that will adapt to veterinary prosthetic devices

Thoracic limb prostheses

- Subtotal mid-shaft radius or ulna amputation (40% antebrachium retention required)
- Subtotal radiocarpal disarticulation
- Subtotal intercarpal disarticulation
- Subtotal carpometacarpal disarticulation
- *Amelia* – a birth defect of lacking one or more limbs
- Congenital limb derangements
- Traumatic limb amputation

Pelvic limb prostheses

- Subtotal mid-shaft tibia or fibula amputation (40% crus retention required)
- Subtotal tarsocrural disarticulation
- Subtotal level intertarsal disarticulation
- Subtotal level tarsometatarsal disarticulation
- *Amelia* – a birth defect of lacking one or more limbs
- Congenital limb derangements
- Traumatic limb amputation

Source: Adapted from Kaufmann and Mich (2014).

---

reliable and robust. The tremendous variability in veterinary patients requires adaptability in socket design, components, and prosthetic limb mechanics to accommodate differences in the degree of injury, body type and condition, species, breed, size, lifestyle, sport or activity, and terrain (Kaufmann and Mich, 2014) (see Box 11.2).

Examples of Successful ITAP Procedures

Some procedures in which ITAP has been used successfully include:

- total hip replacement (Liska *et al.*, 2009; Vezzoni *et al.*, 2015),
- total knee replacement (Mann *et al.*, 2012),
- canine elbow arthroplasty (Burton *et al.*, 2013), and
- titanium partial limb prosthesis in a white crane (Rush *et al.*, 2012).

Follow-Up Care for the Prosthetic Patient

It is critical for the veterinary prosthesis patient to undergo physical rehabilitation. The best way to ensure the highest level of success with a prosthetic device is to follow a rehabilitation plan established by a certified canine rehabilitation professional (certified canine rehabilitation therapist [CCRT] or certified canine rehabilitation practitioner [CCRP]). Sensory feedback extends from the top down rather than from the ground up. Through rehabilitation, the prosthesis patient relearns proprioception, balance, gaiting at different speeds, and ambulation over varied terrain (Mich, 2014). Training companion animals to use socket prostheses is like managing limb disuse. It relies on habituating patients to tolerate the exoprosthesis at rest and loading it (using it) when standing, when walking slowly (indoors), when walking more rapidly (outdoors), when trotting, when galloping, and then during other activities of daily living (e.g., climbing and walking down steps, climbing and walking downstairs, jumping up and jumping down, playing) (Marcellin-Little *et al.*, 2015). Land-based therapeutic exercise is essential. Balance, proprioception, muscle timing (neuromuscular retraining), and coordination lay the foundation for proper device use (Mich, 2014). These must be mastered on land so that the patient can learn to respond to normal ground reaction forces and shifts in their total body force vectors (Mich, 2014).

Complications

Veterinary orthoses and prostheses are considered durable medical devices. As such, they should never be prescribed or dispensed without client training and a comprehensive follow-up plan. Veterinary orthotic/prosthetic patients should be assessed at least annually (see Figures 11.11). Device adjustment and refurbishment are expected to continue meeting therapeutic goals (Borghese et al., 2013).

A recent prospective clinical study (Rosen et al., 2022) over 12 months revealed a high complication rate (mostly skin wounds) in orthoses and prostheses use (91%) and that complication rate was even higher when looking at prostheses alone. What was termed "patient non-acceptance" of the device was a problem in 58% of prostheses patients.

It is beyond the scope of this chapter to discuss the complete process of the veterinary evaluation, defining therapeutic goals, measuring for the mold cast to be sent to the prosthetic fabricator, communication with the fabricator, delivery of the device, and ensuring proper fit. Manufacturing requires skilled modification of the model by hand or using computer-assisted design to build reliefs, which accommodate limb topography and create appropriate corrective forces when the completed device is applied to the limb. The modified model is the structure on which a thermoplastic shell is vacuum-formed. The shell is then hand-cut, trimmed, and ground to the final shape. Materials used to pad and line the shell vary. Hinges, straps, pads, and motion-limiting components complete fabrication. The typical custom veterinary orthotic/prosthetic device cost varies with components and materials but averages $US700–$US1500. This does not include the necessary appointments to ensure proper fit and function along with client education (Mich, 2014).

Where Do I Go?

Professional companies that fabricate these devices are listed at https://tamarackhti.com/resources/animalopdirectory/

Companies that are highly recommended include:

- *OrthoPets*™ (www.orthopets.com/) and partner clinics in many countries (https://www.orthopets.com/find-a-clinic)
- *Bionic Pets, LLC* (www.bionicpets.org)
- *K-9 Orthotics & Prosthetics* (www.k-9orthotics.com)

Summary

The use of assistive devices, orthotics, and prosthetics has enabled many animals to continue to enjoy a high quality of life. Patients who might otherwise be at risk for euthanasia can return to an active lifestyle, reducing the risk of obesity and its associated comorbidities. Secondary or compensatory pain can be minimized by correcting or improving gait mechanics and reestablishing quadruped locomotion.

Video 11.1 UPETS1 device fitting videos made for clients.
Video 11.2 UPETS2 device fitting videos made for clients.

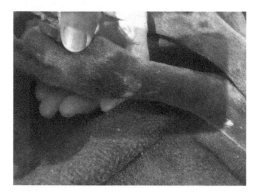

Figure 11.11 A wound complication from an orthosis.

References

Adamson, C., Kaufmann, M., Levine, D. et al. (2005). Assistive devices, orthotics, and prosthetics. *Vet Clin North Am Small Anim Pract* 35: 1441–1451.

Bluebird Care (2015) *Assistive Technology from Ancient to Modern Times*. http://bluebirdcare.ie/assistive-technology-ancient-modern-times/ (accessed January 3, 2015).

Borghese, I., Fair, L., Kaufmann, M., and Mich, P.M. (2013). Assistive devices, orthotics, prosthetics, and bandaging. In: *Canine Sports Medicine and Rehabilitation* (ed. M.C. Zink and J.B. Van Dyke), 201–222. Ames, IA: John Wiley & Sons, Inc.

Burton, N.J., Ellis, R.J., Burton, K.J. et al. (2013). An ex vivo investigation of the effect of the TATE canine elbow arthroplasty system on kinematics of the elbow. *J Small Anim Pract* 54: 240–247.

Case, J.B., Palmer, R., Valdes-Martinez, A. et al. (2013). Gastrocnemius tendon strain in a dog treated with autologous mesenchymal stem cells and a custom orthosis. *Vet Surg* 42: 355–360.

Drum, M., Werbe, B., McLucas, K., and Millis, D. (2014). Nursing care of the rehabilitation patient. In: *Canine Rehabilitation and Physical Therapy*, 2nde (ed. D. Millis and D. Levine), 277–304. Philadelphia, PA: Elsevier/Saunders.

Fitzpatrick, N., Smith, T.J., Pendegrass, C.J. et al. (2011). Intraosseous transcutaneous amputation prosthesis (ITAP) for limb salvage in 4 dogs. *Vet Surg* 40: 909–925.

Goldner, B., Fuchs, A., Nolte, I., and Schilling, N. (2015). Kinematic adaptations to tripedal locomotion in dogs. *Vet J* 204 (2): 192–200.

Hardie, R.J. and Lewallen, J.T. (2013). Use of a custom orthotic boot for management of distal extremity and pad wounds in three dogs. *Vet Surg* 42: 678–682.

Kaufmann, M.W. and Mich, P.M. (2014). Custom external coaptation as a pain management tool: Veterinary orthotics and prosthetics. In: *Pain Management in Veterinary Practice* (ed. C.M. Egger, L. Love, and T. Doherty), 155–160. Ames, IA: John Wiley & Sons, Inc.

Levine, J.M. and Fitch, R.B. (2003). Use of an ankle-foot orthosis in a dog with traumatic sciatic neuropathy. *J Small Anim Pract* 44: 236–238.

Liska, W.D., Doyle, N., Marcellin-Little, D.J., and Osborne, J.A. (2009). Total hip replacement in three cats: Surgical technique, short-term outcome and comparison to femoral head ostectomy. *Vet Comp Orthop Traumatol* 22: 505–510.

Mann, K.A., Miller, M.A., Khorasani, M. et al. (2012). The dog as a preclinical model to evaluate interface morphology and micro-motion in cemented total knee replacement. *Vet Comp Orthop Traumatol* 25: 1–10.

Marcellin-Little, D.J. and Levine, D. (2014). Devices for ambulation assistance in companion animals. In: *Canine Rehabilitation and Physical Therapy*, 2nde (ed. D. Millis and D. Levine), 305–311. Philadelphia, PA: Elsevier/Saunders.

Marcellin-Little, D.J., Drum, M., Levine, D., and McDonald, S.S. (2015). Orthoses and exoprostheses for companion animals. *Vet Clin Small Anim* 45: 167–183.

McDonald, J.W. and Sadowsky, C. (2002). Spinal-cord injury. *Lancet* 359: 417–425.

Mich, P.M. (2014). Topical review: The emerging role of veterinary orthotics and prosthetics (V-OP) in small animal rehabilitation and pain management. *Top Companion Anim Med* 29: 10–19.

Nicolson, A., Moir, L., and Millsteed, J. (2012). Impact of assistive technology on family caregivers of children with physical disabilities: A systematic review. *Disabil Rehabil Assist Technol* 7 (5): 345–349.

Norton, K. (2007). A brief history of prosthetics. *In Motion* 17 (7): 11–13.

Olby, N. (2010). Patients with neurologic disorders. In: *BSAVA Manual of Canine and Feline Rehabilitation, Supportive and Palliative Care*, 168–170. Gloucester, UK: British Small Animal Veterinary Association.

Pancotto TE (2015) Canine wheelchair equivalents. *Clinician's Brief*, http://www.cliniciansbrief.com/article/canine-wheelchair-equivalents (accessed January 7, 2016).

Pazzaglia, M. and Molinari, M. (2016). Review: The embodiment of assistive devices – From wheelchair to exoskeleton. *Phys Life Rev* 16: 163–175.

Prydie, D. and Hewitt, I. (2015). Splints supports and aids. In: *Practical Physiotherapy for Small Animal Practice*, 195–209. Oxford: Wiley/Blackwell.

Rosen, S., Duerr, F.M., and Elam, L.H. (2022). Prospective evaluation of complications associated with orthosis and prosthesis use in canine patients. *Front Vet Sci* 9: 892662. https://doi.org/10.3389/fvets.2022.892662.

Rush, E.M., Turner, T.M., Montgomery, R. et al. (2012). Implantation of a titanium partial limb prosthesis in a white-naped crane (*Grus vipio*). *J Avian Med Surg* 26 (3): 167–175.

Tomlinson, J.E. and Manfredi, J.M. (2014). Evaluation of application of a carpal brace as a treatment for carpal ligament instability in dogs: 14 cases (2008–2011). *J Am Vet Med Assoc* 244 (4): 438–443.

Vezzoni L, Vezzoni A, and Boudrieau, R.J. (2015). Long-term outcome of Zürich cementless total hip arthroplasty in 439 cases. *Vet Surg* 44: 921–929.

12

The Disabled Patient Part 2: The Neurological Patient

Stephanie Kube[1] and Julia C. Tomlinson[2,3]

[1] *Advanced Veterinary Specialty Center of New England, Walpole, MA, USA*
[2] *Twin Cities Animal Rehabilitation & Sports Medicine Clinic, Burnsville, MN, USA*
[3] *Veterinary Rehabilitation and Orthopedic Medicine Partners, San Clemente, CA, USA*

CHAPTER MENU

Introduction

There are three main components to the nervous system: the central nervous system (CNS), the peripheral nervous system (PNS), and the autonomic nervous system (ANS). The PNS consists of the nerves and ganglia located outside the brain and spinal cord. The myelin sheath surrounding the peripheral axons is formed by Schwann cells, whereas CNS axons are myelinated by oligodendrocytes (Thomson and Hahn, 2012). Dorsal and ventral nerve roots attach on each side of the spinal cord and carry sensory and motor axons. Lateral to the spinal cord, the dorsal and ventral roots fuse to form spinal nerves. Adjacent spinal nerves may fuse, in a plexus, to form named nerves in the periphery. There are 12 pairs of cranial nerves that innervate the head and extend

Physical Rehabilitation for Veterinary Technicians and Nurses, Second Edition.
Edited by Mary Ellen Goldberg and Julia E. Tomlinson.
© 2024 John Wiley & Sons, Inc. Published 2024 by John Wiley & Sons, Inc.
Companion website: www.wiley.com/go/goldberg/physicalrehabilitationvettechsandnurses

into the body. Areas of sensory innervation of the skin are categorized as dermatomes, cutaneous zones, and autonomous zones. Somatic lower motor neurons (LMNs) innervating striated muscles of the body have their cell bodies sited in the CNS. Their axons travel in the PNS to connect to the muscle at the neuromuscular junction. A motor unit comprises a single LMN and the group of muscle fibers it innervates.

Healing of Nerves

Nerves are sensitive to oxygen and the glucose level of tissues. More severe injuries first undergo Wallerian degeneration. This is a degenerative process that occurs when a nerve fiber is cut or crushed. Part of the axon is separated from the nerve cell body and degenerates distal to the injury (Coleman and Freeman, 2010).

Wallerian degeneration starts 24–36 hours after injury (a patient can lose more nerve function after the initial injury as the axons degenerate).

Regeneration is slower in the CNS than in the PNS. The myelin sheath in the PNS guides axon regeneration. Aging has been shown to retard the rate of axonal regrowth.

- If conditions are optimal, then nerves will regenerate axons.
  - ➢ First of all, for regeneration, the nerve cell body and any myelin sheath should be intact
- We aim to make conditions optimal with rehabilitation therapy, ensuring;
  - ➢ Adequate capillary bed
  - ➢ Good venous drainage, no congestion
  - ➢ Minimal edema and tissue compression

In more severe nerve injuries where endoneurial tubes are disrupted, regenerating axons are no longer confined to their original myelin sheaths. They can meander into surrounding tissue, thus failing to reinnervate their proper end organs.

The Neurological Examination

The objectives in the management of an animal with a problem that may be related to the nervous system are to (Lorenz *et al.*, 2011a):

1) confirm that the problem is caused by a lesion in the nervous system;
2) localize the lesion in the nervous system;
3) estimate the severity and extent of the lesion in the nervous system;
4) determine the cause or the pathologic process or both; and
5) estimate the prognosis with no treatment or with various alternative methods of treatment.

Patient History

The first step in diagnosis of the neurological problem is taking a history. History can be aided by the use of pre-appointment questionnaires, but a verbal history should be added. History should include length of the disease process/problem, current medications, prior and current treatments/therapies, and goals. Many times, asking the client to bring all medications, the patient is taking (placed in a bag) to the appointment will allow the veterinarian and technician to write down the various drugs and dosages to have this on record. All questions should be framed so that the answer "I don't know" is an acceptable alternative; otherwise, the client may hypothesize rather than relate facts (Lorenz *et al.*, 2011a). The technician/nurse will assist the veterinarian in historytaking. Most likely, the neurological patient who presents for physical rehabilitation will have been previously diagnosed at their primary care veterinary hospital or by a specialist in veterinary neurology.

The client should be asked for an accurate list of current medications or supplements, chronic or recurrent illnesses, and, most importantly, the level of activity to which the animal is expected or needed to return (Millis and Mankin, 2014). A detailed description of housing, including any unique features of the environment and information about the pet's daily routine, is helpful in determining the necessary skill set for a patient's activities of daily living. This description should include types of flooring, presence of obstacles such as stairs or pet doors, feeding and exercise schedules, and any other relevant details (Sims *et al.*, 2015). The patient's current ability to function in the home should be determined with thorough questioning (e.g., can they stand to eat? Is the food bowl raised? Does the surface they stand on to eat have adequate traction?).

Neurological Examination

The physical rehabilitation veterinarian along with the rehabilitation technician/nurse will conduct a thorough neurological examination. The neurologic examination should always be performed in a calm, quiet place with minimal distractions. The aim of the neurologic rehabilitation examination is to assess function (and how that will affect home activities), define current limitations, assess pain, and define goals for treatment. Surfaces of different traction and small obstacles (cavalettis, low steps, etc.) should be available to test stability and function. The rehabilitation veterinarian performs a neurological examination to document the current neurological status and become familiar with the patient's responses to measure progress throughout therapy. Sensation, motor function (including ability to stand and support weight and transition between postures), and bowel/bladder function are noted. The team will document all findings in the medical record.

The general appearance, behavior, posture, and voluntary movements should be documented while the animal can freely move around the examination room. Interaction with the client, behavior that is normal, aggressive, excited, or apathetic, and a change in mentation should be documented because this may indicate cerebral/thalamic localization. Abnormal postures such as head tilts, head turns, kyphosis, or scoliosis are noted. Assessing posture includes transitions.

When evaluating the gait, we first determine if it is normal or abnormal. If it is abnormal, then we describe the patient as ambulatory versus nonambulatory. From this point, further descriptive terminology will let us know the degree of abnormality. Paretic animals have decreased voluntary movement. The animals can be described as ambulatory, para/tetraparetic or nonambulatory, and para/tetraparetic. Tetraparesis is paresis in all four limbs. Hemiparesis is on one side of the body and paraparesis is on the pelvic limbs. If there is no voluntary movement, the patient is described as plegic.

Baseline objective data such as thigh girth, goniometry, body weight, body condition scoring, stance analysis, force plate, and kinematic analysis (when available) may also be collected and recorded in the patient history during this initial assessment (Sims *et al.*, 2015).

Neurological Examination Overview

The factors that should be assessed in a neurological examination are as follows (Rylander, 2013):

1) Mentation
2) Posture and gait
3) Cranial nerves
4) Postural reactions
5) Spinal reflexes
6) Pain on spinal palpation
7) Pain perception.

An assessment of the patient's mentation should be made and recorded. This includes

---

Box 12.1   Neurological Examination

Created by Julia Tomlinson

Basic posture, ability to hold posture, and control of postural transitions. Include degree of assistance needed to complete any transition

a) Standing (e.g., kyphosis, lordosis, scoliosis, abduction of rear limbs). Rear sink into flexion in 10 seconds. Head tilt or turn.

b) Sitting posture: ability to hold sit, rear limb position (e.g., extended or abducted), position of spine (e.g., back arched).

c) Stand–sit–stand (e.g., descends controlled for 50% then falls into sit. When standing, pull with front limbs, head down, and need 3–4 steps forward to gain full rear limb extension).

d) Side laying–sternal: Left and right. Include any limitations in flexibility.

e) Response to perturbations. For example:
   i) Head motion while standing
   ii) Leg lifts
   iii) Side challenge/sway test
   iv) Hop test.

f) Range of motion of spine and limbs, goniometry of limb joints.

g) Voluntary motions.
   i) *Cervical* – extension, lateral flexion, ventroflexion, and rotation
   ii) *Thoracolumbar* – lateral flexion, extension, and ventroflexion
   iii) Squat/sit with full flexion of lower lumbar spine/sacrum.

h) Gait
   i) Grade of ataxia
   ii) *Ground clearance of limbs* – flat surface, small step, or obstacle
   iii) Number of steps before falling (if applicable)
   iv) Knuckling (e.g., intermittent or constant).

i) *Cranial nerve assessment* – I–XII.

j) Eye position, motion, tracking, menace, palpebral, pupillary light reflex (direct and consensual), swallowing, cough reflex to tracheal pinch, and cervical muscle tone.

k) *Myotactic reflexes* – patella, sciatic, tibial, fibular (peroneal), biceps, triceps, extensor carpi radialis, etc., reduced, normal, increased, and clonus.

l) Note tremors while resting or when increasing weight-bearing load (e.g., front leg lifted, rear leg tremor).

---

their mental attitude and response to the immediate environment. The client is the best judge of subtle changes in the patient's behavior in the normal home environment. Be sure to explore this issue when you obtain the history (de Lahunta and Glass, 2009) (see Box 12.1).

Gait is evaluated if the animal can walk. A video of the patient performing a standard set of tasks (walking over ground, on a treadmill or underwater treadmill, trotting, circling, weaving, and stepping over obstacles) is often the most

useful and accurate method for recording gait abnormalities and comparing over time (Olby *et al.*, 2014; Sims *et al.*, 2015). The grade of ataxia (1–4), limb ground clearance, circumduction, dorsigrade placement of the foot (knuckling), ability of an individual limb to support weight in stance phase, or any other abnormal limb motion is noted. Remember to assess the gait using support as necessary to prevent falls. These examinations are performed by the rehabilitation veterinarian with the veterinary technician/nurse.

Neurologic examination

Observation

Mental	Alert	X	Depressed		Disoriented		Stupor		Coma	
Posture	Normal		Head tilt		Tremor		Falling			
Gait	Normal		Ataxia	X	Pelvic limbs	X	All 4		Circling	
Paresis	Pelvic limbs	X	Tetra		Hemi		Mono			
Other										

Postural reactions

Key: 4 = Exaggerated, clonus; 3 = Exaggerated; 2 = Normal; 1 = Diminished; 0 = None; NE = Not evaluated.

	Left forelimb	Right forelimb	Left hind limb	Right hind limb
Wheelbarrow	NE	NE		
Hopping	2	2	0	0
Extensor postural thrust			NE	NE
Proprioooptivo poc	2	2	0	0
Hemistand/walk	NE	NE	NE	NE
Placing–tactile	NE	NE		
Placing–visual	NE	NE		

Spinal reflexes

	Left forelimb	Right forelimb	Left hind limb	Right hind limb
Quadriceps			2	2
Extensor carpi	2	2		
Flexion	2	2	2	2
Crossed extensor	2	2	2	2
Perineal			2	2

Cranial nerves

	L	R		L	R	Comments
II, VII–Vision menace	2	2	VIII–Nystagmus, resting	2	2	Convergent strabismus was evident
II, III–Pupils resting	2	2	VIII–Nystagmus, change	2	2	
Stim L	2	2	V–Sensation	2	2	
Stim R	2	2	VII–Facial mm	2	2	
II–Fundus	2	2	V, VII–Palpebral flex	2	2	
III, IV, VI–Strabismus, resting	2	0	IX, X–Gag	2	2	
III, IV, VI, VIII–Strabismus, position	2	0	XII–Tongue	2	2	

Sensation (Locate and describe any abnormality)

Hyperesthesia	0	
Superficial pain	NE	
Cutaneous reflex	1	Absent caudal to the thoracolumbar junction
Deep pain	NE	

Figure 12.1 Neurological examination form from the Journal of the American Veterinary Medical Association What is your Diagnosis?

A cranial nerve examination should be done, evaluating cranial nerves 1–12 systematically (see Figure 12.1).

Postural reactions are tested. These include (Lorenz *et al.*, 2011a):

- proprioceptive positioning,
- wheelbarrowing,
- hopping,
- extensor postural thrust,
- hemistanding and hemiwalking (see Figure 12.2),
- placing (tactile),
- placing (visual),
- sway test, and
- tonic neck (the tonic neck reaction involves extension of the head and neck so that the nose is directed dorsally).

Spinal reflexes, including myotatic reflexes and flexor reflexes, should be evaluated.

The neurologic examination also includes *palpation for sensation* particularly for areas that are painful. This is not limited to the muscles and joints of the spine but includes the whole body. The skin dermatomes are tested where

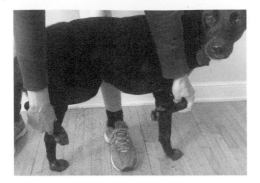

Figure 12.2 Hemistanding. The therapist uses their legs to support the trunk if needed. Hemiwalking is toward the therapist, support as needed. Level of support is noted.

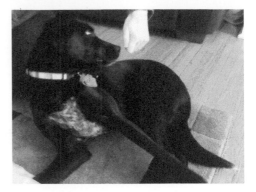

Figure 12.3 Cookie stretch to aid transition. Voluntary movement for a treat is encouraged. Assistance is given as needed and level of assistance.noted.

applicable using a fabric pinwheel or the end of a hemostat (charts can be found in veterinary neurology texts). In general, the ability to perceive *pain* is only assessed in patients with loss of motor function; however, young patients presenting with signs of a sensory neuropathy are an exception (Rylander, 2013). Muscles are palpated for tone both resting and in supporting weight where applicable. Muscle atrophy is noted, along with the innervation of that muscle (for example, atrophy of sciatic innervated muscles of the left rear is noted).

The temperament of the patient often dictates which treatments and therapeutic exercises are realistic. If a patient is aggressive or excessively fearful, it may be difficult for the client or veterinary professional to perform complex exercises (Drum, 2010). Low-stress handling should be used where possible.

Assessment of Transitions

As the patient progresses, the ability to transition, evaluating patient strength and ability to rise independently, should be documented on the form (see Box 12.1). A patient may appear to be incapable of getting up from a down position but with only light support may be able to make the transition, or a patient may need almost full body support to complete the task. These details should be noted on the examination form (see Figures 12.3–12.5).

Examples of transitions are:

- *Lateral to sternal recumbency* – guiding the patient into a sternal position will enable it to strengthen muscles used for this task.
- *Sternal recumbency to sit* – assist them with stifle flexion, limb positioning, and correct foot placement as required.

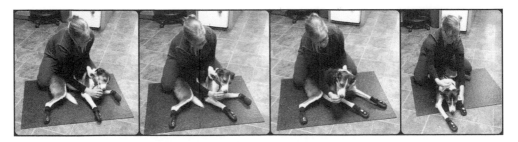

Figure 12.4 Lateral to sternal transition as demonstrated by Jenn Panko. *Source:* Courtesy of NAVTA Journal.

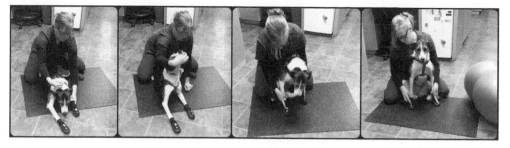

Figure 12.5 Sternal to sit transition as demonstrated by Jenn Panko. *Source:* Courtesy of NAVTA Journal.

- *Sit to stand* – from a sit with stifles in flexion and appropriate support, assist patient to stand and back down into a sit, and guide only as needed.
- *Stand to assisted walking* – assisted sling walking is a great way to provide patients with safe ambulation and weight bearing.

Evidence-Based Information About Neurologic Rehabilitation

Looking at the human literature, conditions that require neurological physical rehabilitation include stroke, traumatic brain injury (TBI), spinal cord injury, and Guillain–Barré syndrome (Jorge *et al.*, 2014). Therapy has been proven beneficial and effective for some of these patients (Brody, 1999).

Neurological diseases present unique circumstances in which veterinary rehabilitation therapy has a critical role in maintenance and recovery of function. Dysfunction of the nervous system can cause loss of motor and autonomic function and a range of sensory abnormalities, including loss of sensation (analgesia), abnormal sensations (paresthesia), and heightened sensitivity to stimuli (hyperesthesia) (Olby *et al.*, 2005). Papers published in the veterinary literature support the usefulness of rehabilitation in recovery from neurological injury and nonsurgical management of neurological conditions (Drum, 2010). Reports of case management with rehabilitation in the veterinary

literature include prolonging survival time for dogs with degenerative myelopathy (Kathmann *et al.*, 2006), having a positive influence on outcomes of dogs with fibrocartilaginous embolism (Gandini *et al.*, 2003), and improving time to return to function in patients with intervertebral disc disease (IVDD) using laser therapy after decompressive surgery (Draper *et al.*, 2012). In addition, electroacupuncture was shown to be more successful than decompressive surgery in a small study of dogs with longstanding severe neurologic deficits from IVDD (Joaquim *et al.*, 2010).

A study on early start to hydrotherapy (within 5 days of surgery for disc extrusion) in 83 dogs found that the majority of recorded complications were unlikely to be caused by the initiation time of hydrotherapy, a possible association was postulated and the authors advised caution with hydrotherapy (Mojarradi *et al.*, 2021). The authors of this chapter usually recommend hydrotherapy not begin until suture removal, about 14 days post-surgery; however, if future evidence finds earlier therapy is not associated with increased risk of complications, then earlier gait patterning may be of benefit.

As part of the veterinary rehabilitation team, the credentialed veterinary technician under the supervision and direction of a licensed credentialed rehabilitation veterinarian is an integral part of caring for hospitalized recumbent and/or neurological patients. Physical rehabilitation during recovery from neurological disorders is important not only for strengthening, gait retraining, and increasing flexibility but also for pain reduction and improvement in quality of life (Lorenz *et al.*, 2011b). Understanding the potential complications and risks, and implementing strategies to minimize these, can reduce the duration of hospitalization, improve patient comfort, and promote faster return to function.

Nursing Care of Neurological Patients in Clinic

Neurological patients often present as recumbent. This usually occurs in patients with severe spinal or generalized LMN disorders (Olby, 2010). Recumbency can cause secondary problems associated with the respiratory system, bladder and bowel function, skin, and musculoskeletal system and can affect the patient's ability to eat and drink and their attitude. The principles of managing such patients include (Olby, 2010):

- awareness of potential complications associated with recumbency;
- regular careful assessment of the patient;
- taking appropriate preventative steps; and
- early and aggressive treatment of developing complications.

Bedding for the recumbent patient should be soft to avoid decubital ulcers. Turning frequently lowers the risk of ulcers and decreases the likelihood of complications such as hypostatic pneumonia or atelectasis (Calvo, 2012).

Ambulatory patients presenting with neurological signs characterized by incoordination (ataxia) or weakness (paresis) have the potential to progress to recumbency. As these patients are not steady on their feet, providing high-traction surfaces for them to move around is essential. The top five care tips for recumbent dogs are listed in Box 12.2.

Box 12.2   Top five care tips for down dogs

1) Provide proper bedding
2) Teach bladder management to the client
3) Rotate, massage, and provide basic therapies
4) Know nutritional needs
5) Monitor for pain and neurologic changes

Source: Adapted from Weber (2016).

Respiratory System

Recumbency on its own can lead to secondary complications, including atelectasis and aspiration pneumonia, which are independent of the disease process causing recumbency. Hypoventilation can occur when a neurological disease process is severe enough to cause recumbency in all four limbs (e.g., cervical myelopathy or a severe encephalopathy). The respiration centers of the brainstem can be affected. Patients with generalized LMN diseases affecting the laryngeal and pharyngeal muscles and the esophagus (e.g., myasthenia gravis) are particularly predisposed to aspiration pneumonia. Preventative nursing care is crucial to the outcome for these patients (Calvo, 2012).

Assessment of respiration includes the following:

- Regular assessment and recording of the respiratory pattern and rate up to every 4–6 hours in severely affected patients; less often in more stable patients.
- If there is a suspicion of aspiration pneumonia, rectal temperature should be taken at least twice daily to monitor for pyrexia.

Measures to prevent respiratory complications include the following:

- Regular turning of the patient (every 4–6 hours), adopting a sternal position as often as possible using appropriate padding (record each time the position was changed: e.g., from sternal to left lateral to sternal to right lateral to sternal).

- Offer water and food only when the patient is in sternal position. Someone should sit with the patient while eating. It is beneficial for the patient to maintain an upright position for 30 minutes after feeding to decrease the risk of regurgitation and aspiration pneumonia.
- Patients who are at high risk of, or have radiographic confirmation of aspiration or hypostatic pneumonia should undergo coupage each time the patient is turned if aspiration or hypostatic pneumonia is suspected; however, this is not always well tolerated.

Coupage is gentle percussion over the thoracic cage using a cupped hand (see Figures 12.6 and 12.7). It is contraindicated in thoracic trauma patients. Thoracic auscultation should be performed at least once daily to identify abnormalities; these should be reported to the veterinarian immediately. Postural therapy with the patient supported in various positions (e.g., sitting, over a therapy ball rolled between head down–rear elevated and head up–rear down) can also be implemented to aid in the removal of excess secretions in combination with nebulization and coupage.

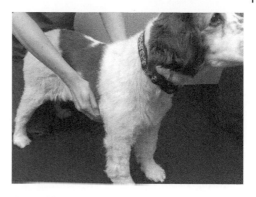

Figure 12.7 Coupage on both sides of chest.

Urination

As a rule, recumbent patients should have general bladder care. If they are paretic, they should not have difficulty urinating, but sometimes cannot move away from the urine adequately. If they are plegic, they are likely unable to urinate voluntarily and require bladder assessment or management in the form of catheterization or manual expression (see Figure 12.8). In neurological patients, urinary function often returns as soon as the patient has voluntary motor function, but this is not a predictable pattern (Olby *et al.*, 2003). A 2018 study found that after intervertebral disc extrusion (Hansen type 1) was treated with surgery, time to return to urinary continence was shorter than time to return to ambulation,

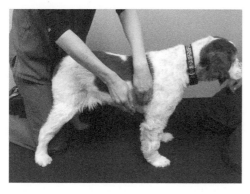

Figure 12.6 Coupage is gentle percussion over the thoracic following the lung field using a cupped hand.

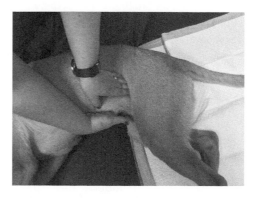

Figure 12.8 Manual expression of the bladder is a learned skill that the rehabilitation veterinary technician should know and can teach.

both correlated to preoperative functional scores (Skytte and Schmökel, 2018). This primarily applies to patients with thoracolumbar disease (only pelvic limbs are affected). Patients with cervical disease (all four limbs affected) may be reluctant to urinate as they are unable to adopt a posture for urination. Diseases of the lumbosacral spinal cord are a slight exception as these patients have urinary difficulties despite retaining voluntary motor function.

An understanding of the urinary function is critical to judge whether urination is voluntary or not. Each time the pressure in the bladder exceeds that of the urethral sphincter, urine will leak out and this may be misinterpreted as voluntary urination (see Box 12.3). Thus, other measures need to be taken to assess the presence of voluntary urination. It is important to teach those caring for the patient how to palpate the bladder and monitor for appropriate urination.

Assessment of the Bladder Includes the Following

- Palpation to assess bladder size before and after urination (training in palpation of bladders is important).

- Recording of all urinations in the medical record, whether voluntary, expressed manually, or via a catheter.
- Preferably, urinalysis on admission and testing urine with a dipstick every 2–4 days for the presence of white blood cells and protein.

Appropriate Bladder Management in Recumbent Patients Includes the Following (See Box 12.4)

- Regular visits outside to encourage the patient to urinate, at least three times daily. A Help 'Em Up Harness™ or similar device can be very helpful for maneuvering the recumbent patient if they are medium to large size.
- If unable to urinate, three bladder management options are available: manual expression every 6–8 hours (depending on bladder size), intermittent catheterization every 6–8 hours (depending on bladder size), or placement of indwelling catheter (urine bag to be checked every 4–6 hours and output recorded).

Box 12.3   Bladder palpation and expression

If the patient is recumbent, then the owner must be taught how to palpate the bladder, as well as how and when to express it.

1) Using one or both hands, depending on the patient's size, place fingers on both sides of the abdomen.
2) Start just below the ribs and squeeze gently inward.
3) Slide fingers caudal until the bladder is located; palpate for size and tone (the bladder has been described as a water balloon in the abdomen).

4) Apply gentle pressure to express the urine.
5) Avoid expression of the bladder if:
   - the bladder is small (this will allow it to fill and the patient is more likely to feel the need to urinate); or
   - the bladder has a strong tone (it may have lost its elasticity from being overdistended for too long or maybe an upper motor neuron bladder that requires medication to relax the detrusor and urethral sphincter muscles).

Note: If the bladder must be expressed frequently then this could be painful.
Source: Adapted from Weber (2016).

<table>
<tr><td>

Box 12.4   Monitoring urine stream and quantity

Owners should be asked to monitor their patient's urination by answering a few basic questions:

- Can the pet posture to urinate?
- Does the stream come out normally (forcefully) or does it come out in dribbles or sporadic?
- Is this a normal amount of urine or has it decreased?
- Does the urine have an odor?
- Is the urine a normal color?

Note: Any patient who cannot urinate should be reported to the rehabilitation veterinarian immediately.
Source: Adapted from Weber (2016).

</td></tr>
</table>

- Medications to improve bladder function will be prescribed by the veterinarian if appropriate.
- Bedding must allow liquid to be absorbed and pass through away from the patient's skin (e.g., acrylic bedding). If incontinence sheets are used directly under the patient's skin, they must fulfill this criterion too.
- Always keep the patient clean and dry, clip long hair if required to enable hygiene management, and to allow accurate assessment of urine scalding developing/progressing.

Defecation

Fecal incontinence can occur because the external anal sphincter has been anatomically disrupted, or the nerves damaged or destroyed. Nerve damage, spinal cord disease, or a degenerative disorder may reduce or stop sphincter function. Fecal incontinence affects dogs with severe lumbosacral disease, leading to a lack of voluntary control over defecation and severe soiling. Cats with neurological problems have a tendency toward constipation. It is important to keep the patient clean and dry always. Lactulose may be used (especially in cats) to aid defecation if constipation is suspected, as manual evacuation is difficult in cats. Patients receiving opioid analgesia should be monitored closely for constipation due to reduced intestinal motility, and pelvic trauma patients should be monitored for tenesmus. In both cases, treatment by the rehabilitation veterinarian to aid in defecation may be needed.

Skin Care

Recumbent patients are at risk of developing dermatitis secondary to urine scald and fecal soiling and the development of decubital ulcers over pressure points. In addition, skin lesions can develop if the patient is dragging themselves or a limb over rough ground.

Complications can be prevented by the use of appropriate soft bedding that absorbs the liquid. This includes using incontinence pads; however, care must be taken to avoid placing the pad directly beneath the patient's skin as the urine will only disperse across the pad, resulting in increased contact time and leading to urine scalds. Acrylic absorbent bedding should be placed directly beneath the patient, followed by the incontinence pad. This prevents multiple layers of bedding from becoming soiled and avoids the recumbent patient from lying in their own urine. Ensure appropriate padding is used around pressure points and perform systematic bony point checks twice daily to monitor for skin redness or early development of decubital ulcers. The patient must be turned regularly (every 4–6 hours) and pressure points massaged to increase local blood flow. If necessary, clip the hair in the perineal region. There should be prompt removal of soiled bedding. See earlier section about appropriate bladder management. The patient must always be kept dry and clean.

Treatment of Skin Complications Includes the Following

- Cleaning of dermatitis with a dilute chlorhexidine solution followed by thorough drying and application of a barrier cream.
- Avoiding excessive moisture around affected areas and applying thick layers of barrier cream, which will only harbor and insulate bacteria. A thin layer of barrier cream that can be easily wiped off is more suitable.
- Applying a dilute solution of bicarbonate of soda and cooled boiled water. This is very effective as it neutralizes the acidity of urine on the skin, reducing scalds or skin irritation. Carefully make sure it is applied to skin folds (for example, those of the testes). The area should be doused and left to dry at room temperature. This can be repeated 3–4 times daily.
- Ensuring that, if decubital ulcers develop, pressure is no longer placed over that region. This can be done by using a doughnut-shaped cushion (in some cases, suturing to surrounding skin).
- Debridement of necrotic tissue.
- Elizabethan collars to prevent the patient from licking or chewing the region.

Care of Toenails

Toenails should be checked and trimmed regularly for the comfort of the patient. Excessively long toenails can hinder the patient from standing/walking when and if they can accomplish this task.

Muscle and Joint Problems

Neurological problems with paralysis can cause muscle atrophy and contracture, and deterioration of joints and their associated soft tissues. Muscle and joint pain can occur secondary to these changes.

Management of These Problems Includes

- Treatment of pain.

- An individualized rehabilitation plan should be started as soon as possible. Exercises for the client at home can be developed.
- Passive range of motion (PROM) and massage to help maintain joint mobility.
- A nutritional plan.

Attitude or Demeanor

Recumbency can contribute to frustration and anxiousness, which can be heightened by pain (Lorenz *et al.*, 2011b).

Demeanor May Be Improved by the Following

- Ensuring the animal's comfort through pain management and appropriate bedding. This includes the amount of contact with humans because some patients prefer to be quiet while others prefer to see and have regular interactions with humans.
- Arranging regular contact with the client.
- Taking the canine patient outside regularly. This is not appropriate for cats unless they are used to harness/leash walking. A cat can have a period of free exploration in a secure cat ward under supervision.
- Placing the patient in a standing position and using support as necessary. Additionally, this helps with pulmonary, musculoskeletal systems, and skin.
- Regular manual therapies (PROM, massage, etc.).

Positioning

The rehabilitation team must be cognizant of the risks facing the recumbent patient. Skin and pulmonary integrity can be compromised if the patient is not on a proper turning schedule. Positioning is important and should be noted on patient charts (Francis, 2007). The patient should be on either side in lateral recumbency or sternal recumbency, sitting and standing, if possible.

Pain

Neurological patients experience pain. Many patients are in pain caused by their primary disease, surgical intervention, or secondary effects of recumbency and spasticity (Lorenz *et al.*, 2011b). The level of pain should be assessed 2–4 times daily depending on the patient. A pain scoring system is most useful for consistency (see Chapter 3).

Manual therapy, ice, heat, electrical stimulation, and therapeutic ultrasound may be used depending on the severity and phase of recovery (acute versus subacute) (Francis, 2007). Because pain-free animals are relaxed and cooperative, recover faster and more completely, and clients are much happier and more compliant with recommendations when their pet is comfortable (Thomas *et al.*, 2014), pain medications should be used to allow for patient comfort.

Nutrition

A recumbent patient's metabolic needs differ from those of a healthy patient (Weber, 2016). The following formula is used to calculate daily needs:

$$\text{Resting energy requirements}\left(\text{RER}\right)\left(\text{kcal/day}\right)$$
$$= 70 \times \text{body weight}\left(\text{kg}\right)^{0.75}$$

Recumbent patients may have reduced appetite or even be anorexic because of pain or depression. The patient needs to be encouraged to eat, although overfeeding of the obese patient needs to be avoided. Extra weight impacts joints and spine when recumbent and can delay return to ambulation because more strength is needed to move a body of higher mass. Do not forget patients' daily water requirements; water intake is important to reduce the risk of cystitis and urinary tract infections in down dogs with bladder impairment. Daily water intake should be 50 mg/kg body weight. Encourage patients to drink by adding small amounts of low-sodium chicken or beef broth to their water. Syringing water or administering subcutaneous fluids may also be recommended in some situations (Weber, 2016).

Risks Affecting Hospitalized Recumbent or Neurological Patients (Abramson, 2009)

The recumbent or neurological patient in hospital is at risk of a range of conditions that the veterinary technician/nurse should be alert to (Abramson, 2009):

- Prolonged or permanent loss of mobility and independence secondary to disuse atrophy
- Chronic pain
- Decubital ulcers
- Urine scald
- Depression
- Self-inflicted trauma
- Reduced lung capacity and compliance
- Obesity.

Key Therapeutic Points (Davidson, 2009)

In addition, the following key therapeutic points should be noted (Davidson, 2009):

- Bladder care must be initiated for incontinent animals to prevent atony and treat infections.
- Attention to bedding and hygiene helps prevent decubital ulcers.
- Neuromuscular electrical stimulation may be used to strengthen muscles.
- Massage can reduce muscle spasms and pain.
- PROM can be used to maintain joint motion and health.
- Assisted standing, balancing, and various types of exercise can be incorporated, depending on the animal's neurologic status.

Types of Neurological Conditions

It is important that the veterinary technician or nurse is familiar with neurological conditions that affect their patients. Being able to discuss the disease with the client, so that the rehabilitation veterinarian's protocols may be carried out, is imperative. Neurological conditions can affect the animal's mobility, balance, strength, and coordination as well as contribute to pain or discomfort (Price, 2014a).

Canine Conditions

Intervertebral Disc Disease (IVDD)

IVDD is a syndrome of pain and/or neurological deficits, resulting from herniation or protrusion of the disc. Although a normal disc can herniate because of major trauma, typically herniation is secondary to preexisting degeneration of the disc (Jeffery *et al.*, 2016). Disc degeneration is associated with decreased water and proteoglycan concentration (Steinberg and Coates, 2013). This dehydration reduces the ability of the disc to function as a hydraulic cushion and predisposes to displacement of a portion of the disc.

There are two types of disc degeneration: chondroid and fibrous metaplasia. Chondroid metaplasia is most common in chondrodystrophic breeds and causes a progressive transformation of the gelatinous nucleus pulposus to hyaline cartilage. This type of degeneration redisposes to disc extrusion, where disc material is displaced beyond the outer edge of the annulus (also called Hansen type I). Fibrous metaplasia is an age-related degeneration process that occurs in any breed but is more common in non-chondrodystrophic dogs seven years of age and older. It is characterized by a fibrous collagenization of the nucleus pulposus and degeneration of the annulus fibrosus. Fibrous metaplasia predisposes to disc protrusion, in which disc material is displaced from the disc space but is contained within an intact annulus (also called Hansen type II). Non-chondrodystrophic breed dogs can also suffer extrusions, and less commonly, chondrodystrophic breeds suffer protrusions (Thomas *et al.*, 2014). Hansen type-III disc disease is also known as "acute non-compressive" or "high-velocity low volume" disc disease. In this case, there is a sudden onset of disease, typically with heavy exercise or trauma, causing a normal nucleus to explode from a sudden tear in the annulus.

Trauma

Automobile accidents, gunshot wounds, falls, and dogfight injuries are common causes of traumatic spinal cord injuries. Spinal injuries may consist of vertebral luxation, vertebral fracture, vertebral fracture/luxation, contusions, concussions, and hemorrhage, as well as traumatic disc herniation.

Peripheral Nerve Injury

Common causes of peripheral nerve injury include fractures (e.g., femoral fracture that damages the sciatic nerve), intramuscular injection (usually affecting the sciatic nerve), traumatic brachial plexus nerve root avulsion, and iatrogenic causes including swelling, trauma to nerve, and hemorrhage that may sometimes occur in surgery.

Neoplastic Disease

Spinal tumors are classified by their location as extradural, subarachnoid (intradural extramedullary), and intramedullary. Extradural neoplasia is most common and includes osteosarcoma, multiple myeloma, fibrosarcoma, chondrosarcoma, hemangiosarcoma, and lymphosarcoma. Extradural lymphosarcoma is the most common spinal tumor in cats and may be secondary to infection with the feline leukemia virus (Thomas *et al.*, 2014). Subarachnoid tumors include nerve sheath tumors, meningioma, lymphosarcoma, and neuroepithelioma. Intramedullary tumors include glioma, lymphosarcoma, and hemangiosarcoma. Metastatic tumors, including metastatic carcinomas and sarcomas, may occur in any location. Spinal neoplasia is more common in middle-aged or older animals (Thomas *et al.*, 2014).

Degenerative Myelopathy

This is a slowly progressive degenerative disease of the CNS that most severely affects the thoracic spinal cord segments. It is inherited as an autosomal recessive trait and is associated with a mutation in the superoxide dismutase 1 (*SOD1*) gene, like the familial form of amyotrophic lateral sclerosis in human patients (Lou Gehrig's disease) (Awano *et al.*, 2009). Degenerative myelopathy affects older dogs, usually more than eight years of age. German Shepherds, Rhodesian Ridgebacks, Pembroke and Cardigan Welsh Corgis, Boxers, and Chesapeake Bay Retrievers are most affected, although cases have been documented in several other large-breed dogs and crossbreeds (Coates and Wininger, 2010). The degenerative myelopathy is mostly caused by a mutation in superoxid dismutase 1 gene (SOD1A); however, a mutation in SOD1B occurs in the Bernese Mountain Dog. Genetic testing is available; however, having the gene does not confirm having the disease.

Myasthenia Gravis

Myasthenia gravis is a neuromuscular disorder (Khorzad *et al.*, 2011) caused by a reduction in the number of functional nicotinic acetylcholine receptors (AChR) on the postsynaptic membrane of the neuromuscular junction. Myasthenia gravis exists either as a rare congenital disease or more commonly as an acquired autoimmune disease, resulting in a deficiency of nicotinic AChR. Acetylcholine is essential for muscle contraction at the neuromuscular junction. The defect in transmission resulting from AChR loss leads to focal or generalized muscle weakness and exhaustion.

Cervical Spondylomyelopathy

Caudal cervical spondylomyelopathy, or wobbler syndrome, is a disorder caused by abnormal development of the cervical vertebrae resulting in compression of the spinal cord. Middle aged (7–9 years) Doberman Pinschers and young (1–4 years) giant-breed dogs (Great Danes, Mastiffs, Rottweilers, Bernese, and Swiss Mountain dogs) are most commonly affected (da Costa, 2010).

Fibrocartilaginous Embolic Myelopathy (FCEM)

FCEM is an acute infarction of the spinal cord caused by a vascular embolus of fibrocartilage, probably originating from the intervertebral disc. Adult large- or giant-breed dogs and miniature Schnauzers are most affected. This disease is less common in small dogs, chondrodystrophic dogs, and cats. The onset is sudden and often associated with activities such as running or playing. Any region of the spinal cord may be affected, and the spinal cord segments involved dictate the specific neurological deficits. In severe cases, there is a loss of deep pain perception caudal to the lesion (Thomas *et al.*, 2014).

Discospondylitis

Discospondylitis is an infection of the intervertebral disc and adjacent vertebral bodies. It is usually caused by hematogenous spread of organisms from sites elsewhere in the body, such as the urinary tract, skin, or mouth. Penetrating wounds, surgery, or plant material migration can cause direct infection of the disc space or vertebra. In certain geographic regions, migrating plant material such as grass awns is a relatively common cause of vertebral osteomyelitis and discospondylitis of the L2–L4 vertebrae (Thomas *et al.*, 2014).

Polyneuropathies

Breed-associated polyneuropathies, such as polyneuropathy of hypothyroidism and laryngeal-paralysis-associated polyneuropathy, are sometimes seen.

Feline Conditions

Intervertebral Disc Disease

IVDD is encountered much more rarely in cats compared with dogs, although both Hansen type I (disc extrusion) and type II (disc protrusion) herniations have been observed (Sharp, 2012b). Type II cases are more common in cats, though they are still rarely found clinically, probably due to the slowly progressive nature of the condition and the lack of obvious clinical signs in this species.

Fibrocartilaginous Embolism

This is rare in cats and, as in dogs, is associated with variable clinical signs and prognosis. A full physiotherapy assessment is essential to identify the specific functional problems of the individual animal and allow the selection of appropriate physiotherapy interventions to treat those problems.

Brachial Plexus Avulsion

This type of traumatic neuropathy is common in cats, with clinical signs including muscle weakness (commonly called "dropped elbow"), proprioceptive deficits (dragging of the foot), absence of spinal reflexes, and deep pain perception. The prognosis is often poor for these animals, but the provision of physiotherapy can help to reduce edema, maintain circulation to the affected area, prevent contractures, and maintain activity in muscles (Bockstahler and Levine, 2011).

Trauma

Automobile accidents, falls, being kicked, abused, or fighting injuries are common (Sharp, 2012b).

Tail Pull Injuries

"Tail pull injury" or sacrococcygeal subluxation is a common neurological condition in cats and can also occur in dogs, albeit rarely (Davies and Walmsley, 2012). It occurs most frequently because of a road traffic accident and results in a varying degree of trauma to the sacral spinal cord segments and cauda equina. The neurological deficits associated with sacrocaudal luxation can include paraparesis, but this is usually transient. The most severe sequelae relate to anal sphincter and bladder dysfunction. ***Never*** lift a patient by their tail.

Establishing Goals

Long-term goals define the patient's expected level of performance at the end of the rehabilitation process. Short-term goals are the component skills established at each phase of rehabilitation that will be needed to attain long-term goals. This plan helps establish the at-home treatment plan that is given to clients (Sturges and Woelz, 2005).

Goals

The goal with neurological patients is to challenge them without causing excess neuromuscular fatigue, pushing them in a positive way with lots of praise and encouragement. The purpose of the exercises is to stimulate proprioceptive tracts to aid body positional awareness and balance, improve muscular strength, and attempt to pattern a correct gait as nerves recover. Typical objectives in rehabilitating patients with neurological diseases are to minimize pain, reestablish normal neural pathways, prevent secondary complications, and, if possible, return the animal to independent function. Therapy also aims to counteract the effects of inactivity. It is essential not to worsen neurologic function or pain in patients with spinal instability (Thomas *et al.*, 2014). A program that is painful or stressful for the patient is unlikely to be effective, may cause the patient to become aggressive, and will potentially damage the human–animal bond between client and patient (Sims *et al.*, 2015).

Passive Manual Therapies for Dogs and Cats

Passive exercises should be performed for neurological patients who lack voluntary movement or strength or whose proprioceptive deficits preclude a normal gait (Olby *et al.*, 2005).

Passive Range of Motion

PROM is commonly prescribed for neurologically impaired patients and is frequently combined with stretching of the periarticular connective tissues and skeletal muscle. The primary benefit of PROM is protection against stiffening or fibrosis of the joint. Other benefits may include prevention of cartilage atrophy, replenishment of the synovial fluid (primary source of nutrients for the cartilage), improved local circulation, and stimulation of sensory and proprioceptive pathways in the synovium and periarticular structures (Sims *et al.*, 2015). Placing each joint through a normal range of motion will help to maintain joint health in patients who have deficits in voluntary movement.

PROM should be performed with the patient lying in lateral recumbency on a well-padded surface. The uppermost limbs should be put through gentle flexion and extension of each joint within the patient's comfort zone. Once each joint has been put through 15–20 cycles, each limb may be put through bicycling movements for another 15–20 repetitions. The patient is then flipped, and the exercise is repeated on the contralateral limbs. This exercise should be performed 3–4 times per day in a recumbent patient.

Massage

Massage is another passive therapy with multiple benefits. It can help alleviate pain and stress associated with recent injury or surgery. Massage aims to improve both local and whole-body circulation and lymphatic drainage, allowing for increased tissue oxygenation and more rapid resolution of edema. Sensory stimulation that could encourage nerve firing in the affected tissues is an added benefit. Massage is clearly pleasurable for most rehabilitation patients, and beginning a therapy session with a whole-body massage in a calming environment may improve patient compliance, thereby increasing the effectiveness of the therapy program. Massage of a mildly contracted muscle group may also be beneficial in restoring its function and should be performed 2–3 times per day after pre-warming the region (Olby *et al.*, 2005).

Acupuncture

Acupuncture can be considered a passive therapy because it does not require the active involvement of the patient and relies primarily on direct mechanical stimulation to achieve its effects. The scientific literature is mixed regarding the therapeutic benefits of acupuncture overall, but the evidence may be more encouraging when examining the benefits of acupuncture specifically for neurogenic pain and the facilitation of nerve signaling (Sims *et al.*, 2015). Electroacupuncture has been shown to improve analgesia and accelerate the recovery of motor functions in dogs with IVDD (Huntingford and Petty, 2022). A study with 80 paraplegic dogs concluded that those dogs treated with prednisone, acupuncture, or electroacupuncture had significantly less pain, recovered to ambulation at a faster rate, and had decreased relapses than those that were treated with prednisone alone (Han *et al.*, 2010). Only a veterinarian certified in veterinary acupuncture may perform this therapy.

Therapeutic Exercise for Dogs and Cats

Therapeutic exercise programs focus on proprioception and balance, muscle strengthening, reeducation of normal posture, and gait training. Proprioception and balance work are important for the neurologically impaired patient. Weight shift training is used following an injury or postoperatively, initially training the patient to use the affected limb and later encouraging appropriate weight distribution during activities of daily living.

Postural reeducation addresses the static postures (stand and sit down) as well as the transitions between these postures; it is often best to start with a sit transition as this is learned early in the life of most dogs and reinforced regularly, meaning the conscious recognition of the command and motor nerve output from the brain should be "strong."

Gait retraining addresses the patient who does not properly use one or more limbs or who has developed an abnormal gait behavior or pattern.

The rehabilitation veterinarian will prescribe which therapeutic exercises will be used for both short- and long-term goals. The rehabilitation veterinary technician or nurse will carry out these exercises with the patient and will be responsible for teaching the exercises to be used by the client at home.

Targeted exercise therapy aids in the management or prevention of many of the consequences of immobility, including atrophy of soft and bony tissues, stiffening, or fibrosis, maintaining proper proteoglycan matrix in the articular cartilage, and stimulating the synovium to replenish the joint fluid (McCauley and Van Dyke, 2013). Exercise therapy stimulates transmission of nerve signals, reinforces proprioceptive and motor pathways, and aids in the restoration of muscle memory for standing, walking, and other activities that require minimal or no conscious effort in the healthy patient (Sims *et al.*, 2015). Exercises that aid in development or preservation of the core muscle groups along the spine and abdomen are particularly helpful in improving a patient's ability to handle transitional movements (Sharp, 2008). The client is often helpful in designing exercises that can be used at home with their own equipment or household items (see Box 12.5).

The neurologically impaired animal may require a cart or sling during active-assisted range of motion and other exercises. A lift can be used in clinics (see Figure 12.9). Support should be used if necessary and may be in the form of splints or orthoses (see Chapter 11).

Therapeutic Modalities for Dogs and Cats

Thermotherapy

Thermotherapy is the use of superficial heat or cold as a therapeutic modality for the treatment of disease or trauma. It may be applied using many different methods (Dragone *et al.*, 2014). It is discussed in detail in Chapter 15.

Therapeutic Ultrasound

The application of therapeutic ultrasound to soft tissues may help to alleviate pain while improving tissue blood supply and speeding up healing. Ultrasound may be

---

Box 12.5   Therapeutic exercises for the neurological patient

- *Neuromuscular facilitation* – Visualize and perform a passive running pattern with the dog's front or hind leg. Be aware of stimuli under the pad of the foot when appropriate in the cycle. This helps to ingrain the pattern of movement and stimulate the neural pathways connected with it. It can be an aid in neural reprogramming and regeneration (Edge-Hughes, 2013).
- *Vibration* – The use of a small electrical vibrator can help stimulate muscle contractions in neurological cases.
- *Ice massage* – Water can be frozen in a styrofoam or plastic cup and then applied to the affected area directly. To perform the massage, the therapist exposes a portion of the ice surface, holds the cup, and applies the ice surface directly to the patient's skin. The ice surface is moved in a continuous, circular fashion across the treatment area for 5–10 minutes (Hanks *et al.*, 2015).
- *Tapping* – Fast and steady tapping over a muscle belly can lead to muscle contractions as well as stimulus of neural receptors in muscles and tendons.
- *Weight-bearing techniques*
- *Postural reactions (these are not reflexes) from perturbations* – Hopping, parawalking, wheelbarrowing, directional rolling over an inflatable therapy ball, and tilting table.
- *Land treadmill exercise* – Active assisted range of motion is possible with the therapist seated over the treadmill behind the patient.
- *Underwater treadmill or supported swimming*
- *Supported standing*
- *Rhythmical stabilizations* – With the animal standing squarely, the therapist places gentle pressure over the pelvis or cranial thoracic region and gently "bounces" the animal up and down. The bouncing motion should be relatively rapid, with only enough recovery time to regain the normal standing position. This generates rapid firing of postural muscles in an isometric fashion, which is ideal for weakly ambulatory or significantly ataxic patients (Drum *et al.*, 2015).
- *Tensor bandaging* – Wrap a bandage loosely around the thoracic and pelvic limbs. This helps to create awareness and connection between the front and hind ends.
- *Joint compressions* (veterinarian or physical therapist only) – Place one hand above the joint and the other hand below the joint. Push the two joints together.
- *Tactile sensory stimuli* – Any sensory stimuli you can provide to the superficial skin receptors can be helpful. Examples include brushing, gently pulling hair, or rubbing the hair in the wrong direction, zigzag petting or tapping, pinching, or picking up the skin, thermal stimulus using ice or a hot pack (with care). *Clapping over body* – Use your hand in a cupped position so that you do not slap the patient. *Wringing the limb* – Gently move your hands circumferentially around the limb of the patient as though you were wringing out a wet towel, up and down the limb (Edge-Hughes, 2013).
- *Acupressure* – This involves application of pressure at acupuncture points. Laser can be used on acupuncture points.

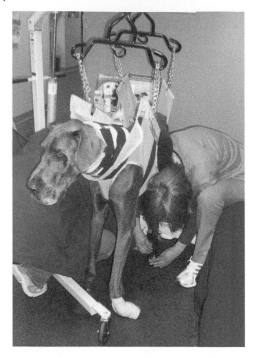

Figure 12.9 Use of a Hoyer lift to support a large patient.

beneficial for epaxial muscles that are experiencing muscle spasms. Its use is contraindicated over an exposed spinal cord, and continuous-mode ultrasound is not recommended at or near the surgical site in postoperative neurosurgical patients (Olby *et al.*, 2005). The modality is very useful in the treatment of contractures when used in continuous mode; extreme care is needed in patients with reduced sensation. This technique is discussed in detail in Chapter 18.

Neuromuscular Electrical Stimulation (NMES)

The application of NMES in patients with acute spinal cord disease may be beneficial to increase tissue perfusion, decrease pain, and delay the onset of disuse muscle atrophy. In patients with LMN disease, stimulation of the affected muscle groups will delay the onset and severity of neurogenic muscle atrophy (Olby *et al.*, 2005). The use of

electrical stimulation is preferred for muscle groups that are not already experiencing spasms. It is contraindicated over surgical sites following a laminectomy or pediculectomy until adequate healing has taken place. NMES should be applied to the muscle groups of affected limbs once a day for 15 minutes each until the patient is ambulating with mild-to-moderate ataxia. This technique is discussed in detail in Chapter 17.

Laser Therapy

Laser therapy has been increasingly incorporated into rehabilitation programs for a variety of conditions, including skin wounds; muscle, tendon, and ligament injuries; neurologic conditions; arthritis; and pain (Millis and Saunders, 2014). This modality is discussed in detail in Chapter 16.

A Special Word About Cats

One must think like a cat to have success. The treatment room must be calm. A peaceful environment encourages a relaxed mood in preparation for rehabilitation treatment. Rehabilitation programs can benefit from using a cat's love of play and its natural hunting instincts. This may allow a more hands-off approach, which is beneficial for cats that are particularly aggressive or fearful (Sharp, 2012b).

Keep It Short

All rehabilitation sessions should be kept short to maintain interest and prevent boredom (Price, 2014b). Activities should be introduced at a level appropriate to the recovery of the cat and progressed to accommodate the cat's improvement.

Make It Fun

Devices that demand activity to variously release food (treat balls), encourage the tracking/hunting instinct (toys and motorized units), or involve reaching observational positions (climbing towers and window sills) can all be beneficial if used appropriately. Placing or hiding food in positions that encourage activity to access it (top of stairs, top of climbing frame, requiring climbing over/under obstacles and/or through tunnels), or simply moving food regularly between rooms can all increase activity levels (Sharp, 2012b). Play combines elements of predatory behavior, including exploration, investigation, stalking, chasing, attacking, pouncing, leaping, swatting, and grasping, and the cat can be provided with a variety of targets. Toys that bounce or move in ways that entice the cat to play can be usefully provided, and successful interactive toys might include zigzag balls, mice on elastic string, or fishing rod toys with fur or feathers. Moving spots of light produced by mirrors, laser pointers, or torches might stimulate some cats to chase, although limiting play just to chasing lights can lead to frustration as the chase is never successfully concluded and the cat is never able to catch and "kill" the target.

Create an Enriched Environment

The development of an enriched environment can provide a valuable means of exercising cats in a "hands-off" manner. Creating a small area (or using a small room) filled with obstacles, as well as hidden treats or toys, may encourage an inquisitive cat to explore and find the hidden "gems" (Sharp, 2012a). A variety of obstacles should be included that require the cat to climb over, crawl under, and creep through them to promote joint mobility, balance, and general activity. Scratching posts can encourage joint flexibility and strength (Sharp, 2012b). The inclusion of various surfaces (bean bags, cushions, and pillows) can provide sensory input as well as promote strength and balance as the cat walks over them to explore the area.

Client Education and Support During Home Therapy

The approach is to teach as much as you can to clients so that the treatment of their pet can be carried over into the home. Time is taken to educate clients about their pet's condition, and home exercises and instructions are given so they can help their pet recover faster at home. The rehabilitation veterinary technician or nurse plays a key role in teaching the client how to manage the needs of a patient with limited mobility, possibly more so than any other clinician involved in the medical management of patients with neurologic injury or disease (Sims *et al.*, 2015). Clients bear the greatest responsibility for patient care once discharged from the hospital. They should be informed about the patient's nursing care needs and signs of complications that need to be addressed by their primary veterinarian. A thorough description, ideally with visual or written aids, of any home therapies will improve the client's confidence and increase compliance.

The technician should help the therapist evaluate the client's ability to understand and safely perform the recommended treatments. Financial, physical, or scheduling restrictions facing the client or pet in the home environment should be discussed because they impact the type, number, and frequency of any prescribed treatments. In cases where the family schedule or home environment cannot accommodate the needs of the patient in the near term, the therapist may recommend hospitalizing or boarding the patient for inpatient care during the initial phases of the physiotherapy program. The use of readily available or inexpensive materials minimizes the burden on the client to seek out or develop equipment for their pet's therapy.

It is important to include information such as a description or demonstration of the activities to be performed, how frequently the treatments should be performed, signs that indicate a treatment is not well tolerated or ineffective, a basic understanding of relevant anatomy, and an approximate timeline for the anticipated results. The rehabilitation team should be prepared not only to provide guidance on medical and nursing care but also to address concerns related to patient welfare, related to the emotional, physical, and financial burdens of managing a pet with special needs, and related to quality-of-life and end-of-life decisions.

Many clients are overwhelmed with the degree of their pet's disability and the tremendous impact of their care on their home routine. Often, clients do not reach a full realization of their new responsibilities until several days or weeks after the diagnosis is obtained and the patient is discharged from the hospital. The therapist needs to set realistic expectations for the client pertaining to recovery or the rate of decline expected. Clients will greatly benefit from referral to a rehabilitation team who can help manage the emotional fallout from caring for a paralyzed or debilitated pet (see also Chapter 14).

Conclusions

Neurological rehabilitation can be among the most challenging and rewarding work for the veterinary rehabilitation team. Determining time for recovery is often the most difficult task. It is important to remember that recovery times can be extremely variable and are intrinsically linked to the neurologic condition, underlying medical conditions, and neurologic status upon presentation for rehabilitation. One must consider time available for treatment, both for the veterinary team and the client, as it is often not feasible to perform all exercises and modalities on a single patient. Some exercises may not be applicable or possible for some patients. Each patient requires a rehabilitation protocol that is specifically designed for that patient's neurologic condition, client expectations and level of participation, and expertise of the veterinary team.

References

Abramson CJ (2009) Nursing care for the "down" dog. In *Proceedings of the American Animal Hospital Association Conference*, Phoenix, Arizona, pp. 721–722.

Awano, T., Johnson, G.S., Wade, C.M. et al. (2009). Genome-wide association analysis reveals a SOD1 mutation in canine degenerative myelopathy that resembles amyotrophic lateral sclerosis. *Proc Natl Acad Sci USA* 106 (8): 2794–2799.

Bockstahler, B. and Levine, D. (2011). Physical therapy and rehabilitation. In: *The Feline Patient*, 4the (ed. G.D. Norsworthy, G.S. Fooshee, M.A. Crystal, et al.), 687–690. Ames, IA: Wiley/Blackwell.

Brody, L.T. (1999). Mobility impairment. In: *Therapeutic Exercise: Moving Toward Function* (ed. C.M. Hall and L.T. Brody), 57–83. Philadelphia, PA: Williams and Wilkins.

Calvo G (2012) Rehabilitation nursing goals. Presented at the WSAVA/FECAVA/BSAVA World Congress, April 12–15, 2012, Birmingham, UK.

Coates, J.R. and Wininger, F.A. (2010). Canine degenerative myelopathy. *Vet Clin North Am Small Anim Pract* 40 (5): 929–950.

Coleman, M.P. and Freeman, M.R. (2010). Wallerian degeneration, Wld, and Nmnat. *Annu Rev Neurosci* 33 (1): 245–267.

Davidson JR (2009) Rehabilitation of spinal cord injury. Presented at the 81st Western Veterinary Conference, February 15–19, 2009, Las Vegas, NV

Davies, E. and Walmsley, G. (2012). Management of tail pull injuries in cats. *In Practice* 34: 27–33.

da Costa, R.C. (2010). Cervical spondylomyelopathy (wobbler syndrome) in dogs. *Vet Clin North Am Small Anim Pract* 40 (5): 881–913.

De Lahunta, A. and Glass, E. (2009). The neurologic examination. In: *Veterinary Neuroanatomy and Clinical Neurology*, 3rde, 487–501. St. Louis, MO: Saunders/Elsevier.

Dragone L, Heinrichs K, Levine D, *et al.* (2014) Superficial thermal modalities. In *Canine Rehabilitation and Physical Therapy*, 2nd edn (eds. D Millis and D Levine). Elsevier/Saunders, Philadelphia, PA, p. 312.

Draper, W.E., Schubert, T.A., Clemmons, R.M., and Miles, S.A. (2012). Low-level laser therapy reduces time to ambulation in dogs after hemilaminectomy: A preliminary study. *J Small Anim Pract* 53 (8): 465–469.

Drum, M.G. (2010). Physical rehabilitation of the canine neurologic patient. *Vet Clin Small Anim* 40: 181–193.

Drum, M.G., Marcellin-Little, D.J., and Davis, M.S. (2015). Principles and applications of therapeutic exercises for small animals. *Vet Clin Small Anim* 45: 73–90.

Edge-Hughes L (2013) *Therapeutic Exercises for the Neurological Patient*. The Canine Fitness Centre, Calgary, Alberta, Canada. www.caninefitness.com.

Francis M (2007) Rehabilitation for patients with neurological diseases. *Proceedings from ACVIM Conference*, June 6–9, 2007, Seattle, WA.

Gandini, G., Cizinauskas, S., Lang, J. et al. (2003). Fibrocartilaginous embolism in 75 dogs: Clinical findings and factors influencing the recovery rate. *J Small Anim Pract* 44 (2): 76–80.

Han, H.J., Yoon, H.Y., and Kim, J.Y. (2010). Clinical Effect of additional electroacupuncture on thoracolumbar intervertebral disc herniation in 80 paraplegic dogs. *Am J Chin Med* 38: 1015–1025.

Hanks, J., Levine, D., and Bockstahler, B. (2015). Physical agent modalities in physical therapy and rehabilitation of small animals. *Vet Clin Small Anim* 45: 29–44.

Huntingford, J.L. and Petty, M.C. (2022). Evidence-based application of acupuncture for pain management in companion animal medicine. *Vet Sci* 9: 252. https://doi.org/10.3390/vetsci9060252.

Jeffery, N.D., Barker, A.K., Hu, H.Z. et al. (2016). Factors associated with recovery from paraplegia in dogs with loss of pain perception in the pelvic limbs following intervertebral disk herniation. *J Am Vet Med Assoc* 248 (4): 386–394.

Joaquim, J.G., Luna, S.P., Brondani, J.T. et al. (2010). Comparison of decompressive surgery, electroacupuncture, and decompressive surgery followed by electroacupuncture for the treatment of dogs with intervertebral disk disease with long-standing severe neurologic deficits. *J Am Vet Med Assoc* 236 (11): 1225–1229.

Jorge, L.L., Mota do Nascimento de Brito, A., and Garcia Marchi, F.H. (2014). New rehabilitation models for neurologic inpatients in Brazil. *Disabil Rehabil* 37 (3): 268–273.

Kathmann, I., Cizinauskas, S., Doherr, M.G. et al. (2006). Daily controlled physiotherapy increases survival time in dogs with suspected degenerative myelopathy. *J Vet Intern Med* 20 (4): 927–932.

Khorzad, R., Whelan, M., Allen Sisson, A., and Shelton, G.D. (2011). Myasthenia gravis in dogs with an emphasis on treatment and critical care management. *J Vet Emerg Crit Care* 21 (3): 193–208.

Lorenz MD, Coates JR, and Kent M (2011a) Neurologic history. In *Neuroanatomy, and Neurologic Examination*. Elsevier/Saunders, St. Louis, MO, p. 2.

Lorenz MD, Coates JR, and Kent M (2011b) Pain. In *Handbook of Veterinary Neurology*, 5th edn (eds. MD Lorenz, JR Coates, and M Kent). Elsevier/Saunders, St. Louis, MO, p. 429.

McCauley, L.M. and Van Dyke, J.B. (2013). Therapeutic exercises. In: *Canine Sports Medicine and Rehabilitation* (ed. M.C. Zink and J.B. Van Dyke), 152. Ames, IA: John Wiley & Sons, Inc.

Millis DL and Mankin J (2014) Orthopedic and neurologic evaluation. In *Canine Rehabilitation and Physical Therapy*, 2nd edn (eds. D Millis and D Levine). Elsevier/Saunders, Philadelphia, PA, p. 193.

Millis, D. and Saunders, D.G. (2014). Laser therapy in canine rehabilitation. In: *Canine Rehabilitation and Physical Therapy*, 2nde (ed. D. Millis and D. Levine), 359. Philadelphia, PA: Elsevier/Saunders.

Mojarradi, A., De Decker, S., Bäckström, C., and Bergknut, N. (2021). Safety of early postoperative hydrotherapy in dogs undergoing thoracolumbar hemilaminectomy. *J Small Anim Pract* 62 (12): 1062–1069. https://doi.org/10.1111/jsap.13412.

Olby, N. (2010). Patients with neurological disorders. In: *BSAVA Manual of Canine and Feline Rehabilitation, Supportive and Palliative Care* (ed. S. Lindley and P. Watson), 169. Gloucester, UK: BSAVA Publications.

Olby, N., Levine, J., Harris, T. et al. (2003). Long-term functional outcome of dogs with severe injuries of the thoracolumbar spinal cord: 87 cases (1996–2001). *J Am Vet Med Assoc* 222 (6): 762–769.

Olby, N., Halling, K.B., and Glick, T.R. (2005). Rehabilitation for the neurologic patient. *Vet Clin Small Anim* 35: 1389–1409.

Olby, N.J., Lim, J.H., Babb, K. et al. (2014). Gait scoring in dogs with thoracolumbar spinal cord injuries when walking on a treadmill. *BMC Vet Res* 10: 58.

Price, H. (2014a). Feline physiotherapy: Part 1. *Companion Anim* 19 (7): 374–378.

Price, H. (2014b). Feline physiotherapy: Part 2. *Companion Anim* 19 (9): 474–478.

Rylander, H. (2013). The neurologic examination in companion animals Part 1: Performing the examination. *Today's Vet Pract* January/February: 18–22.

Sharp, B. (2008). Physiotherapy in small animal practice. *In Pract* 30: 190–199.

Sharp, B. (2012a). Feline physiotherapy and rehabilitation: 1. Principles and potential. *J Feline Med Surg* 14: 622–632.

Sharp, B. (2012b). Feline physiotherapy and rehabilitation: 2 Clinical application. *J Feline Med Surg* 14: 633–645.

Sims, C., Waldron, R., and Marcellin-Little, D.J. (2015). Rehabilitation and physical therapy for the neurologic veterinary patient. *Vet Clin Small Anim* 45: 123–143.

Skytte, D. and Schmökel, H. (2018). Relationship of preoperative neurologic score with intervals to regaining micturition and ambulation following surgical treatment of thoracolumbar disk herniation in dogs. *J Am Vet Med Assocn* 253 (2): 196–200. https://doi.org/10.2460/javma.253.2.196.

Steinberg, H.S. and Coates, J.R. (2013). Diagnosis of and treatment options for disorders of the spine. In: *Canine Sports Medicine and Rehabilitation* (ed. M.C. Zink and J.B. Van Dyke), 311–337. Ames, IA: John Wiley & Sons, Inc.

Sturges BK and Woelz J (2005) Physical rehabilitation for the neurological patient.

Presented at Veterinary Neurology Symposium, University of California Davis, Irvine, CA.

Thomas, W.B., Olby, N., and Sharon, L. (2014). Neurologic conditions and physical rehabilitation of the neurologic patient. In: *Canine Rehabilitation and Physical Therapy*, 2nde (ed. D. Millis and D. Levine), 609. Philadelphia, PA: Elsevier/ Saunders.

Thomson, C. and Hahn, C. (2012). *Regional anatomy Veterinary Neuroanatomy: A Clinical Approach*, 12. Edinburgh: Saunders/Elsevier.

Weber, D.M. (2016). *Care tips for down dogs*, 31–35. *Vet Team Brief.*

13

The Disabled Patient Part 3: Special Considerations for the Geriatric Patient

Mary Ellen Goldberg[1] and Julia E. Tomlinson[2,3]

[1] *Veterinary Technician Specialist- lab animal medicine (Research anesthesia-retired), Veterinary Technician Specialist-*
(physical rehabilitation-retired), Veterinary Technician Specialist- (anesthesia & analgesia) – H, Veterinary Medical Technologist,
Surgical Research Anesthetist-retired, Certified Canine Rehabilitation Veterinary Nurse, Certified Veterinary Pain Practitioner
[2] *Twin Cities Animal Rehabilitation & Sports Medicine Clinic, Burnsville, MN, USA*
[3] *Veterinary Rehabilitation and Orthopedic Medicine Partners, San Clemente, CA, USA*

Introduction

Veterinary geroscience (the biology of aging) does not have a single consensus definition of aging, but it is typically characterized by the increasing risk of disease, dysfunction, and death over time (McKenzie, 2022). On a physiologic level, this entails the loss of robustness (the ability to resist deviation from an original or optimal state) and resilience (the ability to return to this state after deviations induced by external stressors). There is no single pathway or mechanism that causes aging or all age-related health outcomes. There are many relevant pathways, and the importance of each varies by species, genetic background, ontogeny (development of an organism), and environmental context. The goal of geroscience is to understand the biology of aging well enough to extend life and mitigate the

Physical Rehabilitation for Veterinary Technicians and Nurses, Second Edition.
Edited by Mary Ellen Goldberg and Julia E. Tomlinson.
© 2024 John Wiley & Sons, Inc. Published 2024 by John Wiley & Sons, Inc.
Companion website: www.wiley.com/go/goldberg/physicalrehabilitationvettechsandnurses

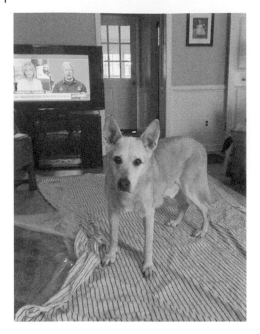

Figure 13.1   Jack, 17-year-old Shepherd cross courtesy Anne Dunnavant Bialkowski.

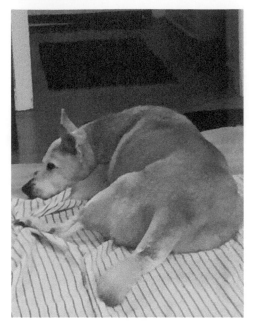

Figure 13.2   Jack, 17-year-old Shepherd cross courtesy Anne Dunnavant Bialkowski. Notice muscle atrophy with geriatric canine patient.

negative impacts of aging on health and function (McKenzie, 2022) (see Figure 13.1).

Telomeres are repetitive noncoding base sequences at the ends of chromosomes that maintain chromosome integrity during cell division and replication. When telomeres become too short, this leads to DNA damage and cellular stress, which can then trigger a dysfunctional, non-replicative cellular state called senescence. These structures are considered a hallmark of aging because telomere shortening accompanies aging, and accelerated aging is associated with telomerase deficiency or induced telomere attrition. Interventions to protect and repair telomeres have extended life spans in experimental animals (López-Otín *et al.*, 2013). Senescence is characterized by decreased function and degradation of the body. These changes cause a slow decline and can lead to functional issues such as reduced fine motor control and weakness. The aging process is not a disease process but a decline in reserves and strength as well as other changes in all body systems which increases the likelihood of a patient developing disease. Changes in the makeup and function of muscles, bones, and joints are common and characteristic aspects of aging. As robustness and resilience decline with age, the capacity of these tissues to regenerate and repair is degraded, and the equilibrium between anabolic and catabolic processes is lost. This eventually leads to the loss of mass and function in these tissues and ultimately clinical disorders such as sarcopenia, osteoporosis, and osteoarthritis (OA) (see Figure 13.2).

Medical issues commonly encountered in geriatric patients include obesity, degenerative joint disease (DJD), neoplasia, and endocrine disease. A comprehensive medical evaluation is an important requirement in planning rehabilitation for geriatric patients regarding expected progression of their physical limitations and how they will respond to physical rehabilitation. In addition to a thorough examination for concurrent disease, nutritional assessment and evaluation of the patient's pain level are important in guiding therapy. Clients with geriatric animals will likely be concerned with quality-of-life issues such as mobility, pain level, fecal and urinary continence, appetite, and maintenance of human–pet interaction within the

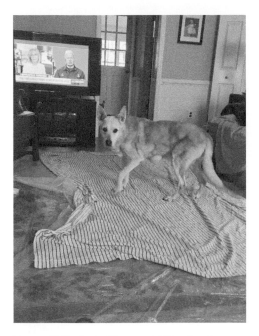

Figure 13.3 Jack, 17-year-old Shepherd cross courtesy Anne Dunnavant Bialkowski. Notice lipomas, grey muzzle, and concerns for urinary incontinence in geriatric canine patient.

household. These issues can be further complicated by behavioral changes or cognitive dysfunction. Physical rehabilitation for the geriatric patient entails addressing issues such as pain with care to avoid exacerbation of weakness and any cognitive signs. Rehabilitation aims to improve mobility and function (via assistive devices and treatments targeted at improving muscle strength and coordination) and address medical and nursing care issues (such as providing adequate bedding and maintaining patient cleanliness in the household). Creating a geriatric wellness program may be beneficial in the physical rehabilitation environment. Marketing aimed at geriatric patients can be targeted to clients interested in maintaining quality of life (QOL) for their elderly pets, patients with DJD, patients with neurogenic issues, and those in need of hospice care (see Figure 13.3).

The Aging Process

Aging is a term that refers to a complex set of biological changes that result in a progressive

reduction of the ability to maintain homeostasis when exposed to internal physiologic and external environmental stresses (Goldston, 1995; Bellows *et al.*, 2015). These changes ultimately lead to decreased vitality, increased vulnerability to disease, and eventually death. Dogs respond to cardiovascular conditioning and strength-training exercises with similar physiologic adaptations as humans, increasing their aerobic fitness and strength (Cerqueira *et al.*, 2018). Cats can respond to strength training with muscle development, but it is unclear whether they adapt to forced aerobic exercise in the same way dogs and humans do (Wyatt *et al.*, 1978). Cats can benefit from strength exercises, flexibility exercises, balance and proprioception exercises, and endurance exercises (Sharp, 2012).

When do Dogs and Cats Qualify as Senior or Geriatric?

Veterinary professionals consider dogs senior at an earlier age than pet owners. Small, medium, and large dogs were all considered senior at around seven years old by veterinary professionals, with giant breed dogs hitting the senior mark around five. Veterinary professionals considered small and medium dogs' geriatric around 11, large dogs near 9, and giant breeds around 7 (Seymour, 2014) (see Table 13.1). The highest percentage of veterinary professionals considered cats' seniors around 9 years old and geriatric around 13 (Seymour, 2014) (see Table 13.2 International Cat Care.org, n.d.). More than 77% of veterinary professionals and pet owners alike said there was a difference between the terms "senior" and "geriatric" (Seymour, 2014).

A study conducted by the American Veterinary Medical Association (AVMA) in 2015 (Bellows *et al.*, 2015) concluded that the major physical and functional changes that occurred in aging patients fell into the following categories:

1) Behavioral changes, such as changes in sleep cycle, responses to verbal commands, and interactions with family and other pets.

Table 13.1 How old is my dog in human years?

Dog's age	0–20 lbs	21–50 lbs	51–90 Bs	>90 lbs
5	36	37	40	40
6	40	42	45	49
7	44	47	50	56
8	48	51	55	64
9	52	56	61	71
10	56	60	66*	78*
11	60	65	72*	86*
12	64	69*	77*	93*
13	68	74*	82*	101*
14	72*	78*	88*	109*
15	76*	83*	93*	115*
16	80*	87*	99*	123*
17	84*	92*	104*	
18	88*	96*	109*	
19	92*	101*	115*	

*geriatric.
Source: Adapted from Tomlinson (2016).

Table 13.2 How old is my cat in human years?

Life stage	Age of cat	Human equivalent
Kitten birth to 6 months	0–1 month	0–1 year
	2–3 months	2–4 years
	4 months	6–8 years
	6 months	10 years
Junior 7 months to 2 years	7 months	12 years
	12 months	15 years
	18 months	21 years
	2 years	24 years
Adult 3–6 years	3 years	28 years
	4 years	32 years
	5 years	36 years
	6 years	40 years
Mature 7–10 years	7 years	44 years
	8 years	48 years
	9 years	52 years
	10 years	56 years
Senior 11–14 years	11 years	60 years
	12 years	64 years
	13 years	68 years
	14 years	72 years
Geriatric 15 years+	15 years	76 years
	16 years	80 years
	17 years	84 years
	18 years	88 years
	19 years	92 years
	20 years	96 years
	21 years	100 years
	22 years	104 years
	23 years	108 years
	24 years	112 years
	25 years	116 years

Source: Adapted http://icatcare.org/sites/default/files/PDF/how-old-is-your-cat-posterweb.pdf.

2) Changes in appearance, such as gray, dull, dry hair coat; loss of muscle mass; and development of cataracts and nuclear sclerosis (see Figure 13.4).
3) Changes in daily function, which could reflect functional changes in the musculoskeletal system (decreased activity and mobility) and special senses (impaired vision, smell, and hearing).

What Physiologic Changes Occur When Dogs and Cats Age? (McKenzie, 2022; Bellows *et al.*, 2015)

Aging affects the entire body and its functions. There is a loss of lung elasticity, and lung capacity is decreased in older pets. The brainstem control of breathing also changes with age, and this results in reduced ability to respond to increased demand – older patients become less tolerant of exercise. Panting tends to become less efficient with age. It is harder for older dogs to cool themselves, and this needs to be considered when exercising an elderly dog. Cardiac output starts to decline in midlife in dogs, and again, ability to respond to the stresses of exercise may be reduced. Chronic heart valve disease is found in around 30% of older dogs (see Box 13.1). The most common cardiac disease in cats older than

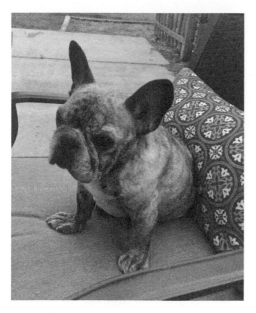

Figure 13.4 McLovin, French Bulldog, approximately 10 years old, courtesy Meredith Pack White.

6 years of age is hypertrophic cardiomyopathy (HCM) (see Figure 13.5).

The integument undergoes changes to skin and nails. Examples include callus formation, resulting in painful weight bearing, altered foot placement, and a tendency to form lumps and bumps such as lipomas and adenomas. Multiple organ systems are known to decline with age, changes occur in the gastrointestinal system (reduced elasticity of the colon and rectum); the liver and kidneys slow drug metabolism and elimination. Aging cats often experience a thinning hair coat, focal alopecia, and increased production of white hairs. Changes in sebum production, along with reduced self-grooming activity, can lead to scaly skin and cause the coat to become dry or oily and dull. Decreased skin elasticity and brittle claws have also been noted in apparently healthy older cats. Some geriatric cats' claws appear to be exposed because they lose the ability to completely retract them into their sheath.

Changes in the immune system result in reduced ability to combat infection. Healing can take longer. Geriatric patients are more prone to develop chronic urinary tract infections. Metabolic systems are more likely to be affected with age; for example, the adrenal glands undergo changes resulting in altered stress response via increased cortisol production, and there may also be changes in electrolyte balance. Other endocrine changes include many dogs showing a dip in thyroid levels as they

---

Box 13.1 Cardiopulmonary changes in geriatric dogs

- Declining cardiac output
- Decreased elasticity of pulmonary tissue
- Increased fibrosis of pulmonary tissue
- Decreased cough reflex
  - Pulmonary secretions have low viscosity
  - Increased chance of respiratory disease
- Monitor for pneumonia
- West Highland White Terriers – pulmonary fibrosis
- Chronic bronchitis – older small breed dogs
- CHF, exercise intolerance and slowly progressive cough
- 75% of dogs over 16 years old have atrioventricular (AV) valve thickening
- *GOLPP* – Geriatric Onset Laryngeal Paralysis Polyneuropathy – can be associated with polyneuropathy, neoplasia, and hypothyroidism
- 32 dogs with idiopathic Lar Par – 100% had esophageal dysfunction
- 1 year later of the 24 dogs evaluated 100% had neurologic signs (ataxia, weakness, conscious proprioceptive (CP) deficits, muscular atrophy)

Source: Adapted from Bellows et al. (2015).

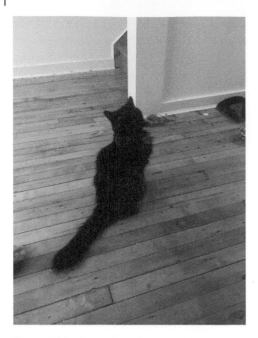

Figure 13.5 Lou, adopted as street cat, age unknown. When adopted became a house cat. Cause of death, congestive heart failure. Courtesy Christian Peter White.

Box 13.2   Hormone excess ("Hyper") disorders in dogs and cats

- Pituitary tumors (most commonly, secrete too much growth hormone or ACTH)
- Hyperthyroidism (secrete too much thyroid hormone)
- Hyperparathyroidism (secrete too much parathyroid hormone)
- Pancreatic insulin-secreting tumor, usually called insulinoma (secrete too much insulin)
- Hyperadrenocorticism, usually called Cushing syndrome (secrete too much cortisol)
- Hyperaldosteronism, usually called Conn syndrome (secrete too much aldosterone)
- Pheochromocytoma (secrete too much adrenaline)

Source: Adapted from Bellows et al. (2015).

Box 13.3   Hormone deficiency ("Hypo") disorders in dogs and cats

- Pituitary dwarfism (secrete too little growth hormone in young animals)
- Diabetes insipidus (secrete too little antidiuretic hormone or vasopressin)
- Hypothyroidism (secrete too little thyroid hormone)
- Hypoparathyroidism (secrete too little parathyroid hormone)
- Diabetes mellitus (secrete too little insulin)
- Hypoadrenocorticism, usually called Addison disease (too little cortisol and aldosterone secreted)

Source: Adapted from Bellows et al. (2015).

---

age. There is an age-related decrease in basal metabolic rate, so obesity risk is higher (Boxes 13.2 and 13.3).

As the nervous system and associated special senses age, changes are commonly seen. Some age-related diminished hearing may occur. As an alternative to behavioral testing for hearing loss in dogs, the brainstem auditory-evoked response (BAER) is one of the most frequently used testing modalities in this respect because the test is objective, reasonably easy to perform, noninvasive, safe, and cost-effective compared with other objective measures of auditory function. The testing apparatus is portable, and test time is brief. Results are reliable, sensitive, anatomically specific, generally independent of the level of consciousness, and resistant to the influence of drugs and yield a comprehensive index of neurologic status (Wilson and Mills, 2005). The current test of choice for identifying cats with congenital sensorineural deafness, and evaluation of other causes of deafness, is the BAER. The BAER is performed in sedated or anesthetized cats and involves the placement of subdermal needle electrodes to measure electrical brain activity in response to auditory stimuli (Cvejic *et al.*, 2009).

There can be age-related retinal degeneration; night vision loss is very common in older dogs, and close questioning of the client can establish this. Home adaptations using lighting can help the pet remain active and healthy. Congenital ocular malformations are uncommon; knowledge about their prevalence is important since they can cause vision impairment or even blindness. Moreover, some human ocular disease phenotypes are like the ones presented by dogs and cats, so they can be used as models to investigate pathophysiology and therapeutic approaches (Saraiva and Delgado, 2020).

It is likely that olfaction decreases with age in dogs and cats. A decrease in a pet's sense of smell may be partial (hyposmia) or complete (anosmia) and can lead to decreased appetite, weight loss, or malnutrition because smell is an important component of "tasting" food. Changes in flavor perception are often caused by changes within the nose, rather than a decrease in the number or function of taste buds (Banks, 2017).

Brain size reduces with age due to atrophy of the cerebral cortex, and this is the part of the brain that controls the body's voluntary actions; patients may be slower to react and slower to learn. There is a loss of fine motor control and decreased body awareness (proprioception). This may result in difficulty with balance and coordination, along with changes in gait. Aged dogs can have slower movements; however, ataxia is never a normal age-related change (see Box 13.4).

Older pets can develop central nervous system (CNS) neoplasia, with meningiomas being the most common primary brain tumor diagnosed in dogs and cats. Other common primary tumors of dogs are gliomas, astrocytomas, and oligodendrogliomas. Lymphosarcoma is the second most common brain tumor in cats, occurring

---

> **Box 13.4   Immune changes in the geriatrics patient**
>
> - Immune compromise
> - Bone marrow proficiency decreases
> - Phagocytic ability of neutrophils decreases
> - Diminished numbers of WBC and peripheral lymphocytes
> - Lymphocytic proliferation response to stimulation declines with age
> - CD4:CD8 (helper T: cytotoxic T cell) ratio decreases with age
> - Decreased cellular immunity
> - Wounds heal slower
> - Changes in hair coat
> - Aged dogs maintain humoral immune response
>   - Respond to vaccines
>   - Respond to novel antigenic stimulation
>
> *Source:* Adapted from Bellows et al. (2015).

---

either as a primary neoplasm or as part of a multicentric disease. Two common neurologic diseases prevalent in older dogs are degenerative myelopathy (DM) and intervertebral disk disease (IVDD).

Mobility and strength naturally decline with age. Sarcopenia is the term for loss of muscle mass due to degeneration with age and this has been confirmed in a study of Labrador Retrievers (Hutchinson *et al.*, 2012). Number and size of muscle fibers decrease, and it takes muscles longer to respond to exercise. Old dogs frequently adopt a movement pattern of either moving or laying down; they rarely stand in one place. The first muscles to atrophy are the slow-twitch postural muscles (e.g., spinal epaxial muscles), as these are very sensitive to reduced load. With atrophy comes decreased ability to maintain a posture, and so the process becomes cyclical. Water content of tendons decreases, muscle fibers are replaced with fat, and the physical loss of

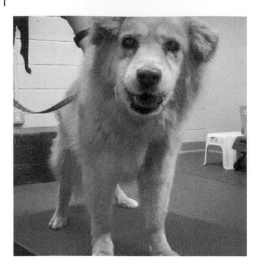

Figure 13.6 Ellie, geriatric canine in Dr Julia Tomlinson's rehabilitation practice. Courtesy Laura Davidson.

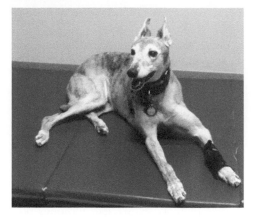

Figure 13.7 A frail canine patient, the patient is 15 years old. She has normal blood work and cognition but is weak and slow to move. Courtesy Dr Julia Tomlinson.

muscle mass causes increased stiffness and loss of strength (see Figure 13.6).

For cats, significant musculoskeletal changes that occur with age include a decrease in lean body mass (LBM) (muscle, bone, skin, and organs), deterioration of joint components, and functional decline (Bellows *et al.*, 2016a, b).

The term frailty has also been used in relation to age-related musculoskeletal deterioration. Frailty is a multisystem impairment associated with increased vulnerability to stressors and describes the condition of individuals that are at increased risk of adverse health outcomes. (Bentov *et al.*, 2019) (see Figure 13.7). Frailty is related to, but not synonymous with, comorbidity and disability. Frailty is characterized by a decline in the body's functional reserve, lower energy metabolism, smaller muscle cells, and altered nervous, hormonal, and inflammatory functions. It is not a disease process, but it leads to increased susceptibility to disease and functional dependency (Qian-Li Xue, 2011).

Cachexia is the loss of LBM, and it affects a large percentage of dogs and cats with age-related diseases, such as congestive heart failure (CHF), chronic renal failure, and cancer. It is characterized by weakness, anorexia, and

perceived poor QOL and is associated with decreased survival (Freeman, 2012; Boxes 13.5 and 13.6; see Figures 13.8 and 13.9).

The specific aging phenotype that emerges in an individual animal is contingent on genetic, ontogenic, and environmental factors, but the underlying physiologic processes are remarkably consistent between tissues, individuals, and even species (see Figure 13.10). The goal of veterinary geroscience is to understand these processes well enough to develop effective preventative and therapeutic interventions. Clinical therapies to mitigate the negative health impact of aging on these species are a realistic long-term goal, and filling in the knowledge gaps highlighted in this review will pave the way to bringing such therapies into the hands of clinicians (McKenzie, 2022).

Cognitive Impairment and Other Behavioral Issues

Cognitive dysfunction is a neurodegenerative disorder of senior dogs and cats that is characterized by gradual cognitive decline over a prolonged period (18–24 months or longer) (Landsberg and Araujo, 2005). Diagnosis of cognitive dysfunction syndrome

---

Box 13.5   Nervous system changes in the geriatric patient

- Coordination and proprioception decline
- Muscle strength declines
  - ➣ Leads to ataxia (increased falls in humans)
- Loss of vision and vestibular input
- Muscle spindle cells provide input on joint position and muscle length for coordinated movement
  - ➣ Muscle spindle cells become less sensitive
  - ➣ Large myelinated nerve fibers that carry the message from the muscle spindle cell to the spinal cord decline
  - ➣ Nerve conduction velocity slow (advanced age)
  - ➣ Tactile sensitivity diminishes in the distal extremities
- Loss of vision
- Lens (cataracts or luxation)
- Corneal issues (KCS) Keratoconjunctivitis sicca
- Trauma
- Retinal issues (degeneration or detachment)
- Loss of hearing
- Decrease in smell

Source: Adapted from Bellows et al. (2015).

Box 13.6   Musculoskeletal changes in the geriatric patient

- Sarcopenia
  - ➣ Muscle fibers are replaced with first fat – no loss of muscle circumference
  - ➣ Then replaced with fibrous tissue – physical loss of muscle circumference
  - ➣ Causes increased stiffness
- Reduced oxygenation of muscle fibers
- Loss of strength of muscles and tendons
- Sarcopenia causes
  - ➣ Decreased support of the joints
  - ➣ Decreased chondrocytes
  - ➣ Reduced ability to respond to growth factors
- With cage rest see significant atrophy of muscles especially at the insertion of the collateral ligaments
- Aging decreases tensile strength of ligaments secondary to loss of collagen
- Fun bone facts
  - ➣ Animals fully change bone content every five years
  - ➣ Lifetime of weight-bearing exercises decreases bone loss normally seen with aging
  - ➣ Weight-bearing training before a bone fracture has faster healing times
  - ➣ Shock wave therapy may aid bone healing specifically in geriatric dogs
- Water content in the cartilage decreases
  - ➣ Thinning of cartilage layer
- Chondrocytes synthesize smaller, less uniform aggrecan molecules and less functional link proteins

- Decreased mitotic activities
- Decrease response to anabolic mechanical stimulants and growth factors
  - ➤ Combined with stress on joints secondary to loss of muscle strength leads to eburnation of subchondral bone and OA
- Do not see osteoporosis in pets, but bones become more brittle due to infiltration of fat into bone marrow and thinner cortexes
  - ➤ Fracture healing is slower
  - ➤ More difficult to form a callus
  - ➤ Obesity and brittle bones exacerbate progression of OA

Source: Adapted from Dowgray and Comerford (2020).

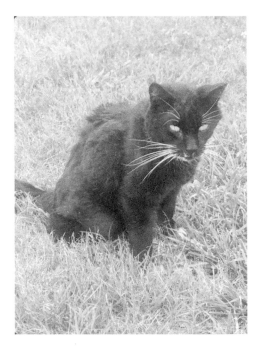

Figure 13.8 Carlton, barn cat, adopted, age unknown. Cause of death abdominal carcinoma. Notice bolus of subcutaneous fluids to assist with dehydration. Courtesy Christian Peter White.

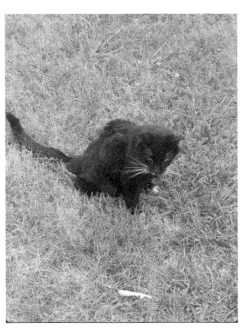

Figure 13.9 Carlton, barn cat, notice lack of grooming as he deteriorated. Courtesy Christian Peter White.

(CDS) is based on recognition of behavioral signs and exclusion of other medical conditions and drug side effects, which in some cases can mimic or complicate CDS. Clinical categories include disorientation, alterations in social interactions, sleep–wake cycles, elimination habits, and activity, as well as increasing anxiety. Deficits in learning and memory have also been well documented (Landsberg *et al.*, 2012) (see Box 13.7). The diagnosis of CDS was initially based on clinical signs represented by the acronym DISH, representing disorientation, altered interactions with people or other pets, altered sleep–wake cycles, and house soiling (Landsberg *et al.*, 2013a).

Signs of Cognitive Impairment

- Confusion
- Altered relationships and social interactions
- Altered response to stimuli

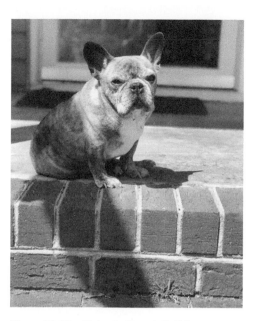

Figure 13.10 McLovin, French Bulldog, approximately 12 years old, courtesy Meredith Pack White.

Box 13.7 Muscle changes in the geriatric dogs

- Geriatric dogs
  - ➤ Lactic acid builds faster
  - ➤ Glycogen depletes faster
  - ➤ Decreased creatine phosphate (used first as a fuel in muscle)
  - ➤ Cannot build muscle strength or endurance as well as younger dogs
  - ➤ Muscle capillarization decreases with age
  - ➤ Decreased oxygen supply to muscles
  - ➤ Decreased endurance
  - ➤ Type II muscle fibers decrease by ~25%
  - ➤ Strength
  - ➤ Type I muscle fibers can increase or stay the same
  - ➤ Endurance and Postural muscles
- *Disuse atrophy* – decrease Type I muscle, especially those that cross one joint, and postural muscles

Source: Adapted from Bellows et al. (2015).

- Changes in activity: increased anxiety, pacing, and repetitive behaviors (vocalizing, pacing)
- Changes in activity: apathy, depression
- Altered sleep–wake cycles; reversed day/night schedule
- Learning and memory problems: house soiling
- Learning and memory problems: deficits in work, tasks, and commands
- Getting stuck behind doors

Behavioral signs are often the first, or only, signs of pain, illness, and of cognitive decline, and so discerning the contributing factors can be a challenge for the family and for the veterinary team. Senior pets may be less able to cope with stress, which may make them more susceptible to changes in their environment (for example, a new cat, a house move). It is the job of the veterinarian and the rehabilitation team members to help discern pain from stress and anxiety, even in a patient with CDS. When in doubt, treat for pain as a trial. Pain assessment, response to pain medications, and the overall well-being of the pet depend heavily on the measurement and assessment of the pet's behavior (Mathews, 2000). A wide range of behavior problems, ranging from avoidance, decreased activity, and inappetence to irritability, restlessness, and aggression, could be due to underlying pain. In fact, any change from normal behavior and the development of new and abnormal behaviors can also be due to underlying pain or disease (Landsberg *et al.*, 2013b).

Monitoring both age-associated cognitive and physiological changes should be conducted at least annually in dogs (starting at 5–8 years for larger breeds and 8–10 years for smaller breeds) and cats (starting at 10–12 years) (Hammerle *et al.*, 2015). Clients with elderly animals will not always mention behavior changes during veterinary visits, so veterinary technicians should be asking clients about any changes in their pets' behavior whenever they see dogs from 8 years of age and cats from 10 years at the latest (ideally, they should do this from puppy- or kitten-hood onward!).

In cats, thorough medical and behavioral history is required for diagnosis. Cognitive and motor performance appears to decline from approximately 10–11 years of age for cats, but functional changes in the neurons of the caudate nucleus in the brain have been seen by 6–7 years (Landsberg *et al.*, 2010).

Signs of Cognitive Dysfunction Syndrome (CDS) Confused with Weakness or Pain Issues

1) *Reduced mobility* – especially negotiating obstacles (thresholds, car entry)
2) Urinary or fecal accidents in the house
3) Change in appetite
4) Decreased alertness
5) Change in interaction with the family

What can Influence Behavior in Geriatric Patients?

- *Anxiety* – CDS can increase anxiety and the likelihood of a patient developing fear- and anxiety-related behavior problems (Overall, 2013).
- *Reduced mobility* – if movement is difficult, this can increase the likelihood of patient's toileting in inappropriate places because they are unable to reach a more appropriate toileting area in time. Animals with reduced mobility also find it harder to move away from people or other animals if they feel threatened, which will further increase the likelihood of them showing defensive aggression (Landsberg *et al.*, 2013b).
- *Restlessness* – CDS patients often find it difficult to rest, which can result in them being unsettled both during the day and at night (Landsberg *et al.*, 2013b) (see Figure 13.11). This can slow progress during rehabilitation.
- *Reduced interaction with owners* – Geriatric patients may not want to play or

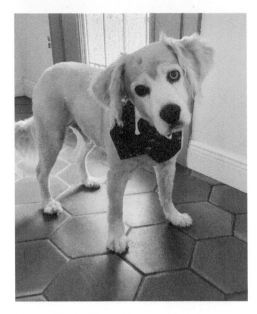

Figure 13.11 Kippy, 18-year-old Cocker Spaniel, courtesy of Linda Silverstein Garrett.

enjoy other interactions with their family, such as petting or going for walks (Overall, 2013). This can negatively affect the pet–client relationship, and if pain is unrecognized and/or untreated this may be a risk factor for relinquishment or euthanasia.

- *Polydipsia and polyuria* – Conditions associated with polydipsia and polyuria such as diabetes mellitus, hyperadrenocorticism, or chronic kidney failure will increase the likelihood of a geriatric patient house soiling or waking their owners at night to ask to be let outside (Landsberg *et al.*, 2013b; Overall, 2013).
- *Neurological and circulatory disorders* – Medical problems affecting the CNS, e.g., brain tumors, or the circulatory system, e.g., hypertension, can cause or contribute to cognitive decline (Gunn-Moore, 2011; Landsberg *et al.*, 2011).
- *Some medications* can also increase the likelihood of animals showing behavior problems, for example, corticosteroids can be associated with increased appetite, urine output, restlessness, and reactivity to stimuli which can increase the likelihood

Table 13.3 Feline Mobility/Cognitive Dysfunction Questionnaire adapted (Gunn-Moore, 2011, 2014).

My Cat...	Yes	Maybe	No
Is less willing to jump down			
Will only jump up or down from lower heights			
Sometimes shows signs of being stiff			
Is less agile than previously			
Shows signs of lameness or limping			
Has difficulty getting in or out of the cat flap			
Has difficulty going up or down stairs			
Cries when they are picked up			
Has more accidents outside the litter tray			
Spends less time grooming			
Is more reluctant to interact with me			
Plays less with other animals or toys			
Sleeps more and/or is less active			
Cries loudly for no reason/to try to gain my attention			
Appears forgetful			

NB. Need to ensure there are no environmental reason(s) for these behavior changes.

of an animal showing problem behaviors, including house soiling, wandering and pacing, and also aggression to owners or other pets (Landsberg *et al.*, 2012).

See Table 13.3 for an example of a Feline Mobility//Cognitive Dysfunction Questionnaire (Boxes 13.8–13.11)

It can be difficult to differentiate between the signs caused by cognitive dysfunction and those caused by OA-related mobility issues. Both conditions often occur concurrently in old cats and many of the treatments for one condition will also help the other.

Management Strategies to Improve Quality of Life

Geriatric animals need to be able to navigate their surroundings easily. This can be particularly challenging for animals with medical problems affecting their mobility, including conditions associated with chronic pain such as DJD and spinal problems. Conditions that reduce sensory abilities, for example, vision and hearing loss or cognitive dysfunction, can be associated with impaired spatial awareness and navigational ability. Important resources which need to be accessible include food, water, comfortable resting places, toilet locations, and for cats' places to withdraw to or hide if they do not wish to interact with people or other animals in the home (Warnes, 2015). Cats like to have food, water, and toilet areas kept separate. These must be easily accessible from the cat's resting area. If a cat spends time on different floors in the home, it is sensible to locate a full set of resources, including a litter tray, on each floor. Once resources have been located appropriately, they should always be kept in the same places so animals can find them easily. If other animals are in the home, then it is imperative that there is no unnecessary competition for these resources (Table 13.4).

Other Considerations for Geriatric Pets

- Introducing a new pet into the household can be extremely stressful for an older animal with mobility problems and especially for one with cognitive dysfunction. Client may be better advised not to do this, especially with cats and any dog that does not have good social skills or is showing severe cognitive dysfunction.
- Play can be associated with a positive emotional response, and increasing

> **Box 13.8 Cognitive dysfunction changes in the geriatric patient (Chapagain *et al.*, 2018; Dewey *et al.*, 2019)**

- Cognitive changes
  - ➤ Increased oxidative stress
- Deposition of B-amyloid plaques (similar to Alzheimer patients) (Prpar and Majdic, 2019)
- DNA fragmentation or damage
- Changes in intracellular signaling leading to a loss of neurotrophic factors
- Anatomic changes in the brain
  - ➤ Cortical atrophy
  - ➤ Increased ventricular volume
  - ➤ Reduced neurogenesis in hippocampus
  - ➤ Responsible for learning and memory
- Progressive neurodegenerative disorder
- Diagnosis of exclusion
- Clinical signs include
  - ➤ Change in sleeping habits
  - ➤ Lack of environmental recognition
  - ➤ Decreased interaction with human and animal family
- Restlessness
- Apathy
- Anxiety
- Altered appetite
- Aggression or irritability
- Vocalization
- Incontinence
- Therapy includes
  - ➤ *Antioxidants* – vitamins B, C, and E; fruits and vegetables
  - ➤ Fatty acid supplementation
  - ➤ Mitochondrial cofactor supplementation – carnitine, alpha lipoic acid (omega 6 FA), Coenzyme Q10
  - ➤ Phosphatidylserine (phospholipid that improves cognitive deficits and memory)
  - ➤ *Ginko Biloba* – a monoamine oxidase inhibitor (MAO-A and MAO-B)
  - ➤ Increases dopamine levels and protects neurons from apoptosis induced by B-amyloid
  - ➤ *Selegiline* – a MAO-B inhibitor (Anipryl®, Ldeprenyl®)

aerobic activity will also boost circulation, increasing oxygen supply to the brain and muscles. Low-impact games such as gentle throw and fetch or search games are appropriate for most elderly dogs, and for dogs with vision loss, search games to find food or toys are particularly suitable. Short play sessions with fishing rod toys or toys that roll and/or make sounds will suit most cats. Older pets can become bored with toys quickly, so the toys need to be rotated every few days.

- Dogs with mobility problems can be taken out in the car and then given a short walk in a new location, or accompany owners on longer walks by riding in a modified baby stroller. Some elderly

---

Box 13.9   Ten steps to make a geriatric health care program successful

1) The practice decision-maker must be convinced that a senior/geriatric health care will become a significant asset to the practice before investing the time, energy, training, and resources necessary in developing and maintaining the program.

2) Convince the entire staff of the significant health benefits the program offers the senior pet. Critical to the success or failure of a senior/geriatric health care program is the involvement and buy-in of your staff.

3) Create a very specific and detailed program, including age of onset, frequency of visits, scheduling periods, fee structure, educational materials, and marketing strategies. Decide exactly which tests are to be included in the program.

4) Convince the owners of the significant health benefits the program offers their aging pet. A percentage of your practice will readily accept the program, but the rest will need repeated convincing. Increased client knowledge usually equates to increased client acceptance and compliance. Early and continued owner education is a long-term investment in a senior/geriatric health care program.

5) A well-designed market strategy correlates with success. Use newsletters, reminder cards, invoices, telephone directory ads, Web pages, and social media to educate your current and prospective clients on age-related problems and solutions. Client marketing efforts should emphasize all the advances in veterinary medicine, including newer diagnostic testing, improved anesthetics and anesthetic monitoring equipment, behavioral drugs, newer arthritis therapy options, leading-edge cancer chemotherapy, more effective cardiac medications, dental care, and nutritional advancements that are available.

6) Bundle the fee structure to include a senior pet discount. Discount the fee for all the services and consider a cost reduction in the senior diets for any patients already on the program.

7) Begin slowly and be patient and the program will grow. A senior/geriatric health care program is a long-term hospital investment. It is much easier to add a test and expand the program than take one away because the cost was considered excessive for the average owner. Unfortunately, an overzealous program coupled with under delivery of value is commonplace. The seeds of program success and client subscription begin when outlining a lifelong preventive health care program the first time a new owner visits the practice, even for puppies or kittens.

8) Since a comprehensive health examination will require more time in the exam room, try to schedule these appointments during slow days or during periods of the day when you can devote the time necessary for a complete evaluation.

9) An attractive three-color trifold brochure for your practice's program is an easy and time-saving marketing tool. The brochure should be uniquely branded to your practice. Highlight the specifics of your program (age of onset, visits per year, etc.), but keep the piece simple for an easy read. Emphasize the advantages of the health program to the older pets and the early warning disease signs to watch for.

10) Periodic program review by your clients and staff is essential in maintaining the consistently high standard of care you have established for your senior patients. Do not be afraid to modify the program to meet the emerging minimum database protocols.

Box 13.10   Medical conditions appropriate for hospice or palliative care

- Terminal diagnosis
- Chronic, progressive disease
- Progressive, undiagnosed disease
- Chronic disability
- Terminal geriatric status

Box 13.11   Teaching bladder expression

1) With your pet lying on its side, place your hands in a prayerlike fashion over the area where you imagine the bladder is located. If your pet is strong enough to support its weight, then this procedure can be done while standing. You may find this procedure works better for you if your hands are facing toward the front of the animal as opposed to the rear.

2) Slowly apply equal and progressively increasing pressure to body wall and by extension the urinary bladder. Slow steady and progressive pressure is the key. This is a skill that your pet likely requires so try to be patient, keep trying, and DO NOT BECOME DISCOURAGED.

Watch for male dog: https://www.youtube.com/watch?v=G8kuOD2Iup4
Watch for female dog: https://www.youtube.com/watch?v=Qyc181o-g0A
Watch cat: https://www.youtube.com/watch?v=9KH_eMDJBC8

---

cats prefer to remain indoors, but if cats do want to go outside, they can do this more safely if the cat wears a harness, or possibly by fencing the garden to prevent the resident cat from leaving and other cats from entering. Screened back porches are excellent for environmental stimulation.

- Animals with severe cognitive dysfunction or anxiety must have an environment that remains stable and unchanging. Highly anxious animals, and especially cats, may cope best when restricted to a single room containing food, water, a litter tray, resting places, and hiding places. It is important to keep furniture and resources in the same places and to avoid big changes in the scent profile of the room, for example, by not using strongly scented cleaning products, as these can be very challenging for cats. It also helps to maintain a consistent routine, ensuring that important events occur in the same order and at approximately the same times every day.

Common Presentation

Geriatric patients often present to the rehabilitation veterinarian because of difficulties performing the activities of daily living (ADLs), for example, difficulty on stairs or getting into and out of the family vehicle. Another often concurrent presentation is for management of chronic pain. The goal of the examination and treatment plan is to explore possible therapeutic options that will effectively improve strength, balance, and comfort without fatiguing the patient, with resultant worsening home mobility problems. Slow, steady progress is the aim of any geriatric rehabilitation plan; the plan must include home assistance and nursing care regardless of the relative stability or functionality of the patient.

Table 13.4 Suggestions for improving the environment and increasing access to resources for elderly cats and dogs adapted (Warnes, 2015).

Resource	Dogs	Cats
Food and water	• Raising bowls off the ground will help dogs with joint and spinal problems to eat and drink more comfortably • Nonslip matting underfoot will prevent dog slipping when eating or drinking	• Need to be in separate locations • Raise bowls off ground by a few inches to enable cats with joint and spinal problems to eat and drink more comfortably • Cats used to be fed on raised surfaces, e.g., windowsills/worktops may need a ramp or steps to enable access or food and water should be provided in more accessible locations
Toileting areas	• Dogs with mobility problems may need to learn to use a toileting area closer to the house, or even be provided with a toileting area indoors, e.g., puppy pads in a large tray, indoor grass • Owners may need to encourage dogs to go to their toilet area regularly because they may no longer indicate when they need to toilet	• Need to be separate from feeding and drinking locations • Cats with mobility problems will prefer large, low-sided litter trays, or equivalents (gardeners' potting trays) • Finer-grained litters are easier to stand on and dig than coarse • Cats that have previously toileted outside may no longer be able to and will need to be provided with litter trays indoors
Sleeping areas and beds	• Beds should be comfortable and supportive, e.g., memory foam, easy to enter/exit, and large enough for them to lie flat • Elderly animals can become cold easily: sleeping areas should be kept warm especially at night in the winter. Heated beds may be welcomed • An Adaptil™ diffuser close to the bed may help reduce anxiety and help dogs settle better at night • Items containing the owner's scent may also help some dogs settle better at night	• Beds should be comfortable and padded, easy to enter/exit, and large enough for them to lie flat • Cats prefer to rest in raised places, but animals with mobility problems may need ramps/steps to access these locations. • Elderly animals can become cold easily: sleeping areas should be kept warm especially at night in the winter. Heated beds may be welcomed • A Feliway™ diffuser close to the bed may reduce anxiety and help cats settle better at night
Moving around inside and outside home	• Nonslip matting or carpet in locations of important resources and on the walkways between important areas can improve accessibility for animals with mobility problems • Nonslip ramps can help dogs navigate steep steps outside the home and also get into and out of cars • Specially designed harnesses can be helpful for supporting dogs with mobility problems to enable exercise and access to toilet areas	• Nonslip matting or carpet in locations of important resources and on the walkways between important areas can improve accessibility for elderly animals with mobility problems • Most cats prefer raised resting places where they can feel safe and observe household activity from a distance. Providing ramps/steps may enable cats with mobility problems to continue to use withdrawal as a way of avoiding things that cause anxiety or fear • Cats with mobility problems may no longer be able to use a cat flap so owners will need to let them in and out unless they prefer to stay indoors.

Health Benefits of Rehabilitation for the Geriatric Patient

The geriatric patient can have many benefits from physical rehabilitation sessions. Their daily function improves as well as their strength (Edge-Hughes, 2009). Pain is generally reduced a great deal. The lungs are better able to transport oxygen, and breathing capacity increases. Joint mobility improves. Usually, patients have reductions in neuromuscular tension and anxiety, along with a tranquilizing effect. Human interaction is usually increased because the patient feels better.

Physical Rehabilitation and Function

Before any physical rehabilitation is undertaken, the patient must have an analgesic plan in place, most likely controlled with analgesic medication(s). There are four key areas of physical rehabilitation available to the geriatric patient: manual therapy; electrotherapy; hydrotherapy; and clinical/home exercise programs (Cottriall, 2014).

Absolute precaution! "The patient should feel better, move better, and have better normal daily function when done with exercises. If they are more lame, sore after resting, or change transitions or posture for the worse after exercises are done, then the plan needs to change." (McCauley, 2016a, b).

Manual Therapy for the Geriatric Patient

Massage can provide relief from pain and spasms of muscles but should be exercised with caution in patients with low muscle mass. Elderly, frail patients may not enjoy massage or even light grooming. Active or passive muscle stretches may be prescribed and performed only in clinic for some patients, at least initially; other patients may be well enough for clients to be taught to use them at home. This can ensure flexibility and muscle length are maintained between treatments. Both joint range of motion and muscle length can also be supported with passive range of motion (PROM) exercises. The PROM should be graded and only carried out after the client is cautioned to work within a limited ROM if pain is likely to be an issue (Cottriall, 2014).

Electrotherapy

Elderly patients may be slower to respond with discomfort during electrotherapy, so these modalities should be used with great caution. Thin skin, less muscle thickness, and body fat can affect absorption of modalities such as laser and therapeutic ultrasound, so watch for discomfort; also reduced special senses and cognitive impairment may mean that patient signals of discomfort will change or be subtler. The therapist needs to be aware of this.

Laser therapy – this photobiostimulation increases cellular ATP and decreases nerve signaling of pain. Caution if the modality heats, patients with thinner skin and less muscle can experience burns more easily. Obese patients can "hold in" the heat of a laser in the fat layer and later fat necrosis may occur.

Therapeutic ultrasound – thermal and non-thermal effects to reduce pain/spasm and increase tissue extensibility. Caution with patients that have low lean body mass, heating the periosteum with resultant damage and discomfort may be more likely to occur.

TENS – transcutaneous electrical nerve stimulation (TENS) is low-level electrical current which disrupts the normal pain perception pathways and can help to manage chronic pain. The first few sessions should always be supervised in clinic, then a home unit can be prescribed with detailed instructions for use. If in doubt about possible discomfort during TENS, cease therapy and reassess with the veterinarian.

Shockwave therapy – high-energy sound waves, stimulate tissue repair and reduce neuropathic pain. This modality is very effective for arthritic pain but causes some discomfort during therapy sessions and temporary exacerbation of pain for a few days in some cases. Be careful about treating multiple joints in one session as mobility at home may become temporarily much worse. Counsel clients about the risks of a pain flare and weigh the pros and cons with them.

PEMF – pulsed electromagnetic field therapy (PMEF) can help with pain, inflammation swelling, and wound healing. PEMF mats are available for home use (purchase or rental). Whole-body PEMF therapy should be avoided in patients with a history of seizures.

NMES – neuromuscular electrical stimulation (NMES) is used to build muscle and has been shown to reduce muscle mass loss, increase its strength, and improve functional muscle use following orthopedic surgery (Cottriall, 2014). It may be painful over a severely atrophied muscle, atrophy due to disuse maintains sensory innervation and so be cautious and err on the side of a lower level of muscle contraction in an elderly patient.

Approach to Exercise Therapy

All patients should benefit from warm-up exercises, but they can be particularly helpful in stiff, elderly patients. The warm-up should aid muscle action and loosen stiff joints while avoiding too much active exercise and resultant fatigue before the targeted therapeutic exercises. The rehabilitation technician/nurse can give a brisk light massage up and down limbs and back to increase circulation and use range of motion to decrease stiffness. If the patient is very stiff, heat packs or warm towels/blankets should be placed on affected joints or whole body.

Once standing, practice cookie stretches and rhythmic stabilization exercises. Assisted standing is utilized if the patient cannot stand on their own.

If the patient has low endurance, then give appropriate rest periods between repetitions and between exercises. Examples of exercise are walk to mailbox and back, rest three minutes to an hour, and repeat, rather than walk twice as far at one time. Sit-to-stand rest example – 1 sit to stand, walk 5′–20′, 1 sit-to-stand, rather than 2–5 in a row. The patient may work up to 10–25 total.

Improving flexibility should be concentrated on this early on in program. Practicing range of motion and stretching is important. It is important to educate the client. Have owner keep a daily diary? Input information such as challenges – walk on uneven surfaces, over broom handles, core strength – sit pretty, diagonal leg lifts, flexibility – treat stretches, range of motion, take special note of how they sit, and get up from the down position.

Make sure the patient stays in the pain-free range.

Some geriatric patients may need assistance with mobility, for therapeutic exercises.

Assistive devices include (see Chapter 10 for more details):

- Harnesses
- Lifts
- Slings
- Carts

Therapeutic Exercises for Geriatric Patients

Weight shifting/postural perturbations help to improve strength, balance, and control; however, the therapist should make sure that the patient is standing on a high-traction surface. Be sure to counsel clients about gentle motions being effective and avoid unbalancing their pets to the point of a fall risk. Gentle more prolonged resistance to perturbation can be incorporated as the patient improves.

Cavaletti or poles placed on the ground will help balance and coordination, even in sight-impaired patients. Go slowly and do the exercise in well-lit areas; avoid bright sunlight as pupil constriction can impair vision further in patients with diminished sight.

Placing paws on targets improves accuracy as well as subtle strengthening, start with low targets, such as a rubber mat, and move on to a higher step, squishy foam pad, or even a balance disc.

Weaving around obstacles in a figure of 8 pattern can improve balance and control as well as spinal flexibility; side steps are another strength and balance exercise – competence with these two exercises can improve ability to turn in tight spaces in the house.

Backing up practice (backward walking) can also help home mobility.

More capable pets can **balance with one or even two legs lifted**.

Transitions practicing sits ranges from assisted transitions (assisting joint motion and strength as needed) to holding a sit. Start with a small, guided squat (half-sit) to standing exercise if needed. A raised platform can help a pet to keep limbs tucked in flexion and good posture for correct spinal alignment and muscle recruitment in a sit.

Active stretches for treats (cookie reaches) will improve flexibility but also challenge balance and subtly strengthen. Stretches, for example, can be nose to hip, down between front legs to arch back from a standing position (crunches) and nose to rear toes.

Tail exercises can help to improve rear awareness and strengthen the pelvic floor muscles, stimulate tail motion by brushing the fur back at the tip of the tail, gentle squeezing, or even with happy talk.

Walking on uneven surfaces can be a challenge for older pets but can also be used as a therapeutic exercise.

Pets can also practice for stair climbing by hill climbing (serpentine up the hill first if easier) combined with step up and over low obstacles and progressing to practicing low stairs in the clinic or at home, finally, steeper steps are an option.

Getting into a vehicle and onto furniture can be broken down into learned steps, a pet can be taught to step their front feet up on a raised level (equivalent of the bed, couch, or car) and wait for assistance in the rear.

Special Considerations for Hydrotherapy

Hydrotherapy for the geriatric canine must be approached with caution due to the medical constraints that may prevail. It can be hugely beneficial, as it will reduce concussive forces on joints and enable standing exercises to be carried out on patients with compromised mobility (Cottriall, 2014). The water treadmill ensures that steady-paced walking is achieved against resistance. Buoyancy aids, limb or body facilitation, and proprioceptive aids can all be applied to enhance the treatment. Only very short periods of therapy may be tolerated, and respiratory rates must be monitored to avoid over exertion, especially in patients with compromised airway function such as those with laryngeal paresis. Muscle building and improvement in cardiovascular and aerobic fitness appear to be slower in elderly veterinary patients, although gains can certainly be made. The goal is to maximize the therapy in terms of physiological and psychological outcomes. Watch for fatigue, both physical and mental. Take care to drain the water more slowly, in short intervals, because the loss of buoyancy/ weight support from rapid drainage of water can cause elderly pets to fall down in response to the sudden increased load of weight bearing.

Elderly patients are more likely to have some level of incontinence, fecal contamination of water is possible, and urinary tract infections appear to be more common as full bladder emptying may not occur. It is a good approach to evacuate and express the bladder before therapy if there is potential for issues. Failure to achieve effective defecation if an elderly patient is too weak to posture can lead to anal gland issues. After hydrotherapy, many dogs need to urinate again. Be sure to allow them to walk outside to relieve themselves.

Increased abdominal pressure in patients with intra or extra abdominal masses can indirectly affect breathing, a full veterinary examination just prior to beginning therapy is needed.

Swimming can be a good therapy for the elderly patient with the same caveats but is probably more suitable for an elderly patient who has been a competent swimmer earlier in life, as the stress and energy consumption levels will be too arduous for the inexperienced swimmer (Cottriall, 2014) (*for more details see Chapter* 21).

Physical Medicine and Rehabilitation for Patients in Palliative and Hospice Care

Veterinary patients in palliative and hospice care experience progressive medical diseases, and these are patients who can benefit from physical medicine and rehabilitation (Downing, 2011; Tinkel and Lachmann, 2002). The patient with a progressive disease can often benefit from the application of physical medicine and rehabilitation techniques, not with the intention of curing the issue at hand, or necessarily reversing the

disease process, but rather to maximize both comfort and function. Comfortable animals are more likely to continue to engage in normal, expected ADLs. In addition, comfortable animals maintain their relationships more easily with their human companions (Downing, 2011). The most applied physical medicine and rehabilitation techniques that lend themselves well to the hospice and palliative care setting include:

- Thermal modalities (cold/heat/therapeutic ultrasound)
- Massage
- ROM
- Stretching
- Chiropractic
- Joint mobilization
- Acupuncture
- Myofascial trigger point release
- Therapeutic laser
- Electrical stimulation
- Targeted pulsed electromagnetic field therapy (tPEMF)
- Therapeutic exercise

Conclusion

Rehabilitation objectives for the geriatric patient include managing pain, improving mobility and strength, providing appropriate assistive devices to promote independent ambulation, and modifying the patient's home environment to provide adequate traction, bedding, and obstacle-free space for ambulation (Starr, 2013).

Aid Graceful Aging

- Manage weight
- Adequate nutrition – macro and micronutrients
- Recognize and treat pain
- Modify environment as needed to assist
- Appropriate exercise – strength, balance, and flexibility

References

Banks, F. (2017). Chapter 7: The nose and smelling. In: *Treatment and Care of the Geriatric Veterinary Patient* (ed. M. Gardner and D. McVety), 51–55. Ames, IA: John Wiley & Sons, Inc.

Bellows, J., Colitz, C.M.H., Daristotle, L. et al. (2015). Common physical and functional changes associated with aging in dogs. *JAVMA* 246 (1): 67–75.

Bellows, J., Center, S., Daristotle, L. et al. (2016a). Aging in cats common physical and functional changes. *J Feline Med Surg* 18: 533–550.

Bellows, J., Center, S., Daristotle, L. et al. (2016b). Evaluating aging in cats how to determine what is healthy and what is disease. *J Feline Med Surg* 18: 551–570.

Bentov, I., Kaplan, S.J., Pham, T.M., and Reed, M.J. (2019). Frailty assessment: From clinical to radiological tools. *Br J Anaesth* pii: S0007-0912(19)30239-9. https://doi.org/10.1016/j.bja.2019.03.034.

Cerqueira, J.A., Restan, W.A., Fonseca, M.G. et al. (2018). Intense exercise and endurance-training program influence serum kinetics of muscle and cardiac biomarkers in dogs. *Res Vet Sci* 121: 31–39.

Chapagain, D., Range, F., Huber, L., and Virányi, Z. (2018). Cognitive aging in dogs. *Gerontology* 64 (2): 165–171. doi: 10.1159/000481621. Epub 2017 Oct 25. PMID: 29065419; PMCID: PMC5841136.

Cottriall, S. (2014). The geriatric canine and physiotherapy. *Companion Anim*, 19 (6): 296–300.

Cvejic, D., Steinberg, T.A., Kent, M.S., and Fischer, A. (2009). Unilateral and bilateral congenital sensorineural deafness in client-owned pure-breed white cats. *J Vet Intern Med* 23: 392e5.

Dewey CW, Davies ES, Xie H, and Wakshlag JJ (2019) Canine cognitive dysfunction: Pathophysiology, diagnosis, and treatment. *Vet Clin North Am Small Anim Pract* 49(3):477–499. https://doi.org/10.1016/j.cvsm.2019.01.013. Epub 2019 Mar 5. 30846383.

Dowgray, N. and Comerford, E. (2020). Feline musculoskeletal ageing how are we diagnosing and treating musculoskeletal impairment? *J Feline Med Surg* 22: 1069–1083.

Downing, R. (2011). The role of physical medicine and rehabilitation for patients in palliative and hospice care. *Vet Clin Small Anim* 41: 591–608.

Edge-Hughes, L. (2009). Physical considerations with exercising the geriatric canine patient. *CHAP Newslett* 12–14.

Freeman, L.M. (2012). Cachexia and sarcopenia: Emerging syndromes of importance in dogs and cats. *J Vet Intern Med* 26: 3–17.

Goldston, R.T. (1995). Introduction and overview of geriatrics. In: *Geriatrics and Gerontology of the Dog and Cat* (ed. R.T. Goldston and J.D. Hoskins), 1–8. Philadelphia: WB Saunders Co.

Gunn-Moore, D.A. (2011). Cognitive dysfunction in cats: Clinical assessment and management. *Top Companion Anim Med* 26: 17–24.

Gunn-Moore, D. (2014). Dementia in ageing cats. *Vet Times* 14–16.

Hammerle, M., Horst, C., Levine, E. et al. (2015). 2015 AAHA canine and feline behavior management guidelines. *J Am Anim Hosp Assoc* 51: 205–221.

Hutchinson, D., Sutherland-Smith, J., Watson, A.L., and Freeman, L.M. (2012). Assessment of methods of evaluating sarcopenia in old dogs. *Am J Vet Res* 73 (11): 1794–1800.

International Cat Care.org http://icatcare.org/advice/how-guides/how-tell-your-cat%E2%80%99s-age-human-years, accessed 8/21/2016

Landsberg, G. and Araujo, J.A. (2005). Behavior problems in geriatric pets. *Vet Clin Small Anim* 35: 675–698.

Landsberg, G., Denenberg, S., and Araujo, J. (2010). Cognitive dysfunction in cats: A syndrome we used to dismiss as 'old age'. *J Feline Med Surg* 12: 837–848.

Landsberg, G.M., DePorter, T., and Araujo, J.A. (2011). Clinical signs and management of anxiety, sleeplessness, and cognitive dysfunction in the senior pet. *Vet Clin Small Anim* 41: 565–590.

Landsberg, G., Nichol, J., and Araujo, J.A. (2012). Cognitive dysfunction syndrome a disease of canine and feline brain aging. *Vet Clin Small Anim* 42: 749–768.

Landsberg, G.M., Hunthausen, W., and Ackerman, L. (2013a). The effects of aging on the behavior in senior pets. In: *Handbook of Behavior Problems of the Dog and Cat*, 3rde, 211–236. Philadelphia, PA: Elsevier.

Landsberg, G.M., Hunthausen, W., and Ackerman, L. (2013b). Is it behavioral, or is it medical? In: *Handbook of Behavior Problems of the Dog and Cat*, 3rde, 75–94. Philadelphia, PA: Elsevier.

López-Otín, C., Blasco, M.A., Partridge, L. et al. (2013). The hallmarks of aging. *Cell* 153 (6): 1194–1217.

Mathews, K.A. (2000). Pain assessment andgeneral approach to management. *VetClin North Am Small Anim Pract* 30: 729–755.

McCauley L (2016a) Overview of exercises, When, What, Why, and How to Treat Geriatric Patients. *Canine Rehabilitation Institute Continuing Education Course*. http://www.caninerehabinstitute.com/Multimodal_Approach_Geriatric.lasso, Lectures from the course.

McCauley L (2016b) Hydrotherapy Considerations with a Geriatric Dog. *Canine Rehabilitation Institute Continuing Education Course*. http://www.caninerehabinstitute.com/Multimodal_Approach_Geriatric.lasso, Lectures from the course.

McKenzie, B.A. (2022). Comparative veterinary geroscience: Mechanism of molecular, cellular, and tissue aging in humans, laboratory animal models, and companion dogs and cats. *Am J Vet Res* 83 (6): ajvr.22.02.0027. https://doi.org/10.2460/ajvr.22.02.0027. PMID: 35524953.

Overall, K.L. (2013). Time to talk about behavioural problems. *Vet Record* 172 (9): 233–234.

Xue, Q.-L. (2011). The frailty syndrome: Definition and natural history. *Clin Geriatr Med* 27 (1): 1–15. https://doi.org/10.1016/j.cger.2010.08.009.

Saraiva IQ and Delgado E (2020) Congenital ocular malformations in dogs and cats: 123 cases. *Vet Ophthalmol* 23(6):964–978. https://doi.org/10.1111/vop.12836. Epub 2020 Oct 15. 33058381.

Seymour K (2014) Aging Pets: Senior, Geriatric and What It All Means to Experts and Readers. *Vetstreet Website*: http://www.vetstreet.com/our-pet-experts/aging-pets-senior-geriatric-and-what-it-all-means-to-experts-and-readers, AUGUST 4, (accessed July 15, 2016).

Sharp, B. (2012). Feline physiotherapy and rehabilitation 1. Principles and potential. *J Feline Med Surg* 14: 622–632.

Starr L (2013) Chapter 18: Rehabilitation for geriatric patients. In *Canine Sports Medicine and Rehabilitation*, 1st edn (eds.MC Zink and JB Van Dyke). John Wiley & Sons, 349–369.

Tinkel, R.S. and Lachmann, E.A. (2002). Rehabilitative medicine. In: *Principles and Practice of Palliative Care and Supportive Oncology*, 2nde (ed. A.M. Berger, R.K. Portenoy, and D.E. Weissman), 968–970. Philadelphia: Lippincott William & Wilkins.

Warnes, C. (2015). Changes in behaviour in elderly cats and dogs, part 2: Management, treatment and prevention. *Vet Nurse* 6 (10): 590–597.

Wilson, W.J. and Mills, P.C. (2005). Brainstem auditory-evoked response in dogs. *Am J Vet Res* 66 (12): 2177–2187.

Wyatt, H.L., Chuck, L., Rabinowitz, B. et al. (1978). Enhanced cardiac response to catecholamines in physically trained cats. *Am J Physiol* 234 (5): H608–H613.

14

The Disabled Patient Part 4: Home Nursing Care

Julia E. Tomlinson[1,2] and Elizabeth E. Waalk[1]

[1] *Twin Cities Animal Rehabilitation & Sports Medicine Clinic, Burnsville, MN, USA*
[2] *Veterinary Rehabilitation and Orthopedic Medicine Partners, San Clemente, CA, USA*

Introduction

People face many challenges when caring for a disabled pet. Challenges can begin on the first day of the injury or disease, or they may develop over time despite the best efforts of both the veterinary team and owner to avoid or overcome them. Clients/caregivers need to gain a thorough understanding of their pet's diagnosis and the prognosis for recovery of function. Accurate prognosis can be very difficult to give in patients with neurologic issues. In our experience, recovery of an injured nervous system tends to be slow, with sporadic improvements, long plateaus, and sometimes regressions (temporary or permanent). The patient that comes out of surgery for a disc fenestration/decompression able to walk when they could not do so before surgery certainly has a good prognosis; however, mild residual neurologic deficits can remain for life. Conversely, studies by Olby *et al.* (Olby *et al.*, 2003, 2020) of dogs with spinal cord compression and loss of deep pain prior to surgery (traditionally thought of as having a poor prognosis; Lawson (1971)) revealed a fair to good prognosis for return to ambulation, though that is dependent on the degree of spinal cord damage and the level of the lesion.

Understanding that some pets are disabled for a brief recovery period, whereas others may remain disabled in the long-term can help caregivers to be equipped mentally and physically at home and to think about home-life adjustments. An optimistic but pragmatic approach to the challenges ahead mentally equips people for the long-term care needs of their disabled pets. Understanding their pet's unique limitations and identifying how to help their pet function maximally with adequate assistance can help minimize the development of additional problems. For example, large dogs that are suddenly unable to support their own weight obviously can present a challenge when moving them around the home, even if the house is only one level. A home with stairs at each exit, along with up to the bedrooms and down to the basement will present significant obstacles. It may be extremely difficult to facilitate even the most basic of activities for the larger pet, whereas a small pet can be lifted and carried when needed.

The caregivers will need some help with caring for themselves. It is physically and emotionally draining to care for a disabled individual, whether human or animal). Proper body mechanics should be explained to guard against injury (e.g., muscle strains).

Proper Body Mechanics

Body mechanics is a broad term used to denote an effort coordinated by the muscles, bones, and nervous system. It can either be good or bad and can be directly related to the occurrence of back pains.

The following rules should be applied when transferring or moving your patients to protect your back:

- Always keep the lower portion of your back in its normal position.
- Move as close to the patient as you can.
- Do not twist your body. Always do a side step or a pivot.
- Set your feet into a comfortable and solid wide base of support when lifting.
- Keep your abdominal muscles contracted, bow slightly using the hips, and squat.
- Keep the head upright and hold your shoulders up.

Pushing up from the knees and using your own momentum will help you lift the patient (see Figure 14.1).

Elderly or disabled caregivers may encounter more challenges when caring for

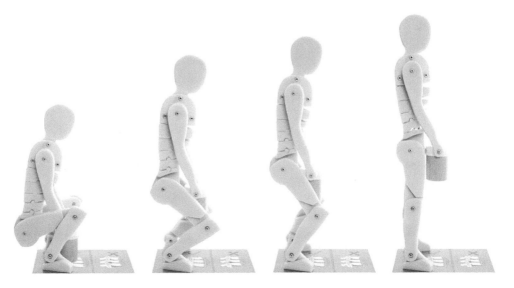

Figure 14.1 Use of proper body mechanics.

even the smallest of pets. Part of our job when providing rehabilitative care is to understand the logistics and limitations of the patient, the home environment, and the caregivers themselves and then to apply this to a realistic home care plan.

Even under the best circumstances and with the most capable caregiver caring for the easiest patient, issues can develop that interfere with caregiver compliance. This, for example, may be a conflict of work schedules, lack of available helpers, or a case of compassion fatigue. It may be other outside influences. Sometimes, friends or acquaintances with strong but well-meaning opinions can have an effect which further burdens the caregiver with pressure to make a decision or to do things differently. Caregivers need friends and family to provide mental and practical support in order to help them care for their disabled pet. When the support system of understanding family and friends is not available, caregivers can quickly become overwhelmed. They may even feel totally absorbed by their pet's problems and, as a result, ultimately guilty for keeping their pet alive in their prolonged disabled state. Compassion fatigue is a natural response to a traumatizing effect experienced by someone close to you: the stress resulting from helping a suffering individual (Figley, 1995). The risk of compassion fatigue increases with ongoing exposure to suffering and with unexpected disruptions to the caregiver's life; this can be particularly common when there is a loss of hope for patient recovery (Sabo, 2011).

Preventing and treating compassion fatigue starts with identifying the risk and providing information to clients. A good place to start is the Compassion Fatigue Awareness Project (www.compassionfatigue.org).

Respite care (see later in this chapter) is a way that the caregivers can take a short break from the constant daily care routine while knowing their pets are well cared for.

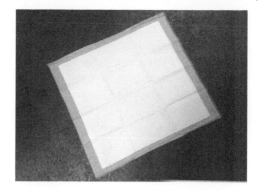

Figure 14.2   Absorbent diaper/potty pads.

Teaching home care techniques can be difficult. Each person learns a little differently and it is important to approach the task with several different ways of teaching care (National Research Council, 2000). Verbal and written explanations are a good start, and handouts with pictures along with video demonstrations can be referred back to later. However, many people learn best by doing the task. Demonstrations should be followed by giving the caregiver an opportunity to go through the motions. This is essential to determine potential success with a procedure and to ease a nervous caregiver into an "I can do it" attitude. Analogies can be helpful. For example, the bladder can be compared to a water balloon when teaching someone how to express it. You can send home samples of materials needed, like absorbent "potty" pads (see Figure 14.2), and this may help to get care started in the right way. A list of resources (websites) should be provided for mobility help, safety confinement, ramps, steps, or other care items.

Goals of Nursing Care

Maintaining Hygiene

This is a continuous process and with an incontinent patient can be viewed as a constant battle. Counsel caregivers that even a continent patient will have accidents, as a poorly mobile pet will not be able to easily signal their need to go outside. Gentle shampoo should be on hand for frequent bathing. Paper towels should be within reach of the caregiver but not the pet. Wet wipes can be useful but can be harsh and contain alcohol. Remember that frequent mechanical wiping can irritate skin, and sometimes rinsing is kinder and gentler. A handheld shower attachment for the tub is a handy thing to have both inside (and outside when the weather is warm enough). Skin protectants and emollients can help to prevent issues and provide a barrier for areas of skin that are frequently wet or soiled. Stacking absorbent pads under the patient can allow for a quick easy cleanup in a time-crunch situation; if an accident happens, simply remove the soiled top pad (see Box 14.1). Multiple waterproof bed liners can help as they can be exchanged and protect underlying padding. Trimming excess hair from the area surrounding the anal opening helps to prevent stool blockage and ultimately constipation.

Box 14.1   Hygiene care for the incontinent pet

Products list for maintaining hygiene:

- Gentle shampoo
- Astringent-free wet wipes
- Absorbable diaper/pee pads (e.g., Chux)
- Emollient or barrier creams (diaper creams)
- Paper towels
- Waterproof bed liners

Diapers can work well provided they stay in place and are changed regularly. A way of keeping diapers up that is available is braces/suspenders (https://pawinspired.com/products/dog-diaper-suspenders). There are reusable washable diapers as well as disposable diapers.

Assisting Mobility

The disabled pet will need varying levels of assistance in order to be mobile. Slings can be helpful and can be purchased in different sizes both with and without padding/linings for comfort. You can also make a sling by cutting the sides from a canvas bag. Simply cut one side of the bag, including the handle, from the top of the bag to the bottom and then the other side of the handle from top to bottom. Keeping the handles intact, you end up with a long strip of canvas with handles at each end (see Figure 14.3). This simple homemade sling is lightweight, inexpensive, and easy to use. However, there is no padding, so it should be used for brief periods only. Harnesses that are padded are much more suitable for long-term use, though they should be removed daily and the skin checked for sores. An example is the Help 'Em Up Harness™ (see Figure 14.4).

It is important to counsel caregivers using any assistive lifting device about how to provide the minimum necessary assistance while allowing for some patient effort (see Figure 14.5, Video 14.1). Carrying the patient like a suitcase is uncomfortable for pet and caregiver and will not aid return of mobility.

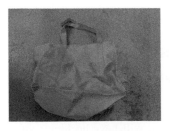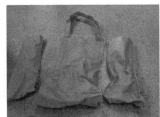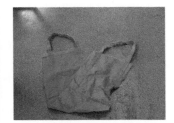

Figure 14.3 Handmade sling.

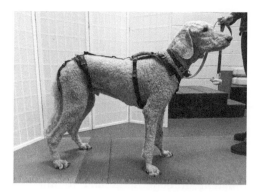

Figure 14.4 Help 'Em UpTM Harness.

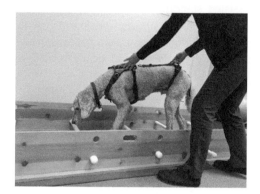

Figure 14.5 Correct way to lift a dog in sling or harness.

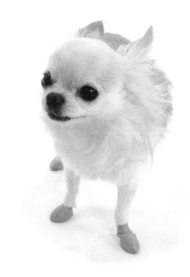

Figure 14.6 PawzTM boots.

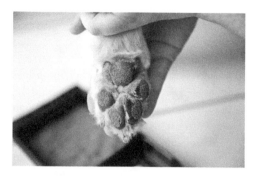

Figure 14.7 Paw Friction by Pawtology.

Providing surface traction is a mobility aid that may be easily overlooked. Caregivers should be questioned about the home environment, including flooring. As a patient starts to regain some functional mobility, traction issues can prevent him or her from getting into a stand or from maintaining the limbs in adduction without slipping. Providing rugs (or the more easily cleanable option of yoga mats) on the floors, trimming nails and hair on feet (as better grip is obtained with foot pads), fitting boots or socks with grip bottoms (see Figure 14.6), adhesive grip "sand" for pads (see Figure 14.7), or toenail grips (see Figure 14.8) can be instrumental in preventing unnecessary falls and allowing some mobility (Video 14.2). Other mobility aids such as carts are discussed in Chapter 11 on assistive devices.

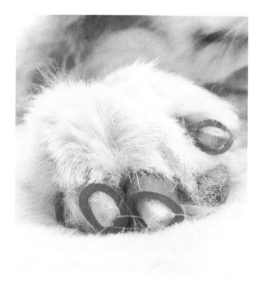

Figure 14.8 Dr. Buzby's ToeGrips™.

Preventing Complications

Benjamin Franklin said, "An ounce of prevention is worth a pound of cure" (Franklin, 1735). This statement can be applied to a disabled pet. The caregiver needs to be mindful of preventing contracture of muscles and connective tissue, including joints, protecting against skin sores and other injuries, and treating pain that occurs from immobility and possible infection. Routine hygiene should always apply, for example, removing feces in a timely manner and washing hands to avoid contamination spread.

When speaking of prevention of injury for the disabled pet, the whole home needs to be examined from the perspective of the patient. Confining the patient to a safe area away from potential falls or other injuries is an important place to start. Remember that as a pet becomes more mobile; low barriers may be inadequate, and further modifications may be needed. Bedding should be kept clean and dry and well padded. Clean dry bedding with waterproof pads beneath it is ideal, or absorbent disposable pads can be placed on top of the bed. Placing mats in the rest of the patient area can help prevent sores from a patient dragging themselves around. Yoga mats or padded play mats are ideal and are easy to keep in place so that they do not slide with the pet. They also wipe clean relatively easily.

One of the plethora of assistive devices for disabled pets is a "bag" which protects the rear limbs of patients who drag their rear around in a sit (scoot). The authors do not condone the use of this bag in most cases, because allowing a patient to gait pattern in a scoot reinforces this pattern as the "normal" gait and makes it harder to encourage walking with assistance (the goal of which is to return to full mobility). However, in patients with no possibility of return to functional gaiting the bag can help to protect the skin of the rear limbs, but it must only be used when the patient is confined to a small space and extra attention needs to be paid to hygiene to avoid a warm bag filled with urine or feces sitting next to the skin.

Recumbent patients should have their position changed, preferably every 4 hours. Prop aids, such as a pillow, rolled up blanket, or towel taped in a roll, can keep a patient in the sternal position to allow full inflation of both lungs and to improve venous return (Lamm *et al.*, 1994; Walther *et al.*, 1998). Upright positioning (sternal or assisted standing) for eating and drinking aids in digestion and can prevent problems with regurgitation and aspiration pneumonia. Food intake should be decreased to avoid weight gain due to less activity. A lower-calorie food with the same micronutrient density and adequate protein intake to prevent muscle loss is ideal. Lower fat, higher fiber diets can provide good satiety while keeping calories low and intestines healthy and regular. Conversely, sometimes, we need to switch the patient to a low-residue food to decrease the number of times stool is passed or the amount of feces in each stool passed by an incontinent patient.

Preventing tissue contracture is achieved with manual therapies both in clinic and for the caregiver to perform at home. Therapies suitable for use at home include passive range of motion (PROM), massage, and stretching. This touch is important as it helps pain management, strengthens the human–animal bond on both sides, and provides the motion that joints and muscles need to maintain health. Therapies such as these should be performed at home a minimum of twice daily, as joint health is dependent on moving through a full range of motion every 8–12 hours (Matsuzaki *et al.*, 2013; Kojima *et al.*, 2014). The importance of these exercises should be stressed to the client, as once contracted, even non-ambulatory patients can run into difficulty and discomfort – some contracted patients may have difficulty fitting in carts.

Maintaining Functional Elimination

A regular schedule is the key to managing incontinence; using the natural gastrocolic reflex to stimulate stool passing can help control accidents. After a patient eats, a caregiver should wait about 10 minutes and then stimulate their pet by gently touching the perineal area with a cotton swab to stimulate anal sphincter contractions. We recommend using a lubricated cotton-tipped swab/applicator and just inserting it into the rectum. The swab does not need to go in very far but just the cotton tip only. It can also be helpful to "circle the drain" to stimulate the whole anal opening all around. This, in turn, will stimulate rectal contractions and passage of stools.

Some dogs need more help, as they may not have the feeling or sensation of the need to void. These dogs would benefit from evacuation assistance versus just stimulation, and this can be taught to caregivers using a hands-on, in-person demonstration, allowing the caregiver to perform the action under your supervision. This technique is also taught to relatives providing home care to humans, and it is safe if taught carefully. The equipment necessary for successful evacuation includes gloves, lubricant, and a bag for the excrement. Caregivers should be instructed to don gloves and to use their dominant hand (for more fine motor control to ensure being gentle as possible), lubricate the index finger, and enter the anal opening. Be sure not to advise to avoid lifting the tail too far putting pressure/discomfort on the lower spine. Once in the anal opening, then feel for stool and gently extract as able using a partially hooked finger or a circular motion while slowly retracting. If weather permits, it is good to take the patient outside to pass stools, even if they are minimally aware of their passing.

Mimicking the old routine, with time of day and location can help to restore some conscious awareness of stool passing, if there is any residual sensation.

You and your supervising veterinarian can discuss changing dietary fiber to modify stools, either to more or less volume and firmer or softer consistency depending on the patient. This option should be tried before laxatives or stool softeners are introduced in the case of constipation, as an unfortunate side effect of loose stools and urgency from treatment with laxatives can cause very difficult problems for the disabled pet.

Bladder emptying needs can vary. It is best to allow as much bladder function (contraction) as possible. For example, the caregiver can initiate urination with gentle pressure on the bladder to stimulate emptying and then allow the patient to continue urination until it slows. Once the stream of urine has slowed and then stopped, the caregiver ensures complete emptying with full expression. Medications can help to improve bladder muscle and sphincter activity in some cases and will be prescribed by the veterinarian. Caregivers need to be counseled about the risk of urinary tract infections due to incomplete bladder emptying (Stiffler *et al.*, 2006). Having good access to drinking water so that urine production is adequate and assisting the flow if the stream is intermittent can help to prevent infections. After initiation of the stream and then allowing the pet to void, the caregiver can express the bladder to remove as much residual urine as possible. Signs of infection or bladder inflammation are not always the same for all pets. Bladder infections can cause an increase in urinary accidents, as the irritation can cause more frequent urination due to spasms of the urethra or bladder wall. The accidents may happen often but usually with less urine output, you may even notice a discharge or an increase in licking of the vulva or penis.

The paralyzed pet may not have the sensation or ability to alert that they are uncomfortable. Consider changes in habits: has the frequency of bladder expression changed? Can you notice more pain or discomfort while expressing the bladder? Can you detect a difference in urine color or odor? Other signs are more subtle, these can range from kicking and jerking to spasm of hind legs. Even a change in demeanor, general malaise, or less excitement for favorite things can be a less obvious sign of urinary issues or bladder infection (Granger *et al.,* 2020).

Bladder expression instructional videos are available at https://www.handicapped-pets.com/blog/how-to-express-cat-bladder/ and https://www.handicappedpets.com/blog/how-to-express-dog-bladder/

Frequent urine samples should be taken in the case of incontinent pets. The provision of test dipsticks for home use is recommended, as an unnoticed infection can cause further problems, including pain and more extensive infections (Ybarra *et al.*, 2014).

Managing Pain and Comfort

Recognizing pain can be difficult for caregivers. Many signs of pain (such as being reluctant to move, stiffness getting up, and restlessness) are not apparent in an already immobile or less mobile pet. Helping caregivers to recognize subtle signs of pain can improve patient advocacy and quality of life. A home pain scoring method is not always necessary, but a checklist of some sort can help caregivers maintain a pet's comfort. Keeping note of appetite, enthusiasm for greetings, sleep patterns, and demeanor in a daily diary is useful, as it can detect patterns of comfort. Sometimes, the most enthusiastic rehabilitation exercises aimed at regaining mobility can result in weakness and pain the next day. The benefits of working hard to regain gait need to be balanced with everyday comfort and adequate pain management. Step one is enlisting the home caregiver to recognize and communicate that.

Pain scoring should be performed at every therapy visit. Do not assume that a patient with poor limb function has no pain just because they have reduced sensation (see Chapter 3 on pain management for more details). After spinal surgery, dogs were found to have some detectable incisional discomfort for about six months (Zidan *et al.*, 2020).

A comfortable environment includes adequate access to food and water, clean padded surroundings, climate control, and good pain management. Bedding can be raised off the ground (hammock bed) to allow ventilation (and drainage if urinary incontinence is present). A chilled gel liner placed under bedding can improve cooling, and a small fan placed just outside the confinement area can also provide some cooling. Be sure to avoid a constant direct breeze. Thin patients with low muscle mass from atrophy can benefit from heat-reflecting blankets or coats to sleep in – care should be taken regarding fit so the patient does not get tangled in the item when shifting positions.

Management of bed sores can be very challenging. Loss of muscle mass will predispose to the issue in addition to immobility. Long-term rehabilitation in nonambulatory patients can minimize muscle loss aiding comfort and reducing the risk of bed sores. Rotational use of multiple different bedding surfaces, including memory foam, textured foam, and mesh hammock beds can help to change pressure distribution and prevent or relieve sores. Counsel caregivers about regularly inspecting the skin over bony prominences and alerting the rehabilitation team about any change, even hair loss. Early intervention can prevent full-thickness wounds. Deep sores (full-thickness skin defect) will need regular veterinary care and careful infection control. Foam pads can be applied or affixed directly to the skin around bony prominences. Bandages need to be changed daily, and education for home bandage changes will be of paramount importance. Digital pictures can be used to communicate progress (or lack of) when the patient is not in the clinic.

Assessing and Improving Quality of Life

It is an unfortunate reality that a disabled patient's life is somewhat restricted when compared to a patient with normal mobility. We have worked with disabled patients who become depressed. The good news is that depression can be relieved with therapeutic intervention and some minor changes in home routine. Your supervising veterinarian may choose to provide antidepressant medications or to change pain medications that have a depressive effect. More importantly, home environment and mental stimulation can be changed (see Box 14.2).

Box 14.2   Questions to ask owners about the patient

Ask the caregiver(s) and their family questions about home behaviors so that you can use this to assess patient demeanor.

- Are they happy and interactive when they greet family members?
- Strangers?
- Does their pet seem to recognize and respond to loved ones, familiar voices and/or touch?
- Do they have normal sleeping habits?
- Are they attention-seeking constantly due to boredom, or are they ignoring most people due to depression?

Mental stimulation is key in preventing depression and boredom. Enriching the home environment is a relatively simple process. Mental stimulation can be improved by keeping the pet in the room which is the main hub of activity or by periodically changing rooms to change the scenery. Visual stimulation can be improved by propping the pet in front of a window. Smaller pets can be taken for walks in a stroller; larger pets in a wagon or cart. We have even had a disabled Great Dane patient who spent a lot of time outside in his large wagon cushioned with a dog bed. Toys can be stimulating for patients (who do not like to eat them). Storing toys and switching them from time to time can make old toys exciting again. Puzzle toys can be mentally stimulating and can be incorporated with mealtime.

Motivation needs to be stimulated both at-home and during in-clinic therapy sessions. Home rehabilitation exercises should include a special treat saved only for this activity, as this can improve motivation. Praise from family is also much needed for patient happiness and motivation. Purchasing a cart for the patient may improve the depressed patient's demeanor because some mobility is restored (see Chapter 11 on assistive devices).

Improving mobility in the neurologic patient can take months or even longer. Neurologic patients usually have plateaus. Look for small triumphs to celebrate and praise. Small achievements are a big deal for neurologically challenged pets, and all of the rehabilitation team members should show enthusiasm to help patients and caregivers through motivation. Rehabilitation can have a great impact on the life of a disabled pet, especially with early intervention, even if return to full mobility is not achieved. The rehabilitation team will need to provide moral support for caregiver and pet. Creativity is key in both at-home and in-clinic therapies, but sometimes, creativity is as simple as making the old new again.

Disabled patients who have orthopedic problems generally return to adequate function more quickly than neurologic patients. The therapy plan should include addressing pain from compensatory issues as well as the primary injury/surgery site. Home therapy can be a large part of this pain management using massage, PROM, and stretching; thermotherapy and other simple modalities such as pulsed electromagnetic field therapy (PEMF) can also be provided at home. Caregivers need to be compliant with both restrictions in activity and with home exercise recommendations. Caregivers of pets with orthopedic problems may be less aware of, and therefore, less careful with subtle disabilities. During therapy visits, the team can help caregivers to understand the need for continued restrictions to prevent further injury or worsening of the existing injury. Counsel caregivers about the importance of following exercise recommendations to progress recovery in a timely manner and to achieve the best possible recovery.

Improving quality of life for the disabled geriatric pet can be challenging (see Chapter 13 – Special Considerations for the Geriatric Patient). Reduced vision or hearing may have already reduced environmental stimulation and interest; loss of sense of smell can affect appetite. Older patients can benefit from learning new behaviors and from changes in environment, even if this means a car ride rather than a walk in a new place. Patients may have been inactive before the onset of their disability and so can lack adequate strength and fitness needed to compensate for even minor disabilities. Muscle loss (sarcopenia) occurs with advancing age and with that strength is also lost (Bellows *et al.*, 2015a). Patients of very advanced age can suffer from frailty syndrome – a decline in the body's natural reserves which results in increased susceptibility to disease and weakness (Bellows *et al.*, 2015b). Inactivity from injury or disability can lead to reduced strength and muscle mass, which feeds into poor mobility and can also lead to obesity. Even a small amount of weight gain can exacerbate lameness or weakness (Mlacnik *et al.*, 2006; Marshall *et al.*, 2010). Loss of functional reserve includes declining cardiovascular and respiratory fitness (Chen *et al.*, 2014). In our practice, we see two main populations of aged patients: the thin, frail pet with poor muscle coverage and reduced appetite and the obese, unfit pet with or without concurrent disease. In both cases, the scales are tipped in the favor of morbidity, and a small problem, such as a low-grade bladder infection, can be enough to result in a marked increase in weakness.

Caring for an aged pet at home involves supporting comfort and mobility. Comfort is addressed in many ways, from adequate footing and bedding, foot and nail care, and managing weight to providing pain relief. Moving water dishes or adding water sources near where a patient is resting can help to maintain adequate water intake. Placing a mat in the kitchen where the pet eats can provide better traction and eliminate some discomfort when eating. Raising the food bowl height can also improve comfort and ensure standing during eating (a good strengthening exercise). Mobility aids range from home environment modifications (ramps and steps to furniture, blocking off difficult stairs) to patient modifications (toe grips, harnesses).

Nursing care includes bowel and bladder care; keeping skin clean and unsoiled is important. Sometimes, elderly pets need to be eliminated more frequently, so they require outside access more often. A geriatric pet may not be able to hold their tail up fully when eliminating and may contaminate their skin. Posturing to eliminate may be difficult, so full evacuation may not occur, which predisposes to bladder infections and constipation. Mobile-disabled cats may have trouble getting into a normal litter box, so using a low-walled structure such as a baking pan can provide easier access. Anal sacs may become full and uncomfortable from chronic inadequate expression. Owners need to be counseled about subtle signs to look for, areas of skin to check, and telltale signs of problems such as urinary tract infections. Improving the quality of life in the geriatric pet is often about the little things. Just having a weak, old pet stand still for a minute can improve stamina, cardiac output, and respiratory function.

Modifying the Home Environment

As stated earlier, environmental enrichment is very important. Home modifications may or may not be necessary to aid mobility depending on pet size and the amount of assistance needed. Preventing slipping in low traction areas is necessary. A simple solution is rugs or runners placed on the floor surface. Ensure that the rug grips the floor and does not slide with the pet. Inexpensive mats and runners are available from home improvement stores. Confining the disabled patient is strongly advised when supervision is not available. A small room with high traction flooring and low to no furniture is ideal if the patient has some mobility. Yoga mats can provide temporary flooring with grip. A crate or kennel is advised for pets with inadequate or no motion in the rear limbs who pull themselves around dragging the rear ("scooting"). This confinement helps to avoid the scooting motion becoming the "normal" efficient gait for the pet, reducing motivation to ambulate on four legs, even with assistance. Baby gates can be used to prevent access to stairs and to confine a pet to a small room. Higher barriers, such as a screen door, may be needed for larger and stronger pets. Ramps can be useful if a home has just a few stairs and can be used for getting into the car. Be cognizant of the incline and choose a suitable length of ramp. Carts are a great way of improving patient mobility; however, owners need to be mindful of the width of the cart and wheels compared to the home hallways and potential limitations of actual space needed to maneuver a cart in the home. It may be better for carts to be used outside only.

Other owners of disabled pets are a great resource for home care tips. In our clinic, we asked owners of long-term disabled pets to help us to prepare an "at home" guide to caregiving. This helped us to gain a fresh perspective, and we prepared a handout for owners (see Box 14.3).

Respite care is the provision of short-term accommodation in a facility outside the home in which a loved one may be placed. This provides temporary relief to those who are caring for family members, who might otherwise require permanent placement in a facility outside the home. Finding such a facility for a disabled pet can be a challenge. We have one boarding facility in our large metro area that provides the necessary level of care; the alternative is a veterinary clinic. This highlights the need for more pet boarding facilities with nursing capacity.

Box 14.3 Guide to caregiving at home

- Make a handout with pointers to help caregivers at home. Recruit previous clients for tips
- Include bowel and bladder care, bedding, and hygiene advice
- Add helpful hints – "keep paper towels in every room for quick clean-up"
- State when a caregiver should contact the clinic for red flags such as bed sores

Administering Medications to the Disabled Patient

Administering pills can be as simple as putting them in the food bowl with daily rations, but sometimes giving medication can be extremely challenging. Some pets can be very creative at avoiding swallowing their medicine. Custom treats designed to mask a pill can be useful. An alternative is to hide the pill in tasty people's food. One thing many people do not know is that fat masks taste: a bitter pill may be easier to give in cheese or peanut butter (take care regarding patients sensitive to fats, such as those prone to pancreatitis). Liquid formulas can help. Medications can also be compounded into chewable taste tablets in some cases. Whole foods stores and coops often sell gel capsules that can be used to disguise a nasty-tasting pill. We often recommend giving two treats – the first treat is untainted by a pill and the second treat contains the medication. This way the pet may be less suspicious. It is best to follow a pill with water or food (especially one administered alone without a treatment) to ensure that the pill does not remain in the esophagus, causing irritation. This is a particular issue with cats but may also be a problem in disabled pets who are immobile and unable to prop themselves up for long periods. A colleague administers pills to cats by following them with a "chaser" of water dripped into the mouth from a gauze sponge, which induces swallowing. If owners can restrain their cats, then this is an excellent method of administration. With dogs, a snack is usually enough following pill administration.

Medication schedules can be challenging for many owners; your supervising veterinarian needs to take this into account. Some medications can be administered 2–3 times daily and maybe the middle-day dose must be skipped on some days due to work or life schedules. Choosing a pain medication considers many factors, one of which should be ease of administration at home, including caregiver schedule. This improves compliance. Making a medication chart that can be checked off or initialed when medications are given is a good idea in a situation where multiple caregivers are involved. Pill cases with daily cups that can be filled for a week at a time can also help. These pill cases can be purchased for once, twice, or three times a day dosing. Both charts and weekly pill cases can help to prevent double dosing. Sometimes, medication will need to be given in injectable form. Caregivers can be taught to administer subcutaneous injections at home, using sterile saline for practice during teaching sessions. A daily dosing chart is advised.

Side effects vary with each medication and caregivers should be given detailed information about potential side effects related to the patient's medications. In the case of rehabilitation patients, the primary care veterinarian, a specialist veterinarian in another discipline, and supervising rehabilitation veterinarian may have all prescribed medications. The patient record needs to be kept up to date with all medications and any medication changes or dosage changes. This way any veterinarian involved in the case will be aware of potential side effects and interactions. As the supervising rehabilitation veterinarian will see the patient on the most frequent basis during in-clinic rehabilitation, this is the person best suited to manage and oversee all medications, and to make changes regarding pain management or other concerns. The rehabilitation veterinarian will always keep the primary care veterinarian informed of any changes.

As a side note, it is best to avoid changing medications just before a weekend, when the clinic staff are not easily available to answer questions about medications and potential side effects. The emergency veterinarian on duty may not be familiar with the case.

In-Home Hospice Care

Hospice care at home is nursing care for a patient in the final stages of life or a disease process that will end in loss of life. Caregivers of disabled pets will be already equipped to provide for their pet's needs when the end of life is near as they have been previously providing nursing care, often including bowel and bladder care. Practical and emotional support through home visits from veterinarians is variably available. The International Association for Animal Hospice and Palliative Care can provide more details (www.iaahpc.org) (see Box 14.4)

Remember that even if it is no longer feasible to transport the pet for regular in-clinic care, recheck visits every 2–3 weeks can be a big help to aid home care. Providing support via remote visits using telemedicine, by telephone, or by email can bridge some of the gap between visits.

Conclusions

Nursing care is a large portion of the rehabilitation veterinary technician's job. As an animal's nurse, you are their advocate and care provider both in clinic and at home through your education of the primary caregiver and their family. A successful rehabilitation plan should always include consideration of the home environment and necessary adaptations and nursing care.

Video 14.1   Instructional video for client on fitting assistive harness.
Video 14.2   Summary of traction aids.

Resources

Back on Track heat reflective mesh sheet or blanket (www.backontrackproducts.com)
Chillow. Soothsoft Innovations (www.chillow.com)
Discount ramps (www.discountramps.com)
Pill Pockets (www.greenies.com)
Pill Pals (https://www.henryscheinvet.com)
Toe grips: www.toegrips.com
Paw Friction: https://pawtology.com/product/pawfriction-kit/

References

Bellows, J., Colitz, C.M., Daristotle, L. et al. (2015a). Defining healthy aging in older dogs and differentiating healthy aging from disease. *J Am Vet Med Assoc* 246 (1): 77–89.

Bellows, J., Colitz, C.M., Daristotle, L. et al. (2015b). Common physical and functional changes associated with aging in dogs. *J Am Vet Med Assoc* 246 (1): 67–75.

Chen, X., Mao, G., and Leng, S.X. (2014). Frailty syndrome: An overview. *Clin Interv Aging* 9: 433–441.

Figley, C. (1995). *Compassion Fatigue: Coping with Secondary Traumatic Stress Disorder in Those Who Treat the Traumatized*. New York: Brunner-Routledge.

Franklin B (1735) Protections of towns from fire. Letters to the editor. *The Pennsylvania Gazette* February 4, 1735.

Granger, N., Olby, N.J., and Nout-Lomas, Y.S. (2020). Canine spinal cord injury consortium (CANSORT-SCI). Bladder and bowel management in dogs with spinal cord injury. *Front Vet Sci* 7: 583342. https://doi.org/10.3389/fvets.2020.583342.

Kojima, S., Hoso, M., and Watanabe, M. (2014). Experimental joint immobilization and remobilization in the rats. *J Phys Ther Sci* 26 (6): 865–871.

Lamm, W.J., Graham, M.M., and Albert, R.K. (1994). Mechanism by which the prone position improves oxygenation in acute lung injury. *Am J Respir Crit Care Med* 150 (1): 184–193.

Lawson, D.D. (1971). The diagnosis and prognosis of canine paraplegia. *Vet Rec* 89 (25): 654–658.

Marshall, W.G., Hazewinkel, H.A., Mullen, D. et al. (2010). The effect of weight loss on lameness in obese dogs with osteoarthritis. *Vet Res Commun* 34 (3): 241–253.

Matsuzaki, T., Yoshida, S., Kojima, S. et al. (2013). Influence of ROM exercise on the joint components during immobilization. *J Phys Ther Sci* 25 (12): 1547–1551.

Mlacnik, E., Bockstahler, B.A., Müller, M. et al. (2006). Effects of caloric restriction and a moderate or intense physiotherapy program for treatment of lameness in overweight dogs with osteoarthritis. *J Am Vet Med Assoc* 229 (11): 1756–1760.

National Research Council (2000). *How People Learn: Brain, Mind, Experience, and School*, expandede (ed. J.D. Bransford, A.L. Brown, and R.R. Cocking). National Academies Press https://www.nap.edu/catalog/9853/how-people-learn-brain-mind-experience-and-school-expanded-edition.

Olby, N., Levine, J., Harris, T. et al. (2003). Long-term functional outcome of dogs with severe injuries of the thoracolumbar spinal cord: 87 cases (1996–2001). *J Am Vet Med Assoc* 222 (6): 762–769.

Olby, N.J., da Costa, R.C., Levine, J.M., and Stein, V.M. (2020). Canine spinal cord injury consortium (CANSORT SCI). Prognostic factors in canine acute intervertebral disc disease. *Front Vet Sci* 7: 596059. https://doi.org/10.3389/fvets.2020.596059.

Sabo, B. (2011). Reflecting on the concept of compassion fatigue. *Online J Issues Nurs* 16 (1): 1.

Stiffler, K.S., Stevenson, M.A., Sanchez, S. et al. (2006). Prevalence and characterization of urinary tract infections in dogs with surgically treated type 1 thoracolumbar intervertebral disc extrusion. *Vet Surg* 35 (4): 330–336.

Walther, S.M., Domino, K.B., and Hlastala, M.P. (1998). Effects of posture on blood flow diversion by hypoxic pulmonary vasoconstriction in dogs. *Br J Anaesth* 81 (3): 425–429.

Ybarra, W.L., Sykes, J.E., Wang, Y. et al. (2014). Performance of a veterinary urine dipstick paddle system for diagnosis and identification of urinary tract infections in dogs and cats. *J Am Vet Med Assoc* 244 (7): 814–819.

Zidan, N., Medland, J., and Olby, N. (2020). Long-term postoperative pain evaluation in dogs with thoracolumbar intervertebral disk herniation after hemilaminectomy. *J Vet Intern Med.* 34 (4): 1547–1555.

15

Modalities Part 1: Thermotherapy

Julia E. Tomlinson[1,2] and Deana Cappucci[3]

[1] Twin Cities Animal Rehabilitation & Sports Medicine Clinic, Burnsville, MN, USA
[2] Veterinary Rehabilitation and Orthopedic Medicine Partners, San Clemente, CA, USA
[3] West Delray Veterinary, Delray Beach, FL, USA

Introduction

Thermotherapy consists of application of heat or cold (cryotherapy) for the purpose of changing the cutaneous, intra-articular, and core temperature of soft tissue with the intention of improving the symptoms of certain conditions. Thermotherapy is a useful adjunct for the treatment of musculoskeletal injuries and soft tissue injuries. Using ice or heat as a therapeutic intervention decreases joint and muscle pain. Heat and cold have opposite effects on tissue metabolism, blood flow, inflammation, edema, and connective tissue extensibility. Thermotherapy can be used in rehabilitation facilities, and there are options that are safe for home use (Brosseau *et al.*, 2003; Nadler *et al.*, 2004; Hurley and Bearne, 2008; Petrofsky *et al.*, 2013a).

Purpose

The goal of thermotherapy is to alter tissue temperature in a targeted region over time for the purpose of inducing a desired biological response. The majority of media used to change temperature are designed to deliver the thermal therapy to a target tissue with minimal impact on intervening or surrounding tissues. The use of superficial thermal agents aims to decrease pain, alter blood supply (e.g., reduce swelling), and temporarily change tissue properties (e.g., extensibility). Extensibility means that muscles can be stretched to their normal resting length and beyond to a limited degree. Superficial agents are often the most convenient modalities as they are readily available, involve minimal expense, and are frequently safe to use as part of a home treatment program (Niebaum, 2013). The primary goal of any thermal modality is to facilitate the rehabilitation plan for regaining maximal function (Dragone *et al.*, 2014).

Heat Therapy

By increasing the temperature of the skin/ soft tissue, the blood flow increases through vasodilation. Heat increases oxygen uptake and accelerates tissue healing. It also increases the activity of destructive enzymes, such as collagenase, and increases the catabolic rate (Kellogg, 2006) (see Boxes 15.1 and 15.2).

Cold Therapy

By decreasing the temperature of the skin/ soft tissue, the blood flow decreases via vasoconstriction. It will be followed afterward by vasodilation. Tissue metabolism temporarily decreases under the influence of cooling, affecting neuronal excitability, inflammation, and conduction rate (see Boxes 15.3 and 15.4). Tissue extensibility also decreases under the influence of

---

Box 15.2 Effects of local application of heat – increases

- Body temperature, respiratory rate, and heart rate if heat is applied for a prolonged time
- Capillary pressure and permeability (which can promote edema)
- Leukocyte migration into the heated area
- Local circulation (promoting healing in subacute and chronic inflammation)
- Local metabolism
- Muscle relaxation
- Tissue elasticity

Source: Adapted from Hayes (1993).

Box 15.3 Effects of local application of cold – decreases

- Blood flow because of vasoconstriction
- Edema formation
- Hemorrhage
- Histamine release
- Local metabolism
- Muscle spindle activity
- Nerve conduction velocity
- Pain
- Spasticity
- Response to acute inflammation or injury

Source: Steiss and Levine (2005). Reproduced with permission of Elsevier.

Box 15.1 Effects of local application of heat – decreases

- Blood pressure (if heat is applied for a prolonged time or over a large surface area)
- Muscle spasm
- Pain

Source: Adapted from Hayes (1993).

---

cooling due to increased tissue viscosity and decreased mobility of nonelastic tissues (Petrofsky *et al.*, 2013b). At joint temperatures of 30 °C (86 °F) or lower, the activity of cartilage-degrading enzymes, including collagenase, elastase, hyaluronidase, and protease, is inhibited. The decreased metabolic rate limits further injury and aids the tissue in surviving the cellular hypoxia that occurs

---

Box 15.4   Effects of local application of cold – increases

- Connective tissue stiffness (with decreased tensile strength)
- Temporary muscle viscosity (with decreased ability to perform rapid movements)
- Activation threshold of tissue nociceptors

Source. Millis (2015). Reproduced with permission of Elsevier.

Table 15.1   Pathophysiologic effects of topical modalities.

	Heat	Cold
Pain	↓	↓
Spasm	↓	↓
Metabolism	↑	↓
Blood flow	↑	↓
Inflammation	↑	↓
Edema	↑	↓
Extensibility	↑	↓

↓, decrease; ↑, increase.
Source: Adapted from Nadler *et al.* (2004).

after injury (Bleakley *et al.*, 2004; Hubbard and Denegar, 2004) (see Table 15.1).

Mechanism of Action

Skin blood flow is controlled by two branches of the sympathetic nervous system: a noradrenergic vasoconstrictor system and a cholinergic active vasodilator system (Charkoudian, 2003). These dual sympathetic neural control mechanisms affect the major aspects of thermoregulatory responses over most of the body's surface. During periods of hypothermia, falling core and skin temperatures lead to reflexive increases in sympathetic active vasoconstrictor nerve activity to reduce skin blood flow and conserve body heat (Sluka *et al.*, 1999). During periods of heat stress, increasing core and skin temperatures lead to reflexive increases in sympathetic active vasodilator nerve activity to increase skin blood flow (Charkoudian, 2003). Heat has an analgesic effect via heat-sensitive calcium channels, which respond to heat by increasing intracellular calcium. This generates action potentials that, in turn, increase stimulation of sensory nerves, causing a feeling of heat in the brain. These channels are part of a family of receptors called TRPV receptors. TRPV1 and TRPV2 channels are sensitive to noxious heat, while TRPV4 channels are sensitive to normal physiological heat (Holowatz *et al.*, 2005). Their multiple binding sites allow several factors to activate these channels. Once activated, they can also inhibit the activity of purine pain receptors (Liu and Salter, 2005). These receptors, called P2X2 and P2Y2 receptors, are mediated pain receptors and are in the peripheral small nerve endings. For example, with peripheral pain, heat can directly inhibit pain. However, when pain originates from deep tissue, heat stimulates peripheral pain receptors which can alter what has been termed "gating" in the spinal cord and reduce deep pain.

Studies have suggested that temperature can affect the exchange between Ca^{2+} and Na^+ in neural cells (Swenson *et al.*, 1996). An increase in both pain threshold and pain tolerance with the use of cooling has been documented. Increased superficial tissue temperature results in the release of chemical mediators such as histamine and prostaglandins, which results in vasodilation and increased blood flow in some tissues. These vasodilatory mechanisms do not significantly affect blood flow in skeletal muscle since skeletal muscle blood flow is heavily influenced by other physiologic and metabolic factors. Exercise is the best way to increase blood flow to skeletal muscle.

Physiologic Effects

Many of the local physiological effects of heat and cold have been studied thoroughly. Heat increases skin and joint temperature, improves blood circulation and muscle relaxation, and decreases joint stiffness. Cold numbs pain, decreases swelling, constricts blood vessels, and blocks nerve impulses to the joints (Oosterveld and Rasker, 1994; Sluka *et al.*, 1999; Brosseau *et al.*, 2003).

Deep heating, such as through thermal ultrasound (Dorn, 2015), is thought to lessen nerve sensitivity, increase blood flow, increase tissue metabolism, decrease muscle spindle sensitivity to stretch, cause muscle relaxation, and increase flexibility. Heat stimulates the cutaneous thermoreceptors that are connected to the cutaneous blood vessels, causing the release of bradykinin, which relaxes the smooth muscle walls, resulting in vasodilation. Muscle relaxation occurs because of a decreased firing rate of the gamma efferents (sending signals away from the central nervous system), thus lowering the threshold of the muscle spindles and increasing afferent activity. There is also a decrease in firing of the alpha motor neuron to the extrafusal muscle fiber, resulting in muscle relaxation and decrease in muscle tone (Prentice, 1982; Peres *et al.*, 2002).

Types of Thermotherapy

Heat

Heating agents are classified as superficial or deep heating. Superficial heating agents penetrate up to approximately 2 cm in depth, whereas deep heating agents elevate tissue temperatures at depths of 3 cm or more (Steiss and Levine, 2005). Heat sources are classified as radiant, conductive, or convective. An infrared lamp is an example of a radiant superficial heating device; a hot pack is an example of a conductive superficial heating device; and a whirlpool is an example of moist heat delivered by conduction and convection.

Superficial Heat

Superficial heating agents may include hot packs, heat wraps, hosing with warm water, whirlpools, paraffin baths, circulating warm water blankets, electric heating pads, and infrared lamps (Dragone *et al.*, 2014). Another common form of superficial thermotherapy is heated beds for dogs, which have been used for comfort or conditions such as arthritis (see Box 15.5).

Deep Heating

Deep heating agents include therapeutic ultrasound and shortwave diathermy. The mechanisms of therapeutic ultrasound are further explained in Chapter 18. Diathermy is a therapeutic treatment most prescribed for joint conditions such as rheumatoid arthritis and osteoarthritis. In diathermy, a high-frequency electric current is delivered via shortwave, microwave, or ultrasound to generate deep heat in body tissues (Giorgi and Crucik, 2013). Diathermy increases blood flow, thereby improving circulation, promoting tissue healing, alleviating

---

Box 15.5   Indications for heat therapy

- Subacute and chronic traumatic and inflammatory conditions
- Decreased range of motion attributable to stiffness and/or contracture (basis for the principle of "heat and stretch")
- Pain relief, because heat may render sensory nerve endings less excitable

Source: From Steiss and Levine (2005). Reproduced with permission of Elsevier.

muscle and joint pain, and increasing connective tissue elasticity (Notarnicola *et al.*, 2017). It has been used as a therapeutic modality in veterinary medicine, mostly in Europe. A report using diathermy on six dogs for either muscle contracture or arthritis used thermography to evaluate the heating effects, this study found a temperature increase of about 1 °C, but it was higher for the short-haired dog at almost 2 °C.

The main contraindications to using diathermy are infection, vascular diseases, neoplasia, and pregnancy (Dragone *et al.*, 2010). Avoid growth plates and reproductive organs. Overweight animals may have more risk of overheating and thermal injury, just as for high-powered laser therapy.

Superficial Heating Agents

Hot packs – Hot packs come in a variety of sizes and shapes. They can be heated sacks with a canvas covering that may be filled with cracked corn, beans, rice, bentonite (hydrophilic silicate gel), or other inert materials. Other hot packs are electric heating pads, damp microwaved towels, or circulating warm water blankets. A hydrocollator unit can also be used to maintain moist heat packs.

Water – Water may be applied directly to the area being treated. Towels heated with warm water may be used, or the affected body part may be immersed in a warm water bath or a whirlpool. If a whirlpool is chosen, be mindful that systemic heating with a warm bath may decrease blood pressure and increase the heart rate (Dragone *et al.*, 2014). Whirlpools have the advantage of also providing increased hydrostatic pressure to submerged body parts, which may reduce edema. Increased hydrostatic pressure helps to increase lymphatic and venous flow from a distal to proximal direction. The temperature of a whirlpool is based on the needs of the individual animal. For example, patients with chronic conditions may be treated with warmer water than patients with more acute disorders.

A combination of heat and electrical stimulation is available via whirlpool therapy. This is a treatment combining the benefits of hydrotherapy using VetSystem's™ warm water whirlpool with the pain management benefits of electrical stimulation using ASP's Omnistim 500 Pro®. The bioelectric whirlpool has assisted in the treatment of animals recovering from orthopedic joint surgeries, osteoarthritis, edema, chronic pain, and acute injuries such as sprains, tears, and muscle fatigue. The warm water and jets from the whirlpool deliver a comfortable massage to the animal, increase blood flow, and promote endorphin release and general relaxation (see Figure 15.1).

Paraffin baths – This procedure is uncommon in veterinary medicine because it is messy. Details can be found in Rothstein *et al.* (2005).

Infrared lamps – Infrared lamps emit infrared light that penetrates the skin to promote increased blood flow and circulation. This method of thermotherapy is used to warm large areas of the body. The lamps are positioned 30–40 cm from the affected area. The therapist should place his or her hand under the heat lamp for several minutes at the desired height to be sure that the temperature is comfortable. Because the patient needs to remain stationary during treatment, this method of heating is uncommon (Dragone *et al.*, 2014).

Ceramic agents – Some products use ceramic to reflect the wearer's body heat and warm a body part. Back on Track® products are used to keep muscles warm in canine or equine athletes, but are also used for the symptomatic relief of painful stiff joints. These products are made from a fabric which contains polyester thread embedded with a fine ceramic powder. They have been used in the authors' clinic to keep the muscles of athletic dogs warm between

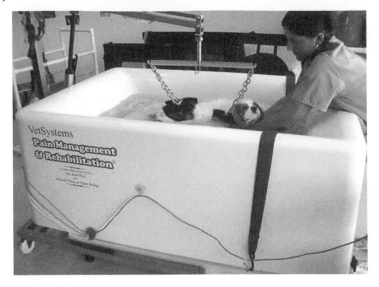

Figure 15.1 Kari Koudelka with a patient in the Bioelectric Whirlpool.

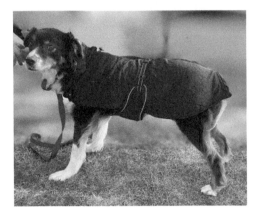

Figure 15.2 Jake the dog in a Back On Track heat reflective sheet.

activities, and some clients have reported pain relief for their older dogs when wearing the products. The company claims that the reflection of body heat is through far-infrared waves (see Figure 15.2).

It has been claimed that far-infrared waves (Masuda *et al.*, 2005; Yu *et al.*, 2006):

- increase blood circulation and oxygen supply to tissues,
- reduce inflammation and swelling in muscles and joints,
- ease muscle pain and tension,
- speed up the healing process, and
- warm the muscles prior to exercise, thereby reducing the risk of strain and injury.

General Recommendations for Heat

Heat should be applied for no more than 15–20 minutes at a time. Hot packs are relatively safe because they cool during treatment, minimizing the risk of burns. Padding is applied around the pack. The pack retains heat for approximately 30 minutes. The heat is absorbed mostly by the skin and subcutaneous fat. Wrapping the hot pack with a towel or drape material is essential so the pack does not come in direct contact with the patient's skin. Heat wraps are marketed for people. Some products provide up to eight hours of continuous low-level heat and could be used for small animals. Whirlpools have the advantage of also providing increased hydrostatic pressure to submerged body parts, which helps to increase lymphatic and venous flow from a distal-to-proximal orientation. Agitation within a whirlpool decreases the thermal gradient so that the temperature of the water in the tank is consistent throughout. The temperature of a whirlpool is based on the needs of the individual animal. For example, patients with chronic conditions may be treated with warmer water than patients with more acute disorders (see Box 15.5).

Precautions When Using Thermotherapy

Test the temperature of the modality you want to use, or have the client test the temperature before applying it to their pets. Heat packs, in particular, can vary in temperature depending on ambient conditions. There is a risk of overheating in dogs immersed in a heated whirlpool. They should be observed, and their rectal temperature measured if in doubt. If there is reduced sensation because of nerve damage or even patient compromise in reaction time (sedation, reduced cognition), then caution should be used. Longhaired animals may heat less quickly than short-coat or clipped patients. A hot or cold pack can be heavy when placed on the animal, so check for this by watching respirations or if the patient becomes irritable. In some instances, the pack can be placed under the area to be treated. Seek the advice of the supervising veterinarian if there are open or infected wounds (see Box 15.6).

Cryotherapy

Cryotherapy is the therapeutic application of cold in rehabilitation and physical therapy. Cold can be applied through a variety of mechanisms, including cold packs, ice massage, cold water baths, mechanical and electrical compression units, and vapocoolant sprays. Cryotherapy can be used throughout the rehabilitative process to mitigate negative effects of inflammatory responses (Hanks *et al.*, 2015). The sensations reported by people after ice application are an initial sensation of cold followed by burning, aching, and eventual numbness (Rintamäki, 2007). Cold penetrates deeper and lasts longer than heat because of the decreased circulation resulting from cold application (Steiss and Levine, 2005). The primary method of providing physical control of pain and inflammation in the immediate postoperative period is cryotherapy (e.g., application of ice). Cryotherapy is used during the acute phase of tissue injury and healing to mitigate the effects of tissue injury. Cryotherapy is also used after

---

Box 15.6 Contraindications for thermotherapy

- Electric heating pads and infrared lamps have a higher risk of burns. Electric heating pads should never be placed under an anesthetized patient or a patient with decreased superficial sensation. In general, a patient should never be left unattended during treatment, and the skin should be monitored frequently
- Do not use heat in an actively bleeding patient
- Acute inflammation

- Cardiac insufficiency
- Decreased impaired circulation in the area to be treated (to avoid overheating)
- Neurologic patients may not feel that it is becoming too hot
- Fever
- Malignancy
- Poor body heat regulation
- Pregnancy

Source: From Batavia (2004). Reproduced with permission of Elsevier.

Box 15.7 Indications for cold therapy

- In animals with acute injury, rest and ice can be readily used. Application of cold to minimize postsurgical swelling is also recommended
- The reduction in pain and inflammation with cryotherapy may lead to increased range of motion in affected joints
- Local cold application may reduce spasticity in spinal cord disorders
- Cooling may inhibit the extension of tissue damage with thermal burns, with greatest benefit occurring when a coolant is applied immediately after burn injury

Source: From Hanks *et al.* (2015). Reproduced with permission of Elsevier.

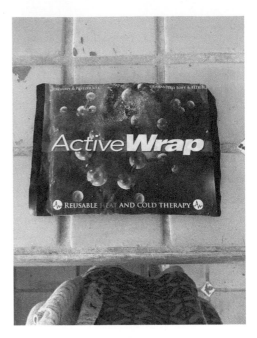

Figure 15.3 Ice Gel Pack. *Source:* Courtesy Mary Ellen Goldberg (author).

exercise during rehabilitation to minimize adverse secondary inflammatory responses (Millis, 2004) (see Box 15.7).

Cryotherapy may be achieved by the following physical mechanisms (Dragone *et al.*, 2014):

- Conduction (ice/cold packs, iced towels, ice massage, contrast bath, and cold compression units)
- Convection (cold baths)
- Evaporation (vapocoolant sprays).

Cryotherapy Agents

Ice or gel packs – Examples of ice packs/cold packs are crushed ice placed in a moist towel; a plastic bag wrapped in a moist towel; or water and rubbing alcohol in a 3:1 ratio in a sealed plastic bag and placed in a freezer (this should result in a slush-type consistency) (Burnett and Wardlaw, 2012). When using a plastic bag filled with ice or a gel pack, cover it before application with a thin, wet layer of fabric to improve temperature exchange between the tissue and cold

agent. Do not use a thick layer of fabric, such as a towel or blanket, because therapeutic temperatures may not be reached in deep tissues. In general, the recommended treatment time for ice packs to target deeper tissue of 1 cm is 20 minutes (Neibaum, 2013; Janas, 2021) (see Figure 15.3).

Ice massage – Freezing water in cups or any other form of cylinder can be used to form an ice massage medium. To apply the massage, the therapist holds onto the cup, exposes the ice surface, and puts it in direct contact with the patient's skin. Treatment time is generally 5–10 minutes or until the affected area is erythematous, slightly pink or red, and numb (assess by pricking with a small gauge needle). This technique can be useful for small, irregular areas (Dragone *et al.*, 2014). Ice popsicles can also be made by placing a handle, such as a tongue depressor, into the water before freezing.

Towels in ice water – Multiple towels must be used because a single towel will not maintain adequate therapeutic temperatures long enough to be effective. An effective method of using towels is to immerse two towels in ice water and alternate applications when the towel being used becomes too warm for therapeutic effectiveness (Bockstahler *et al.*, 2004).

Contrast baths – This technique is used by alternating cold and warmer water. It is generally used to decrease edema because of the alternating vasoconstriction and vasodilation. An example of this would be immersion in cold water for three minutes and then immersion in warm water for one minute (Dragone *et al.*, 2014). The treatment therapy should end with cold.

Cold compression units – These devices are commercially available and use a combination of controlled pressure with a continuous flow of cold water to help minimize swelling and pain postoperatively. The device usually consists of a sleeve with tubing running throughout that alternately circulates cold water and air. The combination of compression and cooling is effective in treating tissues in the acute phase of healing. An example of such a unit is the Game Ready® (which is no longer made). A similar unit is made by https://companionanimal-health.com/page/cold-compression. This technology was developed for canine and equine patients from human technology. Detailed information can be found at www. gamereadyveterinary.com/ (see Figure 15.4).

Cold bath/immersion – In this type of application, the patient typically stands with the affected limb immersed in a container of cold water at 2–16 °C (35–60 °F), and the treatment generally lasts for 10–20 minutes. Rapid and significant tissue cooling occurs but is difficult to apply because of poor patient compliance (Hanks *et al.*, 2015). This therapy is used more frequently with horses, especially for soaking feet that are possibly laminitic. Andrew Van Eps and Christopher Pollitt studied the best methods for adequately cooling the feet of at-risk horses (Van Eps and Pollitt, 2004). It is generally accepted that cold therapy should be continuous for 48–72 hours during the entire developmental phase and for another 24 hours beyond the end of clinical signs of the primary disease. It is important to include the foot, pastern, fetlock, and distal cannon region in the cold therapy for the best results and to maintain intimate cold contact with the limb to achieve therapeutic temperature ranges (see Figure 15.5).

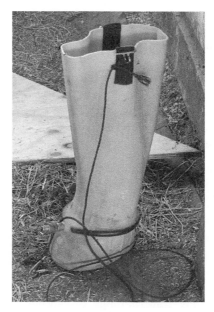

Figure 15.5 Boot for cryotherapy in a horse. *Source:* Courtesy of Dr. Chris Pollitt.

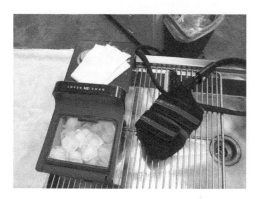

Figure 15.4 GameReady Cryotherapy Compression.

The suggested range for therapy is from 5 to 10 °C (41–50 °F). To achieve intimate contact, crushed ice is preferable to ice cubes. Ice wraps were not suitable because of their size and the air space created between the wrap and the leg. Dry cold therapy provided by a Game Ready® Equine system provided the most intimate contact and also provided intermittent pressure that may aid in blood and lymphatic flow. https://www.recoveryforathletes.com/products/game-ready-grpro-2-1-equine-vet-system-kit A whole body cryotherapy system for horses is available at https://www.equine-cryo.com/ Treatment should continue 24 hours beyond resolution of the primary disease. New studies are demonstrating the benefit of cryotherapy in the early acute phase (Hyman, 2015).

Vapocoolant sprays – These sprays are used for a brief and rapid effect when applied to the skin. An example is ethyl chloride spray. This can be a difficult modality to apply to dogs because of the hair covering the skin surface. Also, some of the commercially available sprays may be harmful to animals if they contact an animal's eyes or are ingested. They are used in humans for treating myofascial trigger points (Dragone *et al.*, 2014). They are excellent for venipuncture once the skin has been shaved.

General Recommendations for Cold Therapy

A general rule for deciding when to apply cold versus heat is that cryotherapy should be used for the first 24–72 hours after acute injury when the acute signs of inflammation are present (swelling, redness, heat, and pain) (Steiss and Levine, 2005). If in doubt, use cold. If range of motion is decreased because of pain, apply cold; if range of motion is decreased because of stiffness, apply heat. Ice packs should be covered with a single layer of wet towel (moisture enhances heat exchange) or nothing between the skin and the ice pack. Otherwise, therapeutic temperatures may not be reached. Application of ice packs is from 10 to 20 minutes. The duration may vary for different types of commercial ice packs. The supervising veterinarian should be asked for instructions concerning application of cold to individual patients.

Precautions for Cold Therapy

The primary precaution is avoidance of frostbite. To be safe and to avoid prolonged application, use a timer and inspect the skin every few minutes. Observe for signs of frostbite during and after cryotherapy application (Millis, 2015).

Caution should be exercised when applying cryotherapy around superficial peripheral nerves because cases of cold-induced nerve palsy of the ulnar and superficial peroneal nerves have been reported in humans (Fox, 2014). It is recommended not to apply cold to open wounds after 48–72 hours because of the vasoconstriction that occurs with cryotherapy. Use caution in applying areas of poor sensation or in very young or old dogs (see Box 15.8). Treatment with ice should not be applied for more than 20 minutes per session to avoid damage to the tissue (Mills, 2015).

Box 15.8 Contraindications for cryotherapy

- If there is a history of frostbite in the area, further cold application is contraindicated.
- Cold should not be used in animals with generalized or localized vascular compromise or who possess an impaired thermoregulatory capacity.

Veterinary Evidence for Both Hot and Cold Therapy

Evidence-based medicine for veterinary physical rehabilitation comments that heat is used to increase blood flow, increase collagen extensibility, and perhaps provide some mild analgesia (Millis and Ciuperca, 2015). A study of 10 healthy dogs that measured tissue temperatures at various depths of the lumbar, and epaxial region found that application of a warm compress should be performed for 10 minutes (Millis and Ciuperca, 2015). A recent study also found that the presence of hair does not have a significant effect on muscle cooling, so hair does not need to be shaved to achieve therapeutic effects (Janas *et al.*, 2021).

Cryotherapy is often applied in the early postinjury or postoperative period to reduce blood flow, inflammation, swelling, and pain (Swenson *et al.*, 1996). Skin and superficial tissues are cooled to the greatest extent. Deeper tissues have a gradual decrease in tissue temperature during time exposed to cold. Rewarming after removal of the cold/ice pack is slower in deeper tissues. The rewarming rate of tissues depends on the duration of therapy and type of cryotherapy application. The greatest decrease in intra-articular temperature in dogs occurred with ice water immersion (Bocobo *et al.*, 1991). Rewarming of the canine stifle also took the longest after ice water immersion. The application of 10–20 minutes of ice water immersion caused a further significant temperature change at only the middle tissue depth; however, for maximal cooling, the minimum time of application should be 20 minutes. For postoperative extracapsular repair for cranial cruciate ligament rupture, cold compression and cold compression with bandaging were found to be equally beneficial in reducing stifle swelling in the first 72 hours. Cold compression was applied for 20 minutes by wrapping the leg from the stifle to the hock with a large cold pack and holding it in place with an elastic bandage once daily. Commercial canvas packs kept in a freezer or Ziploc® bags of ice wrapped in a towel are often used for 10–20 minutes every 6–8 hours while the patient is hospitalized (Corti, 2014). In addition, the application of cryotherapy prior to the administration of a laser treatment will allow deeper penetration into the tissues, as the vasoconstriction will decrease the water and hemoglobin content in the tissue which are the main two laser-absorbing chromophores (Neibaum, 2014).

A Word About Cats

Often, it is assumed that cats will not tolerate rehabilitation due to temperament, lifestyle, or age. In fact, cats respond well to rehabilitation techniques and often enjoy the mental stimulation of therapeutic exercise, stretching, and massage in the hospital and at home (Wright and Rychel, 2013).

Cryotherapy can be applied to regions of inflammation, particularly with an acute or chronic injury, to reduce hyperalgesia and slow local metabolism (Sluka *et al.*, 1999). Heat therapy is also valuable and often appreciated by feline patients. Application of a superficial hot pack over a tense muscle or region of chronic discomfort can help ease muscle spasm, improve blood flow, and reduce pain-associated behaviors (Sluka *et al.*, 1999; Lane and Latham, 2009).

Heat Therapy for Cats

Most cats like the application of heat, especially the use of infrared lamps, whereas the use of hot packs is sometimes difficult because cats often object to lying quietly with a hot pack on a joint or the back (Drum *et al.*, 2015). Many sociable cats prefer to lie in a lap or be held while hot packs are applied. The swaddling technique with a towel is useful as a low-stress restraint technique for hot pack application.

Cold Therapy for Cats

It may be difficult to place the cold pack on the target area because cats sometimes refuse to lie quietly for more than a few minutes. Nevertheless, the therapist should try to use cold, especially in the early phase after surgery.

Conclusion

Selection of the appropriate modality depends largely on an understanding of the diagnosis, an accurate assessment of the stage of tissue healing and repair, an accurate

clinical assessment of the functional limitations, the established treatment goals, and continued reevaluation of the patient. The physical rehabilitation therapist/practitioner will be the one deciding which therapy should be applied and when. The rehabilitation veterinary technician/nurse will be carrying out the instructions that the veterinarian provides. Cryotherapy is most useful during the acute inflammatory stages of tissue healing to cause vasoconstriction and decrease edema and pain (Hanks *et al.*, 2015). Using heat too soon in the inflammatory process may exacerbate the inflammatory process and slow healing. Heating modalities (both superficial and deep) are mostly used to cause vasodilation, increase tissue extensibility, and decrease pain and muscle spasm (Hanks *et al.*, 2015).

References

Batavia, M. (2004). Contraindications for superficial heat and therapeutic ultrasound: Do sources agree? *Arch Phys Med Rehabil* 85: 1006–1012.

Bleakley, C., McDonough, S., and MacAuley, D. (2004). The use of ice in the treatment of acute soft-tissue injury: A systematic review of randomized controlled trials. *Am J Sports Med* 32 (1): 251–261.

Bockstahler, B., Millis, D., Levine, D. et al. (2004). Physiotherapy – What and how. In: *Essential Facts of Physiotherapy in Dogs and Cats: Rehabilitation and Pain Management* (eds. B. Bockstahler, D. Levine and D. Millis), 46–123. Germany: Be Vet Verlag.

Bocobo, C., Fast, A., Kingery, W., and Kaplan, M. (1991). The effect of ice on intra-articular temperature in the knee of the dog. *Am J Phys Med Rehabil* 70 (4): 181–185.

Brosseau, L., Yonge, K.A., Welch, V. et al. (2003). Thermotherapy for treatment of osteoarthritis. *Cochrane Database Syst Rev* 4: 1–25.

Burnett, J.M. and Wardlaw, J.L. (2012). Physical rehabilitation for veterinary practices. *Today's Vet Pract* March/April: 14–20.

Charkoudian, N. (2003). Skin blood flow in adult human thermoregulation: How it works, when it does not, and why. *Mayo Clin Proc* 78 (5): 603–612.

Corti, L. (2014). Topical review: Nonpharmaceutical approaches to pain management. *Top Companion Anim Med* 29: 24–28.

Dorn, M. (2015). Superficial heat therapy for dogs and cats, part 1: Physiological mechanisms and indications. *Companion Anim* 20 (11): 630–635.

Dragone, L. (2010). *Fisioterapia Riabilitativa del Cane e del Gatto*, vol. Vol. 2. Milano, Italy: Elsevier La termoterapia; pp. 21–27.

Dragone, L., Heinrichs, K., Levine, D. et al. (2014). Superficial thermal modalities. In: *Canine Rehabilitation and Physical Therapy*, 2nde (ed. D. Millis and

D. Levine), 312–327. Philadelphia, PA: Elsevier/Saunders.

Drum, M., Bockstahler, B., and Levine, D. (2015). Feline rehabilitation. *Vet Clin Small Anim* 45 (1): 185–201.

van Eps, A.W. and Pollitt, C.C. (2004). Equine laminitis: Cryotherapy reduces the severity of the acute lesion. *Equine Vet J* 36 (3): 255–260.

Fox, S.M. (2014). Physical rehabilitation in the management of musculoskeletal disease. In: *Pain Management in Small Animal Medicine*, 243–265. Boca Raton, FL: CRC Press.

Giorgi AZ and Crucik G (2013) *Diathermy*. http://www.healthline.com/health/diathermy#Overview1 (accessed June 24, 2017).

Hanks, J., Levine, D., and Bockstahler, B. (2015). Physical agent modalities in physical therapy and rehabilitation of small animals. *Vet Clin Small Anim* 45 (1): 29–44.

Hayes, K. (1993). Conductive heat. In: *Physical Agents*, 4the, 9–15. Norwalk, CT: Appleton & Lange.

Holowatz, L.A., Thompson, C.S., Minson, C.T., and Kenney, W.L. (2005). Mechanisms of acetylcholine-mediated vasodilatation in young and aged human skin. *J Physiol* 563 (3): 965–973.

Hubbard, T.J. and Denegar, C.R. (2004). Does cryotherapy improve outcomes with soft tissue injury? *J Athl Train* 39 (3): 278–279.

Hurley, M.V. and Bearne, L.M. (2008). Nonexercise physical therapies for musculoskeletal conditions. *Best Pract Res Clin Rheumatol* 22 (3): 419–433.

Hyman SS (2015) Recent advances in veterinary equine laminitis. *DVM360 Magazine* February:1–4.

Janas, K., Millis, D., Levine, D., and Keck, M. (2021). Effects of cryotherapy on temperature change in caudal thigh muscles of dogs. *Vet Comp Orthop Traumatol* 34 (4): 241–247.

Kellogg, D.L. (2006). In vivo mechanisms of cutaneous vasodilation and vasoconstriction in humans during thermoregulatory challenges. *J Appl Physiol* 100: 1709–1718.

Lane, E. and Latham, T. (2009). Managing pain using heat and cold therapy. *Pediatric Nursing* 21 (6): 14–18.

Liu, X.J. and Salter, M.W. (2005). Purines and pain mechanisms: Recent developments. *Curr Opin Investig Drugs* 6 (1): 65–75.

Masuda, A., Koga, Y., Hattanmaru, M. et al. (2005). The effects of repeated thermal therapy for patients with chronic pain. *Psychother Psychosom* 74: 288–294.

Millis, D.L. (2004). Getting the dog moving after surgery. *J Am Anim Hosp Assoc* 40: 429–436.

Millis, D.L. (2015). Physical therapy and rehabilitation in dogs. In: *Handbook of Veterinary Pain Management*, 3rde (ed. J.S. Gaynor and W.W. Muir III), 383–421. St. Louis, MO: Elsevier/Mosby.

Millis, D.L. and Ciuperca, I.A. (2015). Evidence for canine rehabilitation and physical therapy. *Vet Clin Small Anim* 45 (1): 1–27.

Nadler, S.F., Weing, K., and Kruse, R.J. (2004). The physiologic basis and clinical applications of cryotherapy and thermotherapy for the pain practitioner. *Pain Physician* 7: 395–399.

Niebaum, K. (2013). Rehabilitation physical modalities. In: *Canine Sports Medicine and Rehabilitation* (ed. M.C. Zink and J.B. Van Dyke), 115–131. Ames, IA: John Wiley & Sons, Inc.

Notarnicola, A., Maccagnano, G., Gallone, M.F. et al. (2017). Short term efficacy of capacitive-resistive diathermy therapy in patients with low back pain: A prospective randomized controlled trial. *J Biol Reg Homeos Ag* 31: 509–515.

Oosterveld, F.G.J. and Rasker, J.J. (1994). Effects of local heat and cold treatment on surface and articular temperature of arthritic knees. *Arthritis Rheum* 37 (11): 1576–1582.

Peres, S.E., Draper, D.O., Knight, K.L., and Ricard, M.D. (2002). Pulsed shortwave diathermy and prolonged long-duration stretching increase dorsiflexion range of motion more than identical stretching without diathermy. *J Athl Train* 37 (1): 43–50.

Petrofsky, J., Berk, L., and Lee, H. (2013a). Moist heat or dry heat delayed onset muscle soreness. *J Clin Med Res* 5 (6): 416–425.

Petrofsky, J.S., Laymon, M., and Lee, H. (2013b). Effect of heat and cold on tendon flexibility and force to flex the human knee. *Med Sci Monit* 19: 661–667.

Prentice, W.E. (1982). An electromyographic analysis of the effectiveness of heat or cold and stretching for inducing relaxation in injured muscle. *J Orthop Sports Phys Ther* 3 (3): 133–140.

Rintamäki, H. (2007). Human responses to cold. *Alaska Med* 49 (2 Suppl): 29–31.

Rothstein, J.M., Roy, S.H., and Wolf, S.L. (2005). *The Rehabilitation Specialist's Handbook*, 3rde, 796. FA Davis and Co: Philadelphia, PA.

Sluka, K.A., Christy, M.R., Peterson, W.L. et al. (1999). Reduction of pain-related behaviors with either cold or heat treatment in an animal model of acute arthritis. *Arch Phys Med Rehabil* 80 (3): 313–317.

Steiss, J.E. and Levine, D. (2005). Physical agent modalities. *Vet Clin Small Anim* 35 (6): 1317–1333.

Swenson, C., Swärd, L., and Karlsson, J. (1996). Cryotherapy in sports medicine. *Scand J Med Sci Sports* 6 (4): 193–200.

Wright, B. and Rychel, J.K. (2013). Treatment and assessment of chronic pain in cats. In: *Pain Management in Veterinary Practice* (ed. C.M. Egger, L. Love, and T. Doherty), 289–298. Ames, IA: John Wiley & Sons, Inc.

Yu, S.Y., Chiu, J.H., Yang, S.D. et al. (2006). Biological effect of far-infrared therapy on increasing skin microcirculation in rats. *Photodermatol Photoimmunol Photomed* 22: 78–86.

16

Modalities Part 2: Laser Therapy

Evelyn Orenbuch

Orenbuch Veterinary Rehabilitation, Marietta, GA, USA

CHAPTER MENU

Introduction

The term "laser" started out as an acronym, Light Amplification by Stimulated Emission of Radiation, and has been accepted as a common word. Lasers were first used surgically in high doses to cut or seal tissue. The first report of lasers used for a therapeutic purpose was in 1963 by a team of researchers in Boston led by Paul McGuff. McGuff's group used a Ruby laser to ablate human tumors implanted in hamsters. The team also observed that the irradiated tumors continued to shrink over the course of two weeks, but the mechanism of this action was unknown (Tunér and Hode, 2014). Shortly thereafter, Hungarian scientist Andre Mester and colleagues published several reports describing the ability of nonthermal laser light to stimulate hair growth and promote cutaneous wound healing in rats. In 1967, Carney *et al.* showed that irradiation of skin tissue cultures resulted in increased collagen production. Thousands of other reports have since been published, both supporting and refuting the effects of laser therapy. Often, the studies showing little or no effect of therapeutic lasers can be attributed to incorrect dosage and/or lasers that were not well calibrated. Today, therapeutic lasers have gained wide recognition and use in veterinary medicine (Zein *et al.*, 2018). Although the term "laser" is still commonly used, the correct word is

Physical Rehabilitation for Veterinary Technicians and Nurses, Second Edition.
Edited by Mary Ellen Goldberg and Julia E. Tomlinson.
© 2024 John Wiley & Sons, Inc. Published 2024 by John Wiley & Sons, Inc.
Companion website: www.wiley.com/go/goldberg/physicalrehabilitationvettechsandnurses

photobiomodulation (PBM) (Anders *et al.*, 2015). This is a more accurate term and is defined as any nonthermal application of light that modulates biological processes. The purpose of this chapter is to describe basic physics, discuss the mechanisms and effective dosages, and describe the practical use of photobiomodulation therapy (PBMT) in veterinary rehabilitation patients.

Photobiomodulation Physics 101

Lasers, along with the sun, ordinary light bulbs, X-ray machines, and microwave ovens, emit electromagnetic radiation. Energy from these sources travels at the speed of light in packets known as photons. Photons travel in waves, not unlike sound waves, and the type of radiation is distinguished by its wavelength. Electromagnetic radiation is typically described as a spectrum from very short (gamma rays, 1,000–1 fm) to long (radio waves, 1,000–1 m) wavelengths. Within this spectrum lies visible light (400–760 nm), near-infrared (NIR) (760–1,400 nm), and infrared (1,400 nm–1.0 mm), and laser radiation falls within this band of wavelengths (Robinson, 2015).

In therapeutic lasers, electromagnetic energy is harnessed into an intense, coherent, monochromatic beam of light. The properties of monochromaticity (all waves are same length/color) and coherence (all waves are in phase) are characteristics of all lasers. This is in contrast to LEDs, or "light emitting diodes," which do not emit coherent light. The biomodulatory effects of lasers, particularly in deeper tissues, are believed to be due, in part, to their coherence (Hode *et al.*, 2009); yet, there is some limited evidence to suggest that LEDs and other noncoherent, narrow-waveband radiations are as effective as lasers (depending on the irradiation parameters) in PBM for certain conditions (Heiskanen and Hamblin, 2018).

A laser is made using a material (gas, liquid, and solid) that, when stimulated by an external energy source, such as electricity, will release photons of a single color or wavelength. For example, the most commonly used helium–neon (HeNe) laser emits a wavelength of approximately 633 nm, which falls within the visible light spectrum and produces the color red (green, yellow, and ultraviolet HeNe lasers also exist, and the first HeNe laser emitted NIR at 1,152.3 nm). Gallium arsenide (GaAs) lasers emit a NIR wavelength of 904 nm which is invisible to the human eye.

It is important to note that wavelength is inversely proportional to the energy of a photon. This can be appreciated by recognizing differences between harmless radio waves (long wavelength, low energy) and ionizing gamma rays that are used in cancer radiation therapy (short wavelength, very high energy). Wavelengths between 280–400 nm represent UVA and UVB rays (Robinson, 2015). The wavelengths of therapeutic lasers typically all fall between 405 and 1,064 nm (Robinson, 2015), with those between 635 and 1,064 nm – the so-called "optical window" of living tissue – being used where target tissues are deeper than a few millimeters.

The power of a laser beam – it is "optical output" – is measured in Watts (W) or milliwatts (mW). Therapeutic lasers can range from as much as 25 W to as little as a few milliwatts (mW). At the very low end are laser pointers which have, at times, been sold as therapeutic lasers. Power output is one of the significant parameters to consider when developing treatment protocols.

The ***energy*** delivered by a laser is measured in Joules (J), with one Joule being equal to one Watt of light being delivered over one second; the Standard International Unit for a Joule is the Watt-second (Ws).

A higher-powered laser will deliver more energy than a lower-powered laser over the same amount of time, or the same amount of energy in a shorter period of time. For example, a 0.5 W (500 mW) power setting will deliver 0.5 J per second, or 30 Joules per minute, whereas a 5 W power setting will deliver 5 J/s, or 300 Joules per minute. It is important to note, however, that irradiation time is also an important parameter in relation to how a given amount of light will affect a cellular response, and faster is not necessarily better.

High-powered lasers may deliver energy so quickly that heat is produced in the irradiated tissue, requiring the user to continuously move the handpiece over a large area, spreading the light out and allowing the tissues to thermally relax and dissipate heat, thus avoiding possible tissue damage. Moving the laser has more potential for scattering and reflection of laser light, and appropriate safety measures should be taken. This scattering and reflection of the beam, along with treating an area often much larger than the pathology itself, can reduce the amount of laser energy available to the target tissue, reducing the efficiency of treatment.

Lower-powered lasers with very tightly confined beams can also cause unwanted thermal effects (although the amount of tissue affected is much smaller and, thus, mitigation is easier to achieve); this occurs when the power density of the beam is too high. In addition to its contribution to the potential for thermal effects, power density is a key parameter in the laser treatment equation.

Power density (irradiance or radiant intensity) is the amount of power distributed over a given area and is measured in W/cm^2. A laser beam with 1 W of power may have a very high-power density if the beam spot is very small, but if the same laser beam is spread over a larger area the intensity at each point becomes less (Mester *et al.*, 1968).

Power density is determined by the beam diameter (cm) and thus spot size/area (cm^2) that is **specific to each laser device or handpiece** and the power capability of the device. Some spot sizes/treatment heads can be changed, and some are fixed; similarly, some laser devices can vary the output power, while others have the power capped (see Figure 16.1).

There are several other parameters that differ between lasers. Some lasers can emit energy in a continuous wave (CW) or switched-CW fashion. When a laser is emitting in CW, the beam is on 100% of the time. When a CW laser is switched, the power output typically varies between 100% (peak power) when the beam is on and zero when the beam is turned off. The number of times this happens per second – the pulse rate, or frequency – is measured in Hertz (Hz). Therefore, a laser device that can be "pulsed" or continuous depending on settings is being switched on and off.

Other laser devices, such as the GaAs diode laser, can only operate in a pulsed manner. These devices, often referred to as super-pulsed lasers, typically have very high peak powers (25–50 W) and very, very short pulse widths (<200 ns), so their average output power is very low.

Regardless of the method of pulsing, the total amount of energy delivered in a pulsed manner over time is determined by the average power output of the beam. To calculate the average power, one must know either the peak (or CW) power and duty cycle – the ratio, expressed as a percentage, of the "ON" time of a pulse to the "ON + OFF" time of a full waveform – of the device, or, alternatively, the peak power, pulse duration, and frequency of pulsation.

The average power of a switched-CW laser is, usually, relatively close to that of the CW beam itself, with duty cycles typically ranging from ~10–90% (*switching is one method by which some high-powered*

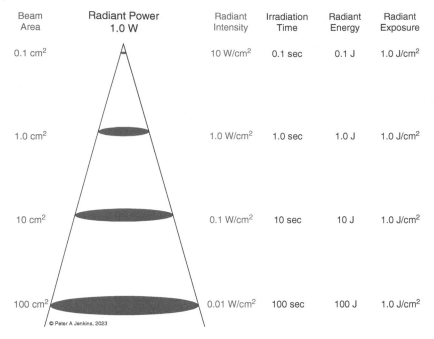

Figure 16.1 The output of a laser may be concentrated in a small spot or spread over a larger area, changing the power density of the beam; this changes the time it takes to deliver a given dose, the total amount of energy delivered during that time, and the effect that dose may have upon and within the irradiated tissue. With thanks to Peter Jenkins for the figure creation.

therapeutic lasers can be held motionless on the skin without causing harm). The average power of a super-pulsed laser, on the other hand, is generally less than 0.1% of the peak power and may vary considerably with changes to the frequency of pulsation; despite having very high peak-powered pulses, these devices seldom produce any increase in tissue temperature.

Laser Safety Classes

Lasers are divided into four safety classes with additional subclasses: I, II, IIIa, IIIb, and IV (alternatively, 1, 2, 3R, 3B, and 4). *A common misconception is that these classes distinguish the efficacy or quality of the laser or the "generation" of technology*. Rather, the classification of a laser is determined by its ability to cause eye injury, considering the beam diameter,

divergence, exposure time, and wavelength, and with the power being measured through a 7 mm aperture (representing a fully dilated human pupil) placed at a distance of 100 mm (the shortest focal distance of the human eye) from the apparent source of the beam.

Class I–IIIa (1–3R) lasers include supermarket scanners, laser pointers, remote controls, and some super-pulsed therapeutic laser devices. Class IIIb (3B) lasers pose a risk of eye injury on direct exposure to the retina, and suitable eye protection is needed. Any laser with greater than 500 mW of average power, measured as described above, falls into class IV (4), which is an acute hazard to the skin and eyes from direct *and scattered* radiation. Note that, due to the specified testing methodology, there are various methods of construction (e.g., safety interlocks, beam diffusers, multiple nonintersecting beams) that may allow a laser with a total power output more than the upper Class IIIb (3B) limit to fall within a lower hazard class.

Dosage

Dosage is described most often in the literature in terms of <u>fluence</u>, measured in Joules per centimeter squared (J/cm^2), which is calculated using the following formula:

$$\text{Fluence} = \frac{P \times t}{A}$$

where
  P = laser's average output power (W)
  t = treatment time (seconds)
  A = total area treated, or the area of the beam spot (cm^2)
  Recall that 1 Joule = 1 Watt per second

The reliance upon J/cm^2 as the measure of dose, however, has led some to believe that it is the most important factor impacting the effect of a laser treatment and that one can, for example, double the power or intensity of the laser and halve the treatment time to achieve the same outcome (delivery of the same amount of joules/cm^2 more quickly). This concept, the Bunsen-Roscoe law of reciprocity, has been demonstrated to not apply in PBM (Jenkins and Carroll, 2011).

Irradiance and time are the important parameters. The effective radiant exposure (J/cm^2) for any given local and/or systemic response to the therapy is consequential, not causative. The same amount of J/cm^2 can produce different outcomes, or the same outcome may be produced by different amounts of J/cm^2, *depending upon the intensity of the light and the time over which it is delivered*. These parameters – time and intensity – accurately and comprehensively define the dose, and so they must both be recorded and communicated.

Other parameters, such as the wavelength, the number and location of treatment points/sites (when using a stationary contact technique) or the total area irradiated (when using a scanning/constant-movement technique), the emission mode (including frequency and duty cycle if switched/pulsed), and the number and timetable of treatment sessions, can all be thought of as comprising the "medicine," as it is the unique combination of each that determines what effect(s) a particular combination of time and intensity will have (Nie *et al.*, 2023). It is, therefore, critically important to record and communicate all these relevant parameters together, not just the J/cm^2 (Jenkins and Carroll, 2011; Tunér and Jenkins, 2016).

Given the great disparity in parameters between the many different PBM devices available and the inability to rely upon J/cm^2 as a predictor of therapeutic effect, *it is important to refer to the guidance of the manufacturer of your laser with respect to the correct application technique and recommended protocols for that specific device*. Lasers that are available commercially and marketed for medical or veterinary use will likely come with recommended doses for various conditions preprogrammed into the unit or listed in the instruction manual. These dosages are determined by the individual laser manufacturers and may not be based on clinical research or be consistent across different companies. *Understanding how each manufacturer calculates their protocols is important*. Ask your laser manufacturer about the spot size of your device (if it is not listed in the user manual or able to be inferred) and/or handpiece so that you can calculate the irradiance you are delivering and/or ask what dosage their automatic protocols are delivering for various conditions.

One last consideration is the depth of laser penetration into living tissue. This depends primarily on the wavelength of the laser, with longer wavelengths within the optical window of the tissue typically penetrating deeper. The mode of operation may also play a role. A GaAs laser (904 nm) can reach tissue depths of 3–5 cm, while a HeNe laser (633 nm) will have more superficial penetration, near 1 cm (Enwemeka, 2001; Corazza, 2007). However, it is unrealistic to believe that there is an absolute barrier in the tissue to keep all energy from going beyond the known penetration depth of a particular wavelength. As energy is applied at the skin surface and interacts with various tissue layers, it attenuates, with 50–90% of the incident light being absorbed and scattered just within the skin (Bjordal et al., 2003). The remaining light then continues to travel into the deeper tissues, giving therapeutic effects once absorbed, well below the known penetration depth of that wavelength (Tedford et al., 2015; Piao et al., 2018). The amount of light attenuation is dependent upon wavelength, tissue characteristics (including pigmentation), method of delivery (on versus off-contact), and the irradiance delivered at the skin surface. Light that is reflected or attenuated due to absorption by nonbiologically active chromophores (i.e., melanin in the skin and hair) does not contribute to the therapeutic effects of PBM and is, essentially, wasted, so device design and application technique should be optimized to minimize these losses. Absorption and scattering in the fat (particularly in overweight animals) must be taken into consideration by the veterinarian when treatment dose is calculated (Zein et al., 2018). Note that, unlike sound waves, laser waves (electromagnetic radiation) can penetrate, and therefore treat, bone.

Photobiomodulation: Proposed Mechanisms of Action

PBM is the application of light to modify a biologic process. Depending on the wavelength, power, and other factors, light can cause beneficial or harmful effects in cells and tissue (Bjordal, 2006a). Therapeutic lasers can be used to stimulate favorable effects in tissue, including enhanced wound healing, reducing inflammation in the gut, and modulation of pain in cases of osteoarthritis, as well as soft tissue injuries such as strains and sprains (Medrado et al., 2008; Alves, 2021, 2022).

Laser therapy can affect each stage of tissue healing (inflammation, proliferation, and maturation) (Mendez et al., 2004). *The role of laser in the inflammatory phase is that of immunomodulation.* Some studies have shown enhancement of the inflammatory response and increased production of growth factors such as TGF-β1, while others show a reduction of inflammatory cytokines such as TNFα and PGE-2 (Callies et al., 2011). Studies have demonstrated acceleration (shortening) of the inflammatory phase, with rapid progression into the proliferative phase of healing (Loreti et al., 2015). Furthermore, laser therapy has been shown to reduce inflammatory mediators, such as COX-2 and PGE2, to decrease inflammatory cell numbers in tissue, and decrease edema (Mester et al., 1970). It is clear from many studies that the proliferative phase of wound healing is greatly enhanced by therapeutic lasers (Loreti et al., 2015). Research conducted on cell cultures has found that various wavelengths and doses are effective at increasing fibroblast proliferation (Wong-Riley et al., 2005). It has also been shown that laser therapy can stimulate epithelialization and collagen deposition in animal models of diabetes and glucocorticoid excess, where wound healing is usually retarded (Woodruff et al., 2004). The final phase of wound healing is maturation or remodeling of scar tissue. Lasers influence this phase by enhancing the organization of collagen fibers within wounds (Montesinos, 1988). These effects have been shown to decrease the healing time and improve the cosmetic appearance of skin incisions post-surgery (Wardlaw *et al.*, 2019).

There are multiple mechanisms involved in the ability of PBM to manage pain. The mechanisms by which laser therapy decreases pain are still being explored. One of the primary means is by decreasing the production of inflammatory products such as PGE2 and TNF α, and inhibiting cyclooxygenase-2 (Viegas *et al.*, 2007; Huang *et al.*, 2020). PBM may also reduce pain through several other mechanisms, including increasing ATP production and stabilizing cell membranes, resulting in the restoration of the cell membrane electrochemical gradient and resting membrane potential of nerve cells (Wakabayashi, 1993; Shurman *et al.*, 2017). This can minimize excessive or inappropriate depolarization of peripheral nociceptors and slow the conduction of pain along C fibers (Sakurai *et al.*, 2000; Shurman *et al.*, 2017). Other potential mechanisms of pain relief include increased release of beta-endorphins and serotonin and enhanced removal of inflammatory mediators from the site of injury due to laser-induced changes in local hemodynamics (Mendez *et al.*, 2004; Huang *et al.*, 2020).

PBM is known to follow a biphasic response curve, with the effects of irradiation determined by the combination of time and intensity (Nie *et al.*, 2023). At subtherapeutic doses, cells will not be stimulated, and no reactions will occur, whereas possible inhibitory effects and damaging photothermal effects may be appreciated if the duration or irradiance is too high (Lam and Wong, 2014). Biostimulation occurs in low doses, but bioinhibition arises at high doses of PBMT (Mester *et al.*, 1985).

Contraindications and Potential Cautions

Because PBM is recognized to enhance neovascularization, irradiation of tumors or wounds that may contain cancer cells has generally been contraindicated. However, there is recent evidence that PBMT has no detrimental effects and/or can also potentially inhibit tumor growth (Robijns *et al.*, 2022; Hamblin *et al.*, 2018; Kiro *et al.*, 2017; Turner and Hode, 2010). In cases in which there is no other treatment for the tumor and laser therapy could potentially ease pain and/or heal the wounds sometimes developed by tumors, it is acceptable to use laser therapy with the informed consent of the owner, knowing it could increase the growth rate of the tumor but also may improve the quality of life or prolong the life of the patient. Laser therapy directly over an open growth plate has been shown experimentally to have detrimental effects. Laser of rat femoral growth plates at 830 nm, 10 J/cm^2 daily for 21 days showed a detrimental effect (Oliveira *et al.*, 2012). Daily laser is impractical in many rehabilitation clinics; however, an increasing number of clients own lasers for home use, so they should be cautioned. Treatment of rat growth plates with an 830-nm laser at two different energy densities (5 and 15 J/cm^2) every other day for 10 days resulted in changes in thickness of the epiphyseal cartilage and increased the number of chondrocytes, but this was not sufficient to induce changes in bone length during the analysis period of only 24 hours after the last laser (Cressoni *et al.*, 2010). Given the growth plate changes at doses given in rehabilitation clinics, though more frequent than most of us treat with laser, the editors advise caution and avoidance of laser irradiation overgrowth plates at this time. Laser therapy over a pregnant uterus is contraindicated since it has not been studied and because the risk is high. Lasers pose a known serious risk to the eye, potentially damaging the retina and/or cornea; therefore, irradiation of or near the eye should be avoided.

Laser Safety in the Clinic

While administering a laser treatment, it is important to take precautions to protect yourself and the patient, as well as being mindful of others in the room. All Class IIIb (3B) and IV (4) lasers should come with their own set of safety glasses. These glasses have lens filters that are specific to the wavelength and intensity of the laser. They will have stamping on the corner of the lens indicating what wavelengths are covered and the level of protection/attenuation provided. Some laser companies provide pet safety glasses as well. These may be specifically made for pets, or they may use modified "Doggles" protective eyewear for pets, in which the usual sunglasses-type lens has been replaced with a lens specific to the wavelength of that laser. Make sure any pet safety glasses used have the same wavelength stamping (optical density [OD] rating) as the human glasses do before relying on them to block laser during emission (see Figure 16.2a and b). It is important to note, too, that no other shaded glasses can block out laser irradiation, including sunglasses or surgical (e.g., CO_2) laser glasses.

If the patient refuses to wear the pet safety glasses, ensure their head is facing away from the laser beam and not facing a reflective surface. A dark towel or opaque e-collar may be useful tools to block the light and keep patients from turning their heads (see Figure 16.3). This is less of a concern for the patient's eyes with a Class IIIb (3B) laser used in a contact method, as the laser would have to be shone directly in the eye of the patient to have a negative effect. The hazard posed by scatter and reflection is greater with noncontact and with higher-powered lasers.

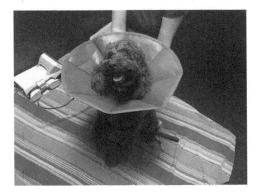

Figure 16.3 This patient could not tolerate safety goggles, so a soft, blue E-collar was used. Keeping the patient comfortable makes for an easier treatment session for both the patient and the person administering the treatment. Many patients do not need an additional pair of hands to keep them still if they are relaxed and comfortable.

(a)

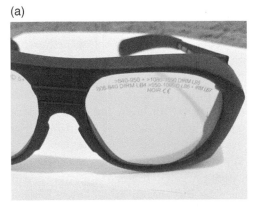

(b)

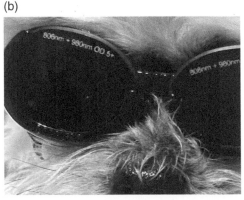

Figure 16.2 (a) and (b) Wavelength-specific safety glasses. The picture on the left is an example of those used for people. On the right, the patient is wearing modified Doggles. Note the stamp in both pictures in the upper corner indicating wavelengths for which the glasses have been tested and approved.

Laser has the ability to reflect once it comes in contact with metal or any other reflective surface. This can be hazardous to others in the room who are not protected. For this reason, treating a patient inside a stainless-steel cage is strongly discouraged, as the risk of scatter is too great for a higher-powered laser. The ideal location for a laser treatment is a small, windowless exam room with a comfortable bed on the ground for you and your patient to sit on. There would be a "Do Not Disturb; Laser in Progress" sign on the door. Everyone present in the room would be wearing safety glasses. If this scenario is impossible in your hospital, make sure the laser operator and everyone within range (determined by the nominal ocular hazard distance [NOHD] of the laser device) of the beam are wearing their protective glasses. Then, look at your surroundings. Are there metallic surfaces inside the safety range, i.e., a "wet" table? If so, cover them with a towel or blanket (see Figure 16.4).

Laser therapy is often performed over metallic orthopedic implants. Since the laser will be reflected back and therefore may increase the total dosage to the tissue between the metallic implant and the laser, the dosage should be reduced, or this tissue should be avoided if possible. It is also important to treat circumferentially around the limb to maximize penetration of light underlying/around the metal implant. It is essential that the technician or veterinarian administering laser therapy have a good understanding of anatomy and the location of orthopedic implants. The supervising veterinarian should give specific guidance in the form of a treatment prescription.

There are not many federal regulations regarding therapeutic lasers. These regulations that do exist regarding lasers are directed toward industrial lasers. At the state level, very few deviate from the federal regulations that are in place for industrial

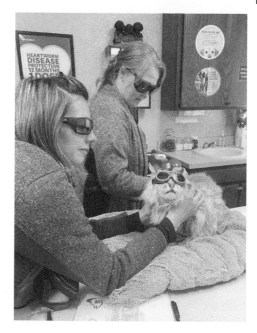

Figure 16.4 This patient is being treated on a table that is not stainless steel, reducing the chance for reflection of the laser beam and the scatter that occurs. Consider covering stainless steel tables with towels or blankets if no other option exists. This patient has also been made very comfortable by doing the treatment on a pet bed. Note that the patient as well as the humans near the laser have appropriate eye protection.

lasers. Your veterinarian should have a clinic policy regarding laser use and will need your help keeping that policy implemented. The Occupational Safety and Health Administration (OSHA) in the United States recommends that a laser safety officer (LSO) be appointed. The LSO would be an employee who is responsible for overseeing the safe use of the lasers within the business location. Veterinary offices with multiple locations that use lasers will need an LSO at each location: https://www.osha.gov/laser-hazards/hazards.

Read the owner's manual for your laser carefully. Many companies will provide their own resources for safe operation.

Veterinary Research

In trying to achieve the same results as those accomplished in the literature, it can be difficult to convert the parameters used into settings that are consistent with the laser used at your clinic. Unless one is certain that the laser in the study is the same one used at the clinic, the power density is likely different, changing what the fluence (dose) should be. If this is not taken into consideration, the outcome will likely be different.

A 2018 study (prospective, blinded, and placebo-controlled) of laser therapy for elbow osteoarthritis showed that 6 weeks of laser therapy significantly improved lameness scores and enabled reduction of non-steroidal anti-inflammatory drug (NSAID) therapy. Laser wavelength was 980 nm, dose (fluence) was 10–20 J/cm^2 (depending on dog size), and irradiance (power density) was 1–2.4 W/cm^2 (depending on dog size). Treatment time was 4–8 minutes (Looney *et al.*, 2018).

A 2020 retrospective study of dogs with osteoarthritis (hip, stifle, and elbow) treated with laser therapy weekly for six weeks for osteoarthritis found that pain scores as assessed by Canine Brief Pain Index (CBPI) were significantly lower at two, four, six, and eight weeks after onset. The therapy laser used was an 808 nm wavelength with a power density of 1 W/cm^2 and energy delivered of 5 J/cm^2 over joints and 4.2 J/cm^2 over muscles, according to laser manufacturer's recommendations. The laser was pulsed, with frequencies of 500–1,000 Hz for joints and 3,000–5,000 Hz for muscles (Barale *et al.*, 2020). It is not clear whether the laser probe was moved or in contact; the treatment area is not defined; and some parameters quoted are contradictory. Although this study has clear benefit to the quality of life of the dogs, as reported by both the owners and the clinicians involved, it may be difficult to repeat in a clinical setting.

They state that the potency was set at 1,000 mW, but that the spot size ranges from 3.5 to 11.5 mm which would produce a power density between 1 and 10.4 W/cm^2. However, in the study, the power density is listed at 1 W/cm^2.

A 2022 study (prospective, double-blinded, and controlled) evaluated the effect of laser therapy on dogs with bilateral hip osteoarthritis; the positive control dogs were treated with the NSAID meloxicam for 21 days to match the laser treatment duration. Improvements in gait and pain scores were seen in the laser group at 8 days following the onset of treatment, started to decline at 15 days post therapy and returned to baseline at 90 days; the control (meloxicam) group returned to baseline lameness by 60 days. The wavelength used was 980 nm for patients with dark coat color and an 80:20% blend of 980–808 nm for light to medium coat color. Irradiance (power density) was 4.2–5.2 W/cm^2 at the skin, and fluence was 14.3–19.5 J/cm^2. In this study, the laser probe was moved continuously in a grid pattern; treatment time was 4.5–5 minutes. Protocol was every other day for three treatments: week 1, week 2 twice, and week 3 once (Alves *et al.*, 2022). The primary study investigator, Joao Alves, confirms via personal communication (June 2023) that the treatment area (cm^2) reported in Table 16.1 of the study is incorrect. It should be 100 cm^2 (instead of 225 cm^2).

One can see how it is difficult to compare studies to each other without a standardized approach. Of the two studies above, two have the same approach and one does not.

In cases of intervertebral disc disease treated with hemilaminectomy, there are two studies on time taken to return to ambulation. One uses a CW emission and shows a positive outcome, and the other is pulsed at 2.5 Hz and finds no difference between lasered and the control group. Unfortunately, both studies have questionable parameters

Table 16.1 Modalities laser.

Indication	Target tissue	Treatment frequency	Dose (J/cm^2)
Cranial cruciate ligament rupture: postsurgical	Incision treated separately	Immediately postoperatively and again daily up to 7 days over the incision	Directly over incision off contact: 4–6 J/cm^2 (Miller, 2017)
	Areas of surgical tissue manipulation, joint capsule (medial and lateral), patellar tendon; sartorius/quadriceps if tight or atrophied	Immediately postoperatively, the following day and then 2–3 times/week for a total of 8–10 treatments based on response, then as needed for maintenance. Repeat loading dose as needed.	8–10 J/cm^2 (Buijs *et al.*, 2017)
CCLR chronic or nonsurgical	Joint capsule, sartorius, quadriceps, and gastrocnemius origin	2–3 times/week for a total of 8–10 treatments, then as needed for maintenance. Repeat loading dose as needed	8–10 J/cm^2 If known OA: 10–20 J/cm^2 at joint capsule
Intervertebral disc disease – surgical (hemilaminectomy; ventral slot)	Incision treated separately.	Immediately postoperatively and again daily up to seven days over the incision.	Directly over incision off contact: 4–6 J/cm^2
	Spinal column over lesion; articular facets surrounding lesion (plus two cranial and two caudal); surrounding thoracic, lumbar, and cervical muscles according to localization; consider treating hypertonic muscles, treat axonal pathways and major nerve tracts leading to site of lesion	Immediately postoperatively daily while hospitalized then 2–3 times/week for 4–6 weeks or as long as needed based on recovery and rehabilitation plan	8–10 J/cm^2
Intervertebral disc disease – nonsurgical	Spinal column over lesion; articular facets surrounding lesion (plus two cranial and two caudal); Surrounding thoracic, lumbar, and cervical muscles according to localization; consider treating hypertonic muscles, treat axonal pathways and major nerve tracts leading to site of lesion	Begin as soon as suspected daily for 3 days then 2–3 times/week for 4–6 weeks or as long as needed based on recovery and rehabilitation plan	8–10 J/cm^2

(Continued)

Table 16.1 (Continued)

Indication	Target tissue	Treatment frequency	Dose (J/cm^2)
Hip dysplasia	Gluteal muscles, pectineus, epaxials, quadriceps, and hamstrings if tight or atrophied; joint capsule (In large dogs, may need to treat from the medial aspect); ±LS space and SI	2–3 times/week for a total of 8–10 treatments, then as needed for maintenance. Repeat loading dose as needed	8–20 J/cm^2
Shoulder tendinopathies	Supraspinatus insertion and musculotendinous junction, origin of biceps tendon ± belly of biceps and insertions at elbow; deltoids, triceps muscles if tight or atrophied	2–3 times/week for a total of 8–10 treatments, then as needed for maintenance. Repeat loading dose as needed	6–10 J/cm^2
Elbow osteoarthritis	Directly over the elbow joint split between the medial and lateral side	2–3 times/week for a total of 8–10 treatments, then as needed for maintenance. Repeat loading dose as needed	10–20 J/cm^2 (Looney *et al.*, 2018)
	Triceps muscles, biceps brachii, flexor, and extensor muscles distal to the elbow		8–10 J/cm^2

Common conditions treated and protocols based on both author's experience and veterinary studies. These can be used as a starting point for each patient. The best protocol should be based on the laser used and the manufacturer's recommendations as well as modifications made for each patient based on response and the user's experience. The best patient outcomes may include nutritional supplements, pharmaceuticals, and additional rehabilitation modalities such as manual therapy, hydrotherapy, acupuncture, and therapeutic exercise. Treatment frequency often starts at 2–3 times/week and then is reduced to "as needed for maintenance." This will be different for each patient. For many patients this is about once a month. For more aggressive conditions such as severe chronic osteoarthritis, maintenance might be every other week or even weekly. The patient should be reassessed regularly, and the treatment plan modified based on response.

that would not be recommended in a clinical setting. Interestingly, the device used in both studies was the same, with the only difference being that the first used CW emission, and in the second, the laser was pulsed at 2.5 Hz.

One study was performed on dogs in hospital after decompressive surgery with a control group and a laser-treated group, treated daily for five days. The laser protocol was 810 nm wavelength. Power 1 W (5 × 200 mW), continuous mode, applied using a stationary contact technique for 1 minute per site over the spinal segment associated with the hemilaminectomy and the two adjacent ones (one cranial and one caudal). The intensity per laser diode was 5 W/cm^2, resulting in a radiant exposure at the skin surface of 300 J/cm^2 (expected dose at spinal cord 2–8 J/cm^2) and a total energy dose of 180 J per session. Laser-treated dogs showed significantly less time to ambulate than untreated dogs (Draper *et al.*, 2012). Although this study shows a positive outcome, we need to learn more about the parameters used. The irradiance, 25,000 mW/cm^2, is likely misreported. This level would cause thermal damage to the tissue (Miller, 2017).

Another study, associated with hemilaminectomy in dogs, was blinded with a sham treatment, controls were two groups, rehabilitation with sham laser, and sham laser only. Laser protocol was 810 nm wavelength, irradiance of 5.5 W/cm^2, and fluence of 329.7 J/cm^2 was used. The laser probe was applied with pressure to each area for 1 minute in a pulsed mode (frequency, 2.5 Hz). The dogs were followed for only 10 days post op. This study found no difference in recovery-related variables among dogs that received PBMT, physical rehabilitation with sham PBM treatment, or sham PBM treatment only. The conclusion was that larger studies are needed to better evaluate effects of these postoperative treatments on dogs treated surgically for intervertebral disk disease (Bennaim *et al.*, 2017). The lack of positive outcomes in this study is likely due to the very low dosage. With a very tiny spot size (0.0364 cm^2) and a non-collimated beam cluster probe (200 mW × 5), delivering a total of 12 J at the skin surface, the amount of Joules reaching the deeper tissue of the spinal cord is likely very small. Additionally, treating for only 5 days postoperatively in a neurologic case, knowing that neuronal regrowth in the best circumstances is quite slow (1 mm/day), is less than is typically recommended.

Using Laser Therapy in Practice

There are many different PBM devices available in the veterinary market today, and while the basic mechanism of action is similar, they all function differently. User competency will affect the outcome of your treatment, so it is important that each operator has been properly trained on the device before administering PBMT. Each laser company should provide some training on the device your practice has purchased. Additionally, one of the veterinarians in your practice should be assigned to training personnel. This person will ensure that all new staff are trained and comfortable with the laser. An excellent knowledge of anatomy is crucial; the veterinarian needs to be able to get a realistic estimate of target tissue depth as well as likely attenuation levels. There are many supportive resources available online. For example, Optimum Pet Vitality offers an in-depth course in the use of lasers in veterinary medicine. This course details the physiology and mechanisms of action of lasers, the treatment of specific conditions, and the use of the most used lasers in the industry (https://www.optimumpetvitality.com/). Additionally, some of the laser manufacturers have good online supportive resources. Take the time to research the options offered by your laser company.

Once all staff have been trained, the next step is implementing the laser into daily practice. Treatments should be first prescribed by a veterinarian. Laser protocol, area(s) to be treated, and number of treatments are decided upon by the overseeing veterinarian and then generally performed by a team member who has been trained on the machine and will adhere to all safety precautions.

Positioning your patient can be tricky since you will often be chasing a moving target. The more comfortable and relaxed the animal is, the easier your job is. Most animals feel more secure on the ground instead of up on a table. Whether you are using the scanning or point-to-point technique, you will want to make sure the probe is kept at a 90° angle to your target area to ensure even and optimal laser emission and penetration (fluence = radiant exposure = Joules per cm^2). Additionally, if it is possible to part the hair and have the laser wand or handpiece directly against the skin or as close to that as possible, it will help to ensure as much of the laser energy is reaching the target tissue as possible. Clipping would be ideal but is not easily accepted by some owners (see Figures 16.5–16.7).

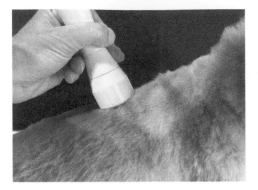

Figure 16.5 The laser probe should always be perpendicular to the target tissue. Lasers that do not generate substantial heat can be used with a point-to-point method to administer treatment. Heat-generating/high-powered lasers should be continuously moved (scanning) to avoid overheating the tissue. Whether scanning or point-to-point, the probe should remain at a 90° angle to the body surface during treatment.

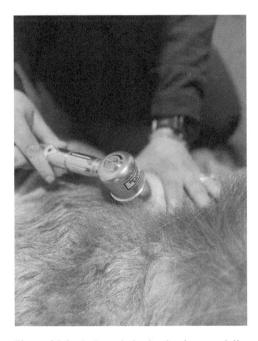

Figure 16.6 In long-haired animals, especially, other than when treating very superficial conditions, it is best to part the hair and place the laser directly against the skin. This is much easier to do with non-heat-generating lasers that can be held in one area. This will help decrease the energy lost to the hair and distance from target tissue.

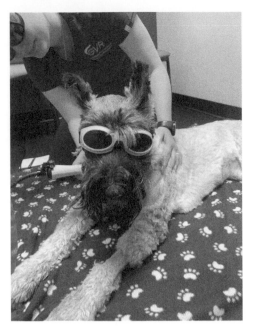

Figure 16.7 This patient is relaxed and enjoying her laser treatment. If possible, treat the patient in a comfortable position on the floor. Having limited reflective surfaces reduces the chance for scatter and potential eye damage.

Having knowledge of muscle anatomy and boney landmarks enables accurate treatment and makes it easier to follow your supervising veterinarian's instructions. A rehabilitation certification course will help you to understand bone and soft tissue anatomy as it applies to laser therapy. For example, a 10-year-old Labrador who had a tibial plateau leveling osteotomy (TPLO) surgery performed when he was 2 years old has now developed moderate osteoarthritis in the joint. The veterinarian has prescribed laser to help with the pain and inflammation and should have given you specific instructions for probe placement, but what if they did not? You have your diagnosis and your treatment plan of action. Now, where to place the probe? First, you should be comfortable palpating and identifying the metal plate used in the surgery. Next, you need to find the joint margins where the joint capsule attaches. The joint capsule is your primary target when treating osteoarthritis because it is the tissue that contains nerve endings and inflammatory mediators (Bjordal *et al.*, 2003). If you were treating a dog within the first few months after TPLO, your target tissues would be the joint capsule, as well as surgical incision and the bone where the TPLO cut was made, remembering to direct your laser around the metal plate. Table 16.1 includes common uses of therapeutic laser in veterinary rehabilitation, the target tissue(s), and protocols used by the author (see Table 16.1).

Conclusions

Integrating laser into physical rehabilitation can be tremendously rewarding. Often, the patient will even enjoy the session. Like other treatments, it can work wonders for some patients, while others may only show mild improvements (see Box 16.1). If the treatment outcome is not as expected, the protocols should be reevaluated. Frequent veterinary reassessment is needed to monitor the effectiveness of laser therapy and modify treatment as needed. The veterinary technician/nurse can help with assessment of therapeutic effect by taking an accurate history of home behavior since last therapy visit and by carefully palpating the affected area to monitor pain level before and after temporary analgesic effect. If the desired

effect is not being achieved in the expected timeframe (usually by 4–5 treatments), note your observations in the record and inform the prescribing veterinarian. If 12 sessions have been prescribed and by the 6th treatment there has been no improvement, do not wait until all treatments are finished to let the veterinarian know. Together, with an understanding of PBMT, the veterinary team can improve the patient's life in quality and quantity.

Box 16.1   Take away points
• Each therapeutic laser device is unique.
• Refer to the guidance of the manufacturer for the correct application technique and recommended protocols.
• Ask your laser manufacturer about the spot size of your device and/or handpiece so that you can calculate the irradiance you are delivering.
• Laser safety classes do not distinguish the efficacy or quality of the laser.
• Irradiance and time are the important parameters. The same amount of J/cm^2 can produce different outcomes, depending upon the intensity of the light and the time over which it is delivered.
• Veterinary research should quote irradiance and treatment time as well as treatment area.

References

Alves, J.C., Jorge, P., and Santos, A. (2022). The effect of photobiomodulation therapy on the management of chronic idiopathic large-bowel diarrhea in dogs. *Lasers Med Sci* 37 (3): 2045–2051. https://doi.org/10.1007/s10103-021-03469-w.

Anders, J.J., Lanzafame, R.J., and Arany, P.R. (2015). Low-level light/laser therapy versus photobiomodulation therapy. *Photomed Laser Surg* 33 (4): 183–184.

Barale, L., Monticelli, P., Raviola, M., and Adami, C. (2020). Preliminary clinical experience of low-level laser therapy for the treatment of canine osteoarthritis-associated pain: A retrospective investigation on 17 dogs. *Open Vet J* 10 (1):

116–119. https://doi.org/10.4314/ovj.
v10i1.16.

Bennaim, M., Porato, M., Jarleton, A. et al.
(2017). Preliminary evaluation of the
effects of photobiomodulation therapy and
physical rehabilitation on early
postoperative recovery of dogs undergoing
hemilaminectomy for treatment of
thoracolumbar intervertebral disk disease.
Am J Vet Res 78 (2): 195–206. https://doi.
org/10.2460/ajvr.78.2.195.

Bjordal, J.M., Couppé, C., Chow, R.T. et al.
(2003). A systematic review of low level
laser therapy with location-specific doses
for pain from chronic joint disorders.
Austr J Physiother 49 (2): 107–116.
https://doi.org/10.1016/s0004-9514(14)
60127-6.

Buijs, S. and Goldbold, J.C. Jr. (2017).
Chapter 9 intra- and postoperative laser
therapy. In: *Laser Therapy in Veterinary
Medicine: Photobiomodulation* (ed.
R.J. Riegel and J.C. Godbold Jr.), 88–99.
Ames, IA: John Wiley & Sons, Inc.

Callies, C., Fels, J., Liashkovich, I. et al.
(2011). Membrane potential depolarization
decreases the stiffness of vascular
endothelial cells. *J Cell Sci* 124 (Pt 11):
1936–1942. https://doi.org/10.1242/
jcs.084657.

Cressoni, M.D., Giusti, H.H., Pião, A.C. et al.
(2010). Effect of GaAlAs laser irradiation
on the epiphyseal cartilage of rats.
Photomed Laser Surg 28 (4): 527–532.
https://doi.org/10.1089/pho.2009.2572.
PMID: 20201664.

Draper, W.E., Schubert, T.A., Clemmons,
R.M., and Miles, S.A. (2012). Low-level
laser therapy reduces time to ambulation
in dogs after hemilaminectomy: A
preliminary study. *J Small Anim Pract* 53
(8): 465–469. https://doi.
org/10.1111/j.1748-5827.2012.01242.x.

Enwemeka, C.S. (2001). Attenuation and
penetration of visible 632.8nm and
invisible infra-red 904nm light in soft
tissues. *Laser Ther* 13: 95–101.

Hamblin, M.R., Nelson, S.T., and Strahan,
J.R. (2018). Photobiomodulation and
cancer: What is the truth? *Photomed Laser
Surg* 36 (5): 241–245. https://doi.
org/10.1089/pho.2017.4401.

Heiskanen, V. and Hamblin, M.R. (2018).
Photobiomodulation: Lasers vs light
emitting diodes? *Photochem Photobiol Sci*
17 (8): 1003–1017. https://doi.org/10.1039/
C8PP00176F.

Hode T, Duncan D, Kirkpatrick S, *et al.*
(2009). The importance of coherence in
phototherapy. Proc. SPIE 7165,
*Mechanisms for Low-Light Therapy
IV*, 716507.

Huang, Y.Y., Lan, C.W., Chen, S.H. et al.
(2020). Photobiomodulation in pain
management: A systematic review and
meta-analysis. *Lasers Med Sci* 35 (2):
269–278.

Jenkins, P.A. and Carroll, J.D. (2011). How to
report low-level laser therapy (LLLT)/
photomedicine dose and beam parameters
in clinical and laboratory studies.
Photomed Laser Surg 29: 785–787.

Kiro, N.E., Hamblin, M.R., and Abrahamse,
H. (2017). Photobiomodulation of breast
and cervical cancer stem cells using
low-intensity laser irradiation. *Tumour Biol*
39 (6): 1010428317706913. https://doi.
org/10.1177/1010428317706913.

Lam, T.K. and Wong, T.K. (2014). Dosimetry
in low-level laser therapy. *Lasers Med Sci*
29 (2): 549–557.

Looney, A.L., Huntingford, J.L., Blaeser, L.L.,
and Mann, S. (2018). A randomized blind
placebo-controlled trial investigating the
effects of photobiomodulation therapy
(PBMT) on canine elbow osteoarthritis.
Can Vet J 59 (9): 959–966.

Loreti, E.H., Pascoal, V.L., Nogueira,
B.V. et al. (2015). Use of laser therapy in
the healing process: A literature review.
Photomed Laser Surg 33 (2): 104–116.
https://doi.org/10.1089/pho.2014.3772.

Medrado, A.P., Soares, A.P., Santos, E.T. et al.
(2008). Influence of laser

photobiomodulation upon connective tissue remodeling during wound healing. *J Photochem Photobiol B Biol* 92 (3): 144–152. https://doi.org/10.1016/j.jphotobiol.2008.05.008.

Mendez, T.M., Pinheiro, A.L., Pacheco, M.T. et al. (2004). Dose and wavelength of laser light have influence on the repair of cutaneous wounds. *J Clin Laser Med Surg* 22 (1): 19–25. https://doi.org/10.1089/104454704773660930.

Mester, E., Ludany, G., Sellyei, M., and Szende, B. (1968). Untersuchungen über die biologische Wirkung der Laser-Strahlen [On the biologic effect of laser rays]. *Bull Soc Int Chir* 27 (1): 68–73.

Mester, E., Ludány, G., Frenyó, V. et al. (1970). Experimental and clinical observations with laser rays. *Langenbecks Arch Chir* 327: 310–314.

Mester, E., Mester, A.F., and Mester, A. (1985). The biomedical effects of laser application. *Lasers Surg Med* 5 (1): 31–39. https://doi.org/10.1002/lsm.1900050105.

Miller, L.A. (2017). Chapter 13: Musculoskeletal disorders and osteoarthritis. In: *Laser Therapy in Veterinary Medicine: Photobiomodulation* (ed. R.J. Riegel and J.C. Godbold Jr.), 132–149. Ames, IA: John Wiley & Sons, Inc.

Montesinos, M. (1988). Experimental effects of low power laser in encephalin and endorphin synthesis. *Laser J Eur Med Laser Assn* 1 (3): 2–7.

Nie, F., Hao, S., Ji, Y. et al. (2023). Biphasic dose response in the anti-inflammation experiment of PBM. *Lasers Med Sci* 38: 66. https://doi.org/10.1007/s10103-022-03664-3.

Oliveira, S.P., Rahal, S.C., Pereira, E.J. et al. (2012). Low-level laser on femoral growth plate in rats. *Acta Cir Bras* 27 (2): 117–122. https://doi.org/10.1590/s0102-86502012000200004.

Piao, D., Sypniewski, L.A., Bailey, C. et al. (2018). Flexible nine-channel photodetector probe facilitated intraspinal multisite transcutaneous photobiomodulation therapy dosimetry in cadaver dogs. *J Biomed Optics* 23 (1): 1–4. https://doi.org/10.1117/1.JBO.23.1.010503.

Robijns, J., Lodewijckx, J., Claes, M. et al. (2022). A long-term follow-up of early breast cancer patients treated with photobiomodulation during conventional fractionation radiotherapy in the prevention of acute radiation dermatitis. *Lasers Surgery Med* 54 (10): 1261–1268. https://doi.org/10.1002/lsm.23608.

Robinson N (2015) Photomedicine Physiology, *Shining Light on Laser Therapy Course*, https://www.onehealthsim.org/education-center/shining-light-on-laser-therapy-2/ (accessed 9/4/2016).

Sakurai, Y., Yamaguchi, M., and Abiko, Y. (2000). Inhibitory effect of low-level laser irradiation on LPS-stimulated prostaglandin E2 production and cyclooxygenase-2 in human gingival fibroblasts. *Eur J Oral Sci* 108 (1): 29–34. https://doi.org/10.1034/j.1600-0722.2000.00783.x.

Shurman, J.R., Zhang, W., and Schmitt, W.M. (2017). Low-level laser therapy reduces hyperalgesia in rats after muscle injury: A randomized controlled trial. *Photomed Laser Surg* 35 (6): 308–315.

Tedford, C.E., DeLapp, S., Jacques, S., and Anders, J. (2015). Quantitative analysis of transcranial and intraparenchymal light penetration in human cadaver brain tissue. *Lasers Surg Med* 47 (4): 312–322.

Tuner, J. and Hode, L. (2004). The laser therapy handbook: A guide for research scientists, doctors, dentists, veterinarians and other interested parties within the medical field.

Viegas, V.N., Abreu, M.E., Viezzer, C. et al. (2007). Effect of low-level laser therapy on inflammatory reactions during wound healing: Comparison with meloxicam. *Photomed Laser Surg* 25 (6): 467–473. https://doi.org/10.1089/pho.2007.1098.

Wardlaw, J.L., Gazzola, K.M., Wagoner, A. et al. (2019). Laser therapy for incision healing in 9 dogs. *Front Vet Sci* 5: 349. https://doi.org/10.3389/fvets.2018.00349.

Wong-Riley, M.T., Liang, H.L., Eells, J.T. et al. (2005). Photobiomodulation directly benefits primary neurons functionally inactivated by toxins: Role of cytochrome c oxidase. *J Biol Chem* 280 (6): 4761–4771. https://doi.org/10.1074/jbc.M409650200.

Woodruff, L.D., Bounkeo, J.M., Brannon, W.M. et al. (2004). The efficacy of laser therapy in wound repair: A meta-analysis of the literature. *Photomed Laser Surg* 22 (3): 241–247. https://doi.org/10.1089/1549541041438623.

Zein, R., Selting, W., and Hamblin, M.R. (2018). Review of light parameters and photobiomodulation efficacy: Dive into complexity. *J Biomed Optics* 23 (12): 1–17. https://doi.org/10.1117/1.JBO.23.12.120901.

17

Modalities Part 3: Electrotherapy and Electromagnetic Therapy

Julia E. Tomlinson[1,2]

[1] *Twin Cities Animal Rehabilitation & Sports Medicine Clinic, Burnsville, MN, USA*
[2] *Veterinary Rehabilitation and Orthopedic Medicine Partners, San Clemente, CA, USA*

CHAPTER MENU

Introduction

Electrotherapy and electromagnetic therapy are the application of electric currents, either directly to the body (electrotherapy) or to produce a magnetic field which is then applied to the body (electromagnetic therapy) in various and specific waveforms and frequencies with the goal of stimulating a tissue response. Goals of electrotherapy and electromagnetic therapy include reduction of muscle atrophy, neuromuscular re-education, pain relief, reduction of inflammation and edema, and facilitation of tissue healing, as part of a comprehensive treatment plan.

Electrical Stimulation

The most used forms of electrical stimulation in veterinary medicine are neuromuscular electrical stimulation (NMES) – a term used interchangeably with electrical stimulation, transcutaneous electrical nerve stimulation (TENS), and functional electrical stimulation (FES). Stimulation of muscle action using an electrical current via the skin usually involves indirect action via first stimulating the motor nerve supplying that muscle (NMES); and when a muscle is denervated and requires direct muscle fiber activation through electrical stimulation, the term EMS is used (Levine and Bockstahler, 2014). FES activates whole nerve trunks innervating extremities to affect more than one muscle generally used in paralyzed people with the aim of restoring function (Delitto and Robinson, 1989). The term TENS in veterinary medicine is generally used to refer to transcutaneous electrical nerve stimulation used for analgesia, although strictly all the above forms of electrical stimulation are transcutaneous.

General Terminology

The **ampere (A)** is the unit of measure for electrical current. **Current** is the speed or rate at which the electrons flow through a tissue. **Volts (V)** are the unit of measure for electrical **voltage** which is the difference in electrical potential, or the number of electrons, between any two points in an electrical circuit. A pair of electrodes placed on a patient with coupling gel to aid conductivity will send electrons from one electrode, through the body tissue and to the other electrode to complete a circuit. You can think of voltage as the pressure of water being pushed through a pipe, and the current is equivalent to the flow rate of the water.

An electrical or electromagnetic **pulse** is a burst of energy, the quantity of a signal changes quickly from its baseline to higher or lower values. The **pulse width** is the time between the leading and trailing edges of an individual pulse of energy.

Frequency (**measured in Hertz or Hz**) is the number of cycles per second of a varying electrical current. Alternating current (AC) that oscillates 50 times in a second has a frequency of 50 hertz (50 Hz).

Electrical waveforms are visual representations of the variation of a voltage or current over time. Each waveform corresponds to a rise in the current of electron flow followed by a drop in flow back to zero. This can be an abrupt cessation or a slow decline in electron flow to zero before the next wave follows. Waves can be uni- or bidirectional. In a depiction of the waveform of a current, the shape of the wave is influenced by the rate of increase and decrease of the current (the ramp), and if the current remains constant at any time. The most common bidirectional waveform is the sinusoidal wave.

Explanation of electrical current waveforms (Canapp, 2007) used in veterinary medicine are summarized in (see Box 17.1).

Medical Terminology

Amplitude or Intensity

Measured in milliamperes (mA), amplitude describes the total magnitude of the electrical wave. A higher amplitude will result in a stronger muscle contraction due to recruitment of a greater number of muscle fibers but can produce discomfort, and as our patient cannot be counseled, it is practical to get the highest amplitude at which the patient remains relatively comfortable. In practice, this means you can feel a contraction and the patient may look at the area being treated or become a little restless, but they can be distracted from it. Higher intensities have been shown to promote strength gains in people (Gondin *et al.*, 2011).

Box 17.1   Current classification

There are three basic waveforms used in commercial therapeutic electrical stimulation units: direct current, alternating current, and pulsed current.

Direct current (DC)

Continuous unidirectional flow of charged particles with a duration of at least 1 s.

One electrode is always the anode (+) and one is always the cathode (−) for the entire event.

There is a build-up of charge since it is moving in one direction causing a chemical effect on the tissue under the electrode.

Alternating current (AC)

Uninterrupted bidirectional flow of charged particles changing direction at least once per second.

Electrodes continuously change polarity each cycle, therefore, no build-up of charge under the electrodes

Often used in interferential commercial stimulators

Pulsed current (pulsed)

Can be unidirectional (like DC) or bidirectional (like AC)

Flow of charged particles stops periodically for less than 1 second before the next event

Pulses can occur individually or in a series

Pulse Duration or Pulse Width

Pulse width is measured in microseconds (µs). The time during which the current flows is known as the pulse duration or width. A longer pulse duration can translate to needing a lower amplitude to stimulate muscle contraction; however, it may stimulate more nerve fibers that mediate pain (Niebaum, 2013). Shorter pulse widths tend to be more comfortable, but a longer pulse width can potentially recruit more muscle fibers to compensate for fatigue (Lagerquist and Collins, 2010). When trying to affect deeper tissue layers, a longer pulse width should be used (Bracciano, 2008). Specific pulse durations have been calculated for comfort and effectiveness in the dog (Sawaya *et al.*, 2008) (see Table 17.1).

Frequency or Pulse Rate

Frequency is measured in hertz (Hz), meaning the number of pulses produced per second **(pps)** during the time the current is flowing. Depending on the NMES unit used, the setting may be quoted as either Hz or pps.

Table 17.1   Recommended pulse duration for neuromuscular electrical stimulation in dogs.

Muscle	Recommended pulse duration in dogs (ms)
Supraspinatus	150–190
Infraspinatus	130–170
Deltoideus	160–200
Triceps brachii	200–240
Gluteus medius	160–200
Biceps femoris	180–220
Semitendinosus	150–190
Vastus lateralis	210–250
Tibialis cranialis	210–250
Erector spinae	180–220

Source: Adapted from Sawaya *et al.* (2008).

The best frequency will vary depending on the goal of therapy. Frequencies as low as 20 Hz will produce tetanic (whole sustained) muscle contractions (Spurgeon *et al.*, 1978; Levine and Bockstahler, 2014), but only submaximal forces of contraction are typically produced in this range. Maximal contraction force is generally achieved at frequencies between 60 and 100 Hz in humans (Duchateau and Baudry, 2014) and 60 Hz reported in dogs (Sawaya *et al.*, 2008). As frequency of the therapy increases, the likelihood of muscle fatigue also increases. A lower frequency (35–50 Hz) will provide strong muscle contractions while reducing muscle fatigue and discomfort (Windsor *et al.*, 1993; Nelson *et al.*, 1999; Levine and Bockstahler, 2014). An alternative for veterinary patients who are not very tolerant of electrical stimulation would be to use a low frequency (<10 Hz), which will provide only a twitch (localized) contraction but will possibly be more easily tolerated while still stimulating some function. This can be helpful when using NMES concurrently with active range of motion. An example of a patient would be a cat that is receiving NMES (see Box 17.2).

On/Off or Duty Cycle

The duty cycle is stated in seconds or in a ratio form of "on-time" and "off-time." Common clinical parameters for on/off times are between 1:1 and 1:5 (for example, 1:3 is 10 seconds on:30 seconds off) but can be modified to accommodate the patient's needs and goals of treatment (Bracciano, 2008; Levine and Bockstahler, 2014). The duty cycle settings can be used to decrease the likelihood of premature muscle fatigue during a therapy session. The "on-time" is when the series of pulses are being delivered. The "off-time" is the time between sequential on-times, and during this no current is being delivered. The off-time phase allows the muscle tissues to recover (relax and reset for next contraction); adequate recovery time decreases the chance of muscle fatigue. During this reset period, the adenosine triphosphate (ATP)/adenosine diphosphate (ADP) is replenished. In the case of neurofatigue, the goal is to avoid lengthening the refractory/hyperpolarization period by providing inadequate off time. Intermittent electrical stimulation is commonly used to increase the comfort level of the patient (Lake, 1992; Doucet *et al.*, 2012). Many clinicians start with duty cycle ratios between 1:2 and 1:5 and watch for signs of fatigue, which indicates the need for a longer off time (Levine and

---

Box 17.2   Typical parameters available in neuromuscular electrical stimulation devices

Waveform: The shape of the visual representation of pulsed current on a current/time plot or voltage/time plot. It can be symmetric, asymmetric, balanced, unbalanced, biphasic, monophasic, or polyphasic.

Amplitude: The current value in a monophasic pulse or for any single phase of a biphasic pulse.

Phase/pulse duration: The duration of a phase or a pulse, usually measured in microseconds.

Pulse rate or frequency: The rate of oscillation in cycles per second, expressed as pulses per second (pps) or hertz (Hz).

Often labeled as pulse rate or pulses per second, or frequency on stimulators.

On/off time: The amount of time the stimulator is delivering current compared with the rest period between contractions, usually measured in seconds.

Ramp: The time in seconds from when the current begins to the peak current (e.g., three-second ramp up, six-second contraction, and two-second ramp down).

Polarity: Electrode may be either the anode (+) or cathode (−) (not relevant when using AC).

Source: Adapted from Levine and Bockstahler (2014).

Bockstahler, 2014). On–off cycles are not a part of continuous flow electrical stimulation (see Box 17.2).

Ramp

This is time taken for the stimulus to reach peak amplitude and to decline again from peak and is usually measured in seconds (Kloth and Cummings, 1991). At the onset of the electric current, a gradual increase in flow is designed to slowly increase the force of muscle contraction. A steady decrease in current at the end of the peak amplitude results in a smooth decline in muscle force. A 1–3 second ramp time is commonly utilized in clinical applications and the amount of time chosen is based on patient comfort. If a patient has increased muscle tone that may create resistance against the stimulated movement (for example, hypertonicity from spastic paresis), then a longer ramp is utilized, a patient with spasticity may need a longer ramp time of 4–8 seconds to avoid stimulating an excess increase in tone (Cameron, 2003). In some situations, using a ramp time may inhibit muscle activity. For example, during NMES use for gait training or standing exercises, the required movement assisted by muscle recruitment from electrical stimulation may be rapid enough to be completed, before the peak amplitude is reached (Knaflitx *et al.*, 1990). Ramp is not a parameter applicable to continuous flow forms of electrical stimulation (see Box 17.2).

Current Types

There are three types of therapeutic electrical stimulation currents: direct (or monophasic) current, alternating (or biphasic) current, and pulsed current (may be mono- or biphasic) (Niebaum, 2013). AC is an electric current in which the flow of electric charge periodically reverses direction, whereas in direct current (DC, also dc), the flow of electric charge is only in one direction.

Direct Current

DC electrical stimulation is used to stimulate denervated muscles, for wound healing, and for iontophoresis. It creates a unidirectional flow of charged particles with a waveform usually using 20–200 μA at a low voltage (Gardner *et al.*, 1999; Cameron, 2003).

Alternating Current

(AC is a bidirectional flow of charged particles – out and back again. The charges are equal in the two symmetrical phases of each pulse, meaning there is no accumulation of charge in the tissues. TENS is an example of an AC therapy. ACs are delivered at various pulse widths depending on the muscle. Recommendations have been made for NMES in dogs based on research (Sawaya *et al.*, 2008) (see Table 17.1).

Pulsed Current

The output of this therapy is one of short, paired pulses with a long interval of no pulses between and is typically delivered at 75–200 V and 80–100 pps. The current flow may be one direction (like DC) or bidirectional (like AC). If one direction, it is referred to as monophasic pulsed current. If current flows in two opposite directions, it is referred to as biphasic pulsed (Gardner *et al.*, 1999; Cameron, 2003) (see Box 17.1).

Evidence Base in Veterinary Patients

There is some evidence in human medicine, but it is not strong, in a meta-analysis the use of NMES for quadriceps strengthening pre- and post-total knee replacement cited the evidence for its use as unclear (Monaghan *et al.*, 2010). However, a meta-analysis cited that NMES may be useful for human adults with muscle weakness from advanced chronic disease (Jones *et al.*, 2016).

The use of NMES has been reported in dogs after extracapsular repair surgery to treat cranial cruciate ligament disease. Studies showed improved gait in treated dogs on subjective scoring; however, objective gait data did not support this. The dogs did show increased thigh circumference and reduced radiographic bone changes in the treated group; however, there was concern at an increased incidence of meniscus damage seen in treated dogs (Johnson *et al.*, 1997).

The use of TENS is currently often practiced in humans with the goal of reversing quadriceps inhibition in cases of anterior cruciate ligament disease (Monaghan *et al.*, 2010). However, there is no evidence of quadriceps inhibition in canine patients. In an experimental model of cruciate disease in dogs, examination of action in the quadriceps, biceps femoris, and gastrocnemius identified no significant changes in muscle function at any timepoint (Adrian *et al.*, 2019). In a clinical study of muscle action in naturally occurring cruciate disease pre and post-stabilization via tibial plateau leveling osteotomy (TPLO), amplitude of muscle contraction of the gastrocnemius and biceps femoris was lower in affected versus unaffected limbs, but no such changes were noted in the quadriceps or semitendinosus (Varcoe *et al.*, 2021). Electromyography of the biceps femoris and semimembranosus muscles in cruciate-deficient dogs (Hayes *et al.*, 2013) found that in both affected and unaffected limbs, there was evidence of delay in muscle activation in both muscles as compared to normal limbs. This leads one to speculate that the positive effects of NMES in dogs post-surgery for cruciate disease is via affecting hamstring activation.

NMES was shown to increase the speed of tibial fracture healing in an experiment on rabbits. However, the treatment was one hour daily for four weeks following fracture stabilization with an external skeletal fixator (Park and Silva, 2004).

TENS was part of the rehabilitation protocol (also included range of motion, massage, and progressive leash walks) in a study on treating overweight dogs with osteoarthritis (Mlacnik *et al.*, 2006) though evidence base for the TENS treatment alone cannot be inferred from this. Studies on the effects of transcutaneous electrical nerve stimulation for analgesia in veterinary patients are (mostly) limited to electroacupuncture. Electroacupuncture is covered in the chapter on acupuncture.

Patient Preparation

Each treatment session generally lasts between 5 and 20 minutes depending on the degree of muscle fatigue (Prydie and Hewitt, 2015).

It is advisable to clip the patient's hair for optimal contact of electrodes with skin. The clip patches also act as a guide for electrode placement in the case of home therapy being assigned using portable electrical stimulation units. The accuracy of electrode placement on clipped patches also depends on the mobility of the skin at the treatment site – even an electrode taped to skin may move with the skin and not stay over the desired muscle. A coupling medium is necessary to transmit the electrical current from the electrodes to the tissues. Some electrodes are carbon silicon–rubber and need to be used with an aqueous gel, while others are coated with a conductive polymer. Commonly used coupling media include gels, moistened sponges, or paper towels; sponges and paper towels tend to dry out, and rewetting is necessary. Conductive performance of any electrode decreases over time. Electrodes should be of the appropriate size to stimulate the desired muscle without stimulating unwanted muscles. The smaller the electrode, the higher

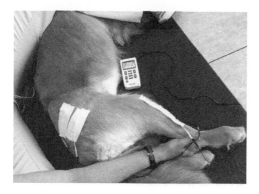

Figure 17.1 A portable NMES unit on a patient. The accuracy of electrode placement is affected by the mobility of the skin at the treatment site – even an electrode taped to skin may move with the skin and not stay over the desired muscle.

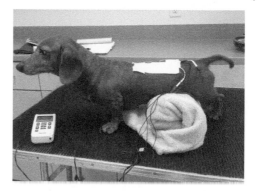

Figure 17.2 The use of NMES following hemilaminectomy surgery. Notice that a rolled towel may be helpful to support the patient if they can stand.

the current density that enters the muscle, and the more uncomfortable the stimulus may be (see Figure 17.1).

Precautions for Electrical Stimulation

The safety of the clinician and patient is of utmost importance when working with animals. A patient who is surprised by a sudden muscle contraction or who is in pain may respond with a bite, scratch, or kick. Most canine patients have bite inhibition and will provide warning; however, it is wise to provide adequate restraint and to keep away from the patient's head (or species-appropriate danger zone). It is our obligation in veterinary medicine to understand and read patient stress, to minimize stress and pain, and to err on the side of caution rather than administering painful therapy (Niebaum, 2013). It cannot be emphasized enough to utilize low-stress handling techniques such as those developed by Dr. Sophia Yin (2009).

Caution must be used always when treating a patient with electrical stimulation because of the potentially harmful effects it may have if applied inappropriately (see Figure 17.2). The canine patient may not be able to communicate the intensity of an electrical stimulus or completely sense the

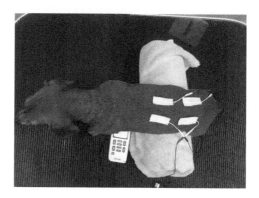

Figure 17.3 Placement of the electrical pads prior to additional tape placement. Notice positive (black wire) and negative pads (red wire) are placed opposite each other.

stimulus in situations where neurologic impairment is present (see Figure 17.3). Burns from electrical stimulation have been reported and are associated with overly high levels of stimulation and usually over areas of diminished sensation or high adipose content. Thus, precautions for the use of electrical stimulation need to be considered when treating such areas (see Figure 17.3) (Hecox *et al.*, 1994; Cameron, 2003; Niebaum, 2013).

Contraindications (See Box 17.3)

One contraindication of electrical stimulation is stimulation directly over the carotid sinus in the neck just behind the vertical ramus of the mandible or over the pharyngeal area.

Box 17.3   Indications and contraindications for electrical stimulation

Contraindications	Where there is instability (i.e., fracture)
Pregnancy	Indications
Wounds	Increasing muscle strength
Malignancy	Increasing range of movement (ROM)
Pacemaker patients	Decreasing acute pain
Over laminectomy site	Decreasing chronic pain
Seizure patients	Reducing muscle spasm
Areas of thrombosis	Promotion of soft tissue healing
Pharyngeal area	Promotion of fracture healing
Carotid sinus	*Source:* Adapted from Hanks *et al.* (2015).
Over eyes	

Stimulation to this area may induce a rapid fall in blood pressure, which could cause syncope. Another area where the placement of electrical stimulation is contraindicated is over the heart. Electrical stimulation in patients with pacemakers may interfere with the functioning of the pacemaker device, altering heart rate or rhythm. Likewise, electrical stimulation should not be used in patients with seizure history as the electrical currents may induce a seizure episode. Since the effects of electrical stimulation on the developing fetus and pregnant uterus are unknown, the use of electrical stimulation over the trunk, abdomen, low back, hips, or pelvis during pregnancy is contraindicated. Areas of thrombosis, suspected thrombosis, or thrombophlebitis should be avoided because of the potential risk of the embolus releasing. This is of importance in cats with rear limb pain or weakness and without a definitive diagnosis; femoral arterial blood flow should be verified with diagnostic ultrasound before considering using electrical stimulation in a cat with weak or painful rear limbs. Also, considering the circulation changes associated with electrical stimulation, it is contraindicated to use over areas of infection because of the theoretical potential to cause systemic spread and sepsis. Another contraindication concerning the circulatory effect is over a malignancy, though occasionally electrical stimulation is used to control pain in patients with malignancies when quality of life (QoL) outweighs the possible risks of the treatment (Hecox *et al.*, 1994; Cameron, 2003; Niebaum, 2013). The use of electrical stimulation should be avoided in any situation where active movement of the area is contraindicated, such as over an unstable fracture. Electrical stimulation should never be used over the eyes.

Adverse Effects

There are very few adverse effects of electrical stimulation, but electrical burns, skin irritation, and pain can occur if the electrical stimulation is applied inappropriately. If there is not enough conduction medium, the risk of a burn increases due to inadequate conduction into the tissues. Electrical burns are most common with the use of DC due to the constant current flow. Skin irritation can occur if the patient has skin sensitivities or is allergic to the contact surface of the electrodes, which is rare. In such cases, a different type of electrode can be tried. Some patients find electrical stimulation painful. In those cases, decreasing the pulse width, increasing the ramp time, and/or increasing the intensity slowly over time may help their tolerance. If it is still painful, other forms of treatment should be utilized (Cameron, 2003).

NMES for Muscle Strengthening

NMES is a non-pharmacological treatment method that can be used to address muscle weakness or atrophy with patients who are unwilling or unable to actively contract a muscle (see Figure 17.4). It is usually applied at higher frequencies (20–50 Hz) with the

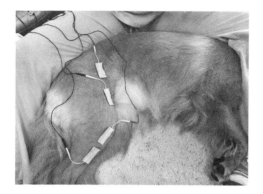

Figure 17.4 Shows use of pads that do not require taping because they have a sticky adhesive on their back.

goal being to achieve muscle tetany and contraction that can be used for functional purposes (Valenti, 1964; Tacker *et al.*, 1991). The goal is to provide an electric potential to a muscle to elicit a non-voluntary contraction. The electrical current creates a muscle contraction by depolarizing the motor nerve (Niebaum, 2013) (see Box 17.4).

Adverse changes in muscle strength and function have been reported following injury or surgery. The primary injury alone will create changes in muscle activity and motor control that are initially thought to be protective, such as spasm and a resultant shorter functional range. There is no evidence of long-term changes in motor control after direct muscle injury. However, if the peripheral innervation is damaged, changes in motor control may persist long after pain has resolved, and tissue healing has taken place. Most studies in human medicine focus on the use of NMES after surgical repair of peripheral nerves and demonstrate success (Gordon and English, 2016). If muscle activity is decreased because of neurological compromise from injury or surgery, the muscle will atrophy, and significant loss of strength and fine motor control will occur. Changes at the cellular level also occur in muscles that atrophy; atrophy is particularly rapid when neurogenic. A reduction in mitochondria,

---

Box 17.4   Current NMES parameters for strengthening

Frequency: Generally between 25 and 50 Hz (<10 Hz will produce twitch contraction for intolerant patients).

Waveforms: Any waveform capable of depolarizing the muscle is acceptable.

Pulse or phase duration: Between 150 and 250 μs – see Table 17.1.

Ramp up/down (rise and decay time): Between 2 and 4 seconds up, for comfort; 1–2 seconds down.

On/off time: 1:3 or 1:4 ratio; 10 seconds on, and 30 or 40 seconds off.

As strength improves, 1:1 or 1:2 ratio is usually used for endurance training.

To prevent atrophy 1:1 (15 seconds each)

Treatment time: 10–20 minutes

Frequency of treatment: 3–7 sessions/week

Amplitude: Sufficient to cause a strong muscle contraction

Position: Initially recumbent but can use functional position which may bring improved strength gains (Niebaum, 2013)

Source: Adapted from Levine and Bockstahler (2014).

glycogen stores, and enzymes is associated with muscle building, and the number of functioning muscle cells is reduced, leaving a smaller, metabolically deficient muscle unit (Bonaldo and Sandri, 2013). The patient will be at a disadvantage when trying to return to normal function, even if resolution of the neurological compromise occurs. Many of the functional problems associated with a neurologically impaired patient can be found to be due to the detrimental changes associated with a lack of normal exercise. If the muscle is not used as much, some atrophy ensues. Immobilization, such as splinting during the healing time of a fracture, causes atrophy and its associated consequences (Henderson *et al.*, 2015).

If the patient is unable to maximally contract a muscle, an electrically induced muscle contraction may create a bigger "top off" force, and therefore, improve muscle activity over patient activity alone (Fitzgerald *et al.*, 2003). However, studies have shown that electrical stimulation is not superior to voluntary strength training and is more effective when coordinated with voluntary muscle activity (Currier and Mann, 1983; Laughmann *et al.*, 1983; McMiken *et al.*, 1983; Selkowitz, 1985; Wolf *et al.*, 1986).

Electrode Size and Placement for NMES

Correct electrode placement is crucial to obtain the best muscle contraction. The technique is to place electrodes over the belly of the muscle(s) to be stimulated, with one of the electrodes placed over a ***motor point***. The motor point is the point over the muscle belly at which the smallest amount of current is required to produce muscle contraction (Lake, 1992). The **distance** between electrodes influences the depth and course of the electrical current. The greater the distance between electrodes, the

deeper the current travels, and conversely the closer together the electrodes are the more superficially the current travels and so fewer muscle fibers are stimulated (Cameron, 2003). This can be a challenge in smaller veterinary patients and electrodes may need to be trimmed down to provide space between electrodes (avoiding the wire). It may be beneficial to have different types of electrodes in the clinic in case a patient demonstrates an allergy to a certain electrode, or there is difficulty keeping one type adhered to the patient. It is recommended to use tape or flexible bandaging to hold the electrodes in place to maintain good contact with the skin throughout the treatment, especially if the patient moves (see Box 17.5).

The size of the electrodes should match the muscle(s) being targeted. Small electrodes are available to accommodate smaller treatment areas, but the current density produced over a small surface area can cause discomfort when used at higher treatment amplitudes. In contrast, electrodes that are too large can cause the current to spread to other muscles. In addition, the electrodes, and their coupling medium, should not encounter each other, as this will result in the current flowing directly from one electrode to the other instead of into the targeted muscle tissues (Niebaum, 2013).

Box 17.5 Criteria for electrodes

- The main criteria in choosing electrodes are as follows:
- Flexible enough to conform to the tissue
- May be trimmed to a specific size
- Have a low resistance
- Are highly conductive
- May be used many times
- Are inexpensive

Source: Adapted from Levine and Bockstahler (2014).

Neuromuscular Electrical Stimulation for Edema

NMES can also help to decrease tissue edema. Muscle contractions during normal movements provide a pumping action, which helps with venous return (Williams *et al.*, 2021). Muscle pumping can be achieved by using low-frequency (1–10 Hz) twitch-like contractions on a continuous setting and is worn for hours in reported human medical protocols (Williams *et al.*, 2021). Electrical stimulation applied to the affected muscles may also generally improve circulation to a compromised area by increasing muscle pumping action. This method is likely impractical in veterinary patients who are not hospitalized, and cold compression has superseded NMES in acute care veterinary settings with strong evidence behind it (von Freeden *et al.*, 2017; Wilson *et al.*, 2018).

When using electrical stimulation to reduce edema, it is best applied to major muscle groups around the edema to promote reciprocal contraction and relaxation of the agonist and antagonist muscles. This alternating contraction will aid in the pumping mechanism that venous return relies upon. The electrode pads can also be placed proximal and distal to the affected area with the same type of intermittent stimulation (Hecox *et al.*, 1994).

Electrical Stimulation for Wound Healing

The use of electrical stimulation is indicated to assist in wound healing if prescribed by your supervising veterinarian. Significant caution needs to be taken when applying electrical stimulation over areas of diminished sensation. The person carrying out the therapy should have a good understanding of the intensity of stimulation provided over a region with neurological compromise. The intensity of electrical stimulation units can accidentally turn up far beyond what may be tolerable to a neurologically intact veterinary patient. High-intensity electrical stimulation will cause burns to the skin. Different waveforms will be tolerated at different intensities. The veterinary technician should have a good understanding of what a specific waveform and intensity feels like before placing it on a patient with sensory compromise to ensure an appropriate and safe intensity is used for treatment. Other modalities indicated for wound healing such as laser and pulsed electromagnetic field (PEMF) therapy are much safer (see Box 17.6).

Remember that adipose tissue is a poor conductor of electricity. This lack of conduction through the fat cells will cause heat to build up in the tissues, predisposing these areas to a higher likelihood of an adverse event occurring with the use of electrical stimulation (Hecox *et al.*, 1994; Cameron, 2003; Niebaum, 2013).

Electrical stimulation at the site of a wound has been shown to be effective in promoting tissue healing by increasing local circulation, retarding bacterial growth, and stimulating tissue repair mechanisms (Ennis *et al.*, 2016).

Physiologically, the effects of electrical stimulation on wound healing can be

---

Box 17.6   Parameters for wound healing

- *Frequency*: 60–125 Hz or pps
- *Pulse* duration: 40–100 ms
- *Amplitude*: High enough to elicit a comfortable sensory response
- *Treatment time*: 45–60 minutes
- *Polarity*: Negative if treating infected area, positive if treating clean area (Cameron, 2003)

explained by the electrical properties of the skin. After an injury to the skin, a DC electrical gradient is present, and it is affecting this which can accelerate wound healing (Ennis *et al.*, 2016). Electrical stimulation is thought to be able to magnify this potentiated normal endogenous biological healing response in the skin, promoting tissue proliferation and improving the rate of healing. In a metanalysis, unidirectional high voltage pulsed current (HVPC) with the active electrode over the wound was the best evidence-based protocol to improve wound healing (Khouri *et al.*, 2017).

Electrical Stimulation for Pain Control

When used for pain control, TENS can be a beneficial modality. It is an alternate form of electrical stimulation that has been historically administered at high frequencies to provide pain relief (Deyo *et al.*, 1990) but is now used at very low frequencies (2–10 Hz) (Sluka and Walsh, 2003). Pulse duration is generally 50–100 ms, short-duration pulses can be used as sensory nerves have relatively low thresholds. Low frequency stimulates sensory nerves instead of motor nerves, which is thought to reduce pain perception through the gate control theory of pain inhibition (Melzack and Wall, 1965; Niebaum, 2013). If a TENS current is applied, the large cutaneous (A-β) fibers are stimulated (Levine and Bockstahler, 2014). The signals from the A-β fibers activate inhibitory interneurons in the substantia gelatinosa of the spinal cord dorsal horn and block the transmission of the slower pain impulses from the periphery to the brain (Melzack and Wall, 1965). Additional mechanisms involve the release of endogenous opioids (Levine and Bockstahler, 2014). Pain relief is provided only while the

> ### Box 17.7 Recommended parameters for pain with TENS
>
> - *Amplitude:* high enough to elicit a comfortable sensory response
> - *Pulse duration:* between 50 and 100 ms
> - *Frequency:* between 2 and 150 Hz
> - *Duration:* of treatment varies according to the activity
> - *Placement of electrodes:* over or around the area of pain, over the peripheral nerve or spinal nerve roots that innervate the painful region, or over acupuncture points
>
> *Source:* Adapted from Nolan (2005).

stimulation is being delivered. However, deactivation of nociceptors can help to reduce the general state of wind up, so over time, TENS can aid in reducing central nervous system (CNS) sensitization (Beckwée *et al.*, 2012). TENS can be used in combination with pharmaceuticals in acute pain situations, such as following trauma or surgery, as well as in chronic pain situations associated with degenerative change (see Box 17.7). Practicalities necessitate the use of a home TENS unit so that the therapy can be performed daily or at least four days a week (video on TENS). These units can be preprogrammed for home use. Remember to clip hair and re-clip as needed to ensure adequate electrode contact. In a metaanalysis for chronic pain in human medicine, no conclusions as to the efficacy of TENS could be drawn (Gibson *et al.*, 2019). No improvement of symptoms, but short-term improvement of functional disability was seen in human patients with lower back pain treated with TENS (Wu *et al.*, 2018). Due to the need to clip hair and lack of evidence in veterinary patients, many veterinarians prefer to use PEMF.

Pulsed Electromagnetic Field Therapy

PEMF is a modality that produces low-frequency pulsed electromagnetic fields. These fields can be applied to the whole body (usually, via a treatment bed or mat) or to a specific target (usually, via a loop in veterinary medicine). PEMF beds, mats, and loops use electricity to produce a magnetic field that in turn results in conduction changes in the tissues (Trock, 2000), as opposed to the electromotive force produced by electrodes applied to the body during EMS.

To understand the effects of PEMF, it helps to first understand that all atoms have an electric field, and the molecules of the body are held together by electromagnetism. It is not just nerve cells that function via flow of ions, all cells will pump ions in and out of the cell body through specialized channels, which provide the means of cellular communication, protein synthesis, and other signaling pathways, resulting in cellular changes to maintain homeostasis. PEMF activates these intracellular processes, it can trigger forced vibration of ions sitting on the cell membrane which then will alter ion channel function, but it can also alter downstream function in cell signaling pathways (Li *et al.*, 2012).

Dose is dependent on intensity, frequency, and time of exposure, just as it is for laser therapy. For PEMF, the dose follows the same inverse square law that applies to X-rays, the further away the target tissue is from the PEMF source, the lower the intensity with that intensity being inversely proportional to the square of the distance from the source. EMF strength is expressed in **Gauss units** (symbol G).

There is increasing use of PEMF as adjunctive therapy for a multitude of musculoskeletal injuries and problems.

Evidence Base in Veterinary Patients

In current clinical veterinary practice, electromagnetic field (EMF) modalities have been shown to have therapeutic benefits for bone and wound repair and pain relief (Gaynor *et al.*, 2018).

Improved incorporation of cancellous bone grafts was found in an experimental study in horses (Canè *et al.*, 1993). In a study on dogs using a gap osteotomy, PEMF produced faster recovery of weight bearing, increased new bone, and a greater strength of the healing site (Inoue *et al.*, 2002).

In a randomized double-blinded placebo-controlled clinical trial of dogs after hemilaminectomy PEMF accelerated healing of the surgical wound and reduced the need for pain supplementation at home during recovery (Alvarez *et al.*, 2019). In another similar clinical trial, PEMF was found to reduce incisional pain in dogs after surgery for intervertebral disc extrusion. The authors also concluded that it may reduce the extent of spinal cord injury, and enhance proprioceptive placing (Zidan *et al.*, 2018).

PEMF has even been used to treat separation anxiety in dogs (Pankratz *et al.*, 2021).

Pulsed Electromagnetic Field Therapy for Wound Healing

A modality applied at home that could assist in healing wounds, especially in high-risk populations for delayed healing, would be advantageous to the pet owner, the veterinary staff, and the patient. Radiofrequency PEMF has been shown to enhance healing of skin wounds (Pilla, 2006). In a study done in 2007, the authors successfully demonstrated that treating wounds with PEMF in very specific settings accelerated early diabetic wound healing in rats. There was increased wound tensile strength at 21 days. The wounds were exposed to a 1.0 G signal for 30 minutes twice daily for 21 days (Strauch *et al.*, 2007). In the canine post-surgical studies, EMF strength and frequency are not revealed, studies used the Assisi Loop® and the manufacturers claim their settings as proprietary information (Alvarez *et al.*, 2019; Zidan *et al.*, 2018).

Pulsed Electromagnetic Field Therapy for Bone Healing

Being a crystalline structure, compression in a long bone will be subject to the piezoelectric effect. The piezoelectric effect states that compressing a crystalline structure results in negatively charged electrons migrating to the side of concavity. It is thought that the electronegative potential creates an environment where osteoblasts can function normally, but osteoclast activity is halted. Thus, the formation of bone tissue exceeds the normal physiologic breakdown of tissue for repair, which results in net bone growth. This is the reason why the trabeculae of the bone are organized in a manner consistent with the stress placed on the bone. This results in trabecular patterns that follow strain patterns in bone and causes greater bone mass to be present in areas of greater physical stress.

PEMF has been shown to increase healing time in non-union and delayed-union fractures. In these cases, it has been theorized that there is an absence of electrical charge to help stimulate osteoblastic activity. A recent meta-analysis found moderate-quality evidence that PEMF increased healing rate and relieved pain of fracture but may not be beneficial in decreasing the incidence of non-union fractures (Peng *et al.*, 2020). PEMF is approved by the US Food and Drug Administration (FDA) for use as an adjunctive treatment to aid in fracture repair (Canapp, 2007; Galkowski *et al.*, 2009).

Pulsed Electromagnetic Field Therapy for Osteoarthritis

Osteoarthritis has been estimated to affect 20% of the US canine population in middle age, and 90% of older dogs have osteoarthritis in one or more joints (Budsberg, 2010). In cats, a report indicated a 26% radiographic prevalence of appendicular osteoarthritis and a 90% prevalence of all types of degenerative joint disease, but the study only included cats older than 12 years of age (Hardie *et al.*, 2002; Bennett *et al.*, 2012).

In 2013, a randomized, controlled clinical trial was published that evaluated the efficacy of pulsed signal therapy (PST), which is the application of PEMF, in dogs with osteoarthritis, as measured by the Canine Brief Pain Inventory (CBPI) (O'Sullivan *et al.*, 2013). The results showed the PST group performed significantly better than the control group, but the objective measures of range of motion and peak vertical force were not statistically significant between groups receiving and not receiving PEMF. It was speculated that the range of motion may have been limited more by mechanical means (i.e., osteophytes and periarticular fibrosis) than by pain (O'Sullivan *et al.*, 2013). A randomized but subjectively analyzed clinical study of dogs with osteoarthritis showed some promise of PEMF for improved outcomes (Pinna *et al.*, 2013).

A 2020 meta-analysis concluded that PEMF therapy has clinically significant effects on pain in human patients with osteoarthritis (Yang *et al.*, 2020).

The theory behind the mechanisms of the effects of PEMF on osteoarthritic pain lies in the anabolic effects that PEMF has on osteoblast and chondrocyte proliferation, which produces healing effects at the cellular level (Diniz *et al.*, 2002) by enhancing regeneration of articular cartilage (Ciombor *et al.*, 2003). Osteoarthritic pain originates from the joint capsule and subchondral bone, not cartilage.

Treatment Protocol for the Assisi Loop

The Assisi Loop (https://assisianimal-health.com/assisi-loop/) offers targeted PEMF in a portable, device that can be used in clinic or in the home/stable. The Loop has been proven to reduce pain and inflammation and has been cleared by the FDA for palliative treatment of post-operative edema and pain in humans (Rohde *et al.*, 2015).

Therapy starts with a minimum of two 15-minute treatments per day for acute and chronic or degenerative conditions. This depends on the animal's progress. When treating following surgery, treatment can begin immediately after the operation and should continue until the surgical site is healed.

With some chronic and degenerative conditions, the patient may get to the point that they would only be treated as needed for pain, particularly, if it is a condition that is prone to flare-ups (see Figure 17.5).

There are no known contraindications with other modalities, however, given that the Loop and other treatment modalities, such as laser, have different mechanisms of action, it is recommended to allow two hours between treatment modalities and not do them concurrently.

Using the Loop over a metal implant or brace will not cause any harm, but it may distract or weaken the signal. If possible, position the Loop so that it is at a 45° angle from the metallic implant. Avoid using over pacemakers or close to people or pets who have an insulin pump.

The use of magnetic fields in pregnant animals should be avoided (Hummel and Vicente, 2019). Caution with fungal lesions and clinical follow-up examination of those lesions should be carried out (Hummel and Vicente, 2019).

Targeted PEMF has no contraindication for the treatment of patients with cancer or for post-cancer surgical healing. Much of the human clinical trial work that has been done has been for patients following mastectomy reconstruction.

Pulsed Electromagnetic Field Therapy Bed or Blanket

PEMF uses pulsing magnetic fields developed by pulsing a small amount of battery current through coils of wire to initiate normal biological cellular reactions that result in improved circulation and provide pain relief. Respond Systems makes three products to provide pain relief for dogs and cats from common problems associated with hip dysplasia, arthritis, muscle, tendon or ligament injury, and old-age stiffness and soreness (https://respondsystems.com/pemf/canine-products/). For horses, they make this product as a blanket, wrap, and mat for the horse to stand upon (https://respondsystems.com/pemf/how-it-works/) (https://respondsystems.com/pemf/equine-products/). Assisi now also makes a PEMF bed (https://assisianimalhealth.com/assisi-loop/) called the Loop Lounge System.

Beds are more feasible for use in patients in which PEMF treatment is indicated for

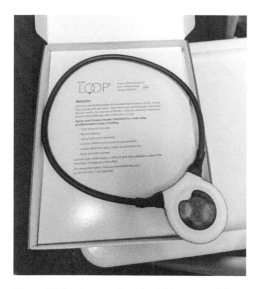

Figure 17.5 Image of an Assisi Loop used for targeted PEMF.

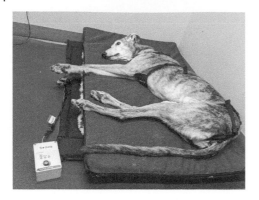

Figure 17.6 A patient on a PEMF bed.

multiple sites, for example, a patient with elbow and hip osteoarthritis, or with thoracic spinal arthritis in addition to lumbosacral intervertebral disc disease (see Figure 17.6). Bed use is not advisable in patients with a history of seizures. Because of the larger PEMF field created by a bed, greater caution is needed regarding owners or pets with pacemakers. As advised for the Loop, it is not advised to use PEMF beds or blankets concurrently with other modalities, wait two hours between different types of modalities to avoid interference due to different mechanisms of action.

Conclusions

Selection of the appropriate modality depends largely on an understanding of the diagnosis, an accurate assessment of the stage of tissue healing and repair, an accurate clinical assessment of the functional limitations, the established treatment goals, and continued reevaluation of the patient under guidance by your supervising veterinarian. Electrical stimulation is mostly used to increase muscle strength. PEMF is used for healing tissues and for pain management.

References

Adrian, C.P., Haussler, K.K., Kawcak CE et al. (2019). Gait and electromyographic alterations due to early onset of injury and eventual rupture of the cranial cruciate ligament in dogs: A pilot study. Vet Surg 48(3): 388–400. https://doi.org/10.1111/vsu.13178. Epub 2019 Feb 13. PMID: 30758853.

Alvarez, L.X., McCue, J., Lam, N.K. et al. (2019). Effect of targeted pulsed electromagnetic field therapy on canine postoperative hemilaminectomy: A double-blind, randomized, placebo-controlled clinical trial. *J Am Anim Hosp Assoc* 55 (2): 83–91.

Beckwée, D., De Hertogh, W., Lievens, P. et al. (2012). Effect of TENS on pain in relation to central sensitization in patients with osteoarthritis of the knee: Study protocol of a randomized controlled trial. *Trials* 13 (1): 1–7.

Bennett, D., Zainal Ariffin, S.M., and Johnston, P. (2012). Osteoarthritis in the cat 1. How common is it and how easy to recognize? *J Feline Med Surg* 14: 65–75.

Bonaldo, P. and Sandri, M. (2013). Cellular and molecular mechanisms of muscle atrophy. *Dis Model Mech* 6 (1): 25–39.

Bracciano, A.G. (2008). *Physical Agent Modalities*. Bethesda, MD: AOTA Press.

Budsberg SC (2010) Medical management of osteoarthritis in dogs. Presented at Central Veterinary Conference, San Diego, November 1, 2010.

Cameron, M.H. (2003). *Physical Agents in Rehabilitation: From Research to Practice*, 2nde. St. Louis, MO: Saunders.

Canapp, D.A. (2007). Clinical techniques in small animal practice. *Clin Tech Small Anim Pract* 22: 160–165.

Canè, V., Botti, P., and Soana, S. (1993). Pulsed magnetic fields improve osteoblast activity during the repair of an experimental osseous defect. *J Orthop Res* 11 (5): 664–670.

Ciombor, D.M., Aaron, R.K., Wang, S., and Simon, B. (2003). Modification of osteoarthritis by pulsed electromagnetic field – A morphological study. *Osteoarthr Cartil* 11: 455–462.

Currier, D.P. and Mann, R. (1983). Muscular strength development by electrical stimulation in healthy individuals. *Phys Ther* 63: 915–921.

Delitto, A. and Robinson, A.J. (1989). Electrical stimulation of muscle: Techniques and applications. In: *Clinical Electrophysiology: Electrophysiology and Electrophysiological Testing* (ed. L. Snyder-Mackler and A.J. Robinson), 95–138. Baltimore, MD: Williams and Wilkins.

Deyo, R.A., Walsh, N.E., Martin, D.C. et al. (1990). A controlled trial of transcutaneous electrical nerve stimulation (TENS) and exercise for chronic low back pain. *N Engl J Med* 322 (23): 1627–1634.

Diniz, P., Soejima, K., and Ito, G. (2002). Nitric oxide mediates the effects of pulsed electromagnetic field stimulation on the osteoblast proliferation and differentiation. *Nitric Oxide* 7 (1): 18–23.

Doucet, B.M., Lam, A., and Griffin, L. (2012). Neuromuscular electrical stimulation for skeletal muscle function. *Yale J Biol Med* 85: 201–215.

Duchateau, J. and Baudry, S. (2014). Maximal discharge rate of motor units determines the maximal rate of force development during ballistic contractions in human. *Front Hum Neurosci* 8: 234.

Ennis, W.J., Lee, C., Gellada, K. et al. (2016). Advanced technologies to improve wound healing: Electrical stimulation, vibration therapy, and ultrasound – what is the evidence? *Plast Reconstr Surg* 138 (3S): 94S–104S.

Fitzgerald, G.K., Piva, S.R., and Irrgang, J.J. (2003). A modified neuromuscular electrical stimulation protocol for quadriceps strength training following anterior cruciate ligament reconstruction. *J Orthop Sports Phys Ther* 33: 492–501.

von Freeden, N., Duerr, F., Fehr, M. et al. (2017). Comparison of two cold compression therapy protocols after tibial plateau leveling osteotomy in dogs. *Tierarztl Prax Ausg K Klientiere Heimtiere* 45 (04): 226–233.

Galkowski, V., Petrisor, B., Drew, B., and Dick, D. (2009). Bone stimulation for fracture healing: What's all the fuss? *Indian J Orthop* 43 (2): 117–120.

Gardner, S., Frantz, R., and Schmidt, F. (1999). Effect of electrical stimulation on chronic wound healing: A meta-analysis. *Wound Repair Regen* 7 (6): 495–502.

Gaynor, J.S., Hagberg, S., and Gurfein, B.T. (2018). Veterinary applications of pulsed electromagnetic field therapy. *Res Vet Sci* 119: 1–8. https://doi.org/10.1016/j.rvsc.2018.05.005.

Gibson, W., Wand, B.M., Meads, C. et al. (2019). Transcutaneous electrical nerve stimulation (TENS) for chronic pain-an overview of Cochrane Reviews. *Cochrane Database Syst Rev* 2(2): CD011890. https://doi.org/10.1002/14651858.CD011890.pub2. PMID: 30776855; PMCID: PMC6379178.

Gondin, J., Cozzone, P.J., and Bendahan, D. (2011). Is high-frequency neuromuscular electrical stimulation a suitable tool for muscle performance improvement in both healthy humans and athletes? *Eur J Appl Physiol* 111 (10): 2473–2487.

Gordon, T. and English, A.W. (2016). Strategies to promote peripheral nerve regeneration: Electrical stimulation and/or exercise. *Eur J Neurosci* 43 (3): 336–350.

Hanks, J., Levine, D., and Bockstahler, B. (2015). Physical agent modalities in physical therapy and rehabilitation of small animals. *Vet Clin Small Anim* 45: 29–44.

Hardie, E.M., Roe, S.C., and Martin, F.R. (2002). Radiographic evidence of degenerative joint disease in geriatric cats: 100 cases (1994–1997). *J Am Vet Med Assoc* 220: 628–632.

Hayes, G.M., Granger, N., Langley-Hobbs, S.J., and Jeffery, N.D. (2013). Abnormal reflex activation of hamstring muscles in dogs with cranial cruciate ligament rupture. Vet J 196(3):345–350. https://doi.org/10.1016/j.tvjl.2012.10.028.

Hecox, B., Mehreteab, T.A., and Weisberg, J. (1994). *Physical Agents: A Comprehensive Text for Physical Therapists*. Norwalk, CT: Appleton and Lange chapters 19 and 21.

Henderson, A.L., Latimer, C., and Millis, D.L. (2015). Rehabilitation and physical therapy for selected orthopedic conditions in veterinary patients. *Vet Clin Small Anim Practice* 45 (1): 91–121.

Hummel, J. and Vicente, G. (2019). Chapter 22: Magnet therapy – static magnetic fields (SMF) and pulsed electromagnetic fields (PEMF). In: *Essential Facts of Physical Medicine, Rehabilitation and Sports Medicine in Companion Animals* (ed. B. Bockstahler, K. Wittek, D. Levine, et al.), 301–305. Babenhausen, Germany: VBS GmbH.

Inoue, N., Ohnishi, I., Chen, D. et al. (2002). Effect of pulsed electromagnetic fields (PEMF) on late-phase osteotomy gap healing in a canine tibial model. *J Orthop Res* 20 (5): 1106–1114.

Johnson, J.M., Johnson, A.L., Pijanowski, G.J. et al. (1997). Rehabilitation of dogs with surgically treated cranial cruciate ligament-deficient stifles by use of electrical stimulation of muscles. *Am J Vet Res* 58 (12): 1473–1478.

Jones, S., Man, W.D., Gao, W. et al. (2016). Neuromuscular electrical stimulation for muscle weakness in adults with advanced disease. *Cochrane Database Syst Rev* 10 (10): CD009419. https://doi.org/10.1002/14651858.CD009419.pub3.

Khouri, C., Kotzki, S., Roustit, M. et al. (2017). Hierarchical evaluation of electrical stimulation protocols for chronic wound healing: An effect size meta-analysis. *Wound Repair Regen* 25 (5): 883–891.

Kloth, L.C. and Cummings, J.P. (1991). *Electrotherapeutic Terminology in Physical Therapy*. Alexandria, VA: American Physical Therapy Association.

Knaflitx, M., Merletti, R., and De Luca, C.J. (1990). Inference of motor unit recruitment order in voluntary and electrically elicited contractions. *J Appl Physiol* 68: 1657–1667.

Lagerquist, O. and Collins, D.F. (2010). Influence of stimulus pulse width on M-waves, H-reflexes, and torque during tetanic low-intensity neuromuscular stimulation. *Muscle Nerve* 42 (6): 886–893.

Lake, D. (1992). Neuromuscular electrical stimulation: An overview and its application in the treatment of sports injuries. *Sports Med* 13 (5): 320–336.

Laughmann, R.K., Youdas, J.W., and Garrett, T.R. (1983). Strength changes in the normal quadriceps femoris muscle as a result of electrical stimulation. *Phys Ther* 63: 494–499.

Levine, D. and Bockstahler, B. (2014). Electrical stimulation. In: *Canine Rehabilitation and Physical Therapy*, 2nde (ed. D.L. Millis and D. Levine), 342–358. St. Louis, MO: Elsevier/Saunders.

Li, X., Zhang, M., Bai, L. et al. (2012). Effects of 50 Hz pulsed electromagnetic fields on the growth and cell cycle arrest of mesenchymal stem cells: An in vitro study. *Electromagn Biol Med* 31 (4): 356–364.

McMiken, D.F., Todd-Smith, M., and Thompson, C. (1983). Strengthening of human quadriceps muscles by cutaneous electrical stimulation. *Scand J Rehabil Med* 15: 25–28.

Melzack, R. and Wall, P.D. (1965). Pain mechanisms: A new theory. *Science* 150: 971–979.

Mlacnik, E., Bockstahler, B.A., Müller, M. et al. (2006). Effects of caloric restriction and a moderate or intense physiotherapy program for treatment of lameness in overweight dogs with osteoarthritis. *J Am Vet Med Assoc* 229 (11): 1756–1760. https://doi.org/10.2460/javma.229.11.1756.

Monaghan, B., Caulfield, B., and O'Mathúna, D.P. (2010). Surface neuromuscular electrical stimulation for quadriceps strengthening pre and post total knee replacement. *Cochrane Database Syst Rev* 1: CD007177. https://doi.org/10.1002/14651858.CD007177.pub2.

Nelson, R.M., Currier, D.P., and Hayes, K.W. (1999). *Clinical Electrotherapy*, 3rde. Norwalk, CT: Appleton and Lange.

Niebaum, K. (2013). Rehabilitation physical modalities. In: *Canine Sports Medicine and Rehabilitation* (ed. M.C. Zink and J.B. Van Dyke), 115–131. Ames, IA: John Wiley & Sons, Inc.

Nolan, T. (2005). Electrotherapeutic modalities: Electrotherapy and iontophoresis. In: *Modalities for Therapeutic Intervention*, 4the. Philadelphia, PA: FA Davis Co.

O'Sullivan, M., Gordon-Evans, W.J., Knap, K.E., and Evans, R.B. (2013). Randomized, controlled clinical trial evaluating the efficacy of pulsed signal therapy in dogs with osteoarthritis. *Vet Surg* 42: 250–254.

Pankratz, K., Korman, J., Emke, C. et al. (2021). Randomized, placebo-controlled prospective clinical trial evaluating the efficacy of the Assisi Anti-Anxiety Device (Calmer Canine) for the treatment of canine separation anxiety. *Front Vet Sci* 18: 1541.

Park, S.H. and Silva, M. (2004). Neuromuscular electrical stimulation enhances fracture healing: Results of an animal model. *J Orthop Res* 22 (2): 382–387.

Peng, L., Fu, C., Xiong, F. et al. (2020). Effectiveness of pulsed electromagnetic fields on bone healing: A systematic review and meta-analysis of randomized controlled trials. *Bioelectromagnetics* 41 (5): 323–337.

Pilla, A. (2006). Mechanism and therapeutic applications of time-varying and static magnetic fields. In: *Handbook of Biological Effects of Electromagnetic Fields*, 3rde (ed. F. Barnes and B. Greenebaum). Boca Raton, FL: CRC Press.

Pinna, S., Landucci, F., Tribuiani, A.M. et al. (2013). The effects of pulsed electromagnetic field in the treatment of osteoarthritis in dogs: Clinical study. *Pakistan Vet J* 33 (1): 96–100.

Prydie, D. and Hewitt, I. (2015). *Modalities. Practical Physiotherapy for Small Animal Practice*, 69–90. Oxford, UK: John Wiley & Sons, Ltd.

Rohde, C.H., Taylor, E.M., Alonso, A. et al. (2015). Pulsed electromagnetic fields reduce postoperative interleukin-1β, pain, and inflammation: A double-blind, placebo-controlled study in TRAM flap breast reconstruction patients. *Plast Reconstr Surg* 135 (5): 808e–817e.

Sawaya, S.G., Combet, D., Chanoit, G. et al. (2008). Assessment of impulse duration thresholds for electrical stimulation of muscles (chronaxy) in dogs. *Am J Vet Res* 69 (10): 1305–1309.

Selkowitz, D.M. (1985). Improvement in isometric strength of the quadriceps femoris muscle after training with electrical stimulation. *Phys Ther* 65: 186–196.

Sluka, K.A. and Walsh, D. (2003). Transcutaneous electrical nerve stimulation: Basic science mechanisms and clinical effectiveness. *J Pain* 4 (3): 109–121.

Spurgeon, T.L., Kitchell, R.L., and Lohse, C.L. (1978). Physiologic properties of contraction of the canine cremaster and cranial preputial muscles. *Am J Vet Res* 39 (12): 1884–1887.

Strauch, B., Patel, M., Navarro, J. et al. (2007). Pulsed magnetic fields accelerate cutaneous wound healing in rats. *Plast Reconstr Surg* 120: 425.

Tacker, W.A. Jr., Geddes, L.A., Janas, W. et al. (1991). Comparison of canine skeletal muscle power from twitches and tetanic contractions in untrained muscle: A preliminary report. *J Card Surg* 6 (1 Suppl): 245–251.

Trock, D. (2000). Electromagnetic fields and magnets. Investigational treatment for musculoskeletal disorders. *Rheum Dis Clin North Am* 26 (1): 51–63.

Valenti, F. (1964). Neuromuscular electrical stimulation in clinical practice. *Acta Anaesthesiol* 15: 227–245.

Varcoe, G.M., Manfredi, J.M., Jackson, A., and Tomlinson, J.E. (2021). Effect of tibial plateau levelling osteotomy and rehabilitation on muscle function in cruciate-deficient dogs evaluated with acoustic myography. *Comp Exercise Phys* 17 (5): 435–445.

Williams, K.J., Moore, H.M., Ellis, M., and Davies, A.H. (2021). Pilot trial of neuromuscular stimulation in human subjects with chronic venous disease. *Vasc Health Risk Manag* 17: 771.

Wilson, J.M., McKenzie, E., and Duesterdieck-Zellmer, K. (2018). International survey regarding the use of rehabilitation modalities in horses. *Front Vet Sci* 5: 120.

Windsor, R.E., Lester, J.P., and Herring, S.A. (1993). Electrical stimulation in clinical practice. *Phys Sportsmed* 21: 85–93.

Wolf, S.L., Ariel, G.B., Saar, D. et al. (1986). The effect of muscle stimulation during resistive training on performance parameters. *Am J Sports Med* 14: 18–23.

Wu, L.C., Weng, P.W., Chen, C.H. et al. (2018). Literature review and meta-analysis of transcutaneous electrical nerve stimulation in treating chronic back pain. *Reg Anesth Pain Med* 43 (4): 425–433.

Yang, X., He, H., Ye, W. et al. (2020). Effects of pulsed electromagnetic field therapy on pain, stiffness, physical function, and quality of life in patients with osteoarthritis: A systematic review and meta-analysis of randomized placebo-controlled trials. *Phys Ther* 100 (7): 1118–1131.

Yin, S. (2009). *Low Stress Handling Restraint and Behavior Modification of Dogs & Cats: Techniques for Developing Patients Who Love Their Visits*, 189–340. Davis, CA: CattleDog Publishing.

Zidan, N., Fenn, J., Griffith, E. et al. (2018). The effect of electromagnetic fields on post-operative pain and locomotor recovery in dogs with acute, severe thoracolumbar intervertebral disc extrusion: A randomized placebo-controlled, prospective clinical trial. *J Neurotrauma* 35 (15): 1726–1736.

18

Modalities Part 4: Therapeutic Ultrasound

Carolina Medina[1] and Wendy Davies[2]

[1] *Elanco Animal Health, Fort Lauderdale, FL, USA*
[2] *Rehabilitation and Regenerative Medicine, University of Florida, Gainesville, FL, USA*

Introduction

Therapeutic ultrasound uses sound waves generated by piezoelectric effect at frequencies greater than 20,000 MHz to stimulate tissues and create physiologic effects. These effects include stimulation of fibroblast activity, improvement of blood flow, increased protein synthesis, increased tissue extensibility, decreased pain, and stimulation of soft tissue and bone healing (Niebaum, 2013; Baxter and McDonough, 2007; Steiss and McCauley, 2004). Therapeutic ultrasound devices may use short bursts or a continuous stream of sound waves to deliver ultrasonic energy to tissues. This modality has been used since the 1950s for indications such as tendon injuries and bursitis (Miller et al., 2012). Based on a National Library of Medicine search, the first clinical report of its use in veterinary medicine was in 2009 (Mueller et al., 2009).

Physical Principles

Sound Waves

Sound waves used for therapy consist of mechanical vibrations that are propagated longitudinally into the biologic tissues via a means of a transducer (a device that converts energy from one form to another) that is placed directly in contact with patient's skin. As sound moves through tissues,

Physical Rehabilitation for Veterinary Technicians and Nurses, Second Edition.
Edited by Mary Ellen Goldberg and Julia E. Tomlinson.
© 2024 John Wiley & Sons, Inc. Published 2024 by John Wiley & Sons, Inc.
Companion website: www.wiley.com/go/goldberg/physicalrehabilitationvettechsandnurses

energy is absorbed and converted to kinetic energy (Niebaum, 2013). Sound waves create pressure and tensile forces on biologic tissues causing them to oscillate. The frequency of the sound waves determines the degree at which oscillations occur. Ultrasonic therapeutic frequencies usually lie between 1.0 and 3.3 MHz (megahertz) (Bockstahler and Levine, 2019).

Absorption of Ultrasound Waves

Factors that affect the travel and absorption of sound waves include the substances traveled through to the target tissue, the components of the target tissue, the coupling media, and the treatment parameters. In general, sound is likely to move faster through solids, and slowest through gases. Therefore, ultrasound transmission is impeded by air between transducer and skin. To reduce sound reflection on the skin resulting from air pockets, it is necessary to use a coupling medium and to clip the hair to eliminate air pockets. Liquids like water and alcohol are suitable but evaporate quickly. A coupling gel is preferred for direct contact of the probe on the skin – gels can be water or lipid based, but the latter are hard to remove after treatment, so water-based gels are more commonly applied. A brand name such as Aquasonic 100™ is a type of coupling gel. Indirect coupling is when the probe does not contact the skin but moves through a medium, most commonly water; this can be useful for applying therapeutic ultrasound over irregularly shaped areas when complete contact with even the smallest treatment probe is not possible.

The patient's body consists of a variety of tissues with different acoustic impedances. Ultrasound is reflected or absorbed differently by each structure within a tissue. Absorption of energy is greatest in tissues with high protein content, e.g., bone, and relatively low in adipose tissue (Steiss and McCauley, 2004; Gamble, 2022).

The prescribing veterinarian and the therapist must be familiar with the composition of the target tissue, and the tissues that the ultrasound waves must travel through to reach the target tissue. Because hair has a high protein content it can diminish ultrasound penetration; therefore, hair coat should be shaved prior to ultrasound therapy in both short and long-haired coats (Steiss and Adams, 1999; Gamble, 2022). Bone surfaces (periosteum) can absorb a large amount of heat resulting in significant pain (Bockstahler and Levine, 2019).

Mechanical Effects of Ultrasound Waves

Cavitation is the most cited mechanical effect of therapeutic ultrasound. Cavitation is the formation of small gas bubbles in tissues that occur when ultrasonic waves vibrate (Bockstahler *et al.*, 2004). Ultrasonic cavitation depends on the pressure amplitude of ultrasound waves; ultrasound transmitted into a tissue may cause pressure amplitudes of several megapascals. The resultant tensile stress is supported by the tissue, and negative tension in the tissue can be several times atmospheric pressure (Miller *et al.*, 2012). Cavitation can affect tissue metabolism by causing temperature elevation, mechanical stress, or free radical production (O'Brien, 2007).

Forms of Cavitation

Stable cavitation is when the gas bubbles remain intact and move with the ultrasonic flux. This form of cavitation is desired to produce therapeutic effects.

Transient cavitation is when the gas bubbles rapidly expand and collapse resulting in high pressure and increased temperature which can damage tissues. It primarily causes local tissue injury in the immediate vicinity of the cavitational activity, including cell death and hemorrhage. To prevent transient cavitation avoid using a high-intensity setting, especially with continuous wave ultrasound.

Cavitation is a secondary effect of transmission of ultrasound waves in tissues. Another secondary effect is acoustic streaming, which is the flow of currents in tissue fluid. The direct mechanical effects of ultrasound waves are compressional, tensile, and shear stresses; when an ultrasound wave moves through tissue, mechanical stress is induced. According to Wolff's law, bones and other tissues remodel in response to stress. Tendon cells produce collagen in response to high-frequency vibrations (Thompson *et al.*, 2015). The therapist aims to use the mechanical effects of ultrasound to stimulate breakdown of abnormal tissue (including scar tissue and mineralization) and to stimulate a tissue repair response. The therapist must also avoid adverse effects (too much tissue breakdown and disruption). Clinical research determining ideal settings (depth, intensity, and time) for treatment of different pathologies is still lacking in both human and veterinary medicine. We do know that the mechanical effects of ultrasound act on the cell membrane, causing mild disruption and increased permeability. Ultrasound has been shown to result in several intracellular events that include triggering biochemical reactions and changes in gene expression. This can result in increased cell proliferation or turnover (Furusawaa *et al.*, 2014). Examples of tissue responses to therapeutic ultrasound include vasoconstriction, ischemia, extravasation, reperfusion injury, and immune reaction (Miller *et al.*, 2012).

Thermal Effects of Ultrasound

Absorption of ultrasound waves by a tissue represents a portion of the wave energy that is converted into heat. If heat is produced by this process at a faster rate than can be removed or dissipated, then a temperature increase will occur in the tissue. The use of unfocused heating can be moderated to produce enhanced healing without injury (Miller *et al.*, 2012). Ideally, tissues should be heated at 4–5 °C for improving tissue flexibility (Levine *et al.*, 2001). Increasing local tissue temperature causes increased enzyme-based reactions, though there is a ceiling effect beyond which too much heat can denature enzymes (O'Brien, 2007). Heat can partially denature (unfold) collagen, by breaking up hydrogen bonds in collagen cross-links, and if temperatures are too high then further denaturation occurs. There is a rebound response after heating, where collagen re-folds (Chen *et al.*, 1998). This may be a mechanism by which ultrasound stimulates tissue remodeling and breaks down scar tissue. Alternatively, the heat produced by therapeutic ultrasound can be deliberately concentrated by a focused beam until tissue is coagulated for the purpose of tissue ablation.

Chemical Effects of Ultrasound

The microbubbles of cavitation are under high pressure and high temperature just before they collapse. These changes are very fast and so have minimal heating effect on surrounding tissues. However, high temperatures can lead to water breakdown and free radical formation. This "sonolysis" in the presence of oxygen leads to the formation of superoxide radicals. These free radicals can stimulate tissue remodeling, just as those produced by white blood cells do. Ultrasound results in an immediate elevation of intracellular calcium ions from the extracellular environment (Furusawaa *et al.*, 2014).

Treatment Parameters

Frequency

Frequency determines the depth of ultrasonic wave penetration and is measured in Hertz (Hz). The frequency selected is based on the tissue to be treated and its depth from the skin surface.

The most common frequencies used in veterinary rehabilitation are 1 and 3.3 MHz. One MHz can effectively penetrate a depth of 2–5 cm, while 3.3 MHz can effectively treat tissues at a depth of 1–3 cm (Bockstahler and Levine, 2019; Bockstahler *et al.*, 2004; Levine *et al.*, 2001; Steiss and Adams, 1999).

Intensity

Intensity is the rate of energy delivered per unit area and is measured in Watts per centimeter squared (W/cm^2). Intensity is important because it describes the force at which the vibrations are applied (how fast the energy is delivered). Too much force could damage the tissue or at the very least result in pain. The higher the intensity, the higher the increase in tissue temperature. When treating an area with thick, soft tissue, e.g., the deltoid muscle, a higher frequency should be selected to heat the tissue. On the contrary, when treating an area with minimal soft tissue e.g., the carpal joint, lower intensity and higher frequency are the parameters of choice as denser tissues heat faster. The most common intensities used in veterinary medicine are between 0.1 and 2 W/cm^2.

Duty Cycle

Duty cycle is the fraction of time that sound is emitted during one pulse period. It refers to whether the vibrations are applied continuously over the course of a treatment, or whether they are pulsed on and off. The ratio of pulse on to pulse off during treatment is referred to as the duty cycle. Most devices offer duty cycles in the range of 10%, 25%, 50%, 75%, and 100%. For example, a 10% duty cycle pulsed waveform would have the ultrasound on for a total of 10% of the treatment time and off for 90% of the treatment time. A 100% duty cycle is considered continuous waveform in which the ultrasound is on 100% of the treatment time. Continuous waveform is used when thermal and non-thermal effects are desired, e.g., muscle spasms, significant scar tissue, and chronic tendinopathies. Pulsed waveform is used when only non-thermal effects are desired, e.g., around bony prominences and in tissues with acute inflammation.

Transducer Heads

There are a variety of sizes of transducer heads (Figure 18.1). The size is selected based on the size of the treatment area. The treatment area should ideally be no more than two to three times the size of the transducer head (Steiss and McCauley, 2004). Treating an area larger than these parameters decreases the dosage and thermal effects; therefore, diminishing the therapeutic effects. An alternative is to divide a larger area into two smaller treatment areas. Common sizes of transducer heads include 1, 3, 5, and 10 cm^2. The transducer head should be held directly over the treatment tissue and perpendicular to the skin. If it is held at an angle above 75°, the ultrasound will travel along the skin instead of treatment tissue (Michlovitz and Sparrow, 2012).

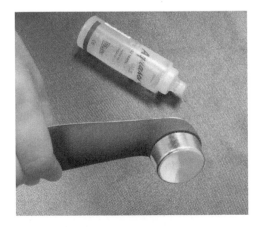

Figure 18.1 A 3-cm sized ultrasound transducer head.

The transducer head should be moved continuously over the skin at a speed of 4–8 cm per second to achieve uniform distribution of the ultrasound and prevent thermal burning and tissue damage (Michlovitz and Sparrow, 2012).

Coupling Techniques

Water-soluble coupling gel must be placed between the skin and transducer head; otherwise, the ultrasound beam is reflected at air–tissue interfaces. Elimination of as much air as possible maximizes tissue penetration of the ultrasound energy (see Figure 18.2).

Direct coupling is placement of the transducer head in direct contact with the skin. It is used when the treatment area is relatively flat and smooth and larger than the transducer head, e.g., gluteal muscles.

Indirect coupling is placement of the transducer head at a distance to the skin. It is used when the treatment area is irregularly shaped and smaller than the transducer head, e.g., digits. The most common form of indirect coupling is submersion, where the treatment is submerged in a

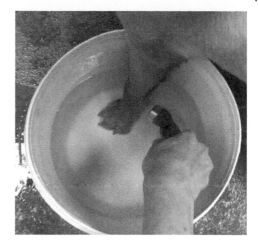

Figure 18.3 Treating a flexor tendon injury with indirect coupling, the patient's limb is immersed in warm water and the transducer head held 2 cm from the skin surface at the level of the lesion.

container water and the transducer head is also submerged and held 1–3 cm from the skin's surface (Figure 18.3). Another type of indirect coupling is coupling cushion where a water balloon covered in coupling gel, or a firm gel spacer is placed between the skin and transducer head.

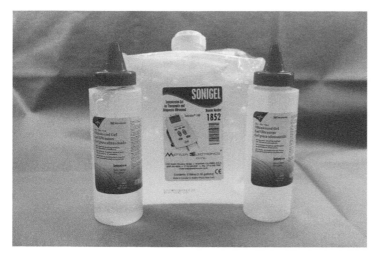

Figure 18.2 Ultrasound gel used a coupling agent. *Source:* Kristen Hagler.

Role of the Veterinary Rehabilitation Technician

A technician who takes courses in veterinary rehabilitation will learn about therapeutic ultrasound and how and when to perform these treatments. If courses are not available to a technician, he/she can learn on the job from their veterinarian. The technician can perform these treatments without the supervision of the veterinarian in some states; however, the treatment must always be prescribed by the veterinarian who employs the technician (legal supervisor). Prescription assigned to a technician by a non-supervising veterinarian is pushing the boundaries of state regulatory laws on the practice of veterinary medicine. After the treatment is completed, the technician should document that the treatment was performed and treatment settings in the patient's medical record (see Figure 18.4).

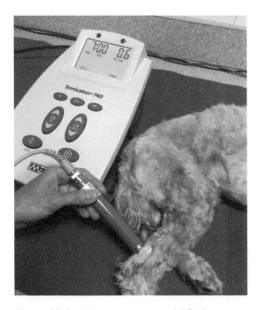

Figure 18.4 Maya, a two-year-old Cockapoo having her Achilles tendon treated. After treatment (in this case, an Achilles tendinopathy), the settings on the machine should be documented in the medical record. *Source:* Bruce Rogoff.

Clinical Applications

Therapeutic ultrasound is primarily used for the therapeutic effects of tissue temperature increase that leads to increased blow flow, improved tissue nutrition, improved elasticity of fibrous structures and collagen, and improved joint mobility (Gamble, 2022).

Conditions that benefit from non-thermal effects include acute soft tissue injuries, fractures, and wounds. Indications that benefit from thermal effects include decreasing pain and muscle spasms, osteoarthritis (except in acute exacerbation), chronic soft tissue injuries, tendinopathies, muscle contracture, scar tissue, and trigger points (see Figure 18.5 and Box 18.1).

Dosage and Treatment Frequency

- Superficial conditions (target depth less than 2 cm) treated with pulsed ultrasound at 3.3 MHz should deliver 0.25–0.9 W/cm^2 (Bockstahler *et al.*, 2004; Bockstahler and Levine, 2019).
- Superficial conditions treated with continuous ultrasound at 3.3 MHz are recommended to be from 1 W/cm^2 to less than 1.5 W/cm^2. This is based on a research study by Levine and Millis in 2001,

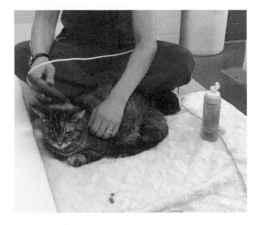

Figure 18.5 A feline patient undergoing ultrasound treatment of her neck muscles.

Box 18.1   Case study: Maya, a two-year-old spayed female Cockapoo

History: Maya was bitten on the right tarsus by her housemate during rough play.

Physical examination: Maya's right tarsus was dropped and hyperextended, and there was a large swelling along distal calcaneal tendon, proximal to base of the gastrocnemius muscle.

Diagnosis: Partial right gastrocnemius and superficial digital flexor tendon avulsion

Treatment: Maya underwent surgical reduction of the right gastrocnemius and superficial digital flexor tendon. A graft using a small portion of the tensor fascia lata was used to fill the 6 mm gap at the end of the gastrocnemius tendon. Protein-enriched plasma was injected into the area of the tendons to help with healing. A bivalve cast was placed on the limb immediately post-operatively.

Two weeks post-operatively, a custom-made orthosis was used to provide stability during the tendon healing phase, and a controlled and secure approach to tendon reloading. Adjustments were made to Maya's orthosis starting at 6 weeks post-operatively, gradually allowing for 10° increase in tarsal flexion up until 14 weeks post-operatively.

Maya received rehabilitation therapy consisting of therapeutic ultrasound to stimulate collagen formation with the goal of allowing tissue formation and eventual stability of the calcaneal tendon.

Ultrasound settings were $0.6 \, W/cm^2$, 3 MHz, continuous wave, 7 minutes using a $5 \, cm^2$ sound head. Low-level laser therapy was used to improve healing, decrease pain and inflammation, as well as alleviate muscle spasms of her paraspinal due to muscle compensation. Massage was performed to alleviate muscle compensation, and manual therapy was performed on all her limbs.

Therapeutic exercises were used to strengthen the muscles of the hamstring complex (semimembranosus, semitendinosus, and biceps femoris), quadriceps, and gastrocnemius. Underwater treadmill was instituted to load the calcaneal tendon in a weight-supported environment.

Outcome

Maya completed 22 weeks of rehabilitation therapy starting 2 weeks post-operatively. Therapeutic ultrasound played an integral role in the healing of the gastrocnemius and superficial digital flexor tendon. At the end of the 22 weeks, she had functional mobility and was able to return to normal activities.

explained in the relevant research section below (Levine *et al.*, 2001).

- Deep conditions are treated with either pulsed or continuous ultrasound at 1 MHz and $1–2 \, W/cm^2$ (Steiss and Adams, 1999).
- Acute conditions are treated in short intervals (e.g., 3 times a week) for a short duration (e.g., 1–2 weeks) (Bockstahler *et al.*, 2004; Bockstahler and Levine, 2019).
- Chronic conditions are treated in long intervals (e.g., 1–2 times a week) for a long duration (2–3 weeks or more if needed) (Bockstahler *et al.*, 2004; Bockstahler and Levine, 2019).

Phonophoresis

Phonophoresis is the use of ultrasound to enhance the delivery and absorption of topically applied drugs such as analgesics and anti-inflammatories to localized areas of muscle, tendon, ligament, or soft tissue (Bockstahler and Levine, 2019). Conditions in which phonophoresis might be of benefit include tendinitis, osteoarthritis, bursitis, sprains, and neuromas (Kleinkort and Wood, 1975). Phonophoresis increases the transfer of fluids and nutrients into the tissues (Bockstahler and Levine, 2019).

Byl conducted a review of human literature and determined that to maximize the clinical effectiveness of phonophoresis the topical drug (both the drug and the carrying agent) should transmit through ultrasound; the skin should be pre-treated with ultrasound, heating, moistening, or shaving; the patient needs to be positioned to maximize circulation during treatment; a dressing that seals the area and prevents the escape of moisture should be applied after treatment; an intensity of $1.5\,W/cm^2$ should be used to capture both the thermal and non-thermal effects; and low-intensity of $0.5\,W/cm^2$ should be used when treating open wounds or acute injuries (Byl, 1995). A study of phonophoresis using hydrocortisone was performed on greyhound stifles. Joint hydrocortisone levels obtained with phonophoresis were extremely low in comparison with those obtained with direct joint injection and the levels were not different from topical application (Muir *et al.*, 1990). Typical parameters for phonophoresis are (Bockstahler and Levine, 2019):

- Non-thermal pulsed
- Duty cycle of 20–60%
- 0.8–$1.5\,W/cm^2$
- 5–7 minutes treatment time

Clinical Reports

Mueller *et al.* published a case report of two cases with partial gastrocnemius muscle avulsion treated with pulsed therapeutic ultrasound (Mueller *et al.*, 2009). The first dog received 13 therapeutic ultrasound treatments (1 MHz, 25% pulsed waveform, 0.7–1 W/cm^2, 10 minutes) for 5 weeks.

During the first two weeks, therapeutic ultrasound was performed three times per week, then decreased to two times per week. The second dog received 12 therapeutic ultrasound treatments (1 MHz, 25% duty cycle, $0.8\,W/cm^2$, 10 minutes), 3 times per week for 4 weeks. The outcome in both dogs was evaluated using ultrasonographic imaging and the measurement of ground reaction forces with a force plate. Both dogs showed an amelioration of the clinical signs within one month after commencement of the ultrasound therapy. The follow-up time for these cases was one year and six months, respectively. Both dogs were free of lameness and returned to their normal amount of exercise. Palpation of the fabella associated with the muscle injury did not produce any signs of pain. Ultrasonographic imaging did not detect any signs of hemorrhage or edema, although scarring of muscle fibers was present. The force–plate analyses revealed an improvement in lameness. These results suggest that therapeutic ultrasound could be a beneficial treatment modality for partial gastrocnemius muscle avulsion (Mueller *et al.*, 2009).

In a clinical study of 124 cases of muscle injury in dogs treated with therapeutic ultrasound, patients were treated with 5 or 6 twice-weekly therapeutic ultrasound treatments. Settings were continuous wave, at a frequency appropriate for the depth of target tissue (most cases 3.3 MHz, a few larger dogs with deeper muscle injury were treated at 1 MHz) and at a power setting of 1.1–$1.3\,W/cm^2$ depending on patient tolerance. A stretching program was instituted at ultrasound treatments number 3–5 (this was decided based on when muscle extensibility improved). Following ultrasound therapy, isometric strengthening exercises were instituted for 2–3 weeks (two- or three-leg stand) followed by sprint practice, and slow return to full activity/sport. Lameness resolved in 91.9% of cases, but a small number recurred, needing long-term management with ultrasound therapy every 4–6 weeks. Lameness improved by 1–2 grades for the remaining cases in which lameness did not resolve. The overall percentage of cases treated for muscle injury with therapeutic ultrasound with resolution of lameness and no recurrence/repeat injury was 85.8%. A total of 93.9% of sporting or working dogs fully returned to sport/work after treatment (Tomlinson, 2015).

Cautions and Contraindications

Thermal burns are a major concern and can be avoided by constantly moving the transducer head over the skin, and by using lowest effective intensity. The transducer head can overheat if held in the air while the unit is emitting ultrasound. Exert caution when using ultrasound over bony prominences, fracture sites, metal implants, artificial joints, irradiated skin, areas of decreased circulation, and areas of decreased pain and/or temperature sensation. Your supervising veterinarian will guide you and should write a specific prescription with treatment parameters; however, this may need to change depending on patient response during treatment sessions. If the patient shows any sign of discomfort, immediately stop the treatment. Palpate the treatment area for sensitivity and resume the same treatment settings only if it is confirmed that the patient was not reacting in pain and was just restless. A good way to determine this is to move the probe head as if treating but with the ultrasound off. This will help to discern discomfort from ultrasound versus discomfort from probe head contact or from restraint. If in doubt, stop and find the supervising veterinarian. The veterinarian will advise you about altering treatment settings (for example, turning down the intensity) and when to cease treatment completely.

Therapeutic ultrasound is contraindicated over the heart in animals with pacemakers, lower abdomen in pregnant animals, eyes, testes, open epiphyseal plates, spinal cord after laminectomy, carotid sinus or cervical ganglia, infection, ischemic tissue, hemorrhage, thrombosis, incisions in the first two weeks post-surgery, malignancy, or acute inflammation (Bockstahler and Levine, 2019).

Maintenance of Equipment

Because ultrasound therapy commonly produces minimal sensation, you must depend on your equipment to ensure appropriate parameters are being delivered. To ensure that your equipment is in proper working order, it should be inspected regularly, e.g., annually, to ensure proper calibration. Often, a local medical company will inspect and calibrate the machine (it does not have to be the machine's manufacturer). Keep the probe heads clean, dry, and protected. The technician should do periodic, i.e., once every 2–4 weeks, maintenance of the equipment by testing the transducer heads. To test the transducer heads, place them in a cup of water and turn the machine on. If the transducer heads are working, a ripple effect will occur in the water (you may also see tiny gas bubbles). If a probe head is dropped or falls, it will need to be checked and calibrated as the crystals in the probe head could have been damaged.

Relevant Scientific Research

In a study of five dogs with induced Achilles injury, tendons were cut and then sutured. A transcalcaneal screw was used to immobilize the tendon. One group received therapeutic ultrasound from the 3rd day after surgery at $0.5\,W/cm^2$ for 10 minutes daily for 10 days. It appears that the ultrasound was used in continuous setting, but it is not directly referred to by the authors. The healing of the Achilles tendon was monitored using clinical observations, ultrasonography, and histology. By day 40, the ultrasound appearance started to improve in the ultrasound-treated group compared to the untreated group. Gross observations suggested that the Achilles tendon in the ultrasound-treated group showed comparatively fewer adhesions than in the untreated group. Histologically, the ultrasound-treated group had better healing across the tendon fibers, and by day 120 the tendon tissue was close to normal. The authors concluded that ultrasound therapy at 0.5 W/cm^2 enhances Achilles tendon healing (Saini *et al.*, 2002).

Ten small (8 kg) dogs underwent bilateral ulna osteotomies resulting in a fracture gap. One side was treated with pulsed therapeutic ultrasound at 1 MHz, 20% duty cycle, and 50 mW/cm^2. Treatment was performed for 15 minutes once a day for 6 days a week for 5 months. The low-intensity pulsed ultrasound enhanced new bone formation and decreased the incidence of non-union (Yang and Park, 2001).

A study of the heating effect of continuous ultrasound was performed on the thigh muscles of 10 dogs (Levine *et al.*, 2001). Treatment intensity was either 1.0 or 1.5 W/cm^2. The temperature of the muscle was measured using thermistors at three different depths (1, 2, and 3 cm). The treatment time was 10 minutes. At the end of treatment, the temperature rises at an intensity of 1.0 W/cm^2 was 3 °C at 1 cm deep, 2.3 °C at 2 cm deep, and 1.6 °C at 3 cm deep. At 1.5 W/cm^2, temperature rose by 4.6 °C at 1 cm deep, 3.6 °C at 2 cm deep, and 2.4 °C at 3 cm deep. Tissue temperatures returned to baseline within 10 minutes or sooner after treatment. The authors stated that research suggests that a 3–4 °C increase in tissue temperature is effective in improving muscle flexibility. Based on these findings, intensity settings below 1.5 W/cm^2 continuous wave are recommended when treating dogs.

A study using 3.3 MHZ continuous wave ultrasound in horses evaluated the effects of temperature on the digital flexor tendons and the epaxial muscles. Ten horses were evaluated, and thermistors were used to measure tissue temperature. One tendon was treated for 10 minutes at an intensity of 1.0 W/cm, and the other at 1.5 W/cm^2. Temperatures rose by 3.5 °C in the superficial digital flexor tendon, 2.5 °C in the deep flexor tendon treated with 1 W/cm^2, and by 5.2 °C in the superficial, and 3.0 °C in the deep digital flexor tendon with 1.5 W/cm^2. The epaxial muscles were treated for 20 minutes with 3.3 MHz (a setting usually used for superficial tissues) at an intensity of 1.5 W/cm^2. Muscle temperature was measured at 1, 4, and 8 cm depths. The temperature rise was 1.3 °C at a depth of 1.0 cm, 0.7 °C at 4.0 cm, and 0.7 °C at 8 cm depth. The authors concluded that the digital flexor tendons are heated to a therapeutic temperature using a frequency of 3.3 MHz and intensity of 1.0 W/cm^2. The epaxial muscles are not heated to a therapeutic temperature using a frequency of 3.3 MHz and an intensity of 1.5 W/cm^2 (Montgomery *et al.*, 2013).

Freitas *et al.* evaluated the effects of therapeutic ultrasound on wound healing in rats. After 10 days of daily therapeutic ultrasound, results showed that therapeutic ultrasound improved wound healing since the wound size had significantly reduced 5 and 10 days after starting treatment. Collagen levels were increased in the 0.6 and 0.8 W/cm^2 treated groups. These authors concluded that therapeutic ultrasound has beneficial effects on the wound healing process, probably by speeding up the inflammatory phase and inducing collagen synthesis (Freitas *et al.*, 2010).

Conclusions

Therapeutic ultrasound is a useful modality in veterinary physical rehabilitation. There is research showing the thermal effects in dogs and horses (at certain tissue depths) and confirming stimulation of bone and tendon healing in dogs. There are also canine clinical reports showing successful treatment of muscle injury with this modality.

References

Baxter, G.D. and McDonough, S.M. (2007). Principles of Electrotherapy in Veterinary Physiotherapy. In: *Animal Physiotherapy Assessment, Treatment and Rehabilitation of Animals* (ed. C. McGowan, L. Goof, and N. Stubbs), 184–186. United Kingdom: Blackwell.

Bockstahler, B. and Levine, D. (2019). Chapter 14: Therapeutic ultrasound. In: *Essential Facts of Physical Medicine, Rehabilitation and Sports Medicine in Companion Animals*, 219–223. Babenhausen, Germany: VBS GmbH.

Bockstahler B, Levine D, and Millis D (2004) Physiotherapy – What and how. In *Essential Facts of Physiotherapy in Dogs and Cats Rehabilitation and Pain Management* (eds. B Bockstahler, D Levine, D Millis). BE VetVerlag, Germany, pp. 88–95.

Byl, N. (1995). The use of ultrasound as an enhancer for transcutaneous drug delivery: Phonophoresis. *Phys Ther* 75 (6): 539–553.

Chen, S.S., Wright, N.T., and Humphrey, J.D. (1998). Heat-induced changes in the mechanics of a collagenous tissue: isothermal, isotonic shrinkage. *J Biomech Eng* 120 (3): 382–388.

Freitas, T.P., Gomes, M., Fraga, D.B., and Freitas, L. (2010). Effect of therapeutic pulsed ultrasound on lipoperoxidation and fibrogenesis in an animal model of wound healing. *J Surg Res* 161 (1): 168–171.

Furusawaa, Y., Hassana, M.A., Zhaoa, Q.L. et al. (2014). Effects of therapeutic ultrasound on the nucleus and genomic DNA. *Ultrason Sonochem* 21 (6): 2061–2068.

Gamble, L.J. (2022). Physical rehabilitation for small animals. *Vet Clin North Am Small Anim Pract* 52 (4): 997–1019.

Kleinkort, J. and Wood, F. (1975). Phonophoresis with 1 percent versus 10 percent hydrocortisone. *Phys Ther* 55: 1320–1324.

Levine, D., Millis, D.L., and Mynatt, T. (2001). Effects of 3.3-MHz ultrasound on caudal thigh muscle temperature in dogs. *Vet Surg* 30 (2): 170–174.

Michlovitz, S. and Sparrow, K. (2012). Therapeutic ultrasound. In: *Modalities for Therapeutic Intervention*, 5the (ed. S. Michlovitz, J. Bellew, and T. Nolan), 85–108. Pennsylvania: F.A. Davis Co.

Miller, D., Smith, N., Bailey, M. et al. (2012). Overview of therapeutic ultrasound applications and safety considerations. *J Ultrasound Med* 31 (4): 623–634.

Montgomery, L., Elliott, S.B., and Adair, H.S. (2013). Muscle and tendon heating rates with therapeutic ultrasound in horses. *Vet Surg* 42 (3): 243–239.

Mueller, M.C., Gradner, G., Hittmair, K.M. et al. (2009). Conservative treatment of partial gastrocnemius muscle avulsions in dogs using therapeutic ultrasound – A force plate study. *Vet Comp Orthop Traumatol* 2 (3): 243–248.

Muir, W.S., Magee, F.P., Longo, J.A. et al. (1990). Comparison of ultrasonically applied vs. intra-articular injected hydrocortisone levels in canine knees. *Orthop Rev* 19 (4): 351–356.

Niebaum, K. (2013). Rehabilitation physical modalities. In: *Canine Sports Medicine and Rehabilitation* (ed. M.C. Zink and J.B. Van Dyke), 122–124. Ames IA: Wiley-Blackwell.

O'Brien, W.D. Jr. (2007). Ultrasound – Biophysics mechanisms. *Prog Biophys Mol Biol* 93: 212–255.

Saini, N.S., Roy, K.S., Bansal, P.S. et al. (2002). A preliminary study on the effect of ultrasound therapy on the healing of surgically severed achilles tendons in five dogs. *J Vet Med A Physiol Pathol Clin Med* 49 (6): 321–328.

Steiss, J. and Adams, C. (1999). Rate of temperature increase in canine muscle during 1 MHz ultrasound therapy: Deleterious effect of hair coat. *Am J Vet Res* 60: 76–80.

Steiss, J. and McCauley, L. (2004). Electrical stimulation. In: *Canine Rehabilitation and Physical Therapy* (ed. D. Millis, D. Levine, and R. Taylor), 324–336. Missouri: Saunders.

Thompson, W.R., Keller, B.V., Davis, M.L. et al. (2015). Low-magnitude, high-frequency vibration fails to accelerate ligament healing but stimulates collagen synthesis in the Achilles tendon. *Orthop J Sports Med* 3 (5).

Tomlinson JE (2015) The use of therapeutic ultrasound to treat muscle injuries. In: *Proceedings of the American College of Veterinary Surgeons*, Nashville, TN. Oct 22–24, 2015.

Yang, K.H. and Park, S.J. (2001). Stimulation of fracture healing in a canine ulna full-defect model by low-intensity pulsed ultrasound. *Yonsei Med J* 42 (5): 503–508.

19

Modalities Part 5: Shockwave Therapy

Melissa Weber and Julia E. Tomlinson

Twin Cities Animal Rehabilitation & Sports Medicine Clinic, Burnsville, MN, USA

Introduction

Extracorporeal shockwave therapy (ESWT), commonly known as shockwave therapy, uses high-energy sound waves called "pulses" or "shockwaves" to stimulate and speed the body's own healing process. ESWT has been used in human medicine since the 1960s for the treatment of urolithiasis, and since the 1980s for many human orthopedic diseases (Gallagher *et al.*, 2012). This technology then emerged as a modality to help with difficult-to-treat orthopedic and soft tissue injuries, including skin wounds. In the late 1990s, veterinary use began in the field of equine medicine (Biggs, 2011). The high-energy sound waves create mechanical stress at a cellular level, leading to a release of growth factors in the body that reduce inflammation and swelling, increase blood flow, and enhance wound healing. ESWT can be used to treat a variety of conditions, including tendon and ligament injuries (Danova and Muir, 2003; Hsu *et al.*, 2004; Hunter *et al.*, 2004; Venzin *et al.*, 2004), osteoarthritis (OA) (McIlwraith *et al.*, 2004; Francis *et al.*, 2004; Dahlberg *et al.*, 2005), wounds (Morgan *et al.*, 2009; Silveira *et al.*, 2010), and non-union fractures (Chen *et al.*, 2004). Shockwave therapy is non-invasive; however, not all patients respond favorably to treatment. Although most studies show significant improvement after treatment, the results are often subjective, and not consistent (Brown *et al.*, 2005). Lack of response may be attributed to an ineffective treatment protocol or technique, or to the patient's individual ability to respond.

A systematic review of ESWT by Boström *et al.* (2022) reviewed literature on horses, cats, and dogs, finding only weak evidence for improved outcomes of bone, ligament, tendons, and muscles. There were no scientific articles on cats found (Boström *et al.*, 2022). With more research, it is hoped that protocols will be refined to provide more consistent results.

General Terminology

Shockwaves are transient, short-term acoustic pulses with a rapid rise (nanoseconds) to a high peak pressure (Mittermayr *et al.*, 2012). To be considered a true "shockwave" the acoustic pulse must travel faster than 1,500 m/s (the speed of sound).

There are three different ways to produce a truly focused shockwave: electrohydraulic, electromagnetic, and piezoelectric. These three methods produce focused shockwaves. Focused shockwave units produce high-energy waves that converge at a point creating maximal pressure at the treatment area. At the treatment area, a specific depth can be achieved and is adjustable (Simplicio *et al.*, 2020). Maximum pressure can rise as high as 80 MPa with a negative pressure wave of 5–10 MPa. The pulse duration is short at around 5 μs (Poenaru *et al.*, 2023). These waves create the effect of cavitation, or microscopic gas bubbles developing and collapsing in the interstitial fluid which provides mechanical stimulation; this is discussed further in the section on mechanisms of action (Poenaru *et al.*, 2023) (see Figure 19.1).

There are some therapy units that use radial pressure waves that travel at a much slower speed (~10 m/s) and therefore do not produce a true shockwave but instead produce a mechanical pressure wave. The field of pressure will diverge once it leaves the unit and reaches maximal pressure at the tissue source rather than a focused treatment point as in focused shockwave (Simplicio *et al.*, 2020). The radial pressure waves treat more superficial tissue (Simplicio *et al.*, 2020). Radial pressure wave machines can be marketed as shockwave machines but are not true shockwaves. Another reason radial pressure wave therapy is not a true shockwave is because the rising time is longer, and maximal peak pressure is much lower than true focused

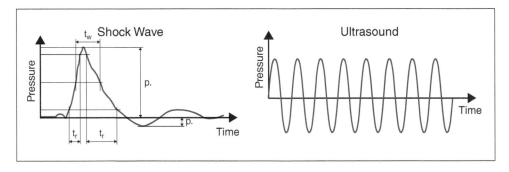

Figure 19.1 A shock wave (left) and an ultrasound wave (right) showing pressure changes over time. In the shockwave, there is a rapid (nanoseconds) rise to peak pressure (*p*). The pressure lasts approx. 0–0.5 μs. Followed by a component of tension (negative pressure) approx. 10% of the peak pressure. The ultrasound wave by contrast is a consistent sinusoidal wave, symmetrical in positive and negative peaks. *Source:* Courtesy of Omar Wess.

extracorporeal shockwaves (Auersperg and Trieb, 2020; Poenaru *et al.*, 2023). Wave pressure persists for as much as 400 μs (Cirovic *et al.*, 2017). The mechanical pressure waves do not deliver focused energy to the treatment site, but instead, the energy is unfocused and dissipates eccentrically at the targeted treatment area (Kirkby, 2013). Cavitation (see later for explanation) will still occur in the tissue (Cirovic *et al.*, 2017). For the rest of the chapter, the main focus will be on true shockwave therapy units including electrohydraulic, electromagnetic, and piezoelectric.

The electrohydraulic principle was used in the first generation of orthopedic shockwave machines. Electrohydraulic shockwaves are generated by an underwater explosion with high-voltage electrode spark discharge. The acoustic waves are then focused with an elliptical reflector and targeted to the treatment area (Wang, 2012). Electrohydraulic shockwave output has a large focal area and deep penetration into tissue up to 40 mm (Leeman *et al.*, 2016).

Electromagnetic generation of shockwaves uses an electric current that passes through a coil, producing a strong magnetic field. The shockwaves are focused using a lens within the device directing the soundwaves to a small focal area (Wang, 2012). The electromagnetic shockwave therapy units have a lower penetration depth compared to electrohydraulic.

The piezoelectric shockwave units have many piezo crystals (>1,000 crystals) mounted within the convex portion of a sphere inside the unit probe head. A rapid electrical discharge causes a pressure change inside the probe head. This causes excitement in the piezo crystals, and they subsequently begin expanding by just a few micrometers thus generating a pulse pressure wave (Chung and Wang, 2017) (see Figure 19.2). The arrangements of the crystals in the spherical shape cause self-focusing of the waves toward the focal area

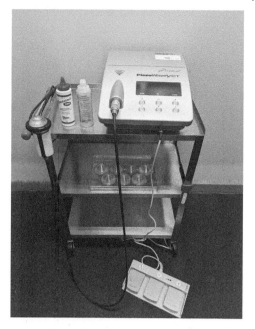

Figure 19.2 PiezoWave Vet shockwave machine and coupling gel. PiezoWaveVet™ machine by ELvation®. This unit has multiple different probe heads to allow precise depths of penetration at the treatment site from 0 to 30 mm. Each probe head increases the depth by 5 mm.

(treatment zone). The focal area for this unit is smaller than the other types of shockwave units. The piezowave is often described as a low-intensity focused shockwave.

Classification of shockwave machines is further described using the properties of the produced energy flux density (EFD), measured in millijoules per millimeter squared. The pressure (bar/KV/Pa) or energy level (low, medium, or high) determines the energy density of the shockwave. The frequency (Hz) is the number of waves produced per second. Higher frequencies can be more uncomfortable for the patient. In veterinary medicine, there is no defined ideal frequency, the authors use between six and eight pulses per second. There is no definitive agreement on what exactly is a low-, medium-, or high-energy ESWT unit.

Ji *et al.* classify a lower energy unit with a produced EFD $\leq 0.28\,\text{mJ/mm}^2$, and a high energy unit can produce $\geq 0.6\,\text{mJ/mm}^2$ (Ji *et al.*, 2016). A systematic review paper by Poenaru *et al.* describes the classification of ESWT as low energy $<0.08\,\text{mJ/mm}^2$, medium $<0.28\,\text{mJ/mm}^2$, and high as $<0.6\,\text{mJ/mm}^2$ (Poenaru *et al.*, 2023). It can be difficult to compare between studies and treatment protocols based on these factors: the type of machine used (i.e., electrohydraulic, electromagnetic, or piezoelectric), and any additional rehabilitation used or not used in any examined study.

Mechanisms of Action

As the shockwaves pass through tissue, energy is dissipated when the wave encounters denser tissue, such as bone, cartilage, tendon, and ligament. The mechanical force of the wave translates to a biological response that promotes healing. The sound waves produce either direct mechanical forces or secondary indirect forces. This has also been described as positive and negative phases, respectively (Simplicio *et al.*, 2020). The direct, or positive forces, occur from the sound waves targeting directly onto the tissue and it can be reflected or passed through and absorbed (Simplicio *et al.*, 2020; Wang, 2012). Indirect forces, or negative phases, produce cavitation between the tissue surfaces, a secondary effect. Cavitation is the effect in which microscopic gas bubbles form and collapse within the interstitial fluid of tissues (Poenaru *et al.*, 2023; Wang, 2012). This second shockwave, or cavitation, is created by the rapid collapse or implosion of the gas/air bubbles (Simplicio *et al.*, 2020), causing local mechanical stimulation of the cells. This similar phenomenon also occurs with therapeutic ultrasound. Currently, the exact mechanism for the action of shockwave therapy in musculoskeletal disorders and

the biological effect on different anatomic structures (bone, cartilage, tendons, and ligaments) is not fully understood.

Neovascularization – Neovascularization is very important in the healing process. As a new blood vessel forms, this allows for removal of byproducts, including via phagocytosis from incoming inflammatory cells, and can help increase oxygen in an area of injury, improving tissue healing (Poenaru *et al.*, 2023). It has been reported by Wang *et al.* in a study using 50 New Zealand rabbits, that one dose of shockwave applied to the tendon–bone interface mediated earlier release of angiogenic markers, including vascular endothelial growth factor (VEGF), endothelial nitric oxide synthase (eNOS), and proliferating cell nuclear antigen (PCNS). In the limbs treated with shockwave, there was a significantly higher number of new vessels and markers of angiogenesis. It was found that VEGF and eNOS increased as early as 1 week post-treatment and remained elevated for 8 weeks before declining at 12 weeks post-treatment (Wang *et al.*, 2003).

Tendon healing – Tendon response to shockwave therapy is a complex process. The goal is for shockwave to aid in tendon remodeling, promotion of the inflammatory phase of healing, and neovascularization. Tendons are relatively acellular, but the few tenocytes present are analogous to a fibrocyte, which is responsible for maintenance of the extracellular matrix (ECM) (Bosch *et al.*, 2007; Poenaru *et al.*, 2023). The ECM contains adhesive components such as proteoglycans in addition to collagen (type I in healthy tissue, type III in healing), and elastin. It is hypothesized that shockwave provides mechanical stimulation causing the tenocytes to release growth factors via a process called mechanotransduction (Poenaru *et al.*, 2023). Mechanotransduction occurs secondary to vibrations in the tissues and leads to the process of tissue regeneration and healing

(Simplicio *et al.*, 2020). There have been in vitro and in vivo studies confirming shockwave treatments can enhance fibroblast proliferation and differentiation (Frairia and Berta, 2011). Activation of transforming growth factor beta 1 (TGF-β1), leads to activating eNOS and VEGF to promote healing (Frairia and Berta, 2011). Shockwave has been shown to downregulate excess inflammatory mediators which are normally found in diseased tendons, which include interleukins (ILs) and metalloproteinases (MMPs) (Leeman *et al.*, 2016).

In a paper by Caminoto *et al.* 10 horses had induced forelimb or rear limb suspensory ligament desmitis. The horses received three shockwave therapy treatments three weeks apart. The ligaments undergoing shockwave therapy produced more new collagen fibers and improved expression of TGF-β1 when compared to the control ligaments (Caminoto *et al.*, 2005).

The effect of shockwaves on normal tendons of ponies has been explored. In a study (Bosch *et al.*, 2007), shockwave was applied to the origin of the suspensory ligament and mid superficial digital flexor tendon (SDFT). Sampling of the tendons was performed three hours after the last treatment. Transient stimulation of tendon metabolism was noted in response to shockwave treatment, with upregulation of growth factors and down-regulation of inflammatory mediators.

Bone healing – The exact mechanism of shockwave-stimulating bone healing is not known. It has been traditionally used in non-healing fractures (including nonunion) but has more recently been used in acute fracture healing (Kieves *et al.*, 2015). The proposed mechanism of action is thought to be related to microfractures caused by the shockwaves. The microfractures then stimulate neovascularization and osteoblastic activity with ultimate stimulation of osteogenic differentiation

within the mesenchymal stem cells (MSC) (Kieves *et al.*, 2015).

Analgesia (pain relief) – The effect of analgesia is thought to occur through hyperstimulation of the peripheral nerves causing release of endorphins and other analgesic molecules, reducing pain. The dose that was reported to be the most effective was the maximum energy density that was tolerated by the patient. There are additional studies that have suggested the reduction of pain originates from reducing pain transmission to the brain stem and this can reduce neurovascular sprouting (Simplicio *et al.*, 2020).

The exact mechanism of analgesia from shockwave therapy has not been fully determined. Some research has shown contradictory results: evidence that shows shockwave therapy has an influence on pain transmission by acting on substance P (Maier *et al.*, 2003; Hausdorf *et al.*, 2008) and calcitonin gene-related peptide (CGRP) (Takahashi *et al.*, 2003), however, findings of Haake *et al.* were no effect of shockwave therapy on release of substance P and CGRP (Haake *et al.*, 2002).

Shockwaves can create hyperstimulation of nociceptors resulting in intense stimulatory input into the periaqueductal gray area (PAG). This "gate control theory," whereby the nociceptive input is dampened by the PAG before it reaches the forebrain, has an abundance of supporting evidence (Rompe *et al.*, 1998; McClure and Weinberger, 2003; Bolt *et al.*, 2004; McClure *et al.*, 2005). Reversible and local pain alleviation has even been hypothesized to be caused by nociceptive inhibition and selective denervation of unmyelinated fibers, without damaging the cell bodies or axons (Souza *et al.*, 2016; Barnes *et al.*, 2019).

Chondroprotection/OA – Unfortunately, there is lack of evidence on the mechanism of action shockwave produces on the articular cartilage and subchondral bone. In a systematic review by Ji *et al.* the paper has many examples of rat and rabbit models showing shockwave therapy may help increase chondrocyte activity and reduce apoptosis. In a study utilizing rats, with consistent use, a chondroprotective effect was seen. Shockwave therapy has been shown to modulate the osteoarthritic disease process in animal models by reducing eNOS, IL-10, and TNF-α levels and decreasing chondrocyte apoptosis, leading to a decrease in cartilage lesions (Moretti *et al.*, 2008; Zhao *et al.*, 2012).

It is important to use caution in the treatment of OA as the cartilage metabolism may be negatively affected, and the formation of osteophytes and joint stiffness may occur (Ji *et al.*, 2016).

Indications

Pain Relief

Research in humans has shown that the analgesic effect of shockwave therapy appears to be more reliable in chronically affected patients rather than those acutely affected (Helbig *et al.*, 2001). Pain relief is quite common for 2–3 days after shockwave therapy (Buch *et al.*, 1998), and in an equine study analgesia was found to be like that induced by local or perineural analgesia, but the duration was 3 days (McClure *et al.*, 2004). Studies in humans suggest shockwave therapy provides bimodal pain relief, an initial effect which wears off, pain returns, and then a gradual waning of pain over time occurs (Ogden *et al.*, 2001). Immediate pain relief (lasting 3–4 days after treatment) is thought to be caused by nociceptive inhibition, and the later (second) pain relieving effect is likely because of angiogenesis and new tissue matrix remodeling as a healing response. This similar bimodal response was seen in an equine study of the effect of shockwave on the thoracolumbar spine of horses (Trager *et al.*, 2020).

An increase in comfort was appreciated in 16 dogs post tibial plateau leveling osteotomy (TPLO) when the shockwave was directed around the joint capsule (Barnes *et al.*, 2019). The shockwave treatment (electrohydraulic, EFD $0.15\,J/mm^2$) was provided to the joint capsule directly after surgery and at the 2-week recheck. Dogs were evaluated with a pain scale and with gait analysis by use of a pressure-sensitive walkway; treated dogs had improved weight bearing (peak vertical force and vertical impulse) versus untreated (Barnes *et al.*, 2019).

There are a wide variety of mechanisms that may allow for pain relief from shockwave therapy. Individual mechanisms may be affected by the type of shockwave generator used, the number of shockwaves performed, energy level, frequency of application, and the area being treated.

Osteoarthritis

Interest in the use of extracorporeal shockwaves to treat orthopedic conditions was started by the observation that patients undergoing lithotripsy had an increase in pelvic bone density (Graff *et al.*, 1987). Souza *et al.* evaluated 30 dogs with hip OA who underwent radial pressure wave therapy. The study design also had a control group of 30 healthy dogs who did not receive any treatment. The dogs diagnosed with OA received radial pressure wave treatment once a week for three weeks. The treatment was focused only on one hip joint, the other limb served as a control for the affected dog. Objective data included a pressure-sensitive walkway and a validated pain scale (visual analogue scale [VAS]). Information was taken at 30, 60, and 90 days after the first treatment session. Dogs receiving treatment had improved VAS scores and improved comfort demonstrated by improved weight bearing (peak vertical force and vertical impulse) (Souza *et al.*, 2016).

In a study, evaluating naturally occurring stifle OA using 14 dogs (7 in treatment group and 7 in control group), an electrohydraulic shockwave machine was used at EFD of 0.14 mJ/mm. The dogs were walked across a force plate, had goniometry performed and a client questionnaire completed. The dogs in the treatment group showed an improvement in peak vertical force as well as range of motion, but the improvement was not statistically different from the control group (Dahlberg *et al.*, 2005).

The evidence that shockwave and radial pressure wave therapy provides pain relief as part of a multimodal treatment plan for OA is growing stronger, and it can be a very valuable tool for managing arthritic pain (Mueller *et al.*, 2007; Souza *et al.*, 2016). Additional research is needed to determine safety and further changes to the articular cartilage and subchondral bone in veterinary medicine.

Tendon and Ligament Injuries
(See Box 19.1)

Learning from our equine colleagues, small animal practitioners have recently started to utilize shockwave therapy as part of the treatment strategy for their patients with tendon and ligament injuries. Evaluation of the bone–tendon interface in both the rabbit and dog model has demonstrated an increase in neovascularization, as confirmed by an increase in the angiogenic markers VEGF and eNOS and the formation of myofibroblasts that leads to healing after being treated with shockwave therapy (Wang *et al.*, 2002, 2003). A study of 15 dogs that underwent electrohydraulic shockwave therapy for issues of shoulder lameness due to shoulder instability or calcifying and inflammatory conditions of this area after failure of conservative therapy. The machine settings were based on the manufacturer's recommendation (not provided directly in the paper). The study found that 64% of the dogs remained improved or were without lameness at long-term follow-up, with a mean follow-up time of 844 days (Becker *et al.*, 2015). Another study looking at shoulder tendinopathy demonstrated improved outcomes after shockwave therapy. This study was a retrospective, owner questionnaire study including 29 dogs. All the dogs had medical records containing radiographs, musculoskeletal ultrasound, or an MRI with no reported medial shoulder syndrome. The dogs underwent one shockwave therapy a week for a total of three weeks using an electrohydraulic unit. There was an 85% reported result of excellent response after treatment (Leeman *et al.*, 2016).

Dogs that developed patellar desmitis after undergoing TPLO were evaluated after treatment with shockwave therapy in a prospective study of 30 dogs. The dogs were divided into a treatment group (15 dogs) and control group (15 dogs). The treatment group received shockwaves at 4- and 6-weeks post-surgery using an electrohydraulic machine (energy flux 0.28 mJ/mm^2, 500–600 shocks). There was a significant reduction in thickness at the most distal aspect of the patellar tendon on radiographs; no ultrasound changes were identified. This study demonstrated the positive effect of shockwave treatment on a radiographically thickened patellar tendon (Gallagher *et al.*, 2012).

Box 19.1 Indications of shockwave for tendon and ligament healing

- Supraspinatus tendinopathy
- Biceps tendinopathy
- Medial shoulder instability
- Calcaneal tendinopathy (in addition to surgery if indicated)
- Patellar tendinopathy

Source: Adapted from Kirkby (2013).

Box 19.1 lists common indications of shockwave therapy for tendon and ligament healing in small animal veterinary medicine.

Wound Healing

Large chronic wounds, especially those on lower limb extremities, can be quite challenging to treat. Research has demonstrated that the use of shockwave therapy may promote soft tissue healing because of neovascularization. Neovascularization will enhance the healing process and reduce pain associated with injury. One human study showed that 75% of patients had 100% epithelialization at a mean follow-up time of 44 days. The findings of this study suggest that unfocused low-energy shockwave therapy is a feasible modality for a variety of difficult-to-treat soft tissue wounds, particularly post-traumatic and post-operative wounds, decubitus ulcers, and burns (Schaden *et al.*, 2007). Currently, there are only experimental studies on equine wounds (Morgan *et al.*, 2009; Silveira *et al.*, 2010; Link *et al.*, 2013) and no published research in small animals. In the study by Silveira *et al.* six horses were utilized, and superficial wounds were created over the forelimbs. Three horses were assigned to either a control group where the wound was treated with just a bandage, and the remaining three were assigned to the treatment group which included shockwave therapy and a bandage. The study found there was no acceleration in wound healing of these wounds but did appreciate reduced granulation tissue proliferation in the treatment group than the control group. In the study by Link *et al.* eight horses had surgical full-thickness biopsy specimens taken on the neck and forelimbs. Expression of growth factors was evaluated pre- and post-skin biopsies. An electrohydraulic shockwave unit was used at an EFD of 0.11 mJ/mm^2 with 100 pulses/cm^2. One group underwent shockwave and bandage application, the other group received just the bandage application. The study found that shockwave therapy caused suppression of TGF-β1 which may help reduce granulation tissue in the horse (Link *et al.*, 2013). Furthermore, research is needed to determine the usefulness of this modality in veterinary medicine in additional species.

Bone Healing (See Box 19.2)

In an experimental canine non-union radial fracture study, four out of five dogs had radiographic evidence of healing six weeks after a single shockwave session. At nine weeks, there was narrowing of the fracture gap and increase in bridging callus. Complete radiographic union was present at 12 weeks (Johannes *et al.*, 1994).

Wang *et al.* demonstrated that shockwave therapy enhanced callus formation and induced cortical bone formation in acute fractures in dogs, and the effect of shockwave therapy appeared to be time-dependent (Wang, 2012). A study of electrohydraulic shockwave on the healing of stifle osteotomies (TPLO) showed that the radiographic healing score in the treated group of dogs was significantly better at eight weeks than in the untreated group (Kieves *et al.*, 2015). Interestingly, another

---

Box 19.2 Indications for bone healing

- Delayed union and trophic non-union fractures
- In conjunction with surgical repair of highly comminuted fractures and/or anticipated slow fracture healing
- In conjunction with external coaptation for non-surgical management of digital, metacarpal, or metatarsal fractures

Source: Adapted from Kirkby (2013).

study using an electrohydraulic shockwave machine on tibial tuberosity advancement (TTA) did not find a difference in their treatment groups on bone healing at the osteotomy site (Barnes *et al.*, 2015). In this study, they treated the TTA site on the day of surgery and once more four weeks later. The treatment groups included dogs who had a cancellous bone graft at the TTA site, bone graft and shockwave, shockwave alone, and no bone graft and no shockwave. They found that at four weeks, there was improvement at the osteotomy site, but no significant differences were appreciated between any treatment group at eight weeks (Barnes *et al.*, 2015).

The overall current research is supportive of the use of shockwave therapy in treatment of delayed union and non-union fractures.

Box 19.2 lists indications for use of shockwave therapy for bone healing conditions.

Enhancement of Biologic Therapies

There has been emerging evidence using shockwave to amplify the effects of both MSC, adipose-derived stem cells (ASC), and platelet-rich plasma (PRP). A study looking at shockwave and MSC indicated there was no detrimental effect to the MSCs, but instead a potential to increase the osteogenic activity of this cell line. In an in vitro study using ASCs, it was shown that focused shockwave therapy to the ASCs showed increased proliferation (Johnson *et al.*, 2022). Lastly, studies showing the use of PRP, and shockwave indicate an increase in platelet-derived growth factors in vitro (Johnson *et al.*, 2022; Seabaugh *et al.*, 2017).

MSC have the capability to differentiate into various cell lines. The MSCs can stimulate chemical factors and signals to help differentiate other cells and reduce inflammation and immune reactions (Salcedo-Jiménez *et al.*, 2020). In an in vitro study by Salcedo-Jimenez *et al.* equine

umbilical cord MSC (CB-MSC) was cultured. There were two groups, one of the cell lines exposed to shockwave treatments and the other serving as a control. The study used an electrohydraulic shockwave generator. They found the cell cultures treated with shockwave had increased metabolic activity, maintained their differentiation potential and had a higher potential for adipogenic cells (which can form many other cell lines) and osteogenic cell lines (Salcedo-Jiménez *et al.*, 2020).

PRP, when injected into a joint or tissue, releases growth factors that can help improve healing and aid in neovascularization (Seabaugh *et al.*, 2017). In canines, administration methods can include using a freeze thaw cycle to help improve platelet activation. In a study by Seabaugh *et al.*, they demonstrated shockwave therapy in conjunction with PRP can help increase the expression of growth factors in the horse. One group of horses served as a control receiving PRP after a freeze thaw cycle, the remaining two groups either received shockwave therapy with a small probe of 20 mm focal width (EFD 0.12 mJ/mm^2) or a 10 mm focal width (EFD 0.28 mJ/cc^2) using an electrohydraulic shockwave unit. Though the freeze thaw cycle sample was superior to either of the shockwave groups, the two shockwave groups had significantly more growth factors as compared to the negative control, with platelet-derived growth factor beta nearly 200% higher (Seabaugh *et al.*, 2017). This study was a nice example of utilizing shockwave therapy as a stall side tool to help improve growth factor release of PRP stall side when a freeze thaw cycle is not feasible.

Equine Use

Shockwave therapy entered veterinary medicine through its use in equine medicine, with the first recorded use in Germany in 1996 (McClure and Weinberger, 2003). The first use in the United States was in 1998 with horses with distal hock joint and navicular pain (McCarroll *et al.*, 1999; McCarroll and McClure, 2002). The research and use of shockwave therapy in equine medicine is vast when compared to that of small animal research. Several studies have shown positive results in the treatment of bone spavin, navicular syndrome, tendonitis, insertional desmopathy of the ligamentum nuchae, dorsal metacarpal disease, incomplete/stress fractures, proximal splint bone fractures, back pain due to "kissing spines" (see Figure 19.3), and muscle pain.

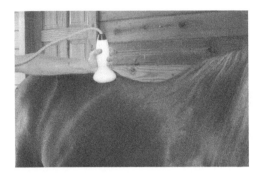

Figure 19.3 Treatment of a horse for kissing spine disease Treating a horse for "kissing spine" disease. The hair coat in this animal was noted to be short enough to allow efficient penetration of shockwave with coupling gel. *Source:* Courtesy of D. Strammel (1ˢᵗ edition).

Back Pain – Equine

In a study by Trager *et al.*, they found reduced pain thresholds in horses with back pain in response to shockwave therapy (see Figure 19.4). Horses with palpable back pain who had been imaged with radiographs were assessed for back discomfort using a pressure algometer, pain was quantified as mechanical nociceptive threshold (MNT). The horses received three treatments of shockwave, two weeks apart. The shockwave in this study was electrohydraulic, depth of 113 mm, EFD of 0.13 mJ/mm^2. Treatment was provided along T12–L5; 83% of treated horses always had improvement in the MNT in the study regardless of radiographic disease. A single shockwave treatment was able to improve the MNT and three treatments two weeks apart were able to improve the MNT over a period of 56 days (Trager *et al.*, 2020).

Tendon and Ligament – Equine

Proximal suspensory desmitis (PSD) is a type of suspensory lameness that often results in poor performance and unfortunately has a guarded prognosis to return to work (Giunta *et al.*, 2019). In the study by Giunta *et al.*, a two-center, randomized, and prospective

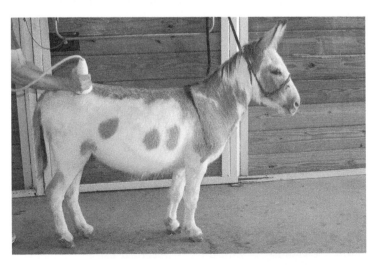

Figure 19.4 Treatment of donkey lumbosacral disease Treatment of donkey for lumbosacral disease. *Source:* Courtesy of D. Strammel (1ˢᵗ edition).

clinical trial using 100 western performance horses to compare the use of shockwave versus PRP alone for clinical improvement in lameness in horses affected with PSD. The horse's lameness was graded using both the American Association of Equine Practitioners (AAEP) scale and a visual analog scale (VAS) to assess for acute and chronic lameness, respectively. Ultrasound of the proximal suspensory was performed and graded (ordinal scale). The horses were randomly assigned to one of two treatment groups, either receiving shockwave therapy or PRP. The shockwave machine was an electrohydraulic machine. PRP was administered using ultrasound guidance. The horses were evaluated at 4 days then phone follow-up at 6 months and 12 months was performed. At the four-day post-treatment evaluation, horses treated with shockwave had a greater reduction in lameness when compared with PRP alone. At the one-year follow-up, the lower ultrasound grades (0–1) responded better to shockwave therapy whereas the higher-grade ultrasound changes (2) responded better to PRP injection according to this study. This study showed less severe ultrasound grades of tendon lesions responded better to shockwave therapy and the higher-grade ultrasound tendon lesions responded better to PRP treatment (Giunta *et al.*, 2019).

In a study by Lischer *et al.* (2006), 52 horses diagnosed with chronic PSD (32 forelimbs, 22 hindlimbs, and 3 both fore- and hindlimbs) were treated with shockwave therapy once weekly for three weeks. The unit was electrohydraulic, with EFD $0.15\,mJ/mm^2$. During the start of treatment, the horses were on stall rest and from weeks 13–24, underwent a 12-week program of controlled exercise. Ligaments were imaged with ultrasound at multiple points, including at one year post-treatment. Of the horses with forelimb desmitis, 61.8% returned to full work by 6 months and 55.9% were still working full-time 1 year later. The overall return to function was 90% for horses with forelimb desmitis. The horses with hind limb desmitis had a lower success rate and a more guarded prognosis with a high chance of recurrence (Lischer *et al.*, 2006).

Equine emerging uses include lung surface treatment for exercise-induced pleural hemorrhage (EIPH), pleural discomfort, thoracic sling discomfort, and sarcoid lesion management (Johnson *et al.*, 2022).

Patient Preparation

Acoustic energy dissipates as it passes from one medium to the next. Energy loss through attenuation is much larger through air than it is through water. The owner should be informed that the area will need to have the hair short or shaved, and a media gel (coupling gel) applied to the skin. Application of gel ensures good penetration of the sound waves, as they pass from the probe head through the skin to the deeper tissues, as any trapped air will reduce transmission of the shockwaves (see Figure 19.5).

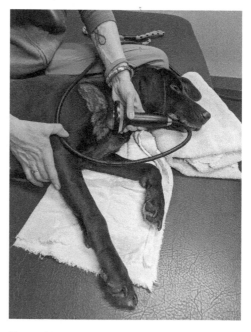

Figure 19.5 An example of Shockwave coupling gel.

It is along the boundaries between different tissue densities such as muscle and bone that the sound field experiences the biggest changes and emits the highest energy, and where the most biologic effects are expected.

After preparing the skin and applying an appropriate coupling gel, apply the probe head to the area being treated and use enough force to ensure good contact between the probe head and the skin. Keep the probe at right angles to the skin surface. Engage the shockwave generator. One method is to move the probe head gently, and slowly over the area being treated, rotating, and gliding the probe head as necessary to reach the intended target of treatment (see Figure 19.5). Another method is to keep the probe head still, especially when treating small areas, apply the prescribed number of pulses, then move 0.5–1 cm before applying a second prescribed number of pulses.

There is no consensus on how best to focus shockwaves to manage a lesion. Some clinicians will use ultrasound guidance when treating a ligament or tendon injury, specifically measuring location, depth, and length of a lesion. Some clinicians will just estimate the area to be treated based on prior radiographic and sonographic diagnosis without a depth measurement. Since focused shockwaves are a locally concentrated therapy without regional or systemic effects, it is necessary to have a clear and concrete diagnosis to define the treatment area (McCarroll and McClure, 2002). A good working knowledge of the anatomical landmarks in the treatment area is essential to delivering the shockwaves to the proper area and to avoid areas that the shockwaves could damage or have less effect on. For arthritic joints, the best patient outcome seems to be obtained from concentrating on the attachments of the joint capsule surrounding the entire joint (see Figures 19.6–19.8).

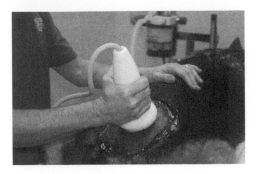

Figure 19.6 Treatment of canine shoulder with probe head Treatment of canine shoulder tendinopathy. The probe head is held in one location until the prescribed pulses are reached. The location and distances can often be determined by previous diagnosis with diagnostic ultrasound or by clinician's knowledge of the patient's anatomy. Often the probe head will be moved 0.5–1 cm for each treatment site.

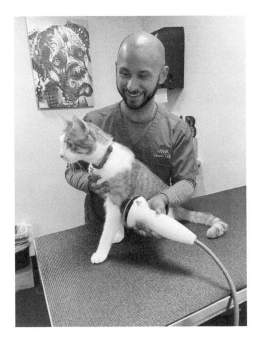

Figure 19.7 Feline treatment of elbow with shockwave. *Source:* Courtesy Dr Carolina Medina (co-author)/Christian Vazquez.

Typically, a loud "clicking" noise is created during the production of the shockwave, and this noise may be startling to the patient, the sound can reverberate through

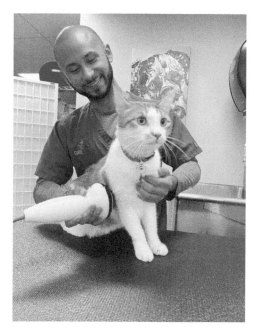

Figure 19.8 Feline treatment of elbow with shockwave. *Source:* Courtesy Dr Carolina Medina (co-author)/Christian Vazquez.

an open-plan building. The piezowave shockwave unit is quieter than the electromagnetic units so far. The intense stimulation from the energy produced by the shockwave may be perceived as uncomfortable to painful, depending on the condition being treated, density of the target tissue or nearby tissues (e.g., tendon over bone), and which shockwave generator is being employed. Therefore, mild to heavy sedation is often used during the treatment sessions. Sedation can range from oral gabapentin and trazodone to injectable with an alpha-2 (dexmedetomidine in small animals; detomidine or xylazine in equine) or a combination of an alpha-2 and opioid (butorphanol, hydromorphone, or morphine). This allows for comfort and stress relief for the patient and has the added benefit of safety for the veterinary staff. Some patients may need earplugs, especially if used in a barn or room where sound

reverberation could be amplified (Johnson *et al.*, 2022).

Treatment Protocol

Treatment protocols have been established by manufacturers for many species, for a wide variety of indications and severity of disease. Because there are several different manufacturers and differences in the shockwave generators, it is imperative to follow the protocols set in place for each individual unit from the manufacturer. Most protocols call for 2 or 3 sessions of shockwave therapy at 1–3 week intervals. Be sure to enter the following information into the patient's medical record for each session: type of shockwave generator used, EFD (mJ/mm^2), pulse repetition frequency, and the number of pulses.

The veterinary technician likely will be carrying out this treatment plan, but the rehabilitation veterinarian will be deciding upon the treatment range and dose. The rehabilitation technician will be instructed by the veterinarian on what and where to initiate shockwave therapy plus the settings used with the machine for each specific patient. A thorough knowledge of anatomy is needed. Pictures and reference texts in the therapy room as well as anatomical models can be very helpful. Veterinarians prescribing treatment should mention proximity to bony landmarks to aid ease of probe placement.

Clinical Indications

The following musculoskeletal conditions have been reported, either through clinical studies or anecdotally, to improve in response to shockwave therapy as the sole method of treatment or as an adjunctive treatment in a multimodal approach (see Box 19.3).

Box 19.3   Common conditions treated by shockwave therapy

- Chronic wounds
- Lick granulomas
- Delayed or non-union fractures
- Non-surgical management of digital, metacarpal, and metatarsal fractures
- Osteoarthritis (OA): hip, elbow, stifle, hock, and shoulder
- Spinal column diseases
  - Intervertebral disc disease
  - Lumbosacral disease
  - Spondylosis deformans
  - Cauda Equina Syndrome
  - Sacroiliac disease
  - "Kissing spine" in equines
- Muscle injuries
- Tendinopathy (patella, calcaneal, and shoulder)
- Equine suspensory desmitis

Box 19.3 lists a summary of common conditions treated by shockwave therapy in small animal and equine veterinary patients.

Adverse Events and Contraindications

When applied according to manufacturer specifications, the adverse events of shockwave therapy are minimal. The most reported side effects are bruising of the skin, soft tissue in the treatment area, or small hematomas and/or swelling may also develop (Johannes *et al.*, 1994; Rompe *et al.*, 2001; McClure *et al.*, 2004; Dahlberg *et al.*, 2005; Speed, 2014). The acoustic impedance of air is distinctly lower than the acoustic impedance of soft tissue; thus, virtually all the energy is reflected at the interface. The phase of the pressure is reversed and the maximum pressure at the interface may turn into rarefaction (reduction of an item's density) pressure, with up to twice the former maximal energy, which may result in considerable tissue damage at the interface. Because of the acoustic impedance, shockwaves used over a lung field can cause the lung tissue to tear or bleed, or worse a pneumothorax (Auersperg and Trieb, 2020). Intestinal perforation has been reported in a human after shockwave therapy, where the colon was in the focal zone (Klug *et al.*, 2001). Large nerves and blood vessels also should not be within the focal zone. Arterial walls develop interstitial damage that can result in rupture, vasoconstriction, or increased permeability (Buch, 1998). Sites with neoplasia and infection have traditionally been avoided because of the potential to develop metastasis or septicemia from the primary site. The mechanical force of the shock wave can release the neoplastic cells and may cause an increase in the rate of metastasis (Oosterhof *et al.*, 1996; McClure *et al.*, 2004).

There have been additional studies in which there is a dose-related effect of ESWT regarding cell viability and ECM viability (Poenaru *et al.*, 2023). In a review paper by Ponearu et al., several study examples were provided. An in vivo study using Achilles tendons of rabbits showed EFD doses up to $0.28\,mJ/mm^2$ were safe and did not indicate damage to the tendon. With an EFD of $0.6\,mJ/mm^2$, there was considerable damage to the tendon and paratenon. The damage included necrosis and inflammatory reactions present in the tendon at four weeks post-treatment. In an in vivo study using quadriceps of rabbits, findings indicated the quadriceps tolerated higher EFD, but still high levels ($1.2\,mJ/mm^2$) created damaging changes in the ECM at 10 days post-treatment. Overall cell death was found to be higher in cases of normal human cell cultures (in vitro) with higher number of pulses (1,000–2,000) versus 500 with the same EFD (Poenaru *et al.*, 2023).

Overall, ESWT is considered safe while following the manufacturer's guidelines. It is important to note, the higher the energy setting, the higher the chance for tissue damage (Auersperg and Trieb, 2020).

According to the US Equestrian Federation, most racing jurisdictions prohibit the use of shockwave therapy within 5–7 days preceding competition, and the Federation Equestre Internationale prohibits shockwave therapy 5 days preceding competition (www.usef.org). This is because shockwave has the potential ability to provide analgesia and would otherwise be considered therapeutic treatment prior to competition. It is recommended to refer to the specific rule book and guidelines for use as there are some exceptions to competing horses.

Conclusion

Shockwave therapy is a unique modality that can be used to treat a wide range of conditions. Shockwaves are high-energy acoustic waves generated under water from a wide variety of generators. The application of shockwave therapy for certain musculoskeletal disorders in veterinary medicine has been around since the late 1990s. This modality is non-invasive and has a low incidence of adverse effects and complications. The current research demonstrates its effectiveness. However, further research is needed to understand the exact mechanism by which it works. Furthermore, due to a wide variety of sound wave generators, protocols need to be researched and developed for each condition treated, including energy level, number of shocks, frequency of pulses delivered, and number of sessions. Shockwave therapy should be considered as part of a multimodal approach to the conditions that have been discussed in this chapter.

References

Auersperg, V. and Trieb, K. (2020). Extracorporeal shock wave therapy: An update. *EFORT Open Rev* 5 (10): 584–592. https://doi.org/10.1302/2058-5241.5.190067.

Barnes, K., Faludi, A., Takawira, C. et al. (2019). Extracorporeal shock wave therapy improves short-term limb use after canine tibial plateau leveling osteotomy. *Vet Surg* 48 (8): 1382–1390. https://doi.org/10.1111/vsu.13320.

Barnes, K., Lanz, O., Werre, S. et al. (2015). Comparison of autogenous cancellous bone grafting and extracorporeal shock wave therapy on osteotomy healing in the tibial tuberosity advancement procedure in dogs: Radiographic densitometric evaluation. *Vet Comp Orthop Traumatol* 28 (3): 207–214. https://doi.org/10.3415/VCOT-14-10-0156.

Becker W, Kowaleski MP, McCarthy RJ, and Blake CA (2015) Extracorporeal shockwave therapy for shoulder lameness in dogs. *J Am Anim Hosp Assoc* 51(1):15–19. https://doi.org/10.5326/JAAHA-MS-6175.

Biggs S (2011) *Update on extracorporeal shockwave therapy*. Veterinary Practice News. https://www.veterinarypracticenews.com/update-on-extracorporeal-shockwave-therapy/.

Bolt, D.M., Burba, D.J., Hubert, J.D. et al. (2004). Determination of functional and morphologic changes in palmar digital nerves after nonfocused extracorporeal shock wave treatment in horses. *Am J Vet Res* 65 (12): 1714–1718. https://doi.org/10.2460/ajvr.2004.65.1714.

Bosch, G., Lin, Y.L., Van Schie, H.T.M. et al. (2007). Effect of extracorporeal shock wave therapy on the biochemical composition and metabolic activity of tenocytes in normal tendinous structures in ponies. *Equine Vet J* 39 (3): 226–231. https://doi.org/10.2746/042516407X180408.

Boström A, Bergh A, Hyytiäinen H, and Asplund K (2022) Systematic review of complementary and alternative veterinary medicine in sport and companion animals: Extracorporeal shockwave therapy. *Animals* 12(22):3124. https://doi.org/10.3390/ani12223124.

Brown KE, Nickels FA, Caron JP, *et al.* (2005) Investigation of the immediate analgesic effects of extracorporeal shock wave therapy for treatment of navicular disease in horses. *Vet Surg* 34(6):554–558. https://doi.org/10.1111/j.1532-950X.2005.00087.x.

Buch, M., Schlangmann, B.A., Lübbers, C. et al. (1998). Results of shock wave therapy of calcaneal spur from the Orthopaedic Hospital in Kassel: Influence of various parameters on the outcome. In: *Extracorporeal Shock Waves in Orthopaedics* (ed. W. Siebert and M. Buch), 30–35. Berlin: Springer.

Buch, M. (1998). Review. In: *Extracorporeal Shock Waves in Orthopaedics* (ed. W. Siebert and M. Buch), 59–88. Berlin: Springer.

Caminoto EH, Alves ALG, Amorim RL, *et al.* (2005) Ultrastructural and immunocytochemical evaluation of the effects of extracorporeal shock wave treatment in the hind limbs of horses with experimentally induced suspensory ligament desmitis. *Am J Vet Res* 66(5): 892–896. https://doi.org/10.2460/ajvr.2005.66.892.

Chen, Y.J., Wurtz, T., Wang, C.J. et al. (2004). Recruitment of mesenchymal stem cells and expression of TGF-beta 1 and VEGF in the early stage of shock wave-promoted bone regeneration of segmental defect in rats. *J Orthop Res* 22 (3): 526–534. https://doi.org/10.1016/j.orthres.2003.10.005.

Chung E and Wang J (2017) A state-of-art review of low intensity extracorporeal shock wave therapy and lithotripter machines for the treatment of erectile dysfunction. *Expert Rev Med Dev* 14(12):929–934. https://doi.org/10.1080/17434440.2017.1403897.

Cirovic, S., Gould, D.H., Park, D.H., and Solan, M.C. (2017). Cadaveric experiments to evaluate pressure wave generated by radial shockwave treatment of plantar fasciitis. *Foot Ankle Surg* 23 (4): 285–289. https://doi.org/10.1016/j.fas.2016.08.006.

Dahlberg J, Fitch G, Evans RB, *et al.* (2005) The evaluation of extracorporeal shockwave therapy in naturally occurring osteoarthritis of the stifle joint in dogs. *Vet Comp Orthop Traumatol* 18(3):147–152. https://doi.org/10.1055/s-0038-1632954.

Danova, N.A. and Muir, P. (2003). Extracorporeal shock wave therapy for supraspinatus calcifying tendinopathy in two dogs. *Vet Rec* 152 (7): 208–209. https://doi.org/10.1136/vr.152.7.208.

Frairia, R. and Berta, L. (2011). Biological effects of extracorporeal shock waves on fibroblasts. A review. *Muscles Ligaments Tendons J* 1 (4): 138–147.

Francis DA, Millis DL, Evans M, *et al.* (2004) Clinical evaluation of ESWT for management of canine OA of the elbow and hip joint. *Proceedings of the 31st Annual Conference VOS Big Sky*, Montana.

Gallagher A, Cross AR, and Sepulveda G (2012) The effect of shock wave therapy on patellar ligament desmitis after tibial plateau leveling osteotomy. *Vet Surg* 41(4):482–485. https://doi.org/10.1111/j.1532-950X.2012.00958.x.

Graff, J., Pastor, J., Senge, T. et al. (1987). The effect of high energy shock waves on bony tissue: An experimental study. *J Urol* 137: 278–281. https://doi.org/10.1016/S0022-5347(17)75848-X.

Giunta, K, Donnell, J.R., Donnell, A.D., and Frisbie D.D. (2019). Prospective randomized comparison of platelet rich plasma to extracorporeal shockwave therapy for treatment of proximal suspensory pain in western performance horses. *Res Vet Sci* 126: 38–44. https://doi.org/10.1016/j.rvsc.2019.07.020.

Haake M, Thon A, and Bette M (2002) No influence of low-energy extracorporeal shock wave therapy (ESWT) on spinal nociceptive systems. *J Orthop Sci* 7(1): 97–101. https://doi.org/10.1007/s776-002-8429-0.

Hausdorf J, Lemmens MA, Kaplan S, *et al.* (2008) Extracorporeal shockwave application to the distal femur of rabbits diminishes the number of neurons immunoreactive for substance P in dorsal root ganglia L5. *Brain Res* 1207:96–101. https://doi.org/10.1016/j.brainres.2008.02.013.

Helbig K, Herbert C, Schostok T, *et al.* (2001) Correlations between the duration of pain and the success of shock wave therapy. *Clin Orthop Relat Res* 387:68–71. https://doi.org/10.1097/00003086-200106000-00009.

Hsu RW, Hsu WH, Tai CL, and Lee KF (2004) Effect of shock-wave therapy on patellar tendinopathy in a rabbit model. *J Orthop Res* 22(1):221–227. https://doi.org/10.1016/S0736-0266(03)00138-4.

Hunter, J., McClure, S.R., Merritt, D.K. et al. (2004). Extracorporeal shockwave therapy for treatment of superficial digital flexor tendonitis in racing thoroughbreds: 8 clinical cases. *Vet Comp Orthop Traumatol* 17: 152–155. https://doi.org/10.1055/s-0038-1632804.

Ji Q, Wang P, and He C (2016) Extracorporeal shockwave therapy as a novel and potential treatment for degenerative cartilage and bone disease: Osteoarthritis. A qualitative analysis of the literature. *Prog Biophys Mol Biol* 121(3):255–265. https://doi.org/10.1016/j.pbiomolbio.2016.07.001.

Johannes, E.J., Kaulesar Sukul, D.M., and Matura, E. (1994). High-energy shock waves for the treatment of nonunions: An experiment on dogs. *J Surg Res* 57 (2): 246–252. https://doi.org/10.1006/jsre.1994.1139.

Johnson, S.A., Richards, R.B., Frisbie, D.D. et al. (2022). Equine shock wave therapy – Where are we now? *Equine Vet J* 1–14. https://doi.org/10.1111/evj.13890.

Kieves, N.R., Mackay, C.S., Adducci, K. et al. (2015). High energy focused shock wave therapy accelerates bone healing: A blinded, prospective, randomized canine clinical trial. *Vet Comp Orthop Traumatol* 28 (6): 425–432. https://doi.org/10.3415/VCOT-15-05-0084.

Leeman J, Shaw K, Mison M, *et al.* (2016) Extracorporeal shockwave therapy and therapeutic exercise for supraspinatus and biceps tendinopathies in 29 dogs. *Vet Rec* 7(1):1–8. https://doi.org/10.1186/1749-799X-7-11.

Kirkby-Shaw K (2016) Cellular mechanisms of shock wave therapy. *Proceedings American College of Veterinary Surgeons*, October 7, 2016, Indianapolis, IN.

Klug, R., Kurz, F., Dunzinger, M., and Aufschnaiter, M. (2001). Small bowel perforation after extracorporeal shockwave lithotripsy of a ureter stone. *Dig Surg* 18 (3): 241–242. https://doi.org/10.1159/000050144.

Link, K.A., Koenig, J.B., Silveira, A. et al. (2013). Effect of unfocused extracorporeal shock wave therapy on growth factor gene expression in wounds and intact skin of horses. *Am J Vet Res* 74 (2): 324–332. Retrieved Jun 22, 2023, from https://doi.org/10.2460/ajvr.74.2.324.

Lischer CJ, Ringer SK, Schnewlin M, *et al.* (2006) Treatment of chronic proximal suspensory desmitis in horses using focused electrohydraulic shockwave therapy. *Schweizer Archiv Fur Tierheilkunde* 148(10):561–568. https://doi.org/10.1024/0036-7281.148.10.561.

Maier M, Averbeck B, Milz S, *et al.* (2003) Substance P and prostaglandin E2 release after shock wave application to the rabbit femur. *Clin Orthop Relat Res* 406:237–245. https://doi.org/10.1097/01.blo.0000030173.56585.8f.

McCarroll, G. and McClure, S. (2002). Initial experiences with extracorporeal shock wave therapy for treatment of bone spavin in horses. *Vet Comp Orthop Traumatol* 3: 184–186. https://doi.org/10.1055/s-0038-1632735.

McCarroll GD, Hague B, and Smitherman S (1999) The use of extracorporeal shock wave lithotripsy for treatment of distal tarsal arthropathies of the horse. *Proceedings of the 18th Annual Meeting of the American Association of Equine Sports Medicine*, pp. 40–41.

McClure, S. and Weinberger, T. (2003). Extracorporeal shock wave therapy: Clinical applications and regulation. *Clin Techn Equine Pract* 2 (4): 358–367. https://doi.org/10.1053/j.ctep.2004.04.007.

McClure SR, Van Sickle D, and White MR (2004) Effects of extracorporeal shock wave therapy on bone. *Vet Surg* 33(1):40–48. https://doi.org/10.1111/j.1532-950x.2004.04013.x.

McClure SR, Sonea IM, Evans RB, and Yaeger MJ (2005) Evaluation of analgesia resulting from extracorporeal shock wave therapy and radial pressure wave therapy in the limbs of horses and sheep. *Am J Vet Res* 66(10):1702–1708. https://doi.org/10.2460/ajvr.2005.66.1702.

McIlwraith, C.W., Frisbie, D.D., Park, R.D. et al. (2004). Evaluation of extracorporeal shockwave therapy for osteoarthritis using an equine model. *Proc Eur College Vet Surg* 257–258.

Mittermayr, R., Antonic, V., Hartinger, J. et al. (2012). Extracorporeal shock wave therapy (ESWT) for wound healing: technology, mechanisms, and clinical efficacy. *Wound Repair Regen* 20 (4): 456–465. https://doi.org/10.1111/j.1524-475X.2012.00796.x.

Moretti, B., Iannone, F., Notarnicola, A. et al. (2008). Extracorporeal shock waves down-regulate the expression of interleukin-10 and tumor necrosis factor-alpha in osteoarthritic chondrocytes. *BMC Musculoskelet Disord* 9: 1–7. https://doi.org/10.1186/1471-2474-9-16.

Morgan, D.D., McClure, S., Yaeger, M.J. et al. (2009). Effects of extracorporeal shock wave therapy on wounds of the distal portion of the limbs in horses. *J Am Vet Med Assoc* 234 (9): 1154–1161. https://doi.org/10.2460/javma.234.9.1154.

Mueller, M., Bockstahler, B., Skalicky, M. et al. (2007). Effects of radial shockwave therapy on the limb function of dogs with hip osteoarthritis. *Vet Rec* 160 (22): 762–765. https://doi.org/10.1136/vr.160.22.762.

Ogden JA, Alvarez RG, Levitt R, and Marlow M (2001) Shock wave therapy (Orthotripsy) in musculoskeletal disorders. *Clin Orthop Relat Res* 387:22–40. https://doi.org/10.1097/00003086-200106000-00005.

Oosterhof GO, Cornel EB, Smits GA, *et al.* (1996) The influence of high-energy shock waves on the development of metastases. *Ultrasound Med Biol* 22(3):339–344. https://doi.org/10.1016/0301-5629(95)02051-9.

Poenaru, D., Sandulescu, M.I., and Cinteza, D. (2023). Biological effects of extracorporeal shockwave therapy in tendons: A systematic review. *Biomed Rep* 18 (2): 1–12. https://doi.org/10.3892/br.2022.1597.

Rompe JD, Kirkpatrick CJ, Küllmer K, *et al.* (1998) Dose-related effects of shock waves on rabbit tendo Achillis. A sonographic and histological study. *J Bone Joint Surg Br*

80(3):546–552. https://doi.org/10.1302/030 1-620x.80b3.8434.

Rompe, J.D., Zoellner, J., and Nafe, B. (2001). Shock wave therapy versus conventional surgery in the treatment of calcifying tendinitis of the shoulder. *Clin Orthop Relat Res* 387: 72–82. https:// doi.org/10.1097/00003086-200106000-00010.

Salcedo-Jiménez R, Koenig JB, Lee OJ, *et al.* (2020) Extracorporeal shock wave therapy enhances the in vitro metabolic activity and differentiation of equine umbilical cord blood mesenchymal stromal cells. *Front Vet Sci* 7:1–11. https://doi. org/10.3389/fvets.2020.554306.

Schaden, W., Thiele, R., Kölpl, C. et al. (2007). Shock wave therapy for acute and chronic soft tissue wounds: A feasibility study. *J Surg Res* 143 (1): 1–12. https://doi. org/10.1016/j.jss.2007.01.009.

Seabaugh, K.A., Thoresen, M., and Giguère, S. (2017). Extracorporeal shockwave therapy increases growth factor release from equine platelet-rich plasma in vitro. *Front Vet Sci* 4: 1–6. https://doi. org/10.3389/fvets.2017.00205.

Silveira, A., Koenig, J.B., Arroyo, L.G. et al. (2010). Effects of unfocused extracorporeal shock wave therapy on healing of wounds of the distal portion of the forelimb in horses. *Am J Vet Res* 71 (2): 229–234. https://doi.org/10.2460/ ajvr.71.2.229.

Simplicio, C.L., Purita, J., Murrell, W. et al. (2020). Extracorporeal shock wave therapy mechanisms in musculoskeletal regenerative medicine. *J Clin Orthop Trauma* 11: S309–S318. https://doi. org/10.1016/j.jcot.2020.02.004.

Souza ANA, Ferreira MP, Hagen SCF, *et al.* (2016) Radial shock wave therapy in dogs with hip osteoarthritis. *Vet Comp Orthop Traumatol* 29(2):108–114. https://doi. org/10.3415/VCOT-15-01-0017.

Speed C (2014) A systematic review of shockwave therapies in soft tissue conditions: Focusing on the evidence. *Br J Sports Med* 48(21):1538–1542. https://doi.org/10.1136/ bjsports-2012-091961.

Takahashi, N., Wada, Y., Ohtori, S. et al. (2003). Application of shock waves to rat skin decreases calcitonin gene-related peptide immunoreactivity in dorsal root ganglion neurons. *Auton Neurosci* 107 (2): 81–84. https://doi.org/10.1016/ S1566-0702(03)00134-6.

Trager LR, Funk RA, Clapp KS, *et al.* (2020) Extracorporeal shockwave therapy raises mechanical nociceptive threshold in horses with thoracolumbar pain. *Equine Vet J* 52(2):250–257. https://doi.org/10.1111/ evj.13159.

Ueberle, F. (1998). Shock wave technology. In: *Extracorporeal Shock Waves in Orthopaedics* (ed. W. Siebert and M. Buch), 59–88. Berlin: Springer.

Venzin C, Ohlerth S, Koch D, and Spreng D (2004) Extracorporeal shockwave therapy in a dog with chronic bicipital tenosynovitis. *Schweizer Archiv fur Tierheilkunde* 146(3):136–141. https://doi. org/10.1024/0036-7281.146.3.136.

Wang CJ, Huang HY, and Pai CH (2002) Shock wave-enhanced neovascularization at the tendon-bone junction: An experiment in dogs. *J Foot Ankle Surg* 41(1):16–22. https://doi.org/10.1016/ s1067-2516(02)80005-9.

Wang, F.S., Yang, K.D., Chen, R.F. et al. (2002). Extracorporeal shock wave promotes growth and differentiation of bone-marrow stromal cells towards osteoprogenitors associated with induction of TGF-beta1. *J Bone Joint Surg Br* 84 (3): 457–461. https://doi.org/10.1302/0301-620 x.84b3.11609.

Wang CJ, Wang FS, Yang KD, *et al.* (2003) Shock wave therapy induces neovascularization at the tendon-bone junction. A study in rabbits. *J Orthop Res* 21(6):984–989. https://doi.org/10.1016/ S0736-0266(03)00104-9.

Wang CJ (2012) Extracorporeal shockwave therapy in musculoskeletal disorders *J Orthop Surg Res* 7(1):8. https://doi.org/10.1186/1749-799X-7-11.

Zhao, Z., Ji, H., Jing, R. et al. (2012). Extracorporeal shock-wave therapy reduces progression of knee osteoarthritis in rabbits by reducing nitric oxide level and chondrocyte apoptosis. *Arch Orthop Trauma Surg* 132 (11): 1547–1553. https://doi.org/10.1007/s00402-012-1586-4.

20

Therapeutic Exercises Part 1: Land Exercises

Janice I. Huntingford[1,2] and Jessy Balc[1]

[1]*Essex Animal Hospital, Essex, Ontario, Canada*
[2]*Chi University, Reddick, FL, USA*

CHAPTER MENU

Introduction

Therapeutic exercises are a crucial component of any patient's rehabilitation program and the cornerstone of veterinary rehabilitation regardless of problem or diagnosis. Exercises need to be tailored to the individual patient considering the clinical diagnosis (a requirement before any exercise prescription), the age of the patient, physical condition, and resources available. Exercises can be used to improve a patient's range of motion (ROM), strength, weight-bearing and gait pattern, flexibility, balance, proprioception, and to decrease pain and improve healing. Exercises also improve strength, aerobic capacity (endurance), and performance and help with weight loss. Therapeutic exercises as part of a home exercise program allow the clients to become involved in their pet's recovery and often strengthen the human–animal bond.

History of Therapeutic Exercise

Physical therapists have been utilizing therapeutic exercises in human medicine since the beginning of physical therapy in the early twentieth century. The aim of therapeutic exercise is to improve function, performance, and disability (Saunders, 2007). Interest in applying these techniques to dogs started in

---

Physical Rehabilitation for Veterinary Technicians and Nurses, Second Edition.
Edited by Mary Ellen Goldberg and Julia E. Tomlinson.
© 2024 John Wiley & Sons, Inc. Published 2024 by John Wiley & Sons, Inc.
Companion website: www.wiley.com/go/goldberg/physicalrehabilitationvettechsandnurses

the mid-1970s with the first publication of a book on canine rehabilitation techniques by Ann Downer MPT (Downer, 1978). Shortly thereafter, national presentations about animal rehabilitation to such groups as the American College of Veterinary Surgeons (ACVS), American Physical Therapy Association (APTA), and the American Veterinary Medical Association (AVMA) led to more interest in canine rehabilitation. A growing interest in canine sports medicine resulted in the formation of the International Racing Greyhound Symposium in 1985. Rehabilitation was a frequent topic at this conference which later included all sporting dogs (McGonagle *et al.*, 2014). In the 1990s, there was the long-awaited publication of two texts: *Care of the Racing Greyhound: A Guide for Trainers* (Craig and Gannon, 1994) and *Canine Sports Medicine and Surgery* (Bloomberg *et al.*, 1998). Today, physical rehabilitation is becoming common in small animal practices. Therapeutic exercises are used not only for recovery but also for wellness care and preventive medicine in the form of weight management and maintenance of muscle strength and conditioning, particularly for athletes and geriatric animals.

The Role of Exercise Physiology

Skeletal muscles perform motions guided by the nervous system. Skeletal muscle performance is dependent on muscle fiber type. Traditionally, muscles are classified as type I (oxidative or slow twitch) or type II (glycolytic or fast twitch) with subclassifications of these two types (Armstrong *et al.*, 1982). However, all muscles consist of a mix of different fiber types, in different ratios depending on the individual muscle and training. Postural muscles (stabilizer muscles) such as the quadriceps femoris are capable of slow and sustained contraction and contain more type I fibers (about 50%) (Lieber *et al.*, 1989) than muscles like the

gracilis, which contain more type II and are speed and power (mobilizing) muscles (Amann *et al.*, 1993). Type I muscle fibers have been thought of as the endurance muscle fibers (found to be more predominant in dogs which run long distances like sled dogs) and type II as the sprinting muscle fibers (for sprinting dogs such as Greyhounds) (Wakshlag *et al.*, 2004). However, when compared to humans, all dogs have a high oxidative capacity in all their muscles and are adapted for endurance activities (Wakshlag *et al.*, 2004). Certain breeds, for example, Greyhounds, do have more fast twitch muscle fibers than others (Guy and Snow, 1981).

When muscles are immobilized, such as in casts or splints, muscle strength decreases rapidly, with as much as 50% of strength lost within the first week (Boyd *et al.*, 2009). With disuse, postural muscles that contain a predominance of type I fibers atrophy more than the mobilizing muscles containing type II fibers. With geriatric sarcopenia (the age-related change in muscles), the epaxial muscles atrophy early in the process in dogs.

A study of live dogs compared epaxial, quadriceps, and temporalis muscle size in aged dogs, and in size and body condition scores matched young dogs. The results showed that epaxial muscles were smaller in aged dogs, but quadriceps and temporal muscles did not differ significantly (Hutchinson *et al.*, 2012). Fiber type loss, however, appears preferential for the large type II (power and strength) fibers (Deschenes *et al.*, 2013), as shown in analysis of cadaver canine biceps femoris muscles (Pagano *et al.*, 2015). This is an important consideration in designing an exercise program for an athlete with muscle loss due to injury, versus a geriatric patient with age-related sarcopenia (Appell, 1990).

Muscle contractions can be described as having two variables: force and length. The force is either tension or load. Load is the force exerted on the muscle by an object and muscle tension is the force the muscle exerts on an object. Isometric contractions occur when muscle tension changes with no change in muscle length. This is a static exercise, for example lifting a front leg so that more weight/load is on the muscles of the contralateral front limb and the rear limbs; these limb muscles are undergoing isometric contractions to support more body weight. Tension bands applied to the standing patient rely on the instinct to lean into pressure. As a patient maintains the same body position under an increased load (whether push or pull), the muscle work has increased without a change in muscle length.

Isotonic contractions occur when the muscle tension remains the same, but the muscle length changes. Isotonic contractions occur as either concentric or eccentric contractions. Concentric contraction occurs when tensions in the muscle increase along with shortening. An example of this would be a human weightlifter performing a biceps curl. Eccentric contraction occurs when the muscle contracts but lengthens because the tension generated in the muscle is insufficient to overcome the load pulling down on the muscle. As the weightlifter slowly releases the biceps curl and extends his elbow to put down the weight the biceps undergoes eccentric contraction. The eccentric contraction controls the movement – it is the natural braking force that occurs during motion (Gillette and Duke, 2014). Eccentric contractions can predispose to injury in untrained individuals (Whitehead *et al.*, 2003). Resistive exercise of all forms leads to the preferential hypertrophy of type II fibers and eccentric contractions render type II fibers more susceptible to damage when compared to type I fibers in humans, rabbits, and rodents (Quindry *et al.*, 2011). In an exercise program, generally, isometric and concentric exercises are performed first to help accustom the muscle to movement. Eccentric

exercises are added later as these have the potential to cause damage to the muscle and delayed-onset muscle soreness, but they help develop greater strength. A balanced program between concentric and eccentric muscle contractions is desired.

Principles of an Exercise Program

When designing an exercise program for a patient the therapist must consider any pathology affecting the cardiovascular, neuromuscular, skeletal, pulmonary, endocrine/metabolic, or integumentary system. These systems can affect muscular performance. As an example, a dog with laryngeal paralysis/polyneuropathy will have some respiratory compromise that needs to be considered during exercise just as a patient with a repaired ligament will have some reduced joint stability early in the healing process. The experience of the client or handler and the willingness of the patient to perform exercises must also be considered. An agility dog with an experienced handler will have a very different exercise program from that of a geriatric companion dog with an inexperienced client.

After evaluating the patient, identifying problems, and the amount of tissue healing that has already taken place (tissue integrity), the therapist must set both long- and short-term goals for the patient. It is important that the client's goals are in line with those of therapist. Each part of the program – proprioception, strength, endurance, and power (speed plus strength) – should have specific goals and these will vary with the patient and with the injury. Exercises should also include relaxation time between bouts, and flexibility exercises specifically tailored to the demands made on the body. It is important for therapists to know as much as we can about the effects of the exercises we use. Although not a lot of information is known about all the exercises we use, where information exists, we should apply it. For example, cross walking (serpentine) on a hill results in a temporary increase in loading of the downside hindlimb, transferring forces off the upside hindlimb, but dogs adapt quickly and compensate – more weight is shifted to the downside forelimb and shorter steps are taken (Strasser *et al.*, 2014). Using a serpentine pattern to start to introduce hills, or to start to increase the workload on a recovering hindlimb may not have the desired effect of significantly increasing the load on that limb beyond the first few steps therefore a different exercise may be more appropriate.

Once the goals are set and the program is designed, it is important for the therapist to evaluate the patient at each visit. Asking and documenting questions about soreness and level of home activity after the last session is crucial. The rehabilitation technician/nurse is instrumental in acquiring this information. This allows the therapist to adjust the program as needed so the patient continues to progress through the rehabilitation process. Therapists should ensure proper, efficient mechanics in motion for their patients. Faulty patient body mechanics must be corrected wherever possible and good fundamentals ingrained. Use a hand or an assistive device to guide as needed. Watch for decline of movement patterns (in gaiting and during transitions) as signs of fatigue. Do not continue an exercise once body mechanics degenerate from the best possible for that patient at that time (even if that best had initially required some assistance). Rest for a period (usually a few minutes), then attempt to resume the exercise. If the exercise cannot be performed to the level it was earlier in the session, then end the session. Ask for an easy motion to end on a good note.

At no time should the patient be harmed or uncomfortable. Chronic overexertion and fatigue can increase susceptibility to injury. According to the International Associations of Athletics Federations, online medical manual (IAAF, 2016) muscular overexertion may present as muscle soreness, muscle stiffness, and muscle spasm. Adaptation to the demands of strengthening exercises occurs gradually, over long periods of time. Efforts to accelerate the process may lead to injury. Conversely, an inadequate training load will not provide an adequate stimulus, and a strengthening of tissues will not occur.

Certain activity patterns are especially likely to cause overtraining (IAAF, 2016). These include a sudden increase in training volume and/or intensity without a gradual build-up and the use of a single, monotonous training format which fatigues one muscle group or energy system. Early warning signs of overtraining include a longer recovery time needed between exercise bouts (patient is tired and stiff for longer than two hours after exercise). In this case, the exercise may be too intense, or the patient may need re-evaluation. Icing post-exercise and prophylactic pain control will be needed, particularly for postoperative patients. In weak, ataxic, or non-ambulatory patients, assistive devices must be used for exercise, and this can include booties to protect feet from scuffing the floor or harnesses or slings to assist in ambulation.

According to McCauley and Van Dyke (2018), there are five variable parameters in any exercise program:

1) Frequency of work done (multiple times per day, daily or weekly)
2) Speed/intensity
3) Duration of work (time or number of reps)
4) Environment (terrain, footing, and substrate)
5) Impact (low, high, or no impact).

As the patient heals, the frequency, intensity, and duration of the exercise are increased to further challenge the patient and to strengthen the muscles. Tendons, bones, and articular cartilage also remodel and "strengthen" with a correctly targeted exercise program. It is usually safe to increase the activity by 10–15% each week if the patient does not experience an increase in pain or a loss of function (Millis *et al.*, 2014).

Canine Rehabilitation Equipment

Physioballs/Peanuts/BOSU® Balls

Exercise balls come in many shapes and sizes and have many different uses. Peanut balls look exactly like a peanut shell, with an indent in the middle providing two separate points of ground contact for added stability over an oval ball. A physio roll is like a peanut ball but lacks the middle indent. Egg-shaped balls have less stability, which makes exercises on these more challenging. Round balls are the most challenging as they allow movement in all directions. A BOSU® ball is flat on one side and has a half-ball attached, allowing the patient to balance on the half-ball side or when flipped over to balance on the flat side (see Figure 20.1).

In general, most ball work will start with an underinflated peanut for the most stability. The therapist should stabilize the

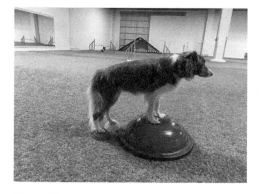

Figure 20.1 Patient on a BOSU® ball working on proprioceptive training.

peanut and allow for only small motions. Make sure the patient has good posture, avoid strengthening one muscle group predominantly over another (e.g., spinal flexors over extensors and resulting in kyphosis), and always follow with a stretch to reverse the motion. As the patient progresses, more air is added for an additional challenge; later, more challenging ball shapes, along with more challenging postures, are used. When introducing a patient to the ball, make it a positive experience by using treats (see Chapter 9). When using balls for exercises, remember that time can be lengthened for sustained muscle contraction, and transitions on the ball can be used for improving both strength and control further. Be cognizant of the type of muscle contraction you are asking for, and hence the muscle fiber type you are targeting. An old dog with weak spinal stabilizing muscles will benefit more from standing still in good posture on a challenging surface, rather than attempting transitions.

- Physioballs can help build strength while also increasing balance and proprioception.
- Peanut balls and BOSU balls are used for beginners as they allow more stability due to increased ground contact. BOSU balls are particularly good for core strengthening. The back legs can be placed on additional equipment to reinforce proprioceptive training.

Cavalettis

Cavaletti poles or ground poles have been used extensively for training horses. In the small animal patient, these poles are used to train gait, improve proprioception, and strengthen the forelimb and hindlimb flexor muscles (see Figure 20.2). They are also used to improve active ROM – specifically, they increase flexion and extension of stifle and flexion of the carpus and elbow along

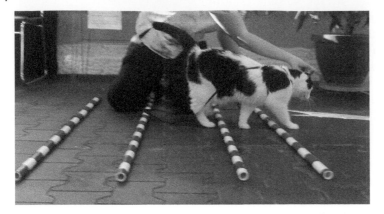

Figure 20.2 Cavaletti poles are a great strengthening exercise for dogs and cats.

with flexion of the tarsus (Holler *et al.*, 2010). Cavalettis are placed in a series and are adjustable in height. They are placed low or on the ground when the patient begins the exercise or has significant muscle weakness. The height can be adjusted as the patient progresses through rehabilitation. They can also be placed in a circular pattern for jumping or as a series of "bounce" jumps for more advanced patients or athletes (Millis *et al.*, 2014). Spacing is patient-dependent; it depends roughly on height and body length, but most importantly on stride length.

Cavalettis are very easy to make using pylons (cones) with holes and PVC pipe or crushed aluminum cans and 2×4-inch planks. For home use, clients can use anything from PVC pipe to broomsticks or even pool noodles, depending on the size of the dog. The cavalettis are spaced so that only one paw at a time is placed between the poles in gaiting over them, thus challenging proprioception as the dog avoids touching the pole. The height of the pole determines how much flexion occurs; more flexor strengthening occurs with higher poles.

- Cavalettis are used for improved proprioception and strengthening. They are a good exercise for dogs and cats ranging from weak geriatric to athletes. They are easy for the client to make at home.

Weave Poles and Cones

These poles and cones are used for circling, walking in figure eight, and weaving (in a serpentine). Weaving in and out of cones creates lateral flexion of the spine, aims to strengthen the adductor and abductor muscles, and improves balance and proprioception. Six to eight traffic cones can be used to make up an obstacle course for the dog to weave in and out of. Alternatively, multiple objects such as bowling pins, water bottles, or a line of trees can be used if they are lined up evenly spaced so the dog can weave in and out of the objects. Vertical weave pole agility sets can be used. An alternate is traffic cones with a pole at the top. The distance between the poles needs to be adjusted so that sufficient lateral bending occurs.

- Weaves can be used to visualize any discrepancy in the patient's gait. The objects can be anything that is lined up in a straight line. Weaves are used to help build core muscles and improve proprioception.

Planks/Blocks/Stairs

Planks are 2×8inch (5×20cm) or 2×10inch (5×25cm) pieces of wood that are 8–10feet (2.5–3.0m) in length. The planks are initially placed on the floor and the dog walks along it while maintaining balance. The plank is then raised up onto cinder blocks. The dog is further challenged by placing blocks as obstacles on the plank.

Blocks are smaller, thicker pieces of wood with a 4×6 inch (10×15 cm) non-slip area. Grip tape can be added (skateboard product). They are made in sets of 2-, 4-, and 6-inch (5, 10, and 15 cm) heights. Alternatively, commercial blocks can be purchased. The dog stands with one foot on each block or any combination of diagonals or front or back paws. Strengthening of the stabilizer muscles of the trunk is emphasized by this exercise.

Stairs can be made of any material and many different types of stairs exist in a home or clinical setting. Climbing stairs is good for proprioceptive training, core muscle strengthening, improved hindlimb weight bearing, and improving ROM of pelvic limb joints (improved extension of hip and hock and improved/increased flexion of stifle and hock) (Durant *et al.*, 2011). Descending stairs is also good for balance and proprioception and should increase forelimb weight bearing.

- Planks, blocks, and stairs strengthen and target proprioception (see Figure 20.3)

Balance Discs or Boards

Balance discs are rounded on both sides, not as curved as a ball, with a side rim of about an inch (2.5 cm) high. Each surface has a different texture. One is smooth, and the other is textured and can provide more grip. Balance discs create an uneven surface that helps to improve balance and strength, in both the digital flexors and in the stabilizer muscles that are activated by the uneven stance the balance disc creates. Balance discs are easier to stand on than balls and can be used alongside other stabilization exercises.

Balance boards are created by laying a piece of plywood over a pillow, water bottle, or ball, thus creating an unstable surface. These can be made by gluing a half tennis ball to the bottom of a piece of plywood that has been covered in indoor/outdoor carpeting, making a non-slip surface.

Limb Weights

Limb weights are small weights that can easily be secured to the limbs. Normally they have a Velcro strap attached to them. With some creativity, limb weights can be manufactured for patients of different sizes. For some dogs, we have used stainless steel washers of various sizes that are readily available in the hardware store. These are wrapped in vet wrap and placed on the limb. Curtain weights also work. The advantage of these small structures is that you can use numerous ones of varying weights to slowly increase the weight on the limb. Limb weights are for more advanced rehabilitation, and they promote natural weight shifting on the diagonal. Commercially available weights are available (e.g., from Canine Icer™).

Elastic Resistant Bands

These (e.g., TheraBands) are 6-inch-wide (15 cm) latex resistance bands that are color-coded for different resistance levels, which are determined by the thickness of the material. They can be used in both

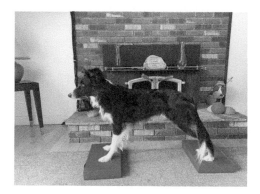

Figure 20.3 A dog working on core strength on blocks.

beginner and advanced therapy and can also be used as a means of pulling a paralyzed leg forward, mimicking regular gait. They can also be used to increase tension and resistance to facilitate muscle development.

Trampoline (Mini)

This is a very useful tool for training proprioception and balance in small dogs and cats (see Figure 20.4). The trampoline causes an uneven surface area that in turn causes multiple muscle firings. It is an excellent tool to increase core strength in small dogs recovering from back surgery and to build up core strength to help prevent back problems in this same group of dogs.

Land Treadmills

Land treadmills provide a great workout for dogs and cats, improving limb strength and increasing cardiovascular endurance. Neurological patients can benefit from treadmills for gait patterning during recovery from paralysis. A board placed across the front of the treadmill allows the front feet to be elevated off the belt while hindlimb gait retraining is concentrated. Small patients can be placed in their carts on a treadmill. Most treadmills can be inclined (or in some cases down to a decline) to work on improving strength or reducing the force placed on front or hind legs. It has been reported that dogs walking on a treadmill with a 5% incline had increased hamstring activity, but that gluteals and quadriceps were not affected (Lauer *et al.*, 2009).

The speed and length of time can be varied to build up endurance and for conditioning. Canine athletes can be conditioned on treadmills with various inclines and various speeds for intervals of

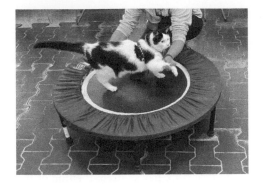

Figure 20.4 A cat on a Mini Trampoline.

20–30 minutes at a fast trot. Most medium to large dogs will comfortably walk at a rate of approximately 2 mph (3.2 km/h) whereas neurological patients must be started at 0.1–0.5 mph (0.2–0.8 km/h). It is important that the therapist evaluate each dog on the treadmill to determine optimal speed and effort while maintaining a normal gait (see Box 20.1). What works for a Golden Retriever may not work for a Border Collie!

Dogs that are leash walked can be easily trained to walk on a treadmill (see Box 20.2). A variety of treadmills can be used for exercising dogs. Specific dog treadmills such as Jog a Dog (inclined treadmills) or Dog Pacers can be purchased, or a human treadmill can be used. If a human treadmill is used, the belt length needs to be long enough to accommodate the dog's stride. An easy guide is to measure the dog laying on their side, forelimbs and rear limbs placed in slight extension at the shoulder (~45° from the line of the spine), measure front foot to rear foot, and add 10 inches. Many medium and large dogs have too long a stride length for the traditional treadmill, especially at trot. Remember that during normal gaiting on land, speed varies. Also, a treadmill has the potential to retrain a patient into an undesirable pattern. Land treadmills can be used for feline patients if the cat is taught slowly (Figure 20.5).

Box 20.1   Treadmill safety

- Always use a leash and harness with the patient. Collars can be dangerous
- Never tie the patient to the treadmill or leave the patient unattended. Stand next to the dog throughout the entire workout
- Do not face the treadmill into a wall – the dog will resist walking "into" the wall
- Lead the patient onto the treadmill using an incentive such as a treat or toy, and then the treadmill can be slowly turned on
- If your treadmill does not have safety walls you may need assistance to keep the pet's attention looking and walking forward. Place one side against the wall so the patient does not fall off the side

- Short intervals are important until the patient gets accustomed to the treadmill. Go slowly and let the patient get acclimatized to the routine
- Always monitor the amount of panting, the pet's gait, body language, and signs of fatigue (excess or rapid panting, glazed eyes, change to gait, (wobbling, staggering) and drooping tongue) the entire time
- Allow rest periods where stretching, massage, and ROM can be performed
- A water dish can be offered during intermission time as well
- Remember that each session should be positive and time on the treadmill should be dictated by the patient's condition and response

Box 20.2   Treadmill introduction

- Walk the dog into the room and around the treadmill while it is off
- Walk the dog up onto the treadmill while it is off, giving treats while on the treadmill. Practice walking on at the back and off at the front. You may want to start to introduce commands for getting on the treadmill and getting off so that the sessions are controlled
- Have the dog sit by the treadmill when it is on, giving cookies so that he or she remains calm and becomes accustomed to the noise
- Place whatever device you will be using while doing the treadmill on your dog (harness/safety vest/leash) and have them get back onto the treadmill
- Never tie the dog to the treadmill. Always hold the leash and stand next to the treadmill in case of emergency
- Slowly turn the treadmill on while feeding cookies to make it a positive experience. Remember that in the beginning taking one step should be

rewarded. As time passes, reward for longer sessions
- You may need to hold the harness so the dog feels comfortable or show a favorite toy to motivate him or her to walk forward
- Unless you know if your dog can chew and walk at the same time (which many cannot) you should reward with praise and pats until the treadmill stops
- Increasing speed and time is not crucial until the dog is comfortable with being on the treadmill. Increasing speed can cause the dog to misstep and cause injury. Increased time can cause fatigue muscle soreness and therapy setback
- The whole point is to have the dog walking on the treadmill in order to strengthen muscles, and increase endurance, as well as a multitude of other reasons. However, the most important thing to remember is – make it fun!

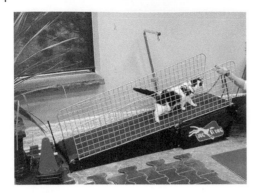

Figure 20.5 Land treadmills can be used with feline patients.

Desirable features for a land treadmill include (McCauley and Van Dyke, 2018):

- belt length long enough to accommodate expected size of dog (minimum 6 feet/2 m)
- incline/decline capacity
- ability to go in reverse direction (hence decline?)
- one button push-start/stop or turn of a knob
- exact speed visible (this allows consistent exercise intervals)
- starting speed of 0.1–0.2 mph (0.2–0.3 km/h)
- side rails.

Control, Supportive, and Assistive Devices

Harnesses, safety vests, and leashes should be used to control the patient during exercise. Harnesses that do not restrict shoulder motion are used for rehabilitation. For patients that are not ambulatory or ataxic, front and rear-end harnesses are used to assist both the patient and the therapist. Booties are used if the surfaces are slippery or if the dog is weak and dragging of the feet may be a problem. Doing exercises over balls, foam rollers, peanuts, or while in a sling can be very useful for neurological patients (see Chapter 11 for more details about this topic).

Walking

Controlled leash walking is an excellent therapeutic exercise. It is easy to do, and dogs usually enjoy it. Health benefits should include increased endurance, strength, cardiovascular fitness, and good mental stimulation. According to Fry et al. obese patients who combined a restricted calorie diet with an exercise program lost more weight and had improved fitness. All dogs can benefit from regular controlled exercise.

Unless the dog is confined for safety and only allowed outside for bathroom privileges, most dogs can start walking soon after surgery. Leash walks generally consist of 5 minutes of activity 2–3 times daily at first and progress each week by 1–5 minutes per walk depending on the patient. Be sure to specify the relative speed of the walk, and the need for continuous walking rather than the stop-and-sniff of a leisure walk. During inclement weather or cold winters, land treadmill walking may be preferable to walking outdoors. Treadmill walking, although it provides exercise, weight-bearing, and strengthening, does not give the dog (or client) any mental stimulation (Saunders, 2007).

Exercise Categories

In the following sections, various exercise categories are discussed:

- Balance and proprioceptive exercises,
- Core strengthening,
- Hindlimb exercises,
- Forelimb exercises,
- Neurological rehabilitation exercises, and
- Exercises for cats.

Balance and Proprioceptive Exercises

Cavaletti Course
This helps with proprioception, strengthening, and gait retraining. Pole heights can

vary, and the distance is case-dependent. The poles are evenly spaced and the animal walks over the poles very slowly. The slow pace allows the animal to step over the poles one paw at a time and recognize their paw location. The goal is to walk over the poles without touching them. It is best to start exercises with five minutes or less twice daily. The pace can be progressed to a trot as patient strength increases, and distance between poles can be lengthened to encourage more limb extension in protraction (longer stride length).

Balance Boards or Balance Discs

These are used for balance, proprioception, and muscle strengthening. Place the targeted legs on the board, elevate the other limbs to the same height to equalize weight bearing, or elevate the other limbs above the board level to increase weight bearing through the affected limb(s). Control the patient with a harness. The board can initially be stabilized to allow only a small ROM in rocking as the patient learns to balance, then as the patient becomes more competent the board can be rocked back and forth. Balance discs or BOSU balls can also be used for this, and at home a firm cushion or air mattress. To increase the balance challenge, the patient take treats from different locations on the board so they will have to shift position while maintaining balance. Start with a small amount of time twice daily and progress as the patient strengthens. Determine amount of time based on in-clinic observations. Watch out for fatigue and postural compensation as a guideline for when to stop and give the client a time limit for home exercise, as well as red flags to look out for (see Figure 20.6).

Weave Cones

Weave cones are generally used to improve proprioception and increase core strength. The exercise can also be pattern-improved for weight bearing when a limb is being

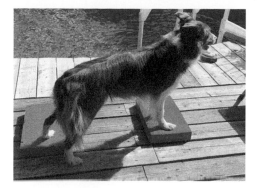

Figure 20.6 Dog working hind limb muscles on uneven surface.

protected after long-term adaptations to pain. Objects, normally 6–8 of them, are lined up about 1–3 feet (30–90 cm) apart (depending on patient size), and the dog is weaved in and out of the objects. Work to have an even number of bends in each direction. The dog needs to learn to pivot sharply at the end of the pattern, and the therapist or client can use their body as a guide to prevent excess lateral motion and to keep the turns tight. Normally, this exercise lasts about five minutes twice a day but based the amount of time on observations in-clinic, looking closely for signs of fatigue (reduced control in the tight turns, reluctance to bend, slowing down, etc.).

Figure Eights

This exercise is also performed using cones and is used to increase balance, coordination, spinal ROM, and weight shifting from one limb to another. It is completed by walking the outline of the number "8" around two cones. The length of figure eight normally is twice the height of the dog and the activity should be performed at a slow speed. The slow speed allows for an increase in spinal ROM. This should be done a few minutes at a time to avoid dizziness.

Blocks

These are used in developing proprioception and core muscles. The animal places one paw on each block in a standing position and holds the stance for increasing periods of time. The blocks can be moved closer to mid-line or both paws can be on one block.

Balance Beam

This is a length of plywood elevated as described above (in the section on Planks/Blocks/Stairs) that the dog walks along and sits on while maintaining their balance or posture. The goal is to have the dog walk along and not step off the beam.

Trampoline, Cushions, Air Mattress

These uneven surfaces help improve weight bearing as well as proprioception. This exercise can be done in many ways. Start with two paws on the uneven surface and move the patient around it, then have the patient walk across the surface. Progress to standing on the surface while the therapist applies gentle pressure to each hip or shoulder in a back-and-forth motion to challenge balance. Be sure to use a harness to control the patient so they do not lose their balance and fall.

Rhythmic Stabilization and Weight Shifting

Weight shifting is used to increase weight bearing and balance. Weight shifting should be done while the dog is standing. Place your thumbs over the dog's pelvis bones and your hands down their sides. Slowly sway side-to-side or front-to-back, making sure both legs are weight-bearing. Do not use enough force to cause the dog to lose their balance. This can also be performed in a supported stance, on a therapy roll, etc.

Ball Work

This targets proprioception, allows for advanced strengthening and balance, and increases core and trunk stability. Most exercises can be performed on a Theraball™. Once the dog has mastered exercises on solid ground, balls can slowly be introduced. To work on balance and proprioception, a large, egg-shaped ball should be used. The goal is to have the dog balance on the unstable surface and eventually perform transitions such as sit-to-stand exercises. More ball work is described in other sections.

Core Strengthening

Crawling

This exercise is great for core strengthening, improving spinal mobility, ROM, and limb strengthening, especially digital flexors. It can be done anywhere and with anything; dogs can crawl under chairs, beds, boxes, and agility tunnels, or they can just learn to crawl along the floor. The higher the "crawling tunnel" that is created, the easier the exercise is for the patient. Begin with short distances and put treats along the tunnel to encourage the patient to move forward. Gradually increase the distance. Remember to add a command word and always reward, while they are learning.

Sit Up and Beg

This helps core strengthening and hind leg strength. Initially, the dogs sit squarely and then get up onto their back legs as though they were begging. Treats will help make this easier to teach. The dog may be unstable, and the therapist may need to hold one front leg until the dog is stronger (higher is easier for the dog). Once, the dog can hold the beg position, asking the dog to stand on their hind legs will strengthen the pelvic limbs. This is done while holding a treat higher. The dog is then asked to get back into the beg position. The up and down from beg to stand is like performing squats for humans. Eventually, work up to two sets of 8–10 twice daily. This exercise should not be done if the dog has significant spinal or hip issues. Monitor for discomfort after this exercise.

Diagonal Leg Lifts

This exercise helps with core strengthening but also balance, weight shifting, and leg strengthening. The stance is achieved by lifting one leg off the ground along with the diagonal leg. Both legs are to be lifted at the same time and minimal support to the limbs should be provided so the dog can balance (see Figure 20.7). Hold this pose for 10–30 seconds and repeat 8–10 times. When this exercise is easy for the dog, progress to having the dog stand on four blocks and then lift the diagonal legs. Finally, add some weight shifting to cause the dog to balance further.

Diagonal leg lifts on a therapy ball are another possibility and these can be done as further challenge for the dog.

Planking on a Ball or BOSU

There are many ways this exercise can be done depending on the focus of the exercise. The dog may stand with their front legs on one peanut ball, their back legs on

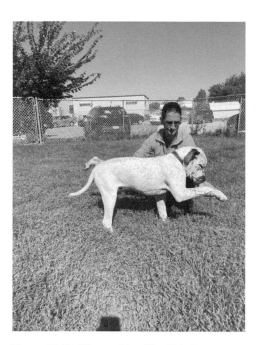

Figure 20.7 Diagonal leg lifts: This is a core strengthening exercise. As the patient's balance and core muscles improve, the legs can be lifted higher.

another ball, or front legs on a BOSU or ball and back legs on a balance disc or on the ground. The ball may also be moved while the dog is on it, rolled forward, or side to side while the dog balances. Alternatively, the dog may be asked to keep its front legs on the ball and walk around the ball.

Side Sit-Up

This exercise builds core strength but also increases spinal ROM. The dog should lie laterally. Using a treat, lure the dog up sideways, as if they were doing a sit-up sideways. Try to hold for five seconds then return to lateral. Do up to 10 reps per set. Dogs with spinal problems should be cleared before doing this exercise.

Hindlimb Exercises

Sit-to-Stand

This exercise aims to improve strength in the pelvic limbs. When performing this exercise, it is important to ensure that the dog sits squarely and that on transition to standing, both pelvic limbs are used to propel the rear into extension. The patient should not pull themselves forward with the front limbs. A square sit occurs when the hips, stifles, and tarsi are in a straight line with the shoulders. The shoulders are perfectly aligned with the carpal joints. If the dog kicks one leg out to the side the therapist should have the dog stand again and sit while the therapist places their leg against the dog's paw, thus ensuring a square sit. Alternatively, the dog could be asked to sit against the wall with the affected leg against the wall, thus preventing the leg from moving laterally. This exercise can be repeated over and over for increased strengthening.

Backward Walking

This exercise aims to strengthen the pelvic limbs and increase balance, coordination, and proprioception. We do not know the effects on specific muscles, only that the stance and swing phases of all four limbs are shorter with backward walking but that hip, stifle, shoulder, and elbow ROM are similar for forward and backward motion. There is some reduced ROM in carpus and tarsus, although this varied between the dogs studied (Vilensky and Cook, 2000). This exercise is easier to start with the dog parallel to a wall, a sofa, or anything straight. The therapist should hold a treat at their chest level and walk toward the dog saying "Back." Most dogs will try to turn while they are learning to walk backward, so it is important to give a reward when the dog takes a step backward. Another way of training this is to have a couch parallel to the wall just far enough from the wall that the dog cannot turn around. Lure the dog in forward with a treat, then say "Back" and encourage the dog to walk backward for another treat. This is an important exercise to teach all dogs and puppies at some time in their lives. All dogs need good hindlimb awareness.

Side Stepping

This exercise aims to improve both forelimb and hindlimb strength as well as proprioception and balance. The therapist stands facing the side of the dog, grasps the dog's collar in one hand, and holds the other hand on the dog's opposite hip. The therapist then walks toward the dog, encouraging the dog to sidestep. An alternate method is to use a treat to keep the head focused forward, one hand on the hip, and gently walk into the dog. If there is a problem controlling the back end of the dog during this exercise, a front and back-end harness can be used for extra back-end control. This exercise needs to be performed in both directions to target the muscles symmetrically.

Incline Walking

Incline walking helps build muscle in the rear legs due to the weight being shifted toward the back. On a treadmill, an incline has been shown to predominantly increase hamstring muscle activity versus gluteal and quadriceps activity (Lauer *et al.*, 2009). Incline walking increases stifle joint flexion (Holler *et al.*, 2010). This exercise should be started with shallow inclines and then steeper inclines can be added when the pet is comfortable and adjusting well. Serpentine or cross-hill walking can also be incorporated, where the patient walks in a zigzag pattern across the hill up and down (see section on Principles of Exercise Program). Start with 5 minutes and gradually work up to 20 minutes twice daily, incorporating hills.

Stairs

Stair ascent increases extension of the hip (coxofemoral) and hock joints and results in reduced stifle extension when compared with level walking (see Figure 20.8). The stairs also increase maximal flexion of the stifle and hock with each stride

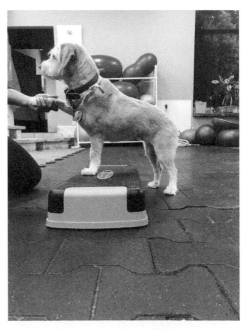

Figure 20.8 Stairs can work many different muscle groups.

(Durant *et al.*, 2011). An example of therapeutic use would be for a patient with reduced flexion ROM in the hock (e.g., postsurgical osteochondritis dissecans) therapy would include stair ascent starting with low-rise steps at the appropriate time in recovery. Descending stairs increases ROM in the hip, stifle, and tarsal joints versus walking on a decline slope (Millard *et al.*, 2010).

Loving on Stairs/Couch

This exercise is used to improve rear leg weight bearing and strength, ROM, and hip extension. The client sits on the stairs/couch. With the dog's back legs firmly on the ground, lift up the front legs and place them one/two stairs up or on the couch cushion (height is dependent on dog's body length). This causes the dog's weight to be shifted to the pelvic limbs, and the weaker back legs must support most of the body's weight. While the pet is standing up on their back legs, praise them and give love or treats so that the time passes quickly.

Crawling or Tunnels

This exercise has been described in the section on Core Exercises.

Cavaletti

Cavaletti walking results in increasing flexion of the stifle and tarsal joints and increases extension of the stifle joint (Holler *et al.*, 2010). This exercise has been described in the section on Balance Exercises.

Zink-Zeus Get Up

This exercise was created by Dr. Christine Zink as an exercise she used with her patient Zeus. It is one of the most challenging hindlimb exercises and one that many dogs dislike performing. With the dog lying in lateral recumbency, the therapist holds the top paw. While holding the paw so it cannot be used to assist the movement, a treat is used to lure the dog into a standing position. If the dog will not lay laterally, the exercise can be started with the dog in sternal recumbency. Initially, most dogs can only do 1–2 reps of this exercise (Zink, 2018). It is important to do this with caution and make sure the dog is not overcompensating with another limb or a truncal twist.

Ladder Walking

This exercise aims to strengthen the legs and improve ROM, balance, coordination, and proprioception. The exercise is performed with a ladder placed flat on the ground. This exercise is like cavalettis but can change in difficulty. Initially, the dog walks forward over the rungs but can be taught to walk backward and sidestep through the ladder. This exercise should start at five minutes twice daily and work up in frequency.

Front Limb Exercises

High Five Salute

High five salute helps with ROM and strengthening of front legs. To perform this exercise, the dog should be sitting. The dog then brings the paw up to their head and away as though saluting. This exercise does take some training for most dogs. When "giving a paw," dogs usually only move their forelimb distal to the elbow. In this exercise, they need to move their shoulder, which allows the paw to get up to their head. In this way, the extensors of the shoulder and limb protractor muscles are targeted, and if the paw is placed in various locations, then abductors and adductors can also be strengthened. Start by holding a treat in your hand. When the dog paws at the treat, the reward is given. Move the hand higher and into the position you wish the dog to stretch.

Wheelbarrow

Wheelbarrow targets the front limbs and the core. This may seem like an easy exercise, but it is quite challenging and needs to be done slowly and cautiously. First, never just pick the dog or cat up with their pelvic limbs, as that is a great deal of load on them and you need to assess patient compliance. Start with lifting the patient by the caudal part of the abdomen or under the pelvis so that the rear legs are a few inches off the ground. Observe contractions of the core muscles. Keep the stationary position for a while until the dog is comfortable with being lifted. Second, slow movement forward and backward can be added, making sure that the animal's spinal alignment is monitored. Advancing the exercise, the rear legs can be lifted, and the patient balances on the front limbs. Use treats to lure the patient. The spine should be perfectly straight to prevent injury. Do not push the patient too quickly; this can cause tripping, leading to the dog's head hitting the ground. Do not perform this exercise with a patient with significant spinal issues, shoulder pain, or carpal hyperextension.

Stairs

This exercise (as discussed earlier) is like walking on a decline and the stairs or decline should start out shallow and gradually become steeper as the patient progresses. Changes should only be added when the pet is comfortable and adjusting well. Time may be increased as the patient becomes stronger.

Crawling or Tunnels

This exercise has been described in the section on Core Exercises.

Cavaletti

Forelimbs show increased flexion of the carpus and elbow over cavalettis (Holler *et al.*, 2010). This exercise is described in the section on Balance Exercises.

Play Bow

This exercise aims to increase forelimb strength and flexibility and to promote core strengthening. The therapist holds a treat in one hand and the other hand is under the abdomen. The treat is moved to the floor and the dog's head and shoulders follow while the abdomen is being held up so back legs are standing, and front legs are down.

Digging

This exercise aims to strengthen the front limbs, improve ROM in flexion, improve proprioception, and increase core strength. When performing this exercise, it is beneficial to have a command and a designated area where digging can occur. Sand, soft soil, or snow when in season are good substrates when they are not too packed down. Stones can hurt their paws and should not be used. A treat or favorite bone can be buried and dug up. Caution: some clients do not wish to encourage digging!

Ladder Walking

This has been described in the section on Hindlimb Exercise but also works well for forelimbs.

Neurological Rehabilitation Exercises

See also Chapter 12 for more information.

Assisted Standing

This exercise is important to build and maintain muscles needed for balance, proprioception, and locomotion. These muscles become atrophied if not used frequently, for example, in a paretic patient (see Figure 20.9). A therapy ball, rolled towel, cushion, foam roller, or other device (depending on the size of the dog) is placed under the dog's abdomen. While performing assisted standing, it is crucial to keep the pet's feet in normal anatomically correct standing position without knuckling. Larger dogs normally require additional abdominal support from a sling or back-end harness. Frequently, the feet need to be positioned by two people. Smaller dogs and cats generally require only one person if

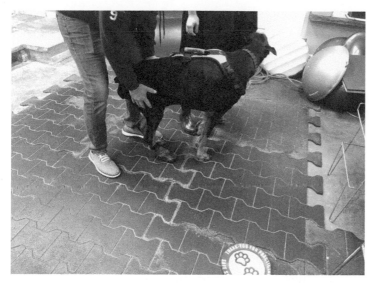

Figure 20.9 Assisted standing is a good exercise for neurological patients.

their abdomen is supported by a Theraball™. Aim to keep the patient's spine as close to a normal standing posture as possible, not kyphotic. Assisted standing should only last until the first signs of fatigue. After a brief rest, it can be repeated, but do not exhaust the patient.

Physioball Work

Balls are particularly important for rehabilitation of neurological patients. They can be used for assisted standing as described earlier, as well as for assisted walking and to regain balance and coordination. Frequently, the front end of the patient is placed on the ball and the ball is rocked back and forth. Foot placing by a second therapist may be required.

Weight Shifting

Neurological patients need to practice balancing on three limbs to mimic the transient unloading of a limb during ambulation. To perform this exercise, the therapist places the dog or cat in a standing position and lifts one limb. When they start to sway, the limb is replaced. All four paws are rotated through this exercise.

Treadmill Gait Training

Land treadmills are used for gait retraining for neurological patients. Many times, the patient must be supported with a sling. The therapist moves the dog's legs in a walking gait pattern: RR to RF, LR to LF (Zink, 2018). Skin sensation stimulus (vibrations, scratching, or even e-stim) can be used to overcome spasticity. As the gait becomes more normal, incline can be added.

Proprioceptive Neuromuscular Facilitation (PNF) Patterns

PNF has been around since the 1930s when neurology physician Herman Kabat began to use the technique on his patients. He found that by stimulating the distal segments, the proprioceptive nerves in more proximal segments became stimulated. His purpose was to enhance and create movement in areas where the neurological system has been compromised. His techniques were based on the principles that describe the rhythmic and reflexive actions that lead to coordinated motion. PNF uses the body's proprioceptive system to facilitate or inhibit muscle contraction (Stillman, 1966). PNF patterns mimic the dog's running motions and other normal functions of daily living (scratching and digging). To perform a PNF pattern for running, lay the dog on their side and mimic the running pattern, then mimic in a supported stance if possible. The therapist should use one hand to mimic the ground contact at the appropriate part of the gait cycle (Edge-Hughes, 2012).

Tactile Stimulation

Tapping or using a vibrating massager over a muscle belly aims to elicit muscle contractions and stimulate the neural receptors (muscle spindle cells and Golgi tendon organs) in muscle and tendon. This should be done for 3–5 minutes a few times a day as part of the nursing care for animals recovering from paralysis. Keep moving the stimulus as mechanoreceptors quickly damp. Brushing, scratching, pinching, or using a vibrating massager provides additional sensory stimulation to skin receptors to increase input into the nervous system.

Tensor Bandaging, Thundershirts™, or Snuglis™

The principle of using tensor bandages or Thundershirts for neurological dogs is to increase sensation in cutaneous and deeper tissues and so increase body awareness. The increased sensation input to higher centers can help with neurological coordination.

Exercises for Cats

Cats can be challenging when it comes to rehabilitation. The principles of exercise are the same for cats as for dogs, but the personality of the cat may limit what the therapist can do. Cats are commonly presented for rehabilitation due to chronic pain from injuries, obesity needing weight loss, or because of osteoarthritis, which is common in cats. Cats can require rehabilitation following surgery for such conditions as cruciate rupture or patellar luxation. A few examples are listed here.

Proprioceptive Exercises

These may include balance and rocker boards standing on a therapy ball or using a rocking chair or glider as the uneven surface (see Figure 20.10). Initially, some cats will only tolerate 30 seconds of exercise but may work up to 2 or 3 minutes as they become more comfortable. It is important that the therapist understand cat body language and discontinue the exercise, as soon as the cat starts to become agitated.

Treadmill Training

Cats can be trained to walk on land or underwater treadmills. If the cat is amenable to wearing a harness, then leash walking and use of a land treadmill with assistance can be used to improve weight bearing and limb function (Millis *et al.*, 2014). Movement can be encouraged by attaching a feather or small toy to a string and pulling it in front of the cat.

Cavaletti Rails

Some cats can be trained to walk over cavaletti rails, particularly if they are food motivated. Some cats will respond to treats – others need to be encouraged by toys or by chasing a laser pointer over the rails.

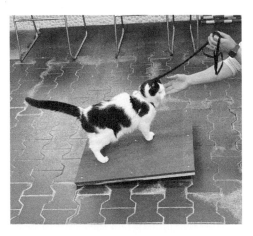

Figure 20.10   A cat on a rocker board.

Case Studies

Case Study 1   Post T12–L1 Hemilaminectomy

Signalment/History

A five-year-old, male neutered Dachshund, Apollo, presented three weeks post hemi-laminectomy surgery with weakness in hind legs (paraparesis). Radiographs and blood work were not presented for evaluation. Dog was not currently on any pain medication and had been cage rested since surgery. Client had installed yoga mats and ramps at home where needed to prevent slipping. Apollo was classified as motor but non-ambulatory at this time.

Clinical Signs

- Non-ambulatory weakness in the rear causing diffuse muscle atrophy.
- Unable to sit/stand squarely without support, unable to transition from down to stand.
- Panniculus/cutaneous trunci reflex cuts off at L1 on the right and L2 on the left.
- Absent conscious proprioception in the pelvic limbs. Sensation and reflexes to the pelvic limb are normal. There is motor function when stimulated.
- Left pelvic limb weaker than right, moderate muscle atrophy of the hamstring group, quadriceps, biceps femoris, tensor fascia latae, and gracillis.
- Shoulder muscles have high tone with myofascial trigger points in triceps and deltoid muscles.
- Normal ROM of all joints and symmetrical muscle mass measurements.

Goals

Improve neurological function, muscle mass, muscle strength, and regain ability to ambulate properly.

Therapy

Therapies that were recommended were acupuncture and electro-acupuncture (ACUP/EAP), therapeutic laser, underwater treadmill (UWTM), home exercises, and supplements.

Client left pet at the clinic for two weeks allowing the following therapies to be performed: in hospital-exercise, ACUP/EAP, and UWTM.

Daily exercises included PNF patterning for walking, PNF patterning for scratching the ear, and square sit-to-stands with assistance, along with assisted standing, stretching, and massage.

ACUP/EAP with points GV-14, BAIHAI, BL-11, BL-18, BL-25, JIN JIAO, SHEN SHU, SHEN PENG, SHEN JIAO, BL-40, BL-54, BL-60, KID-1, and BA FENG for dry needle and GV-14 TO BAIHAI, BL-11 to BL-25 for EAP.

UWTM was performed every other day with the parameters of 6.5″ water height and 0.2 mph speed. The three sessions were three minutes long which allowed for gait patterning to be performed that decreased over time due to tail pinching.

ACUP/EAP occurred twice weekly, while at the clinic and exercises were done daily. Once the owner returned, she continued home exercises daily and brought Apollo in for therapy initially twice weekly then decreased to once weekly.

The left hind required more stimulation as it was weaker. PNF patterning for walking was taught to the client and was performed in clinic. PNF patterning for scratching the ear was also demonstrated. Square sit-to-stands with assistance were performed along with assisted standing.

Gait patterning was performed on the underwater treadmill.

A re-evaluation performed 11 weeks post-surgery indicated improvement in muscle mass, daily performance, and function. Recommended increase of protein intake to help rebuild muscle and continue doing daily exercises at home while continuing ACUP sessions every other week and UWTM weekly.

Home Exercise Program

- *Sit-to-stands assisted 10 reps 3 times each* – twice daily.
- *Cavaletti course with pool noodles* – work up to five minutes twice daily.
- *Weave poles – 10 reps* – twice daily.
- Walking on a non-slip surface is slow enough that the patient can correct their foot placement. Start walking five minutes a day and increase weekly by five minutes if no issues or new paw sores. It is recommended to break the walks up into twice daily.
- *Abdominal bandage walking* – walk for 5–10 minutes with a belly band around the dog's abdomen and tie it fairly snug (For urinary incontinence).
- *Dog kegels* – stimulate the area between the anus and the testicles with an electric toothbrush. While doing this lift one of the back legs and watch to see if the anus puckers. Do this 5–10 times twice daily (For urinary incontinence).
- *Treat stretches* – 8–10 reps of each exercise we added later.

Outcome

Fifteen weeks post-surgery, therapy goals were within reach however therapeutic exercises will need to continue long-term to help build and maintain muscle mass. Re-evaluation in a month would be the next step.

Case Study 2   Iliopsoas Injury and Partial Cranial Cruciate Ligament Tear

Signalment/History

A six-year-old male neutered Golden Retriever presented for rehabilitation one week after tentative diagnosis of a partial cranial cruciate tear and an iliopsoas muscle injury. Radiographs and musculoskeletal ultrasound were performed to confirm diagnosis. The dog had been injured by falling from an A-frame during an agility run three weeks prior to presentation.

Clinical Signs

- Iliopsoas pain and spasm on right side.
- Slight drawer in flexion right stifle with very mild restricted ROM in flexion.
- Partial weight bearing and mild muscle atrophy right pelvic limb (1 cm discrepancy in circumference).
- Pain on ambulation, particularly extension of right pelvic limb and in left sacroiliac joint.
- Shoulder muscles have high resting tone and myofascial trigger points in triceps.

Goals

Relieve pain, normalize ROM, improve ambulation, strengthen muscle, and improve weight bearing.

Therapy

Therapeutic ultrasound, passive range of motion (PROM), and stretching helped relieve pain. Pain medication and herbs were also prescribed. Hydrotherapy was used to aid with strengthening.

Therapeutic exercises in hospital and at home were used to aid recovery.

Exercise Plan

Warm-up right pelvic limb with hot packs applied for 10 minutes to iliopsoas and biceps femoris muscle. Massage and stretching were performed before exercise to improve circulation and help with pain relief.

Exercise sessions up to 20 minutes. Icing was done post-exercise for 5–10 minutes. In hospital, exercises consisted of cavaletti course (cones with poles 4 inches [10 cm] high) for 5 minutes total with a few 10- to 30-second breaks. Weave poles 30 inches (76 cm) apart 6 cones in total; figure eights, slow circles, and turns for 5 minutes total with a few 10- to 30-second breaks; rhythmic stabilization on a rocker board 3 sets of 30 seconds each; side-stepping initially 3 sets of 30 seconds each; 5 sit-to-stand exercises; backward walking 8–10 feet (2.4–3 m) 3 times; and treat stretches and twists. In hospital, exercises were to be done 2–3 times weekly.

Home Exercise Plan

Client was instructed to hot pack the pelvic limbs for 10 minutes before exercising and ice for 10 minutes following exercise. After hot packing the limbs, stretching was performed with the dog standing and one leg stabilized above the stifle, mimicking sitting position with a stretch and hold of 15 seconds. After that, the leg was moved in a bicycling motion. Lastly, the limb was stretched gently in adduction and abduction. Stretches were performed five times before the exercise session.

Home Exercises

- *Loving on the stairs with a twist* – This patient had pressure added to each side of the body to sway him back and forth while he was standing on a cushion. This increased the firing of the muscle that allowed him to improve his overall balance even more since he was standing on an uneven surface. This was to be performed twice daily for 10 repetitions.
- Cavalettis, weave poles, and figure eights were to be done twice daily and at a slow pace.
- *Challenged standing* – This exercise was performed at least twice daily with 10–15 repetitions per performance.
- *Play bow* – This exercise was done twice daily and worked up to 15 repetitions each session.
- *Side-stepping* – This dog had a lot of obedience training and already knew how to walk sideways, so the duration was increased to 20–30 feet (6–9 m) 5 times twice daily.
- *Sit-to-stands* – This dog sat to one side on their left hip and abducted their right hip. To correct this the client needed to position the dog against a fence/wall with their right leg touching the wall while he sat. This removed the ability for the hip to abduct and the patient sat. Repetition was set at 15 sit-to-stands 3 times a day every day and the emphasis was on square sitting.
- *Treat stretches or twists* – Twice daily for five minutes combined.
- Backward walking and backward walking upstairs/hill – In this case, he was already able to walk backward and was trained to do so previously, so the length was increased to 20 feet (6 m) 3 times a day with 5 repetitions each session.

Three weeks after the initial rehabilitation consult the client was having a few issues with the at-home exercises. The client was also finding it hard to keep the dog rested, as there was more than one dog in the house.

- *Walking backward* – There was a complication with the backward walking as the dog started to turn while walking backward since he was still favoring the right rear leg. It was recommended to walk along the fence line instead so that the dog was unable to turn.
- *Walking backward up hills* – The dog would only do two stairs backward and then stop. The easiest solution would be to continue doing the two stairs multiple times per day if the dog was not willing to walk backward up more than those two steps.
- Leash walks were allowed for 10 minutes 2–3 times daily. The duration could be increased by 10 minutes each week but no off-leash running/play was allowed.

Five weeks after the rehabilitation consult the dog was doing much better. The iliopsoas muscle did not have any trigger points and muscle mass started to rebuild in hind right leg. The dog was sitting squarely almost every sit and the restriction of leashed bathroom break was removed.

Home exercises were continued with the addition of 30-minute walks and zig-zag hill walking.

Outcome

By 10 weeks the dog had normal ROM and even muscle girth with no visible lameness and was discharged from rehabilitation.

References

Amann, J.F., Wharton, R.E., Madsen, R.W., and Laughlin, M.H. (1993). Comparison of muscle cell fiber types and oxidative capacity in gracilis, rectus femoris, and triceps brachii muscles in the ferret (*Mustela putorius furo*) and the domestic dog (*Canis familiaris*). *Anat Rec* 236 (4): 611–618.

Appell, H.J. (1990). Muscular atrophy following mobilization – A review. *Sports Med* 10: 42–58.

Armstrong, R.B., Sauber, C.W.T., Seeherman, H.J., and Taylor, C.R. (1982). Distribution of fibertypes in locomotory muscles of dogs. *Am J Anat* 163: 87–98.

Bloomberg, M.S., Dee, J.F., and Taylor, R.A. (1998). *Canine Sports Medicine and Surgery*. St. Louis, MO: Saunders/Elsevier.

Boyd, A.S., Benjamin, H.J., and Asplund, C. (2009). Splints and casts: Indications and methods. *Am Family Phys* 80 (5): 491–499.

Craig AM, Gannon JL, and Blythe LL (1994) *Care of the Racing Greyhound: A Guide for Trainers*. American Greyhound Council.

Deschenes, M.R., Gaertner, J.R., and O'Reilly, S. (2013). The effects of sarcopenia on muscles with different recruitment patterns and myofiber profiles. *Curr Aging Sci* 6 (3): 266–272.

Downer, A. (1978). *Physical Therapy for Animals: Selected Techniques*. Springfield, IL: Thomas Publishers.

Durant, A.M., Millis, D.L., and Headrick, J.F. (2011). Kinematics of stair ascent in healthy dogs. *Vet Comp Orthop Traumatol* 24 (2): 99–105.

Edge-Hughes, L. (2012). Conservative management of chondrodystrophic dogs with thoracolumbar intervertebral disc disease (IVDD). *CHAP Newsl* 12: 4–6.

Gillette, R. and Duke, R.B. (2014). Basics of exercise physiology. In: *Canine Rehabilitation and Physical Therapy*, 2nde (ed. D.L. Millis and D. Levine), 155–161. Philadelphia, PA: WB Saunders.

Guy, P.S. and Snow, D.H. (1981). Skeletal muscle fibre composition in the dog and its relationship to athletic ability. *Res Vet Sci* 31 (2): 244–248.

Holler, P.J., Brazda, V., Dal-Bianco, B. et al. (2010). Kinematic motion analysis of the joints of the forelimbs and hind limbs of dogs during walking exercise regimens. *Am J Vet Res* 71: 734–740.

Hutchinson, D., Sutherland-Smith, J., Watson, A.L., and Freeman, L.M. (2012). Assessment of methods of evaluating sarcopenia in old dogs. *Am J Vet Res* 73 (11): 1794–1800.

IAAF (International Associations of Athletics Federations) (2016) Official Documents: Medical. http://www.iaaf.org/about-iaaf/documents/medical (accessed May 9, 2016).

Lauer, S.K., Hillman, R.B., Li, L., and Hosgood, G.L. (2009). Effects of treadmill inclination on electromyographic activity and hind limb kinematics in healthy hounds at a walk. *Am J Vet Res* 70: 658–664.

Lieber, R.L., McKee-Woodburn, T., and Gershuni, D.H. (1989). Recovery of the dog quadriceps after 10 weeks of immobilization followed by 4 weeks of remobilization. *J Orthop Res* 7 (3): 408–412.

McCauley, L. and Van Dyke, J.B. (2018). Therapeutic exercise. In: *Canine Sports Medicine and Rehabilitation* (ed. M.C. Zink and J.B. Van Dyke), 132–157. Ames, IA: John Wiley & Sons, Inc.

McGonagle, L., Blythe, L., and Levine, D. (2014). History of canine physical rehabilitation. In: *Canine Rehabilitation and Physical Therapy*, 2nde (ed. D.L. Millis and D. Levine), 1–7. Philadelphia, PA: WB Saunders.

Millard, R.P., Headrick, J.F., and Millis, D.L. (2010). Kinematic analysis of the pelvic limbs of healthy dogs during stair and decline slope walking. *J Small Anim Pract* 51: 419–422.

Millis, D.L., Drum, M., and Levine, D. (2014). Therapeutic exercises: Joint motion, strengthening, endurance and speed exercises. In: *Canine Rehabilitation and Physical Therapy*, 2nde (ed. D.L. Millis and D. Levine), 506–525. Philadelphia, PA: WB Saunders.

Pagano, T.B., Wojcik, S., Costagliola, A. et al. (2015). Age related skeletal muscle atrophy and upregulation of autophagy in dogs. *Vet J* 206: 54–60.

Quindry, J., Miller, L., McGinnis, G. et al. (2011). Muscle-fiber type and blood oxidative stress after eccentric exercise. *Int J Sport Nutr Exerc Metab* 21 (6): 462–470.

Saunders, D.G. (2007). Therapeutic exercise. *Clin Tech Sm Ani Pract* 9 (3): 155–159.

Stillman, B.C. (1966). A discussion on the use of muscle stretch in re-education. *Aust J Physiother* 12 (2): 57–61.

Strasser, T., Peham, C., and Bockstahler, B.A. (2014). A comparison of ground reaction forces during level and cross-slope walking in Labrador Retrievers. *BMC Vet Res* 10: 241.

Vilensky, J.A. and Cook, J.A. (2000). Do quadrupeds require a change in trunk posture to walk backward? *J Biomech* 33 (8): 911–916.

Wakshlag, J.J., Cooper, B.J., Wakshlag, R.R. et al. (2004). Biochemical evaluation of mitochondrial respiratory chain enzymes in canine skeletal muscle. *Am J Vet Res* 65: 480–484.

Whitehead, N.P., Morgan, D.L., Gregory, J.E., and Proske, U. (2003). Rises in whole muscle passive tension of mammalian muscle after eccentric contractions at different lengths. *J Appl Physiol* 95 (3): 1224–1234.

Zink, M.C. (2018). Conditioning and retraining the canine athlete. In: *Canine Sports Medicine and Rehabilitation* (ed. M.C. Zink and J.B. Van Dyke), 132–157. Ames, IA: John Wiley & Sons, Inc.

21

Therapeutic Exercises Part 2: Hydrotherapy (Aquatic Therapy)

Pádraig Egan

East Neuk Veterinary Clinic, Scotland

CHAPTER MENU

Introduction

Principles of Hydrotherapy

The definitive goal of aquatic therapy is ultimately to make the patient more functional on land in a faster time frame in comparison to land-based therapy alone. Swimming and underwater treadmill (UWTM) walking remain the most commonly encountered aquatic therapies in veterinary medicine.

Physics of Hydrotherapy

To gain an understanding of how aquatic therapy differs from land-based therapy, you must understand the properties of water and how those properties act on the patient during hydrotherapy.

Density and Buoyancy

The density of an object determines whether it will sink or float when placed in water. In hydrotherapy, we look at the relative density of an object, which is described as a ratio between the object's weight and the weight of an equal volume of water. If an object's density is less than that of water it tends to float and if an object's density is greater than that of water the object tends to sink. The relative density of an object, or in our case a

Physical Rehabilitation for Veterinary Technicians and Nurses, Second Edition.
Edited by Mary Ellen Goldberg and Julia E. Tomlinson.
© 2024 John Wiley & Sons, Inc. Published 2024 by John Wiley & Sons, Inc.
Companion website: www.wiley.com/go/goldberg/physicalrehabilitationvettechsandnurses

patient, is dependent on the patient's body composition and it is related to the patient's skeletal mass, muscle mass, and body fat percentage (Prydie and Hewitt, 2015). When a patient is immersed in water there are two main forces acting on them – gravity and buoyancy. Gravity is attempting to submerge the patient, while buoyancy provides upward thrust, which counteracts gravity. A patient's center of buoyancy depends on their body conformation, and on the volume of fat and muscle that makes up their body. The water level of a UWTM can be changed as required, and the percentage of bodyweight carried by a dog's limbs while using the treadmill can be changed by varying depths. Basically, the deeper the water, the less bodyweight is loaded onto the limbs (Tomlinson, 2013).

Hydrostatic Pressure

Hydrostatic pressure is the sum of pressure on a body surface exerted by the fluid that it is immersed in (Connell and Monk, 2010). The hydrostatic pressure exerted on the patient is directly proportional to the depth and density of the water that they are standing in. Hydrostatic pressure increases with increased depth and density of water. Density of water is temperature-dependent. Increased hydrostatic pressures during hydrotherapy can reduce edema by moving tissue fluid from the extravascular space to the intravascular space. Increased hydrostatic pressure also has a direct effect on cardiac function; peripheral blood flow venous return has been shown to increase as hydrostatic pressure increases, and this can lead to a 10–15% drop in heart rate (Levine *et al.*, 2014). It has also been established that increased hydrostatic pressures during aquatic therapy can reduce pain during exercise. The elevated hydrostatic pressure of water blocks the pain response by acting on mechanoreceptors in the skin, which send signals to the cerebral cortex, downregulating pain pathways (Prydie and Hewitt, 2015).

Viscosity and Resistance

Water molecules are attracted to each other and objects moving through them. This attraction generates frictional resistance to movement of an object through water. Marine animals are adapted to have streamlined bodies that enable lower friction (drag) when moving through water. Our canine patients lack these adaptations and we can use this to our advantage; the drag of movement through water provides more resistance to muscles than walking through air (Prydie and Hewitt, 2015). Viscosity is a measure of fluid friction, with more viscous substances generating more resistance to movement. We can alter the viscosity of the water in a pool or UWTM by altering the temperature of the water. Cold water is denser than warm water and is therefore more viscous and vice versa. The friction created by moving through water helps provide sensory feedback to patients via their skin. This may help, particularly in the rehabilitation of neurological patients who have damaged sensory positional awareness. Gait is exaggerated and gait speed is slowed by water viscosity. This is of benefit in patients recovering from neurological injury and is also useful as it allows more accurate assessment of a patient's gait, especially when walking on a UWTM.

Surface Tension

The attractive force exerted between water molecules on the surface of a body of water is described as surface tension. Water molecules stick to each other with more force at the surface of a body of water than underneath the surface. This means that there is higher resistance to movement at the surface of a body of water in comparison to below the surface. For patients, this means that it requires more effort to move a limb in and out of water ("break the surface of the water") than if the limb remains submerged 100% of the time. As therapists, we can use this to increase force of motion on a joint (or limb segment) by adjusting where the surface of the water lies.

Refraction

The path of light is altered as it passes across the boundary between two substances of differing density (e g , air to water). This is known as refraction. It alters the patient's depth perception, which can make animals misjudge their foot placement on steps and ramps during water entry and exit. Care must be taken when transferring patients into and out of water. The refraction of light may also alter the therapist's perception of a patient's limb movement under water.

Clinical Evidence

There is a paucity of evidence-based literature within the field of veterinary aquatic rehabilitation in comparison to human rehabilitation. There is currently a need for well-constructed research projects to evaluate the benefits of aquatic therapy across an array of orthopedic and neurological conditions. The main areas of research so far have revolved around using aquatic therapy to rehabilitate patients after cruciate ligament surgery and have largely been driven by the economic importance of cruciate disease (Wilke *et al.*, 2005). One study (Preston and Wills, 2018) evaluated the effect of a single hydrotherapy session on dogs with elbow osteoarthritis and found an improvement in range of motion and stride length.

More details about biomechanics are included later in this chapter, but it is worth noting here that water level at mid-thigh increased muscle work in the quadriceps, and biceps femoris of dogs compared to no water in healthy dogs using an UWTM;

water at the stifle or hock did not significantly increase work in these muscles over no water (Vitger *et al.*, 2021).

In humans, underwater exercise has been shown to generate less cardiovascular and respiratory demand than equivalent land-based activities (Yoo *et al.*, 2014). This is of use in patients with coexisting disease or in obese patients who have low levels of athletic capability. Water temperature plays an important role in human aquatic therapy. Cold water temperatures have been shown to increase the energy expenditure of patients during aquatic therapy (Versey *et al.*, 2013), but the same evidence cannot be assumed to be directly transferable to veterinary aquatic therapy.

Which Patients Will Benefit?

There is substantial research available which indicates that muscle atrophy begins within 24–48 hours following immobilization. The muscles first affected are the postural muscles, which contain a large proportion of type I muscle fibers (Randall, 2010) (see Box 21.1).

Box 21.1 Aims of hydrotherapy

- Enhance preoperative fitness and conditioning (e.g., before a hip replacement)
- Complete resolution of clinical signs (e.g., after cruciate surgery)
- Postoperative restoration of some function (e.g., in cases of intervertebral disc disease)
- Merely palliative (including analgesia)
- Increase cardiovascular fitness
- As an adjunct to obesity management
- As a "fun" form of exercise

Source: Prankel (2008)/John Wiley & Sons.

The Orthopedic Patient

The most common orthopedic conditions treated with aquatic therapy are cranial cruciate disease, hip dysplasia, and osteoarthritis (Goldberg, 2015). Patients visiting your clinic for aquatic therapy will either present for non-surgical management of their orthopedic disease or for post-surgical rehabilitation.

Non-surgical management of veterinary orthopedic disease compromises pharmaceutical management of pain, weight management, and rehabilitation therapy (Waining *et al.*, 2011). Patients with degenerative joint disease suffer from loss of muscle mass, reduced joint range of motion, and joint pain. These are all problems which can be effectively managed with aquatic therapy. Orthopedic disease of the canine coxofemoral joint is often managed with rehabilitation. Research has highlighted that between 70% and 90% of patients with hip dysplasia will have clinical signs attributed to the disease process and therefore most patients with hip dysplasia could benefit from aquatic therapy (Farrell *et al.*, 2007). Research has confirmed patients with degenerative joint disease benefit from hydrotherapy. Twice-weekly hydrotherapy over an eight-week period has been proven to improve the function of joints affected by degenerative joint disease (Nganvongpanit *et al.*, 2014b). The benefits of even a single session of pool-based aquatic therapy in dogs with elbow dysplasia have been shown with increases in elbow range of motion and forelimb stride length (Preston and Wills, 2018).

Aquatic therapy is an integral component of the post-surgical rehabilitation of patients undergoing surgery for orthopedic disease. Research has shown that over US$1.32 billion dollars a year is spent on the treatment of cranial cruciate disease in canines (Wilke *et al.*, 2005). Results of a study suggested that following surgical management of cruciate disease in dogs, swimming resulted in greater extension and flexion of the stifle and tarsal joints than walking alone, which helps accelerate a return to normal function (Marsolais *et al.*, 2003).

Neurological Patients

Intervertebral disc disease and degenerative myelopathy are the two most common neurological diseases treated using aquatic therapy in our practice. Aquatic therapy should be the cornerstone of rehabilitation in neurological patients and in patients with loss of deep pain sensation evidence suggests rapid initiation of aquatic therapy may improve the likelihood of recovery from ambulation (Olby *et al.*, 2022). It can be tailored to accommodate patients with varying degrees of neurological disease from quadriplegia to mild muscular weakness. Standing in water is assisted by buoyancy, which provides a simple and comfortable means to maintain a standing position in non-ambulatory patients (Prydie and Hewitt, 2015). Standing can benefit lung inflation and cardiovascular fitness in a patient who has been nonambulatory for some time. Pool- or UWTM-based aquatic therapy is also more likely to encourage limb movement earlier in the recovery period than similar therapeutic exercises carried out on dry land. The resistance provided by the water helps to strengthen muscles while the buoyancy of the water assists patients in reaching and maintaining a standing position with less exertion (Prydie and Hewitt, 2015).

Therapy in the UWTM may be more appropriate than a pool for neurological patients once they begin to develop a partially coordinated gait pattern, as the treadmill will provide a more controlled movement during which the gait pattern can be assisted to correct motion. The controlled motion provided by UWTM-based exercise places less strain and torque on the spine and encourages normal gait (the action of the treadmill belt drawing the limb caudally in stance phase along with the exaggerated flexion needed to bring the limb through swing phase in the water). Patients with neuromuscular disease are also likely to benefit more from UWTM-based therapy in comparison to free swimming, as the UWTM will help reinforce a proper gait pattern and provide vital tactile feedback during footfall onto the treadmill belt. Water level and treadmill speed can be adjusted to achieve an optimal gait pattern along with the ability to provide an assisted active range of motion as needed. The UWTM can also allow the impaired patient to perform movement against gravity earlier during therapy than they would be able to during assisted exercise on a land treadmill.

Aquatic therapy also has several ancillary benefits for the immobile and weak neurological patient. Hydrostatic pressure and elevated water temperatures can help to ease muscle pain, reduce edema, and promote lymphatic drainage (Prydie and Hewitt, 2015). When carrying out aquatic therapy on patients with neuromuscular disease it is important to bear in mind that these patients fatigue very rapidly, and they should have their head and neck fully supported to prevent aspiration of water during therapy (you can use a pool float or an inflatable neck pillow). Swimming in a pool is often limited to very short periods of time (60–120 seconds) in these patients every 2–3 days, as this is the best way to avoid fatigue and exacerbation of weakness at home from this fatigue. It is best to have the patient wear a life vest (buoyancy aid) for their own safety. Hands-on support to the chest or abdominal areas can bring about a more comfortable swimming position, putting less strain on the spine.

There remains a debate regarding the ideal time to initiate aquatic therapy in the post-surigcal neurological patient with some evidence suggesting initiating therapy within five days of surgery may increase the risk of post-operative complications (Mojarradi *et al.*, 2021) while other research suggests early initiation of therapy is safe (Zidan *et al.*, 2018). Careful assessment of the patient and consultation with the operating surgeon is vital to account for variables which may preclude early rehabilitation and remains the safest way of deciding when aquatic therapy should commence.

Athletes

There is a wide variety of sports in which canine athletes currently compete; a few examples include obedience, agility, herding, dock-diving, disc-dog and flyball, coursing, hunting and field trial, sledding, and skijoring. Working dogs such as those in police protection and detection work and search and rescue dogs also fall within the category of athletes. These sports (and jobs) require strength and aerobic fitness. Some activities require endurance. Aquatic therapy can provide vital post-injury strengthening and conditioning in rehabilitation of the canine athlete. Aquatic therapy can also play an integral role in training of canine athletes (strength and endurance). It can be used in the off-season to maintain condition. Maintaining a level of fitness during the offseason helps to prevent injury when the patient returns to competition, though it should be emphasized that sports-specific training (for example jumping) is still needed.

Aquatic therapy engages and trains muscle groups that are difficult to recruit during land-based exercises, and therefore helps add to the overall fitness of the patient. Water-based therapy is less strenuous on the patient as it does not cause the same repetitive concussive forces on a patient that training on dry land does. An increase in joint flexion during aquatic therapy helps to increase a patient's active range of motion during land-based activities (Marsolais *et al.*, 2003).

Equipment

Pool Design

Prefabricated pools offer an "off-the-shelf" option to centers wishing to introduce pool-based aquatic therapy. Prefabricated pools are manufactured in a variety of sizes and tend to command less space than a custom-built pool. They can be surface-mounted or sunken to meet the design constraints of the facility. One key advantage over a custom-built pool is that prefabricated pools can be moved if the facility decides to move and they tend to have water management plant systems incorporated into the product (or plant systems that can be easily moved). Decking can be built around an above-ground pool to provide ramp access from ground to pool level.

Custom pools provide a permanent solution to introducing aquatic therapy to a facility. The financial commitment associated with installing a custom-built pool means the facility must not be planning on moving in the medium- to long-term future. Custom pools give design flexibility in comparison to prefabricated pools, and they can be designed to fit into the available space. A custom pool also allows for the internal design of the pool to be tailored to the needs of rehabilitation unit. Different methods of entry and exit (i.e., ramp and steps) down into the water can be added (see Figures 21.1 and 21.2). Working platforms of varying depths can also be added to provide areas on which to rest animals and provide static water-based therapy. Custom pools also add flexibility when it comes to water management plant design. If a custom-built pool becomes so busy the water management system is unable to

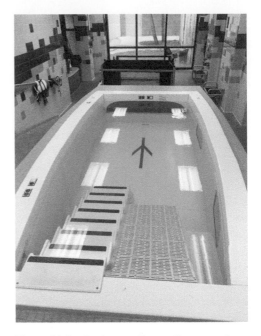

Figure 21.1 Pool entry. *Source:* Courtesy of Wendy Davies.

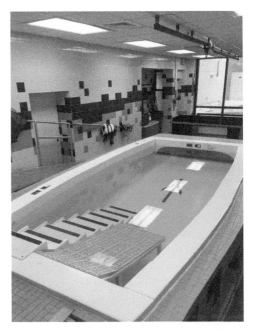

Figure 21.2 Pool entry side view. *Source:* Courtesy of Wendy Davies.

Box 21.2 Benefits of swimming
• Totally non-weight-bearing • Maximum active range of motion of joints • Nonambulatory patients with paraparesis/paralysis • Improved core and trunk strength • Cardiopulmonary conditioning • Endurance for cross-training • Fun for patient • Facilitates passive range of motion/ all bodywork *Source:* From Chiquoine *et al.* (2013). Reproduced with permission of John Wiley & Sons.

maintain water quality, the systems can usually be easily upgraded.

Pool jets are an option that can be added at the time of pool installation. Underwater jets generate turbulence in the water that increases the amount of drag and consequently increases the amount of work being done by a patient (see Box 21.2).

As pool size increases it should be kept in mind that specialist air-handling equipment may be required to manage the air quality in the therapy suite. Humidity levels and temperature must be controlled to maintain patient and therapist comfort as well as prevent damage to the fabric of the building due to excessively high humidity levels.

There are large costs associated with heating a pool/UWTM every day. To conserve energy and control heating bills careful consideration should be made when planning how to retain and maintain the temperature of the water in the pool/UWTM. Pools tend to circulate water 24 hours a day to maintain water quality, so ensuring all pipework is lagged with proprietary heat-retention products can help retain a lot of heat in the pool. In addition, it is recommended to use a pool cover to maintain the heat in the pool while it is not in use. The pool cover should be insulated with foam or similar material to ensure as much heat as possible is retained. UWTM differs from pools in that the water used in the treadmill tends to be stored in a tank. Non-insulated tanks expend a lot of energy keeping the water to temperature even when the treadmill is not in use, so it is recommended to insulate the water storage tank to save energy.

Underwater Treadmill

There are several companies manufacturing UWTMs across the globe. When looking to invest in a UWTM first explore all the options available to you in your geographical location. Second, aim to visit rehabilitation centers that are using the treadmills you are considering and ask the therapists using the machines to give you all the positives and negatives regarding that unit (see Box 21.3).

When investing in a UWTM one should examine the minimum and maximum speed of the unit and what is the smallest incremental speed change that can be made on the unit during a therapy session. To effectively rehabilitate small patients after

Box 21.3 Benefits of the underwater treadmill
• Improved active range of motion compared to land • Permits partial weight-bearing • Proprioceptive gait training • Improved balance while walking • Cautious fracture loading • Builds lean muscle in limbs • Helps timid/new swimmers get started • Speeds gait retraining *Source:* From Chiquoine *et al.* (2013). Reproduced with permission of John Wiley & Sons.

neurological injury you need to be able to alter belt speeds by small increments (0.1 mph) so that small changes in belt speed can be made to tailor therapy to the exact needs of the patient. It should be noted that treadmill speeds are usually not calibrated to actual speed so if the facility has two UWTM, they may differ in actual speed. Before committing to a unit ensure you check whether speed can be altered during the therapy session. Does the machine need to be stopped, the belt speed adjusted, and then the belt restarted? The ability to add an incline during therapy is an important addition that many treadmills offer. Some units automate adding inclination to the belt via the control unit, allowing you to change the angle of inclination during a therapy session (see Figures 21.3 and 21.4). Most units available on the market require the inclination of the belt to be set manually prior to commencing the therapy session and do not allow the inclination to be altered once the UWTM has had water added.

UWTMs are complicated mechanical machines that require daily maintenance in the clinic and regular maintenance from the manufacturer. Ensure you purchase a product that has good availability for ongoing maintenance or repair at your location, as needed. Cleanliness is incredibly important to keep a UWTM running effectively and daily maintenance protocols should be established to maintain the machine.

Ancillary Equipment

A buoyancy jacket, or life vest, helps a patient to float in the pool or in the UWTM if the treadmill is filled to the patient's shoulder blades. Buoyancy jackets allow the therapist to remain in control of patients via handles and straps. A jacket also helps the patient maintain a level stance in the water. An exception to the use of a buoyancy jacket to keep a patient level is the amputee. The rotational instability which is already a

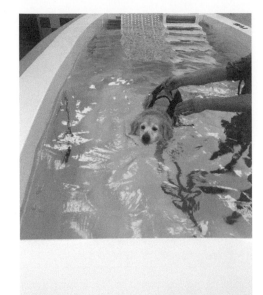

Figure 21.3 Dog swimming in pool.
Source: Courtesy of Wendy Davies.

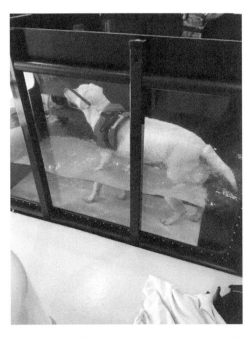

Figure 21.4 Weight bearing is reduced by 15% if the water is filled to the level of a patient's stifle in an underwater treadmill.
Source: Courtesy of Wendy Davies.

Box 21.4 Equipment used with therapeutic swimming

- Life vest
- Harnesses
- Slings
- Head wraps
- Balance equipment
- Leg weights
- Resistance swim mitts
- Pool noodles
- Toys
- Food

Source: From Chiquoine *et al.* (2013). Reproduced with permission of John Wiley & Sons.

problem for the amputee in the water can be made worse by increasing buoyancy (see Box 21.4). Buoyancy jackets are very useful in patients who are fearful or lack confidence in the pool as they help the patient maintain their head well out of the water (see Figure 21.5). The jackets must be carefully sized for the patient to ensure they do not restrict limb or neck movement.

Once a patient no longer requires a buoyancy jacket during therapy, use a non-flotation jacket or a robust harness during their therapy session. Harnesses or jackets provide the same patient control benefits as buoyancy jackets without providing flotation.

Patients with neurological conditions affecting limb strength may require additional flotation for therapy to be beneficial. Long foam cylinders, commonly called pool noodles, are useful for both pool and UWTM therapy and can be placed under the thorax or abdomen to provide additional flotation during treatment sessions. These foam cylinders make excellent bumpers for use in the UWTM to prevent patients from placing their limbs on the static side panels on either side of the treadmill belt. An alternate bumper for this latter use is a fender float (see Figure 21.6).

Motivation is key to ensuring a patient remains focused and attentive during therapy. Owners should be encouraged to bring along toys that the patient enjoys playing with. Toys can be used to encourage a patient to swim laps or lengths of a pool and can be used to promote consistent gaiting during UWTM therapy. Toys should be cleaned prior to use to minimize pool contamination and should be in good repair to prevent the patient from possibly swallowing broken pieces. Toys should also easily fit in a patient's mouth; excessively large toys that require the patient to open their jaws to the maximal extent may put the patient at risk of aspiration of water into the respiratory tract.

There are various therapeutic aids that can be used to make aquatic therapy more

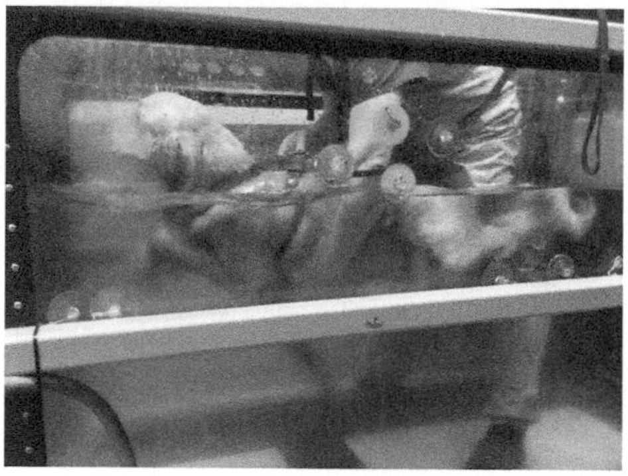

Figure 21.5 Harness for controlling patient in underwater treadmill and keeping head above water. *Source:* Courtesy of Dr Julia Tomlinson.

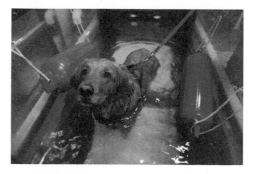

Figure 21.6 Fender floats prevent patients from placing their limbs on the static side panels on either side of the treadmill belt. *Source:* Courtesy of Dr Julia Tomlinson.

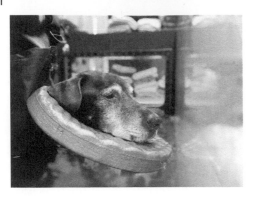

Figure 21.7 A flotation device is used to support the patient's head during therapy. *Source:* Courtesy of Julia Callaghan CCRVN.

challenging for the patient. Flotation devices for the head should be used in patients that need this support (see Figure 21.7). Velcro weights can be placed around the carpus and tarsus to increase the work a patient must carry out to move their limbs during therapy. A source for pre-made leg weights is Canine Icer (www.canineicer.com/), or use curtain weights to make your own weighted wraps. Weights must be used with caution to prevent patient fatigue. Additional flotation can also be added to a patient's lower limbs using either children's air-filled water wings, modeling balloons, or foam piping insulation cut into short strips. The added flotation means the patient must use more effort to bring their paw down to the tread-mill belt during movement as the added buoyancy draws the limb upward.

Safety and Maintenance

Microbiological contamination of UWTM and pool water can result in pathological organisms causing infections in both patients and therapists. Contamination is introduced into the water largely by our canine patients, with skin and fecal bacteria causing most bacterial contaminations. Pathogens can also be introduced into the water from poorly maintained water filters and occasionally from defects in the pool design. The regional legislation regarding water quality in UWTM and pools should be consulted to ensure local health and safety legislation is being adhered to. Microbiological assessment of UWTM and pool water is largely directed at identifying markers of fecal contamination and assessing the levels of *Pseudomonas aeruginosa*, as these bacteria have been associated with ear and skin infections in both dogs and therapists. The presence of significant colony numbers of *Ps. aeruginosa* during microbiological testing or the presence of *Escherichia coli* indicates poor water management and remedial action must be taken. Cultures should be taken from a dry treadmill, so resident bacteria can be identified without dilution. Allow the treadmill to dry overnight (empty the bottom water, under the belt) then swab corners and under the belt. It can often be submitted to a diagnostic laboratory as an environmental culture so they look for a wider range of potential pathogens including opportunistic ones. If a positive culture of a pathogen is identified then cleaning should include thorough scrub with a degreaser, then a disinfectant (safe for skin when diluted), rinse, and then steam cleaning. Reculture after the treadmill dries out. Use of treadmill with an identified pathogen should be limited to systemically healthy patients with no skin irritation until the clean culture has been received.

Water management is an integral part of running a safe aquatic therapy unit. Poor water quality or inappropriate use of water management chemicals can have a major impact on the health and safety of therapists and patients. Poor water quality can also lead to staff sickness, staff injuries, and staff absences. From the patient's point of view, poor water quality can also lead to sickness and injury which will lead to client dissatisfaction and have a detrimental effect on your business success. The complexity of the water management protocol will be dictated by the size of the UWTM or pool and the number of patients using the pool daily. Protocols for water management should be tailored to meet the exact needs of the unit and there must be records outlining when, and by whom, water management tasks are carried out. Water treatment can be aided with an ozone machine or UV light machine within the storage tank as well as the baseline salination with chlorine, bromination, or chlorination for water management.

All owners should be instructed to bring their pets to an area to encourage defecation and urination prior to commencing an aquatic therapy session. Despite the best efforts of owners and therapists our canine patients will challenge the therapist from time to time by defecating during an aquatic therapy session. Fecal contamination of the pool water must be dealt with swiftly and safely. Nets and sieves can assist in removing formed fecal matter and, if carried out in a timely fashion, the UWTM or pool can likely be kept open. If loose feces are passed in the UWTM or pool, it is likely the unit must be shut down for 3–4 hours and a decontamination cycle run to maintain water safety. This highlights the importance of the owner answering pre-hydro questions regarding the recent toilet habits of their pets. In the case of patients who have fecal incontinence or who are "repeat offenders" contaminating the water, manual evacuation of the rectum and a bath before hydrotherapy is recommended.

Protecting Staff and Clients

When working in and around pools and UWTM all staff and clients must be made aware of the risks of being in an aquatic therapy unit. Local legislation regarding health and safety around a pool or UWTM should be carefully researched, including the appropriate guidelines regarding safe working practices and rules within the unit to ensure the safety of clients, patients, and therapists. There should be clear protocols to deal with emergencies such as clients becoming unwell and it is advisable that staff members are trained in first aid techniques to assist both their colleagues and clients in the event of an injury on the premises.

Patient Assessment

Initial patient assessment should occur prior to the patient arriving for hydrotherapy. Paper or email referral forms should be sent to both the client and the primary care veterinarian. Question the client to ascertain a patient's prior experience with water. Patient and therapist safety is paramount and dogs that have a serious fear of water or are reluctant to swim may pose a danger to themselves and to therapists. When a patient panics, the natural reaction of a therapist is to try to restrain the patient and remove them from the water. This can lead to injury and, in extreme cases, the loss of bite inhibition caused by panic may lead to the therapist receiving serious bite injuries. Low-stress handling should be used and slow introduction to the environment performed. Client questionnaires should also ask about the best way to motivate a patient (e.g., food or toys) and establish whether the patient is safe to be around other canines. The questionnaire should be accompanied by a set of therapy guidelines, health and safety guidelines, and terms and conditions. The veterinary referral form should focus on why the patient is being sent for aquatic therapy and what the supervising rehabilitation veterinarian is hoping to achieve from therapy. There should be declarations regarding coexisting diseases that may interfere with aquatic therapy and the patient's vaccination status should be confirmed on the referral form.

Client Questionnaires

Upon arrival at the therapy unit, the client should be asked a standard set of questions which are designed to assess the patient's immediate suitability for aquatic therapy. The pre-session questions should ascertain if the patient has emptied their bladder and bowels prior to the session. The therapist should also focus on identifying how the patient was in the hours after the last aquatic therapy session. This information should be used to form a basis for whether the therapy session needs to be made more challenging.

Coexisting Disease

Understanding why a patient is presenting for aquatic therapy and how preexisting medical conditions affect their ability to safely engage in aquatic therapy is vital. Preexisting medical conditions such as heart, respiratory, kidney, or liver disease do not preclude a patient from engaging in aquatic therapy. Each patient should be evaluated as an individual and a tailored plan created. It is unsuitable for a patient with concurrent clinical cardiac disease to engage in strenuous swimming or treadmill activity, but they may benefit greatly from water-based massage therapy and water-based range of motion exercises. They may be able to walk for a short period, if their heart rate is monitored before exercise, during exercise (in a break), and after to ascertain return to resting heart rate. The key to creating tailored aquatic therapy plans for patients with multiple disease processes is gaining a complete understanding of the patient's limitations and understanding the risks that water-based therapy may present to that individual. The rehabilitation veterinarian will perform a

thorough examination determining the patient's abilities to carry out aquatic therapy. Gaining a complete medical and orthopedic history for every patient is key; a close working relationship with referring veterinarians is also vital for creating patient-centric treatment plans.

Surgical Wounds

Although historically, patients with surgical (sutured) wounds were excluded from aquatic therapy, new advances in surgical wound management are challenging this concept. There are a variety of wound sealant products that can be applied in theatre to theoretically completely seal a surgical wound to allow early aquatic rehabilitation (Baranoski and Ayello, 2012). The performance of such products has been evaluated in human medicine and studies will continue in animals to validate the use of these products in animals receiving aquatic therapy in the early postoperative period. Patients with open wounds or infected surgical wounds should not receive aquatic therapy until the wound is fully healed.

Contraindications for Hydrotherapy

Although every effort should be made to create a treatment plan that accommodates a patient's coexisting disease, there are several presentations that exclude a patient from aquatic therapy either temporarily or permanently. For the protection of staff members, and in the interest of water hygiene, dogs with acute or chronic gastrointestinal disease that leads to either vomiting or diarrhea should be excluded from aquatic therapy and should see the veterinarian. Patients who are obviously unwell with evidence of an elevated body temperature or signs of malaise should not receive therapy and instead should be directed to their supervising veterinarian

---

Box 21.5 Contraindications to hydrotherapy/aquatic therapy

- Unhealed surgical incisions
- Skin irritation or infection
- Emesis
- Diarrhea
- Untreated cardiac, liver, or kidney disease
- Incontinence
- Uncontrolled epilepsy
- If the dog has an external fixator, as there is a risk of infection associated with open wounds

Source: Adapted from Tomlinson (2013) and Connell and Monk (2010).

---

for assessment. The chemicals used in water management have been shown to irritate damaged skin, and therefore patients with acute dermatological problems (e.g., acute moist dermatitis) should not swim (Nganvongpanit and Yano, 2012). Patients with chronic dermatological conditions should only swim under the clearance of the supervising veterinarian and attention should be paid to post-therapy management (see Box 21.5) if the patient has had a positive skin culture for a pathogen then they need a negative repeat culture (swab around ears and mouth as well as axilla) before entering hydrotherapy equipment. Patients with signs of infectious diseases, such as kennel cough, should be excluded from the clinic until the infectious period has passed. Lastly, patients with a history of uncontrolled epileptic activity should not engage in aquatic therapy until their condition is medically controlled.

There are patients that you will encounter who are simply not suitable to engage in aquatic therapy. Although it is recommended to try at least 2–3 sessions to acclimate and get a patient used to either pool-based or UWTM activity, some patients find the experience too stressful or use their limbs in a counterproductive fashion and are at risk of making their particular condition worse.

Managing the Incontinent Patient

Opinions will remain divided on whether the urinary incontinent patient should receive aquatic therapy due to the risk of pool contamination and ascending urinary tract infection. The most commonly encountered urinary incontinent patient is the neurological patient suffering from intervertebral disc disease. Aquatic therapy plays a key role in the rehabilitation of these patients and withholding such therapy could prolong the patient's recovery time. Several strategies can be applied for managing the urinary incontinent patient. The first involves pretherapy bladder emptying to ensure the patient has an empty bladder prior to starting aquatic therapy. Technicians/nurses who have received veterinary training in bladder expression can empty the bladder using manual expression. This should provide a 30- to 60-minute window where the patient will produce a negligible volume of urine and should be able to receive UWTM or pool-based rehabilitation without urine contamination. Specially designed canine incontinence pants can also be used to minimize leaking urine. Infant swimming diapers can also be used in small dogs.

Patients with urinary incontinence can also be managed with a Foley catheter in situ. This remains a controversial strategy, with some believing it predisposes the patient to ascending urinary tract infection. If the catheter is meticulously managed during aquatic therapy, there should be no reason why its presence should prevent a patient from receiving therapy. The bladder should be actively emptied via the Foley catheter prior to therapy. The catheter should then be sealed using an appropriate bung to prevent water from entering. At this point, the patient can begin therapy. On completion of therapy, the external portion of the Foley catheter and the prepuce should be flushed and cleaned with dilute chlorhexidine solution. The bung should be disposed of and the patient reconnected to a closed collection system.

Patients with fecal incontinence may be presented for aquatic therapy. Incontinent patients can be accommodated only if the bladder is expressed prior to exercise and the patient has an anal tone so once manually evacuated will not pass further stools. It is the author's opinion that these cases should not receive aquatic therapy unless an appropriate swim diaper is placed after evacuation of the rectum. Many times, patients can have a bowel movement stimulated by using a "Q-tip" around the anal sphincter. This helps to stimulate evacuation. If a patient has persistent liquid feces or cannot be managed using a swim diaper the patient must not swim because of the risk to the health and safety of the therapist.

Patient Conformation

Although almost any size and shape of dog or cat can be taught to swim in a pool or use an UWTM there are some considerations that should be made for individual breeds, and the challenges that their specific conformation and breed personality present to the therapist. The conformation, or size and shape of a patient, affects a patient's ability to swim. Brachycephalic breeds, such as Bulldogs and Pugs, with shortened faces, have narrowed nasal passages. This conformational change is often accompanied by an excessively long soft palate and a small trachea in comparison to overall body size. These changes restrict these patient's athletic capability, as they simply cannot effectively move enough air in and out of their lungs to maintain strenuous athletic exertion. These dogs may also struggle to carry

toys in their mouth during therapy and protect their airway at the same time. With these breeds, careful attention should be paid to providing enough flotation in the form of jackets and ancillary flotation devices to maintain the patient's head above the surface of the wateralways. The therapist must also pay careful attention to the early signs of fatigue.

Pool Versus Underwater Treadmill

There are distinct differences in the therapeutic benefits of pool-based aquatic therapy and those of UWTM rehabilitation. The choice of pool-based therapy or UWTM therapy is tailored to the problem that is being treated. Many patients can benefit from a combination of pool-based therapy and UWTM therapy. It should be remembered that many small and medium patients can swim in the UWTM.

Pool-based therapy allows the patient to be rehabilitated without bearing any weight; this is ideal for patients who are painful when weight-bearing; or are unable to weight-bear due to neurological disease or an unstable limb. Rehabilitating patients in a non-weight-bearing environment can be continued until these patients start to show improvement; they can then be transitioned to UWTM therapy to help retrain the patient to gait normally and slowly return to weight-bearing. Patients who lack flexion when gaiting on land can benefit from swimming versus UWTM activity as the limbs are in flexion during swimming (Marsolais *et al.*, 2003).

Research on normal dogs swimming revealed that the propulsion (power) phase for each limb is when the limb is accelerated ventrally and caudally in an arc and was about 34% of each stroke; the rest was the recovery phase where the limb is moved forward, this applies for both fore- and hindlimbs. Shoulder flexion and elbow extension (hip, stifle, and hock extension for the rear) provide the power stroke. Supination and pronation ability of the carpus appears important (a consideration for rehabilitation of carpal injuries or cases with radius and ulnar fusion as they may need more assistance). The recovery phase needs elbow, shoulder then carpal flexion (hip and stifle for rear limb). The forelimbs move a lot more into the water vertically than the rear, this means the therapist should take extra consideration for how early swimming (and perhaps walking in water) should be used in cases of forelimb soft tissue injury. Each limb is moved individually in order left hindlimb, right forelimb, right hindlimb, and left forelimb (Fish *et al.*, 2021).

The water height in a UWTM can be adjusted to tailor the amount of weight a patient is bearing during therapy (Levine *et al.*, 2002, 2010). As a patient improves during therapy the water level can be lowered to allow more weight bearing, and then upon completion of the therapy program the water can once again be deepened to allow the patient's athletic capabilities to be challenged (see Box 21.6).

The UWTM provides some distinct advantages over pool-based therapy in certain scenarios and vice versa. Most UWTMs have clear plastic sides which allow the patient's gait (and joint extension and flexion) to be assessed during motion. This can be very difficult to assess when using pool-based therapy. UWTMs provide a more controlled environment in which to introduce animals that have never encountered water to paddling and even swimming. Patients bear weight during training on a UWTM, which may benefit patients that are recovering from fracture repair, tendinopathies, and other conditions in which weight bearing can stimulate healing. The controlled weight bearing offered by a UWTM can be advantageous during rehabilitation of

---

Box 21.6 Assessment of anxiety and fatigue when swimming

Anxiety

- Anxious facial expression (lips pulled back)
- Rapid breathing/pulse
- Thrashing forelimbs
- Inability to rest
- Attempting to exit the pool

Fatigue

- Tired body posture
- Deep or irregular breathing
- Slowed swim pace
- Reluctance to swim
- Change in tongue color/shape

Source: From Chiquoine *et al.* (2013). Reproduced with permission of John Wiley & Sons.

---

fracture patients or those recovering from joint instabilities. Pool-based therapy is more suited for strengthening a patient's core and trunk muscles as the rotational forces encountered during swimming help build these muscle groups. A pool allows the patient's whole body to be treated and enables massage and manual therapy to take place in the water environment; this is very difficult to do in a UWTM because of space limitations.

Pool-Based Exercises

Static Therapy

Static therapy ideally takes place on a platform within the pool, allowing as much of the patient's body to be submerged with the patient's paws on a solid surface. Static therapy is used to help treat specific areas of muscle pain, improve patient comfort, and increase the range of motion of a joint. In addition, static pool-based therapy helps reeducate patients in maintaining a normal standing posture. It should be noted that although patients are often referred to treat a specific joint or problem, it is imperative to take a holistic approach to aquatic therapy (the meaning of holistic is to look at the patient's whole body). For example, a patient recovering from cruciate ligament surgery may have muscle fatigue and pain in the contralateral non-operated limb due to transitioning weight in adapting to operative limb pain and weakness. Water-based massage therapy can help to reduce muscle pain, reduce postoperative edema, improve flexibility, and greatly improve a patient's comfort and well-being.

The pre-therapy examination should focus on identifying areas of pain, discomfort, and tightness in major muscle groups. Therapy should then focus on massage of these muscle groups by a qualified individual along with gentle stretches aimed at improving flexibility (see Chapter 5). Joint mobilization aims to improve joint motion and reduce joint pain, thus improving joint function. Carrying out joint mobilizations underwater adds the warming and hydrostatic benefits of the aquatic therapy to this modality. It should be noted that joint mobilizations should only be carried out by suitably qualified rehabilitation veterinarians or physical therapists. Postural exercises such as three-legged standing can be used in the pool to encourage a patient to actively load a specific limb.

Active Therapy

Pool-based active aquatic therapy aims to improve muscle strength, improve aerobic fitness, increase flexibility, and improve range of motion. It tends to involve either swimming lengths or laps of the pool depending on the size of the pool. In an endless pool, the patient will swim against the water flow, which provides resistance. In the early stages of therapy, the patient must be supported and guided by a technician/nurse. Active therapy does not mean simply allowing a patient to swim uncontrolled. An active role is taken by the handler during the session and ensures the patient is using their limbs as normally as possible during therapy. Patients who have limb paresis and paralysis have their affected limbs cycled through a swimming motion (active assisted range of motion) during therapy to stimulate neural pathways and encourage volitional limb movement. In large patients, two handlers may be required – one to guide and support the patient and a second to carry out the therapeutic exercises. Toys make excellent motivational aids for patients engaging in pool-based aquatic therapy and are often a necessity to ensure patients engage with therapy and get the most out of a session.

During assisted swimming the technician/nurse can challenge the patient by gently rolling the patient from side to side while swimming. This rolling movement, described as a perturbation, stimulates the patient's righting reflex. Stimulating this postural reaction evokes limb extension mediated through neural feedback pathways with stepping responses in the patient, which, when translated onto land, helps patients with balance, bending, and turning. These perturbations also help build and strengthen a patient's core stabilizing muscles. A point may be reached with some patients where little support or guidance is required during swimming due to the patient having a high level of proficiency. A technician/nurse should remain in the pool with these patients; however, little input is required.

The patient who becomes adept at swimming can be transitioned to a lake and swimming with companions (see Figures 21.8 and 21.9). This technique can be used for maintaining cardiovascular fitness.

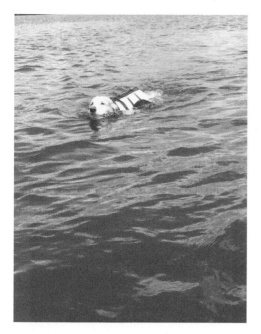

Figure 21.8 Swimming in open water – in this case, a lake. *Source:* Rick Tucker.

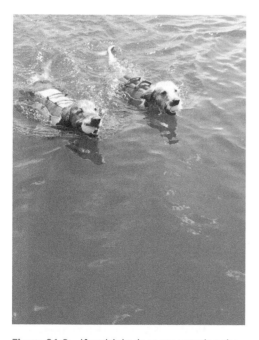

Figure 21.9 If multiple dogs are entering the pool/lake at the same time during a fun swim session it is important that all the dogs are confident in the water and are wearing appropriate jackets or other flotation aids.

Treadmill-Based Exercises

Speed

There is a lack of research to determine exactly what belt speed is most appropriate for patients with specific conditions and for specific breeds. However, there is a wealth of experienced aquatic therapists that have established the most useful treadmill belt speeds for a variety of breeds and conditions. Leg length and stride length must be taken into account when deciding upon a belt speed. It should be noted that smaller dogs often walk relatively faster than larger dogs (Voss *et al.*, 2010). It was stated earlier that treadmill belt speed is not calibrated to miles per hour (or km/h) by most UWTM manufacturers; therefore, advice regarding speed is not given in this chapter. It is best to say the speed should be adjusted to the most comfortable-looking gait in each patient, whether that gait is walk, trot, or, in some cases, faster. Pacing should be avoided unless the dog has always paced naturally. Doubling belt speed from the walk should in most patients initiate a trotting gait. If a patient fights the transition into a trot it may start to use a pacing gait. Patients can be moved out of a pace into a trot by encouraging them forward on the belt, using a leash or toy.

Patients with neurologic issues may have a dissociative gait where the forelimbs move at faster tempo with shorter strides than the rear limbs (Gordon-Evans *et al.*, 2009). A platform can be added over the front of the treadmill belt so that the patient can stand with the forelimbs and gait with the rear limbs. This has been successful in practice for gait retraining these types of patients (Tomlinson, personal communication).

Water Depth

The depth/height of the water has a great impact on the amount of work being carried out by the patient during UWTM aquatic therapy. Studies have examined how water depth affects the amount of weight a patient is supporting during therapy. Filling the UWTM to the level of a patient's tarsus reduces the weight bearing of the patient by 9% (Levine *et al.*, 2010). Weight-bearing is reduced by 15% if the water is filled to the level of a patient's stifle. If the treadmill is filled to the level of a patient's great trochanter (hip joint) we see the greatest reduction in weight bearing, with a maximal reduction in total weight bearing in the region of 62% (Levine *et al.*, 2010).

Filling the UWTM to different levels on a patient's body not only affects the total weight bearing but also influences the ratio of weight being supported by the forelimbs in comparison to the hindlimbs. Unaided by the buoyancy of water, dogs support approximately 60% of their weight through their forelimbs. This is largely unchanged as water is brought up to their hock and stifle joints (Levine *et al.*, 2014), but as water is filled up to a patient's great trochanter we see the forelimbs supporting up to 71% of the patient's weight (Levine *et al.*, 2010). Remember that overall weight bearing is reduced by 62% when the water is this high, but this weight redistribution may still be of significance in patients who have forelimb disease as UWTM therapy with deep water levels may in some patients exacerbate fore-limb weight load. Patients who have an adaptive weight shift to the forelimbs due to hindlimb insufficiency may be better served by being exercised in the UWTM at a maximum water height of the stifle to avoid exacerbating the forward postural shift.

Altering the depth of water in the UWTM also alters limb kinematics and the amount of muscle activation occurring. Improving joint range of motion involves challenging the current range of motion; depending on which joint/joints are being focused on the correct depth of water is required to achieve this. Elbow and carpal flexion are increased in all depths of water with an increasing depth bringing about an increased flexion. To achieve an increase in shoulder extension water depth must be at least at the level of the stifle. Tarsal and stifle flexion is increased in all depths of water with an increasing depth bringing about an increased degree of flexion. Significantly increasing hip ROM is challenging unless water levels reach the level of the hip joint. It should be noted that achieving increased extension during UWTM therapy is challenging; carpal and tarsal extension tend to be significantly reduced during UWTM use (Bliss *et al.*, 2022). Water depth also affects the degree of muscle activation occurring during rehabilitation. Research has shown that the muscle activity required to walk in water at a depth above the stifle joint is greater than that required to walk at shallower water levels (Vitger *et al.*, 2021).

Water Temperature

Pool and UWTM water temperature is an important variable to control during aquatic therapy. Studies have investigated the ideal water temperature for patients undergoing therapy. Water temperatures between 30 and 34 °C were examined and the effects of different temperatures on heart rate, respiratory rates, rectal temperature, and patient exertion were measured. Research showed that all patients undergoing therapy showed increased vital parameters during therapy, but there were no significant differences in parameters between different water temperatures. This research demonstrates that water temperatures between 30 and 34 °C (86–93.2 °F) are considered safe for canines (Nganvongpanit *et al.*, 2014a).

Maintaining the water temperature of a pool or UWTM represents one of the largest expenses for an aquatic therapy business and water temperature should be thermostatically controlled to control energy expenditure.

Inclination

Exercising on an incline on land changes joint kinematics in dogs (Bockstahler *et al.*, 2012). Increasing the incline of the UWTM belt during therapy likely increases the work for the patient but the effects on joint motion are unknown. Most neurological and orthopedic patients will not require the addition of an incline to the UWTM belt during therapy, but those patients who have recovered fully from their injury and canine athletes may benefit from the addition of an incline to the belt during therapy to challenge their fitness during therapy.

Session Duration

It is imperative to build the duration of activity in a patient's aquatic therapy slowly. A patient's first few UWTM sessions may not progress beyond 2–3 intervals of walking for 45–60 seconds. Patients should be given 90–120 seconds to recover by standing still in the water between training intervals. This recovery time frame may need to be shortened in animals with a high level of fitness or lengthened in very unfit animals. As a patient becomes more confident on the UWTM the interval length should be increased session by session. At the end of a session, a patient should be evaluated to determine how difficult they found a session. If they are excessively exhausted by the session it should be made less intense at the next appointment. If the patient obviously coped with the session well, it should be made tougher at the next appointment.

Developing Patient Programs

The patient's first session in the pool or on the UWTM is often more of an acclimatization session rather than a true therapeutic session. It is important to get the patient as comfortable as possible and get them used

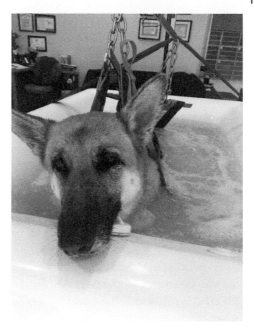

Figure 21.10 Whirlpool bath for a neurologically impaired dog.

to the sensation of water moving up their body as well as to the movement of the treadmill belt prior to engaging in useful therapy sessions. Engaging in static therapy in the pool or UWTM during the first session is a very useful acclimatization tool (see Figure 21.10). A whirlpool bath can be used for the neurological patient at the beginning of rehabilitation therapy.

A patient's treatment program must have specific goals. The goals of a program dictate the ideal number of sessions a patient should engage in on a weekly basis. Patients early in their recovery from a neurological or orthopedic injury benefit from more frequent sessions. Both UWTM and pool-based therapy revolve around repetition of training intervals. In the pool, an interval may be a single length or lap of the pool. As a patient progresses through an aquatic therapy program, the number of repetitions will be slowly increased during the session, while at the same time, the rest period between intervals is slowly decreased. In the UWTM, the number of intervals for a given time is increased, as is the length of the training interval as the patient progresses in an aquatic rehabilitation program.

There are some parameters that can be examined to determine if a program is meeting the goals of a patient. The recovery of a patient in the hours after a pool or UWTM session is one of the best guides of whether a program is suitable or requires adjustment. If a patient recovers rapidly and does not appear tired after a rehabilitation session, it is possible that the session was not demanding enough and at the next session the duration or speed should be increased. When a patient appears tired for 4–6 hours after a session one must consider that the session was too demanding for the patient and the next therapy session should be adjusted so that the session is less demanding on the patient. This advice is all subjective and you should be guided by your supervising veterinarian as fatigue needs to be carefully avoided in some patients.

Once rehabilitation has been completed the patient should ideally be transitioned to a maintenance program that focuses on maintaining the improvements that have been achieved. This maintenance program may include hydrotherapy. Maintenance therapy should consistently bring a patient to the edge of their ability to maintain cardiovascular fitness, preserve muscle mass, and, most importantly, retain the improvements gained during an aquatic therapy program.

Canine athletes are common visitors to aquatic therapy centers, not only to treat specific orthopedic problems but also to maintain and improve cardiovascular fitness during the off-season to maintain fitness and improve athletic prowess. Once a patient can easily achieve a level of continuous exercise in a pool, it can be difficult to apply further challenges to patients in the pool apart from increasing the length of the session. The UWTM may be a more versatile tool for canine athletes aiming to maintain fitness, as it allows an array of parameters to be adjusted to challenge the patient during their session. Resistance jets (may also be available in some pools), incline, water height, and speed can be adjusted. The aim for canine athletes who are engaging in UWTM should be to reach a point where they can maintain a single interval on the UWTM of between 20 and 30 minutes at a brisk walk without a break. Once a patient can maintain a brisk walk for 20–30 minutes the session should be interspersed with a small number of brief 20- to 30-second intervals at the fastest pace the canine can maintain.

Business Diversification

There are significant costs associated with running a UWTM or swimming pool. To maximize income, any rehabilitation center offering these therapeutic options should examine how they can make these assets pay for themselves. Adapting opening hours to suit client needs is a basic strategy that can help increase bookings; evening and weekend openings offer appointments outside of the usual daily working hours and are very popular. In addition to flexible opening hours, diversifying away from pure aquatic rehabilitation and exercise therapy can assist in increasing UWTM/pool revenue and ensure maximal use of the facilities.

Obesity Clinics

While aquatic therapy is unlikely to be successful in achieving weight loss in the obese canine/feline if used alone, if combined with dietary restriction and lifestyle modifications it can be a very effective means of achieving weight loss. The veterinary technician or nurse should remain in the UWTM or pool with the patient (see Figures 21.11–21.14). Accelerated weight loss has been reported in patients that have

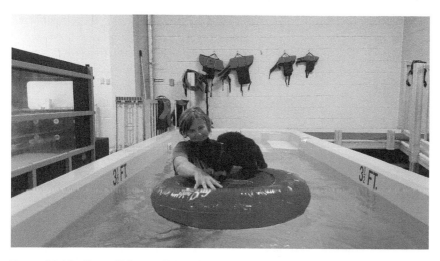

Figure 21.11 Dawn H. Rector, LVT, VTS (physical rehab), CCRP, CVPP, CCFT says this is the best way to do balance exercises with a cat.

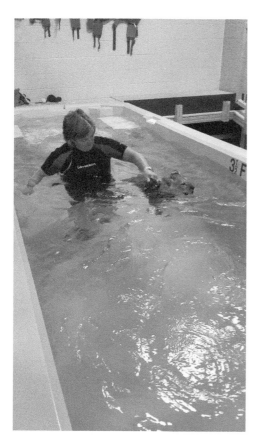

Figure 21.12 Dawn H. Rector with a liliger swimming.

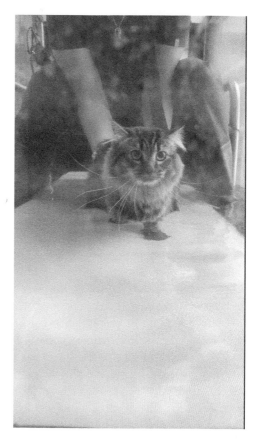

Figure 21.13 Wendy Davies BS CVT, CCRVN, VTS-Physical Rehabilitation in underwater treadmill with a cat.

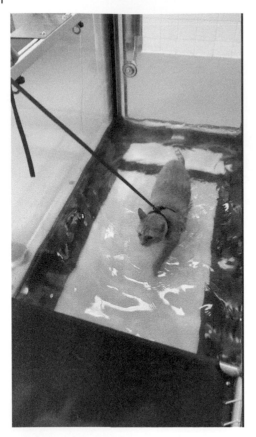

Figure 21.14 Wendy Davies supervising a cat walking in an underwater treadmill.

results are seen early and these results can only be achieved if a holistic approach to weight management is taken. Once a target weight has been achieved, owners can be encouraged to continue aquatic therapy on a maintenance basis to help the patient maintain their target weight.

Developing the "Fun" Swim

The nontherapeutic aquatic session or "fun swim" can prove an important revenue stream for rehabilitation centers with a pool. Fun swims need to be supervised to ensure dog and client safety, but they are less labor-intensive than therapeutic sessions. If multiple dogs are entering the pool at the same time during a fun swim session, it is important that all the dogs are confident in the water, they are wearing appropriate jackets or other flotation aids, and that there are sufficient staff members to evacuate the animals from the pool in a timely fashion. Legal disclaimers need to be incorporated in the United States.

Puppy Water Introduction Classes

As previously discussed, there is a subset of dogs that have not experienced swimming or being partially submerged in water. This can lead to fear and aversion to water in dogs. Puppy water introduction classes are aimed at exposing young dogs to water in a controlled and safe fashion in either a UWTM or a pool. Buoyancy aids should be worn in the early sessions. Some dogs can be safely introduced to water over a single session, but some may require multiple sessions to become confident in water. One should first introduce a puppy to water of a depth level to the patient's carpus and use positive reinforcement, either verbal or treat-based, to put the dog at ease. The water should be gradually deepened over the session while ensuring the dog feels comfortable and reassured. This is where

hydrotherapy incorporated into a weight loss program. Weight loss of up to 1.5% body weight per week was reported in a study that saw patients exercising on a UWTM for up to 30 minutes once a week (Chauvet *et al.*, 2011). This is compared to reported weekly weight losses of 0.75% per week with dietary modification alone.

If you are going to promote UWTM or pool swimming as a weight loss tool, it is important that you involve the supervising veterinarian in the development of the exercise program as well as details of dietary management. Client education, dietary management, and additional home-based exercises are key to successful weight loss and one cannot rely on aquatic therapy alone. Owner compliance will be better if working "pods" in a pool come into their own, as you have a static platform on which to work with the dog. Over the water introduction session in a pool with a platform, the dog should be encouraged to lift its feet off the platform and begin to swim. If the dog becomes distressed, return to a solid surface and work on building the dog's confidence prior to attempting swimming again.

Water Safety Courses

Older dogs can be safely introduced to water in a similar fashion to puppies. Water safety classes are something that can also be utilized in working dogs, such as army and police dogs, who currently rarely receive water safety lessons during their training. Police and army dogs, as well as other working dogs such as gun and trial dogs, may unexpectedly enter water of varying depths in their working life and should be trained to cope with this. Handler involvement is paramount to success in effectively training working dogs and if insurance permits, the handler should be directly involved, ideally being in the pool with their working dog. One particular area of training that can assist working dogs is training dogs to exit water unassisted, which could prove a lifesaving skill if a working dog enters water without supervision.

Promoting Your Business

Successful promotion of an aquatic rehabilitation business can be the key to accelerating a rehabilitation clinic's growth and the onus for this frequently falls on the veterinary nurse/technician rather than the supervising veterinarian. All investments in advertising should focus on reaching clients and referring veterinary surgeons within a sensible geographical radius. Investing in a quality waterproof camera will help you generate engaging and interesting images and videos to use in promotion of the business. Underwater videos can also be used to document a patient's session-by-session progress.

Building relationships with referring veterinarians is key to maintaining a steady flow of rehabilitation cases and a lot can be said for visiting possible referring clinics to discuss what you can offer. Face-to-face communication can build business relations that can support the growth of a rehabilitation center in its early years and build security by providing a steady stream of referrals. Having a physical presence at local community events and sponsoring local community teams and events all help to build community bridges that build the clinic's profile. Your veterinarian should join you.

Social media provides a cost-effective platform through which you can engage with clients, potential clients, and referring veterinary surgeons. A Facebook business page can provide a fledgling aquatic therapy unit with an excellent platform on which to advertise the business prior to making the investment in a webpage and domain. Publishing regular, interesting, and succinct articles about the conditions that aquatic therapy can assist with is an excellent starting point to gain confidence in writing and publishing social media content. Twitter can be used in a similar way to Facebook to generate client interest and promote aquatic therapy. Encouraging current clients to engage with your social media platforms is paramount if a venture into social media is going to work. Publishing daily updates about the patients you are treating is an excellent way of growing interest in an aquatic therapy business. When venturing into social media it is vital that client confidentiality is protected always and permission needs to be gained from all clients prior to publishing pictures of their pet, or any images of the actual client.

Conclusion

Aquatic therapy remains a cornerstone of rehabilitation for many orthopedic and neurological conditions. When the approach taken to therapy is regimented, individualized, and responsive to a patient's progress and when it considers the holistic needs of the patient, the impact on a patient's life can be hugely positive. This sphere of therapy will continue to mature as research helps us to define specific benefits that aquatic therapy has for a spectrum of specific conditions.

References

Baranoski, S. and Ayello, E.A. (2012). Wound dressings: An evolving art and science. *Adv Skin Wound Care* 25 (2): 87–92.

Bliss, M., Terry, J., and de Godoy, R.F. (2022). Limbs kinematics of dogs exercising at different water levels on the underwater treadmill. *Vet Med Sci* 8 (6): 2374–2381.

Bockstahler, B.A., Prickler, B., Lewy, E. et al. (2012). Hind limb kinematics during therapeutic exercises in dogs with osteoarthritis of the hip joints. *Am J Vet Res* 73 (9): 1371–1376.

Chauvet, A., Laclair, J., Elliott, D.A., and German, A.J. (2011). Incorporation of exercise, using an underwater treadmill, and active client education into a weight management program for obese dogs. *Can Vet J* 52 (5): 491–496.

Chiquoine, J., McCauley, L., and Van Dyke, J.B. (2013). Aquatic therapy. In: *Canine Sports Medicine and Rehabilitation* (ed. M.C. Zink and J.B. Van Dyke), 158–175. Ames, IA: John Wiley & Sons, Inc.

Connell, L. and Monk, M. (2010). Small animal postoperative orthopaedic rehabilitation. *The Vet Nurse* 1 (1): 12–21.

Farrell, M., Clements, D.N., Mellor, D. et al. (2007). Retrospective evaluation of the long-term outcome of non-surgical management of 74 dogs with clinical hip dysplasia. *Vet Rec* 160 (15): 506–511.

Fish, F.E., DiNenno, N.K., and Trail, J. (2021). The "dog paddle": Stereotypic swimming gait pattern in different dog breeds. *Anatom Rec* 304 (1): 90–100. 10.1002/ar.24396.

Goldberg ME (2015) Top 5 most common orthopedic conditions in dogs. *Veterinary Team Brief* August:27–30. http://www.veterinaryteambrief.com/article/top-5-most-common-orthopedic-conditions-dogs (accessed March 21, 2016).

Gordon-Evans, W.J., Evans, R.B., Knap, K.E. et al. (2009). Characterization of spatiotemporal gait characteristics in clinically normal dogs and dogs with spinal cord disease. *Am J Vet Res* 70: 1444–1449.

Levine D, Tragauler V, and Millis DL (2002) Percentage of normal weight bearing during partial immersion at various depths in dogs. In *Proceedings 2nd International Symposium on Rehabilitation and Physical Therapy in Veterinary Medicine* Knoxville, TN, pp. 189–190.

Levine, D., Marcellin, D.J., Millis, D.L. et al. (2010). Effects of partial immersion in water on vertical ground reaction forces and weight distribution in dogs. *Am J Vet Res* 71: 1413–1416.

Levine, D., Millis, D.L., Flocker, J., and MacGuire, L. (2014). Aquatic therapy. In: *Canine Rehabilitation and Physical Therapy*, 2nde (ed. D.L. Millis and D. Levine), 526–542. Philadelphia, PA: Elsevier.

Marsolais, G.S., McLean, S., Derrick, T., and Conzemius, M.G. (2003). Kinematic analysis of the hind limb during swimming and walking in healthy dogs and dogs with surgically corrected cranial cruciate ligament rupture. *J Am Vet Med Assoc* 222 (6): 739–743.

Mojarradi, A., De Decker, S., Bäckström, C., and Bergknut, N. (2021). Safety of early postoperative hydrotherapy in dogs undergoing thoracolumbar hemilaminectomy. *J Small Anim Pract* 62 (12): 1062–1069.

Nganvongpanit, K. and Yano, T. (2012). Side effects in 412 dogs from swimming in a chlorinated swimming pool. *Thai J Vet Med* 42: 281–286.

Nganvongpanit, K., Boonchai, T., Taothong, O. et al. (2014a). Physiological effects of water temperatures in swimming toy breed dogs. *Kafkas Univ Vet Fak Deg* 20: 177–183.

Nganvongpanit K, Tanvisut S, Yano T, *et al.* (2014b) Effect of swimming on clinical functional parameters and serum biomarkers in healthy and osteoarthritic dogs. *ISRN Vet Sci* 459809. doi.org/10.1155/2014/459809.

Olby, N.J., Moore, S.A., Brisson, B. et al. (2022). ACVIM consensus statement on diagnosis and management of acute canine thoracolumbar intervertebral disc extrusion. *J Vet Intern Med* 36 (5): 1570–1596.

Prankel, S. (2008). Hydrotherapy in practice. *In Practice* 30: 272–277.

Preston, T. and Wills, A.P. (2018). A single hydrotherapy session increases range of motion and stride length in Labrador retrievers diagnosed with elbow dysplasia. *Vet J* 234: 105–110.

Prydie, D. and Hewitt, I. (2015). Modalities. In: *Practical Physiotherapy for Small Animal Practice* (eds. D. Prydie and I. Hewitt), 69–90. Chichester, Sussex, UK: John Wiley & Sons, Ltd.

Randall, X. (2010). Principles and application of canine hydrotherapy. *Vet Nurs J* 25 (12): 23–25.

Tomlinson, R. (2013). Use of canine hydrotherapy as part of a rehabilitation program. *Vet Nurse* 3 (10): 624–629.

Versey, N.G., Halson, S.L., and Dawson, B.T. (2013). Water immersion recovery for athletes: Effect on exercise performance and practical recommendations. *Sports Med* 43 (11): 1101–1130.

Vitger, A.D., Bruhn-Rasmussen, T., Pedersen, E.O. et al. (2021). The impact of water depth and speed on muscle fiber activation of healthy dogs walking in a water treadmill. *Acta Vet Scand* 63 (1): 46.

Voss, K., Galeandro, L., Wiestner, T. et al. (2010). Relationships of body weight, body size, subject velocity, and vertical ground reaction forces in trotting dogs. *Vet Surg* 39 (7): 863–869.

Waining, M., Young, I.S., and Williams, S.B. (2011). Evaluation of the status of canine hydrotherapy in the UK. *Vet Rec* 168 (15): 407.

Wilke, V.L., Robinson, D.A., Evans, R.B. et al. (2005). Estimate of the annual economic impact of treatment of cranial cruciate ligament injury in dogs in the United States. *J Am Vet Med Assoc* 227 (10): 1604–1607.

Yoo, J., Lim, K.B., Lee, H.J., and Kwon, Y.G. (2014). Cardiovascular response during submaximal underwater treadmill exercise in stroke patients. *Ann Rehabil Med* 38 (5): 628–636.

Zidan, N., Sims, C., Fenn, J. et al. (2018). A randomized, blinded, prospective clinical trial of postoperative rehabilitation in dogs after surgical decompression of acute thoracolumbar intervertebral disc herniation. *J Vet Intern Med* 32: 1133–1144.

22

Troubleshooting as a Team

Amie Lamoreaux Hesbach[1], Julia E. Tomlinson[2,3], and Erin White[4]

[1] *EmpowerPhysio, Maynard, MA, USA*
[2] *Twin Cities Rehabilitation & Sports Medicine Clinic, Burnsville, MN, USA*
[3] *Veterinary Rehabilitation and Orthopedic Medicine Partners, San Clemente, CA, USA*
[4] *SportVet Canine Rehabilitation and Sports Medicine, Tallahassee, FL, USA*

Introduction

The collaborative goal of the veterinary rehabilitation team is to improve quality of life (QoL), relieve pain, and maximize function of the animal patient, even considering physical limitations and impairments. The primary veterinary rehabilitation team may consist of a veterinarian further educated in physical rehabilitation (often with training in acupuncture and manipulative therapies), a veterinary technician/nurse educated in rehabilitation, and a physical therapist further educated in physical therapy for animals. Adjunct team members might include chiropractors with further training in chiropractic on animals, massage therapists who have had animal-specific training, and physical therapist assistants, also with further education in physical therapy for animals. Collaboration with primary care veterinarians, veterinary specialists (e.g., neurologists, surgeons, oncologists, etc.), other veterinary clinic staff, and the owner/handler/caregiver is integral to the success of rehabilitation. This collaboration is especially vital when troubleshooting patient problems, exacerbations, red flags, or a plateau.

The Role of the Rehabilitation Veterinarian

The rehabilitation-trained veterinarian will examine the patient with a rehabilitation focus but with evaluation techniques inclusive of the general health of the patient, pain (including pain score), integrity of injured tissues, presence of concurrent disease, evaluation of physical impairments, including posture, strength, range of motion (ROM), balance, sensation and proprioception, and neurological status, functional mobility, and gait. The rehabilitation veterinarian may order further diagnostics and then develop a rehabilitation treatment plan, based on the pathological diagnosis, which might include at-home and in-clinic therapies, medications, and nursing care. The veterinarian may perform or prescribe manual therapies and other specialized treatments. Other professionals, if part of the team, will contribute to this plan. The rehabilitation veterinarian may be a specialist in veterinary sports medicine and rehabilitation (DACVSMR) or certified in veterinary rehabilitation.

The Role of the Rehabilitation Veterinary Technician

The rehabilitation veterinary technician or nurse will assist the rehabilitation veterinarian, physical therapist, and any other adjunct professional with the evaluation and treatment. The technician will assist in handling the patient and in taking and recording measurements and observations, such as vital signs and pain scoring. The rehabilitation technician will contribute to the education of the client and explain the recommended home care and in-clinic rehabilitation plans. Mobility questionnaires may be part of the information that clients need to regularly fill out (see Boxes 22.1 and 22.2). The rehabilitation veterinary technician will also complete or carry out in-clinic therapies under the supervision of the rehabilitation veterinarian and should have received specific training in (if not certification in) veterinary rehabilitation. There is now a veterinary technician specialty (VTS) in rehabilitation in the United States (see Chapter 2). It is important to understand that in most states, veterinary technicians cannot work independently of a supervising veterinarian and, therefore, cannot be supervised by a physical therapist.

The Role of the Physical Therapist

The physical therapist, educated and trained in animal rehabilitation beyond the entry-level degree, whether master's or doctorate, preparing them for practice with human patients, will evaluate the patient after veterinary diagnosis, and document impairments in strength, ROM (including accessory joint motions), flexibility, balance, sensation and proprioception, neurological status, which impact functional limitations in postures, functional mobility, and gait, and which might be associated with acute or chronic inflammation or painful conditions. Together with the rehabilitation veterinarian, the physical therapist will develop and implement the treatment plan and will perform treatments including manual therapy, facilitation techniques, therapeutic exercises, and physical modalities. Physical therapists might also be integral in the fitting of assistive devices, including orthotics, prosthetics, and wheelchairs. Physical therapists practicing in animal rehabilitation hold a master's degree or certification in animal rehabilitation, depending upon rules and regulations of the state, province, or country of practice. Additionally, a physical therapist in animal rehabilitation may supervise a physical therapist assistant. This is an individual with an associate or bachelor's degree who can provide many therapies under the supervision of a physical therapist. It is important to understand that in most states, physical therapist assistants cannot work independently of a physical therapist and, therefore, cannot be supervised by a veterinarian. As with all team members, the physical therapist assistant will have training (including certification) in animal rehabilitation and should be proficient in low-stress handling of the patient.

Box 22.1   Feline mobility questionnaire. Courtesy today's veterinary nurse

CLIENT HANDOUT

Feline Mobility Questionnaire

1. Mobility

Tell me about your cat's behavior. _____

Does your cat still want to interact by jumping to the table, chair, etc? _____

Tell me about your cat's ability to jump up to or down from higher places. _____

Does your cat jump to the chair first and then to a higher or lower place? _____

Tell me about any changes in toileting behavior. _____

Please describe your litterbox:

- Height _____
- Width _____
- Cleaning frequency_____
- Type of litter used_____

2. Activity Level

Describe your cat's sleeping behavior. _____

Does your cat frequently adjust his/her position to try to be more comfortable? _____

Tell me about your cat's playing/interacting with members of the family._____

- Human or animal?_____
- Have you noticed any changes? _____

3. Grooming

Describe your cat's grooming behavior. _____

Describe your cat's coat/fur. _____

Does your cat have difficulty reaching certain areas to groom or clean? _____

Have you noticed if your cat's claws are overgrown? _____

How often do you clip your cat's claws? _____

4. Temperament

Is cat hiding from family members?_____

Does the cat appear to be "grumpy" and irritable? _____

Weight of cat: _____

Body condition score: _____

Muscle condition score: _____

today's veterinary
nurse

An Official Journal of the NAVC ● todaysveterinarynurse.com

Box 22.2   Canine mobility questionnaire. Courtesy today's veterinary nurse

CLIENT
HANDOUT

Canine Mobility Questionnaire

1. Behavior

Tell me about your dog's interaction with you and the rest of the family. _____

Does your dog enjoy car rides? _____

- Describe how he/she gets into the vehicle. _____

- What changes in toileting have you noticed? _____

- Give me examples of changes in your dog's behavior that are unlike his/her normal behavior. _____

2. Activity Level

Describe your dog's exercise regimen. Has it changed over time? _____

Tell me about your dog's play behavior. _____

- Has your dog appeared to be less interested in playing/interacting with human or animal members of the family? _____

Does it seem your dog's enjoyment of activity has changed? _____

- What is preventing your dog from taking walks? _____

- What is preventing your dog from interacting with you? _____

Does your dog appear to tire easily? _____

- Is your dog lying around more than in the past? _____

- Demonstrate how your dog rises from rest. _____

- Tell me how this differs from prior behavior. _____

3. Eating and Sleeping

Tell me about your dog's appetite. _____

- Have you noticed any changes in your dog wanting to eat? _____

- Is your dog able to finish their meal? _____

Tell me about your dog's sleeping behavior _____

- Tell me how this differs from prior behavior. _____

- Does your dog frequently adjust his/her position to try to be more comfortable? _____

4. Environment

Tell me about the flooring in your home. _____

How many stairs are in your house? _____

Weight of dog: _____

Body condition score: _____

Muscle condition score: _____

today's veterinary
nurse

The Role of Other Team Members

Other team members might include veterinarians trained in acupuncture or spinal manipulative therapy (e.g., the veterinary term for chiropractic) and other specialty veterinarians (i.e., surgeon, oncologist, neurologist, and primary care veterinarian). Chiropractors as well as massage therapists who have received additional training and certification in animal therapy may be involved in the care of the rehabilitation patient.

Case Management

Each case will differ; two dogs with similar medical history and signalment with the same problem, undergoing the same surgical procedure at the same facility, will have differing resultant levels of pain, function, and recovery rates, regardless of the plan, highlighting the need to avoid applying a set protocol (or recipe) to groups of patients and the need for continuous evaluation and re-evaluation by the rehabilitation team.

The foundation of the therapeutic plan is the evaluation. Patient evaluation should continue throughout the rehabilitation process; evaluation of patient function, and objective measures such as pain score and goniometry. Examination for concurrent disease should occur at every rehabilitation visit. The veterinary technician should immediately report to the supervising rehabilitation veterinarian any changes that have occurred from one visit to another so that appropriate measures may be taken. The therapeutic plan is altered accordingly and might include changes in medications, progression of home exercises, relaxation of restrictions, or, in the worst case or red flag scenario, referral back to the veterinary specialist.

Communicating with Specialists and the Primary Care Veterinarian

It is essential that communication with the primary care or specialty veterinarian be on a frequent and regular basis, and, in the case that there is a sudden change in patient status, immediate. The rehabilitation veterinary technician may be facilitating this communication via phone or electronic communications. In the case that a client self-refers their own pet to rehabilitation, the rehabilitation facility staff must continue to inform the client that communication and collaboration with the primary care veterinarian is required, both prior to rehabilitation evaluation, but also intermittently and regularly during the rehabilitation episode of care.

If the patient develops a new issue that requires further diagnostics or treatment that is not available or feasible within the rehabilitation clinic, it is the responsibility of the rehabilitation veterinarian to refer the patient back to the primary care veterinarian, specialty veterinarian, or a different specialist. The American Animal Hospital Association Referral Guidelines (www.aaha.org) state that, "A referral should be considered when there is a need for additional expertise/advanced training, additional services to provide further diagnostic testing or an unresolved or worsening medical condition." All veterinarians involved in the care of the patient should be made aware of the change in condition and of any subsequent referral. Communication between the rehabilitation team and all veterinarians involved in patient care should include updated medication lists and medical records from the rehabilitation facility.

The rehabilitation veterinary technician fulfills an important role as the patient and client advocate and should be proactive in communication when recognizing changes in patient status. The ultimate advice in any case is, when in doubt, ask your supervising veterinarian.

Communicating with Team Members

With team members of varied educational and experiential backgrounds involved in rehabilitation, many points of view regarding treatment decisions will be advocated. A rehabilitation-trained veterinarian should be the supervisor, but it may be a specialist in sports medicine and rehabilitation (DACVSMR) or a surgeon (DACVS) who is the supervising veterinarian. Team member input should be solicited and considered in every case while maintaining respect professional ethics and courtesy.

Daily rounds (see Figure 22.1) including the entire rehabilitation team, in which

patients are discussed (both inpatients and outpatients) and the therapy plan is adjusted are strongly recommended. Alerting your supervising veterinarian about concerns regarding the patient may take a few moments because they are overseeing several patients at one time yet is essential and provides an efficient solution. In a red flag situation, owners should be counseled on the need to wait for veterinary intervention before progressing with therapy for that day. Troubleshooting should always involve the supervising veterinarian as the veterinary technician is not the case manager and should not be determining the therapy plan.

Collaboration is a simple process when all team members are physically located at the same facility and have immediate access to the patient. Problems can arise when members of the veterinary care team (including the rehabilitation team) interact with the patient and client at different times or in different facilities as patient status can

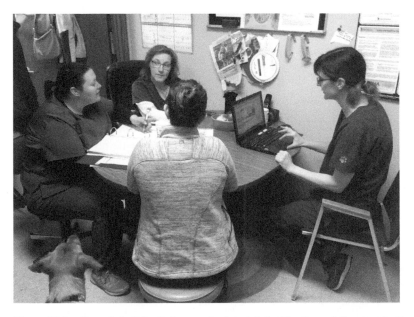

Figure 22.1 Rounds in this clinic are scheduled daily (Tomlinson). Communication is enhanced via "rounds sheets" which are prepared prior to the meeting and contain written descriptions of the daily therapy plan as well as copies of the digital records of the most recent rehabilitation session. This allows for productive and efficient discussion of cases between and among members of the rehabilitation team.

differ from day to day and recommendations may be made that counter those made by other team members. Team members should avoid making recommendations to the client that contradict previous recommendations made by other team members and the case should first be discussed with the team leader. Team members who are not qualified to make a diagnosis or recommend a treatment should avoid doing so, especially with regard to nutrition, supplements, medications, assistive devices, or home instructions. For example, though a pet store employee can make recommendations with regard to diet and supplements without legal consequences, these recommendations might have consequences for the health and well-being of the animal. Non-veterinarian members of the rehabilitation team should not make such recommendations. Though supplements and food are not tightly regulated, recommendations can do harm. Regardless, all members of the rehabilitation team should strive to avoid the effect of "too many cooks spoiling the broth" and refrain from making unilateral decisions.

Examples of Case Management

Case 1: Unexpected Diagnosis

A five-year-old intact male Labrador retriever, who is a competitor in both field trial and agility, presented to the rehabilitation clinic with a primary concern of him having become slower on his retrieves. The main sport he trained for was field trial. Field trial competitors are elite athletes who need to train for speed, strength, and stamina. The patient had been seeing a specialist (DACVSMR) every 4–6 months for an evaluation of his general sports preparedness, and maintenance of toe function due to osteoarthritis secondary to a previous sprain. Two years prior, he had been treated by the specialist for biceps tendinopathy

with a series of platelet-rich plasma (PRP) injections and shockwave therapy.

The massage-trained veterinary technician that the patient sees monthly noted tightness in the lumbar paraspinal muscles that would not fully resolve in response to her treatment. The therapist had suggested chiropractic (or veterinary spinal manipulative) therapy, which is a service that his veterinarian acupuncturist also provides. On evaluation by the veterinarian who was certified in acupuncture and spinal manipulation, spasm was noted in the iliopsoas and longissimus muscles with discomfort in the periphery of the L5 vertebra. Manual therapies were performed at L3–L6 and sacroiliac joints, followed by electroacupuncture. Following this appointment, the patient returned to training with a normal level of enthusiasm for retrieving drills. After the first week, he started to show the previous symptoms again. Per the owner, when he was loaded into the truck post-training, he was noted hesitating to jump up. He had a repeat treatment with the veterinary acupuncturist, with relief of symptoms for two weeks. After three more visits, the resulting duration of relief was not increasing and, in fact, was declining.

The patient was referred to the American College of Veterinary Sports Medicine and Rehabilitation (ACVSMR) specialist veterinarian for a non-routine evaluation.

Physical examination by the specialist revealed discomfort in passive motioning of the L4–5 and L5–6 intervertebral joints. There was also discomfort on tail hyperextension (tail raise) test. Internal (rectal) examination was performed for evaluation of pain in the intrapelvic portion of the iliopsoas muscle, the lumbosacral disc space, and/or a portion of the sciatic nerve. There was a mild pain response on pressure over the right lumbosacral facet but not over the sciatic nerve or the iliopsoas. The urethra and prostate were also evaluated, and the prostate was thought to be enlarged; the surface felt irregular. On a more targeted client interview, the specialist learned that the dog had not been fully voiding feces in one static squatting position but had been walking forward while defecating. The prostate and bladder were imaged via diagnostic ultrasound and radiographs were taken of the lumbar spine and hips with the goal of identifying potential causes of the pain.

Diagnostic results – The prostate was found to have a small pocket of fluid within the parenchyma; however, the urethra was patent. The size of the prostate was measured and compared to normal ranges, but there was no in-clinic information available regarding the relation of prostate size to body mass, given the scope of the clinic library. Radiographs showed remodeling of the right articular facet of the lumbosacral joint and of the left and right L5–6 articular facets; however, there was no apparent narrowing of disc spaces or the intervertebral foramina therefore static nerve compression was not suspected. The rectal temperature was within the normal range.

Plan – The rehabilitation specialist referred the patient to an internal medicine specialist veterinarian for further evaluation of possible prostatitis versus benign prostatic hyperplasia, considering that prostatitis is a cause of pain. Photobiomodulation therapy (laser) (500 mW continuous, contact probe) was also initiated to treat the lower back discomfort (whether due to referred pain or locoregional) and performed by a veterinary technician therapist at the specialty clinic, twice weekly for three weeks. Prescription for all therapy was written by the ACVSMR specialist.

Light field training under the specialist's prescription (short single bumper retrieves, no swimming) was resumed with an oral anti-inflammatory prescribed for use as needed following training. Injectable polysulfated glycosaminoglycans (PSGAGs) were prescribed for spinal facet joint osteoarthritis

due to being a disease-modifying osteoarthritic agent. Following communication with the veterinary acupuncturist, manual therapies were resumed in the form of joint mobilizations and manipulations along with acupuncture. Generalized massage by the technician was discontinued until prostate infection could be ruled out (given the theory of possible lymphatic spread of localized infection after massage). The technician instead focused on the forelimbs and thoracic and cervical regions.

Case progression – The dog continued training to tolerance to avoid a generalized loss of fitness. The client was educated to modify training activities to avoid back-to-back training days and to reduce the next training session by 25% if post-training stiffness was seen and lasted more than a day (note the post-training stiffness had so far only manifested as occasional reluctance to jump into the vehicle immediately after training).

The dog's tolerance for training improved with no apparent loss of speed during training drills. A month later, the dog and handler participated in a field trial (back-to-back days) which was well-tolerated until the third day of the trial during which the dog lost enthusiasm and speed and was pulled from further competition. "Lumbar discomfort" was reported by the field veterinarian at the trial. The prescribed anti-inflammatory was given daily along with the muscle relaxer, methocarbamol, which was prescribed by the field veterinarian.

A post-trial visit for massage three days later revealed ongoing tightness in the lumbar paraspinals which resolved in response to passive and active stretching techniques (direct massage continued to be avoided). The technician performing massage and client emailed an update to both the veterinary acupuncturist and the ACVSMR specialist. An acupuncture treatment followed and resulted in a subjective improvement in comfort.

The internal medicine specialist evaluation was performed six weeks after the referral and ultrasound imaging, biopsy, and internal examination confirmed benign prostatic hyperplasia. The patient was prescribed finasteride, and a recheck examination was scheduled for eight weeks later. The plan was to discuss neutering, if needed, at that appointment. The internal medicine specialist forwarded medical records to the ACVSMR specialist and primary care veterinarian. Neither the veterinarian acupuncturist nor the massage therapist received communication from the internal medicine specialist. The client and ACVSMR specialist informed these members of the team, and the patient was cleared for full massage.

The patient continued to train and work at a lighter-than-usual level. Approximately, four weeks into finasteride therapy, the patient was rechecked by the DACVSMR, he had been performing well and the report from the massage therapist was that the lumbar paraspinal tightness was minor, resolving quickly with massage. The client noted that the dog was up to full speed during training and trials with no signs of tiring. The dog had also been voiding feces in one static squatting posture. Physical examination by the ACVSMR specialist revealed improved response to palpation with minimal discomfort on passive motioning of the L4–L5 intervertebral joints and no pain response to L5–L6 motioning. There was no discomfort on tail hyperextension, an improvement since the evaluation. Internal (rectal) examination was not performed due to the upcoming appointment with internal medicine (a decision for low-stress handling).

At the internal medicine appointment, the prostate was noted to be smaller on ultrasound imaging but still enlarged. A decision was made for long-term use of finasteride due to the breeding potential of the dog (see Box 22.3).

Box 22.3   Case 1: Discussion

1) Regional discomfort can be multifactorial and a thorough clinical examination is recommended, with appropriate referral as needed.
2) In this case, a large team of individuals cooperating was needed to help this patient return to function.
3) Why did the technician avoid the lower lumbar area during massage?

   Prostatitis is a deep-seated infection; caution is needed due to theoretical risk of infection spread secondary to increased lymphatic drainage during massage

---

Case 2: Virtual Consultation

Arrow, a 9.5-year-old male Nova Scotia Duck Tolling Retriever had a laceration injury to bilateral hindlimbs, immediately proximal to the calcaneus on the caudal aspect, in March 2022. The pet's wounds were sutured under anesthesia at the primary care veterinary hospital. Fortunately, the wounds involved only the epidermis and subcutaneous adipose layer with fascia and deeper layers intact and closed without complication prior to the suture removal 10 days later.

At four weeks post-injury, the owner noted right hind limb lameness and that the right wound and common calcaneal tendon looked and felt thicker than the left. Arrow was seen by the traveling surgeon who suggested that there was scarring over the tarsal joint (but not within the joint capsule) and suggested a consultation with an ACVSMR specialist. Unfortunately, the initial appointment was unable to be scheduled immediately and was over 10 weeks after the original injury due to a high volume of cases at that rehabilitation clinic.

In the meantime, the owner consulted a Certified Canine Rehabilitation Practitioner/Certified Canine Rehabilitation Therapist (CCRP/CCRT) Doctor of Physical Therapy who was able to perform an online consultation focusing on instructing the client in ROM, stretching, and exercise which might assist in Arrow's recovery in preparation for his in-person rehabilitation consultation with the ACVSMR specialist. This consultation was scheduled for six weeks post-injury and was performed via a Zoom link after a review of medical records and owner-submitted videos of Arrow's posture, functional mobility, and gait.

The owner's primary complaint at the time was right hind limb weight-bearing lameness with an early toe-off and shortened stance phase, which was also observed in videos and during the online consultation.

The owner's concerns included:

- Right hind limb lameness (apparent especially when descending stairs, when fetching/running, with a shortened stride length) The right hind is seen with external rotation/toeing out and increased tarsal extension bilaterally.
- Right hind limb "twitching"
- Right hind limb guarding after exercise/activity
- Arrow pulls himself up on furniture with his forelimbs rather than jumping up
- Arrow will not fully extend the right hind when stretching
- Arrow sits "wide" with his hind limbs toed out/externally rotated/abducted
- Per the owner, he has tightness in his right hindlimb paw, especially

During the online video consultation, the owner was instructed in passive range of motion (PROM), massage, and stretching techniques to reduce the potential that scar tissue (increased thickness of the tissue) was restricting mobility along the Achilles/common calcaneal tendon and

mobility throughout the hindlimb. The hope was that these conservative techniques might increase mobility of the skin and scar tissue relative to the deeper tissues, improve ROM, functional limb mobility and postures, and improve strength and motor control so as to reduce the risk of injury to other limbs, joints, and the spine, especially.

Further instructions included: continued activity/mobility restriction including restriction of stair climbing and activity on hardwood flooring, short leash walks, passive heating with a heating pad, massage, skin rolling, stretches, therapeutic exercises to promote muscle contractions and weight bearing, and, finally, ice application. The therapist also educated the client on the benefits of photobiomodulation (laser) therapy and instructed him to follow-up with the ACVSMR specialist for a full manual evaluation. Follow-up was unremarkable and by electronic mail and messaging only.

At the 10-week post-injury date, the ACVSMR specialist examined Arrow and found evidence of luxation of the right superficial digital flexor tendon with limited tarsal flexion and compensatory discomfort in the cervical and glenohumeral regions. Limited rehabilitation was initiated, and a referral was made to a local surgeon for potential repair of the luxation. The ACVSMR specialist communicated the physical examination findings directly with the Doctor of Physical Therapy.

The luxation was repaired, and postoperative recovery was uneventful. Arrow was referred back to the ACVSMR specialist at three weeks post-surgery for rehabilitation therapy (see Box 22.4).

Case 3: In Over Your Head

Daisy, a one-year-old Goldendoodle, had acute onset rear paralysis (deep pain present) and was referred to Animal Specialty

---

Box 22.4   Case 2: Discussion

1) What red flags are suggested by this case?
   The proximity of the wound to the calcaneal tendon, and the thickening of the calcaneal tendon. Calcaneal tendon injuries can progress slowly and can result in loss of use of the affected limb

2) Has pain been managed adequately?
   There is twitching and guarding after activity but overall there is no consistent lameness. Pain is mostly managed

3) Without a manual examination, what conclusions can be made? **Only that there is regional thickening of tissue and some restrictions in motion.**

4) What activities can the client perform without potentially harming her pet?

   Active range of motion as long as any avoidance by the pet is noted and allowed (until physical examination can clear for more difficult exercises) gentle passive range of motion and massage

5) What assistive devices or home modifications might be helpful in protecting him and his injury? **Ramps to furniture, avoid stairs until physical examination**

6) If the client is unable to physically access a rehabilitation professional, what options does the primary care veterinarian have? **Refer to orthopedic surgeon to assess why progress in healing has stopped.**

Center emergency department. She had an magnetic resonance imaging (MRI) and subsequent hemilaminectomy to treat intervertebral disc extrusion at L1–L2. She was examined post-operatively and found to still have deep pain but no motor function. Rehabilitation therapy was instituted by the adjacent primary care clinic, Skye Veterinary, which had an underwater treadmill, photobiomodulation (laser) therapy equipment, and a veterinary technician certified in rehabilitation. On rehabilitation examination, Daisy was found to have excess extensor tone and would try to bite any individual attempting to perform PROM. The veterinary technician at Skye Veterinary contacted the neurologist who had performed Daisy's surgery, and she advised sedated examination to explore how much ROM the patient had. The patient was on analgesics at the time, a nonsteroidal anti-inflammatory drug (NSAID) and gabapentin. The neurologist also put the veterinary technician in contact with the veterinary technician

specialist (VTS) at Animal Specialty Center to provide further rehabilitation guidance.

Daisy was sedated at Skye Veterinary once weekly for several weeks and had PROM performed multiple times. The sedation protocol did not include any analgesics in addition to the oral medications she was on. Daisy underwent underwater treadmill therapy with gait patterning in the rear performed by the rehabilitation veterinary technician. Some return of motor function was noted in the medical record, slight initiation of protraction in the right rear.

Daisy continued to be aggressive in response to PROM exercises at home and in a clinic, so this exercise was stopped unless Daisy was sedated. Despite therapy, Daisy continued to get stiffer and to lose flexion ROM in her hocks and stifles. The technician with a VTS in rehabilitation had continued to remotely advise the technician at Skye Veterinary. It is unclear whether the neurologist was aware of Daisy's status. The treatment duration was three months.

The client became concerned that Daisy was in continued pain and contacted Garden Veterinary Rehabilitation clinic, an examination was scheduled and performed later that month. The rehabilitation-certified veterinarian examined, and pain-scored the patient using the Glasgow Pain Scale (see Chapter 3 in this textbook). The pain score was 13 out of 20 on the modified scale allowing for lack of mobility. Examination revealed quadriceps contracture and stifle and tarsal joint contracture. The digits could be manually flexed with no discomfort response. The patient had both superficial and deep sensation, but superficial sensation was likely altered due to self-inflicted trauma wounds over the hocks bilaterally. The patient was prescribed a higher dose of gabapentin, and amantadine was added in addition to the gabapentin and NSAID. Under the supervision of the rehabilitation-certified veterinarian, a rehabilitation technician performed the following prescribed modalities. Photobiomodulation (laser) therapy three days a week (810 nm 500 mW continuous) was started over the spine at the surgery site extending two vertebrae above and below, and a pulsed electromagnetic field (PEMF) device was sent home for use over the distal limb wounds and over the spine and thigh muscles. After four days on the new regimen, therapeutic ultrasound three times weekly over the contracted tissues was started. The ultrasound settings were continuous wave 1.0–1.1 W/cm^2 at 3.3 MHz, the hock was treated using a gel offset given the contours of the joint (could be immersed in water but this was avoided due to the wounds). After a week, Daisy stopped vocalizing when resting at home and began to allow in-clinic flexion of her rear limbs. Clinic notes were sent to the neurologist and to Skye Veterinary.

After 6 weeks of in-clinic rehabilitation, stifle flexion was improved from 150° to 110° but with muscle-spasm end feel. Hock flexion was improved to 90°. The rehabilitation veterinarian and technician at Garden Veterinary Rehabilitation noted some motor function (weak withdrawal), but that the ongoing contracture was preventing protraction. Options discussed with the client were to try gait patterning in a cart on a land treadmill or in an underwater treadmill, or to fit a cart with the rear limbs suspended off the ground. The client was principally concerned with pain control and QoL after what was viewed as a long recovery period involving multiple veterinary visits.

A cart was fitted, enabling Daisy to move independently outside of the house and to go on walks. Daisy's demeanor was much improved in response to this treatment. An attempt was made to reduce her medications slowly; however, Daisy began to chew at her hocks again, so the full dose and range of medications were resumed.

Daisy continues to visit Garden Veterinary Rehabilitation every six months to check on her comfort and mobility (see Box 22.5).

Case 4: Activity Restrictions

Luke, a four-year-old, neutered, Belgian Malinois was referred to Fit Furry Friends Animal Rehabilitation Center, six weeks after surgery to repair an Achilles tendon rupture. Initially, Luke had presented to the orthopedic surgeon following four weeks of non-weight-bearing lameness after a laceration to his left tarsus. The laceration had been repaired by his primary care veterinarian, but a week after surgery he began walking with an almost fully plantigrade stance (see Figure 22.2). Surgery was performed and the identified tendon tear was apposed with sutures. The surgeon noted that there was an increased amount of tension on the repair since the tendon had retracted proximally. A calcaneotibial screw was placed to lock the tarsus in hyperextension during healing. A full bivalved cast was also placed

---

Box 22.5   Case 3: Discussion

1) What red flags are suggested by this case? **Concern for tissue contracture and permanent loss of range of motion. Lack of guidance for the technician therapist in a complex case.**

2) Was pain managed adequately? **The patient was biting during attempts at range of motion, regardless of temperament this should be first considered as a sign of pain.**

3) How soon should signs of contracture be addressed? Is there a time window where this issue could have been resolved? **Contracture should be immediately addressed; however, it is not always possible to completely correct or to prevent progression in a patient who has no motor function.**

4) Sedation requires the presence of a veterinarian and whole veterinary team, should analgesia have been part of the protocol considering that flexion was painful while awake? **Analgesia should have been part of the sedation protocol, an opioid is recommended.**

5) When should the neurologist have been informed? Should they have taken different action? Should the neurologist have given advice and warning about potential contracture? **The neurologist in this case was surprised and unaware of the contracture, they had not experienced this issue before and so had not given any warning. The neurologist should have been informed immediately via written report of therapy session.**

6) Is it appropriate for a technician to advise another technician at a different clinic on treatment protocols? **Technicians can of course share advice but a veterinarian with rehabilitation training and experience should have been consulted.**

7) Should the technician at Skye Veterinary be treating this patient without supervision of a rehabilitation veterinarian? **No, the potential for severe complications in rehabilitation cases like this indicates the need for knowledgeable supervision from a qualified individual who can take the case further.**

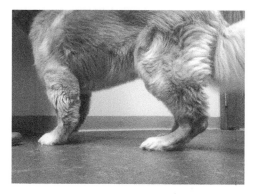

Figure 22.2 A dog with an almost plantigrade stance of the left rear due to Achilles tear.

over a bandage to restrict movement of the stifle and distal limb. Luke returned for weekly bandage changes until four weeks after surgery when removal of the calcaneotibial screw was performed and his cast was changed to a soft padded bandage with a lateral splint. Bandage changes continued weekly for two weeks, at which time he was referred to the rehabilitation team for orthosis prescription and rehabilitation consultation (six weeks after surgery).

During Luke's initial consultation with the physical therapist, he was non-weight

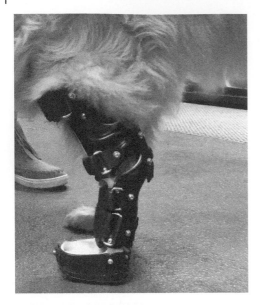

Figure 22.3 An articulating tarsal and foot orthosis (Orthopets) placed on the patient from Figure 22.2.

bearing on his left hindlimb. He had moderate atrophy of his left gluteals, quadriceps, and hamstrings with severe restriction of left tarsal flexion ROM. After taking measurements and a fiberglass impression for an articulating tarsal and foot orthosis (see Figure 22.3), the physical therapist consulted with the surgeon regarding the implementation of other modalities that would help facilitate Luke's healing. The surgeon was not a "fan of rehab" and elected to keep Luke in a soft padded cast and declined any further therapies at present.

Two weeks later, Luke returned for his orthosis fitting and adaptation exercises. Upon consultation with the surgeon again, the physical therapist was advised not to begin additional therapies. The rehabilitation technician reviewed orthosis care instructions and recommendations with the client, who was advised to return to the surgeon for a recheck (see Box 22.6). The following week, the surgeon contacted the physical therapist and reported that a skin sore had formed, so the surgical staff replaced the orthosis with a soft padded lateral splint. The owner was frustrated with this "step back" in healing and wanted more assistance with orthosis use once the wound had healed. The surgeon then contacted the physical therapist and advised that it would be acceptable to initiate rehabilitation modalities and take over care of the orthosis after a week in the bandage splint to allow sores to heal.

At the next rehabilitation visit, the bandage splint was removed, the orthosis was reapplied and photobiomodulation (laser) therapy of the left Achilles tendon, quadriceps, and hamstrings was initiated. Neuromuscular electrical stimulation (NMES) was applied to the quadriceps and hamstrings (for a co-contraction). The orthosis was to always be worn. The client was given specific instructions regarding permissible activity and exercise in the orthosis to reduce the risk of skin sore development. Luke was to continue outpatient therapy once weekly and the client to follow a specific home exercise plan. An orthosis recheck evaluation at the rehabilitation facility was set up for two weeks later.

Ten days later, 21 weeks following the repair and a few days before the scheduled orthosis recheck and weekly therapy visit, the surgeon called and reported that Luke had jumped off the bed and was not wearing his orthosis at the time of the incident. Upon examination, it was determined that Luke's Achilles repair had failed. The owner stated that Luke could not wear the orthosis for more than 20 minutes without his skin reddening and due to concerns about a sore, she had been removing it at home. She always took Luke to therapy in the device, however.

Several options were discussed with the owner: first, repair of the tendon, with the risk of it being a weaker repair and, therefore, more prone to re-injury; second, a pantarsal arthrodesis; and third, amputation. The owners elected to perform the arthrodesis.

Box 22.6   Case 4: Discussion

1) Would a rehabilitation veterinarian as team leader have made it easier to use other prescribed therapies? On referral, treatment choice is at the discretion of the receiving veterinarian. The surgeon was team leader but had no rehabilitation training. **A rehabilitation veterinarian may have been able to consult with and convince the surgeon with a different approach but this is not guaranteed. Treatment should have been the choice of the receiving rehabilitation veterinarian even if the client self-referred.**

2) An orthosis is a medical device; the individual prescribing and fitting should monitor and evaluate orthosis use and complications as they have the most suitable skill set. Some orthotics companies will only work directly with a veterinarian

3) The orthosis was reapplied but why had the sores occurred in the first place? Did the orthosis need refitting or changing? **A thorough examination by an individual trained in the use of orthoses would have been able to locate the level of the wound and match it to any constrictions or roughening of the surface of the orthosis. Also, evaluating fit as fitted by the owner is very valuable, applying the orthosis too loose can result in severe friction wounds.**

4) An owner may be non-compliant. Careful, repeated counseling about the risks and importance of proper device use is needed.

Case 5: Direct Versus Indirect Supervision

Sam, a 10-year-old male neutered Labrador, presented to Jane Doe who was a certified veterinary technician and had completed a certification course in canine rehabilitation. Sam had just had a tibial plateau leveling osteotomy (TPLO) on the right stifle. The rehabilitation facility was housed next to a primary care veterinary clinic. State law read that a technician could work under indirect supervision by a veterinarian, which was interpreted by Jane as meaning a veterinarian could refer directly to her for rehabilitation care and that she would manage the case. Jane owned her own business and was paid by clients directly.

Sam was sent to Jane by a local surgeon for routine postoperative rehabilitation. Sam was otherwise healthy. He started on a program of twice weekly hydrotherapy on an underwater treadmill followed by balance and proprioceptive work. Home exercises recommended by Jane were flexion and extension ROM of both stifles and rhythmic stabilization.

Sam progressed well until week 6 after surgery when he developed a grade 4/5 lameness while exercising on the underwater treadmill. Jane immediately terminated therapy, drained the tank, and brought Sam out. After quickly drying him, she examined him closely for signs of heat, swelling, and pain. Jane noted pain on palpation over Sam's cranial thigh muscles on the right. Sam was not painful when his right stifle was extended, but he was painful at end-range flexion. He was not painful on pressure medially over the surgical implants (see Box 22.7).

Jane iced Sam's cranial thigh muscles, his stifle, and advised his owner to do the same that evening. Jane's business was not connected to the adjacent primary care clinic, nor was Sam a patient of that clinic. Jane called Sam's surgeon and his primary care

---

Box 22.7   Case 5: Discussion

1) The term "indirect supervision" is interpreted in the relevant State/Province or Country's Veterinary Practice Act. In the case of a veterinary technician working in veterinary medicine under the indirect supervision of a veterinarian, the technician needs to be under the employ of that veterinarian who would carry the liability insurance

2) Recommending a treatment plan is the same as prescribing a treatment, this can be interpreted as the practice of veterinary medicine

3) It is not clear whether the primary care veterinarian or the surgeon is Jane's supervising veterinarian. Jane was right to contact them both, but what if recommendations from each were different? **In general, it is important to defer to the specialist. If more than one specialist is involved then deferring to the individual with knowledge in that particular field (e.g., sports medicine and rehabilitation versus surgery) is recommended. It can be challenging for individuals like Jane to navigate case decisions.**

4) Sam's veterinarian(s) who were supervising Jane should have informed her of the plan and outlined their instructions for her in management of the case

5) Jane cannot legally make a diagnosis or prescribe a treatment for that diagnosis

---

veterinarian to facilitate an examination at either the primary care or surgical clinic. The primary care veterinarian saw Sam the next day, prescribed a nonsteroidal anti-inflammatory (the same one that Sam was previously on for two weeks immediately after surgery), and took radiographs of the stifle. The radiographs were checked by the surgeon and no new pathology was noted. Sam's owners were instructed by the surgeon to confine him to a crate and to rest him for two weeks with leash walks to the bathroom only. Jane was informed of the plan for Sam by his owners and despite her concerns, she had no legal power to modify the veterinarian's recommendations. Following the two weeks of rest, Sam went back to Jane's rehabilitation facility. He was no longer on the anti-inflammatories, but exercise was still being restricted to leash walks. On examination, Sam had a grade 3/5 lameness on the right rear which was an improvement since the most recent onset of acute lameness, but prior to that time, Sam's postoperative lameness had been only a grade 2/5. Jane had concerns about persistence of pain. On further examination, Jane found that Sam was painful during direct palpation over his quadriceps muscles on the right, and slow stretch of these muscles produced resistance and pain, the left quadriceps had normal stretch with no pain (see Figure 22.4). Jane was concerned about a quadriceps strain but had not examined the quadriceps specifically before the acute onset of lameness Jane applied photobio-modulation (laser) therapy to the quadriceps and then gently massaged the muscle group. Sam's owners were instructed to massage at home twice daily. Sam visited for laser therapy five times over two weeks with improved muscle tone and pain relief noted following each session, but on each return visit the muscle spasm, shortening, and pain had returned. Sam's grade 3/5 lameness persisted.

Jane encouraged Sam's owners to make a recheck appointment with the surgeon so that she could re-evaluate Sam. Sam's treatment notes were sent to the owners so that

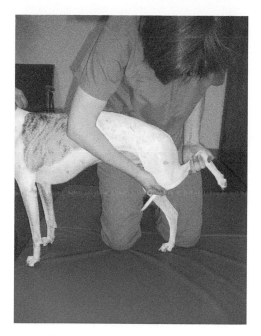

Figure 22.4 Quadriceps stretch.

the surgeon could understand Jane's examination findings. Jane could not write a diagnosis of a quadriceps muscle strain anywhere in the medical record as diagnosis or prescription of treatment was outside of her scope of practice. Jane was aware that even changing to a therapeutic modality for a new problem was technically illegal without a veterinarian prescribing this therapy. The medical record was carefully worded "pain on palpation over muscles of right cranial thigh, mostly limited to the quadriceps muscle group. Quadriceps stretch shortened compared to the left side. Applied laser therapy for symptomatic relief. On return to the rehab center, Sam still had the same pain and shortening of his right quadriceps. It was recommended to have an evaluation by a surgical specialist."

Sam was brought to the surgeon for examination. She confirmed muscle pain but said that it was likely secondary to relative overload from too much activity and recommended a further two weeks' rest with leash restriction. A follow-up visit was

booked for then. The anti-inflammatory medication prescribed by the primary care veterinarian was resumed for another two weeks. Sam's lameness persisted and on repeat examination and radiographs, the surgeon recommended implant removal as his osteotomy was healed but there was a small amount of bony reaction around the distal screw. The medical notes also indicated some progression of Sam's stifle arthritis.

Following implant removal, Sam was rested for two weeks. His lameness appeared to have resolved and so exercise restrictions were lifted by the surgeon. The surgeon recommended returning to Jane for therapy as Sam's right rear leg had "lost muscle." The anti-inflammatory was continued to help manage pain from arthritis. It would be "reduced to lowest effective dose once Sam was back to full fitness."

Sam returned to the rehabilitation center and resumed therapeutic exercises including hydrotherapy, balance work, and cavaletti rails. Jane measured Sam's thigh circumference and the right was 2 cm less than the left. The home exercise plan was altered by Jane, adding isometric strengthening of the rear limb muscles using front leg lifts (three-legged stands) in addition to his ROM and rhythmic stabilization exercises.

Sam's first two therapy sessions went well. Jane palpated his quadriceps before and after each therapy session and there was no pain response, although she did not evaluate his response to stretch. Sam returned for the third session with a grade 3/5 right hindlimb lameness. On examination, Jane found pain over the right quadriceps muscle group and shortened stretch, which was painful. Jane treated the muscle spasm and pain with laser therapy and massage and recommended a home heat and stretch exercise. She informed Sam's primary care veterinarian, who recommended leash restriction along with continuing

Jane's plan for laser therapy. After six more laser and massage treatments Sam was feeling better, and the stretch of the right quadriceps had improved. Jane decided that hydrotherapy might be "too much" for Sam and so continued the home exercise plan of front leg lifts progressing to diagonal leg lifts. She added sit-to-stand exercises. Leash walks twice daily were started on the second week of the exercise plan and increased incrementally by five minutes each week.

Sam's owners followed the plan and returned for a recheck four weeks after the home-only plan was started. Sam appeared comfortable and his thigh circumference measurements were 1 cm different now – an improvement of 1 cm. Jane removed Sam's leash restriction, allowing short periods of time in the backyard.

Sam's owners called to cancel his recheck appointment which had been scheduled for two weeks after removal of restrictions. Sam was lame again. He was going to see the orthopedic surgeon. Sam also went to a sports medicine and rehabilitation clinic where he saw a rehabilitation veterinarian and a physical therapist. A grade II quadriceps strain was diagnosed and was treated by the team with therapeutic ultrasound, myofascial trigger point therapy (dry needling), and manual therapies including cross-friction massage and mobilization of the coxofemoral and stifle joints. Sam's lameness resolved and he was slowly returned to full activity. His non-steroidal anti-inflammatory medication was discontinued.

Case 6: Working with Adjunct Professionals

Sophie, a seven-month-old female Irish Wolfhound presented to the Piney Animal Rehabilitation Clinic for an intermittent rear lameness that had suddenly progressed to ambulatory paraparesis in the rear. It was winter and the puppy had been outside on snow and ice with other dogs when the lameness had first been seen.

The owner had initially consulted her chiropractor who was trained with certification in animal chiropractic. The chiropractor had examined the patient and had concerns about working with a neurologic patient with no veterinary diagnosis. A recommendation was made to seek veterinary advice, particularly from a specialist rehabilitation veterinarian (DACVSMR). Following the chiropractor's advice, the owner self-referred her dog to Piney Animal Rehabilitation for initial examination. After the client made the appointment, a technician at the rehabilitation clinic contacted the primary care veterinarian to inform them of the self-referral and to ask for patient records (pending owner release).

A review was made of the medical notes from both the primary care veterinarian and the chiropractor. It was apparent that the patient had not been seen by the primary care veterinarian since she had developed neurologic signs. The patient had been clinically normal at the last veterinary examination. The chiropractor's records noted a mentally alert but ataxic patient, palpation of the spine revealed atlanto-occipital joint restriction in motion. No spinal adjustments were performed, but manual therapy techniques were applied to the muscles of the neck. After two visits and no improvement in gait or comfort, the recommendation for veterinary examination was made. It was noted in the chiropractor's medical record for the dog that it is "customary for chiropractors to advise clients that three chiropractic visits should take place before drawing conclusions about how much change we will be able to make through adjusting however concerns about patient status raised a concern before this. It was becoming clear that imaging should be performed. An evaluation from a rehabilitation veterinarian will help to narrow the specific area to be imaged."

The review of the notes produced a tentative differential diagnosis list. Top of the list was spinal cord compression. It was the rehabilitation veterinarian's opinion that cervical vertebral malformation was the primary differential diagnosis, but that other forms of spinal compression, congenital issues with central nervous system development, or infectious/inflammatory disease of the nervous system were possible (see Box 22.8).

As the patient's condition was stable, an examination at the rehabilitation clinic was performed as requested. Referral to a neurologist would then be discussed with the owner after the physical and functional examination findings were explained.

Rehabilitation veterinarian examination findings included grade 2/4 ataxia of the rear limbs with low ground clearance in swing phase and wide-based stance which became wider on turning. On turning, the patient swayed in a frontal plane but did not fall. Transitions between postures (sit, down, and stand) revealed reduced eccentric control of motion with some tendency to fall into a sit or a down after initiation of movement. The sitting position was with the forelimbs placed in abduction and the rear limbs extended to one side. The head position was forward with the neck in slight flexion. Stance posture was head-low and wide-based rear limbs. The patient could rise from a down or sitting position without assistance but relied on forward motion of the head, neck, and front limbs. Rear extension was partial until the patient moved forward several steps after a stand was achieved. Voluntary motion of the cervical spine using treat motivation revealed

---

Box 22.8   Case 6: Discussion

1) The animal chiropractor had not manipulated the patient's joints in the areas of concern. Although manipulations have been shown safe and effective in the management of discomfort due to nerve compression (Lisi and Bhardwaj, 2004) and to safely provide symptomatic relief in cervical disc herniation (Peterson *et al.*, 2013), it was clinically advisable to use caution as hypomobility may be a protective response to hypermobility/instability, or to spinal cord impingement.

2) Acute progression from lameness to paresis indicates spinal cord compression. A patient with these signs should be fully evaluated by a veterinarian as soon as possible. Advanced imaging of the spinal cord is advised.

3) A young, large-breed dog with neurologic signs may have cervical vertebral spondylomyelopathy/instability (wobblers syndrome) or other congenital abnormality

4) A patient who has a potential diagnosis of instability may have intermittent exacerbation of spinal cord compression with some motions – in this case, avoid full range neck movements. Rapid motions involve more force in muscles, with more compressive forces on the vertebral joints.

5) A patient may improve in strength and coordination with rehabilitation, but this does not mean the underlying disease is completely managed or resolved. Age-related progression in cases of vertebral instability are due to degenerative changes in the discs, hypertrophy of ligaments and of other soft tissues which can increase compression of the spinal cord. Owners should be cautioned about this, and the need for regular monitoring.

normal ROM in lateral and ventral flexion of the neck but reluctance to extend the neck beyond the neutral (in line with thoracic spine) position. Palpation of the spine revealed restriction in motion of the C4–C5 intervertebral joints and the atlanto-occipital joints. Neck musculature was noted to be high in tone, but no specific areas of pain were identified. Segmental spinal reflexes were within normal limits, and there was minor weakness in the withdrawal reflexes of the rear limbs. Tail motion was normal.

Radiographic findings (tipping at vertebral end plates, narrowing of spinal canal) were consistent with signs of cervical spondylomyelopathy, and advanced MRI along with consultation with a neurologist was recommended by the rehabilitation veterinarian. The owner declined as she was not prepared to "put her animal through subsequent surgery" based on previous experiences she had undergone with a dog who had had the same disorder.

A therapeutic/management plan was developed. The patient would undergo in-clinic and home exercises aimed at working on strength and coordination while preventing overload and excess motion in the cervical spinal cord as much as possible. A cervical collar (neck brace) was custom-ordered from a veterinary supply company (see Figure 22.5) and was used to prevent

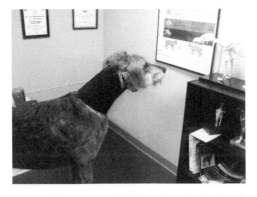

Figure 22.5 Custom cervical brace (Therapaw).

large motions of the cervical spine. The patient was changed to a diet with relatively low energy intake, correct calcium: phosphorus balance, and adequate protein to prevent developmental orthopedic disease. Daily caloric intake was calculated by the rehabilitation technician who was responsible for nutritional counseling as well as home care advice and teaching home therapeutic exercises. The rehabilitation veterinarian explained the disorder to the owner at length and advised about the potential for progression and management of that progression. Every team member was also educated about progression, precautions, and activity contraindications.

The rehabilitation technician carried out in-clinic therapeutic exercises under the supervision of the rehabilitation veterinarian. Clinical signs indicating fatigue or relative overload of the cervical spine were discussed as signals to stop or change therapy, and daily rounds ensured that the case was discussed with the team each time the patient visited for therapy. The animal chiropractor used manual therapies to maintain normal joint motion in the thoracolumbar spine and took time to counsel the owner about the condition. Communication with the primary care veterinarian was through biweekly updates. Communications also occurred after any significant reevaluation and/or status change. Sophie did have intermittent episodes of pain that arose from a prone (down) position. These episodes were associated with higher levels of activity the previous day. Pain was managed with a nonsteroidal anti-inflammatory and gabapentin. The owner was counseled about consistency of activity level. However, this was difficult in a multi-dog household. Sophie improved in coordination slightly, and her strength improved markedly. She could turn more easily and had improved control of transitions. Sophie was transferred to a home-only exercise plan for maintenance and coped well with no decline in clinical signs. She continued to see her chiropractor monthly and had rechecks at the rehabilitation clinic every 4–6 months.

Conclusions

Through a collaborative team approach, incorporating the strengths of each of the team members, best practices and patient outcomes can be achieved in the rehabilitation setting. Regular communication, re-evaluation including measurement of objective outcomes, and respect for the rehabilitation team roles and legal scope of practice of each team member is essential, especially when an unexpected problem, exacerbation, or urgent situation is encountered. The complement and overlap of the skill set provided by each individual team member can benefit the patient and client by ensuring comprehensive and safe patient care. The integrity of the team can be challenged through unprofessional behaviors and conduct, including a lack of inclusivity. Ensuring provision of the best possible patient-focused collaborative rehabilitation service while maintaining open communication will preclude these limitations. Each team member should feel safe, heard, and able to contribute.

References

Lisi, A.J. and Bhardwaj, M.K. (2004). Chiropractic high-velocity low-amplitude spinal manipulation in the treatment of a case of postsurgical chronic cauda equina syndrome. *J Manip Physiol Ther* 27 (9): 574–578.

Peterson, C.K., Schmid, C., Leemann, S. et al. (2013). Outcomes from magnetic resonance imaging-confirmed symptomatic cervical disk herniation patients treated with high-velocity, low amplitude spinal manipulative therapy: A prospective cohort study with 3-month follow-up. *J Manip Physiol Ther* 36 (8): 461–467.

23

Equine Rehabilitation

Steve Adair[1] and Dawn Phillips[2]

[1] Equine Performance and Rehabilitation Center, University of Tennessee Veterinary Medical Center, Knoxville, TN, USA
[2] University of Tennessee, College of Veterinary Medicine, Knoxville, TN, USA

Introduction

The process of rehabilitating a horse after an injury or surgery is neither cookbook nor inflexible. Horses must be treated as individuals. The goal of a rehabilitation program is to achieve as close to the level of pre-injury physiologic and psychological fitness as possible in the shortest amount of time.

Physiotherapy is common in human medicine. In the human field, there are many studies that have been performed on the different modalities that have demonstrated efficacy for specific conditions. An example would be the use of cryotherapy to decrease post-operative pain and swelling. However, there are some modalities that have limited or no proven efficacy.

In the horse, there is even less information available in the form of evidence-based medicine. However, research into the tissue effects and efficacy of therapeutic modalities has been increasing. The quality of the research that has been performed recently is improving though most are dealing with effects and not efficacy for a condition. Just because there is an effect does not mean a particular therapy is efficacious.

There is minimal work that has been done on the horse to validate the efficacy of different therapeutic modalities. Many of the treatment protocols have been adapted from human medicine for which there is better evidence of efficacy. There are clinical technique reports that address specific conditions or modalities; however, these reports utilize techniques that have been adapted from human medicine or personal experience. Now, there is no reason not to use modalities that have been proved to be efficacious in the human; however, efficacy determination needs to be performed in the equine.

Therapeutic Plan Development

A "shotgun" approach to developing and implementing a treatment plan should be avoided. Rehabilitation programs need to address pain, proprioception, flexibility, strength, endurance, and functional demands (Haussler *et al.*, 2021a). It is important to realize that this is a team approach. The team consists of the veterinarian, veterinary technician/nurse, therapist, owner, as well as other professionals (trainers, farriers, etc.). All members of the team should be involved in all aspects of the treatment to ensure the best possible outcome.

There are several things one must look at while developing a rehabilitation program for an individual horse. The first is to understand success with patients that your teams have treated for a similar condition. How have they progressed during the treatment period? The second is to establish some outcome goals. Where should this patient be during a certain time in the rehabilitation process? Third, the team should determine therapist capabilities and the resources/facilities you have available. If a specific modality is indicated and you do not have it, then the patient should be referred to a clinic that does possess this capability, or alternatively a different plan should be developed. Fourth, there should be a full assessment of the patient. What is the nature of the injury? What type of therapy or surgery has been done? How amenable is the patient to therapy? What are the owners' expectations? These questions should be answered prior to initiating therapy. The team should develop a plan specifically for the patient based on the answers to the above questions.

Any plan will depend on the stage of the injury. The initial stage after injury is from the time of injury or surgery until all acute inflammation has resolved (Prentice, 2014). This may be as short as a few days to as long as or longer than 3–4 weeks. The goal during this initial stage is decreasing pain and inflammation, preserving range of motion (ROM), and prevention of muscle atrophy. Typically, cold therapy, supportive wraps, and passive motion are all utilized in this period.

The second stage begins after injury as the acute inflammation is resolved (Prentice, 2014). The goal of this stage is to gradually increase the stress being placed on the healing tissues. This aids in structural healing and preventing or revising scar tissue. Therapies that could be considered include therapeutic exercise, aquatic therapy, and modalities such as therapeutic ultrasound, shockwave, as well as others.

The choice of which modality to use and in which stage is dependent upon the veterinarian, the therapists' experiences, and the exact goal for the modality. For instance, laser therapy may be used in stage 1 to help relieve tissue edema or inflammation and in stage 2 to help in epithelial migration during wound healing.

Therapeutic Monitoring

It is extremely important to develop methods for evaluating the effects of therapy and the response of the disease or injury to therapy – the distinction should be made between these two things. In addition, one must be able to document these changes. Ideally, one should use quantifiable methods (see Figure 23.1). There are fairly simple methods available. A tape measure may be used to measure limb circumference. Goniometers can be used to measure joint angles. Pressure algometry may be used to

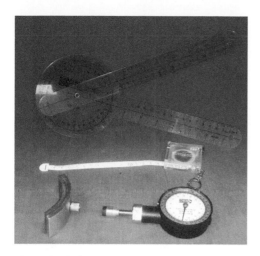

Figure 23.1 Therapeutic monitoring equipment. From top to bottom: goniometer, tape measure, and pressure algometer.

evaluate for lessening pain in an area. More sophisticated methods can also be used, including but not limited to radiographs, diagnostic ultrasound, thermography, or lameness evaluation (Paulekas and Haussler, 2009). Inertial sensor systems are also an excellent method for objective evaluation of changes in gait (see Figure 23.2a and b).

It is important that measurements be taken at the onset of therapy and frequent re-evaluations be performed. Early in the therapy period re-evaluations may need to be performed daily or weekly, while later they may need to be done at monthly or longer intervals. If worsening or no improvement of the condition is noted the therapeutic plan must be modified.

Facilities, Equipment, and Personnel

Prior to the development of a rehabilitation practice, it is important to read the state veterinary practice act. In most states performing animal rehabilitation is considered the practice of veterinary medicine. As such, if a person is not a veterinarian, then they will need to be a full-time employee of a veterinarian. If a person is a full-time employee of a veterinarian, then the level of supervision required will need to be determined. In most states a licensed veterinary technician/nurse can work under indirect supervision, meaning that the licensed veterinarian need not be on the premises, has given either written or oral instructions for treatment of the patient, is readily available by telephone or other forms of immediate communication, and has assumed responsibility for the veterinary care given to the patient by a person working under his or her direction. However, laws vary from state to state and need to be reviewed for each state in which a person is working.

It is important that individuals who will be developing rehabilitation plans, performing therapies, and monitoring progression should be thoroughly trained. This should be more in-depth than the technical service training provided by equipment manufacturers. Individuals should seek out advanced training in the form of certification courses or by spending time training at a veterinary equine rehabilitation center. One of the major problems in the field of equine rehabilitation today is the lack of formal training and education. Often therapies are provided that are of no benefit to the patient or in some cases are detrimental. Depending on what services are going to be provided advanced training is available for equine rehabilitation, hyperbaric oxygen therapy (HBOT), therapeutic taping, and massage to name a few.

When planning a rehabilitation service, the demographics of the area need to be evaluated. Types of, and concentrations of horses in the area need to be determined. Additionally, the equine disciplines (dressage, cross country, hunter/jumpers, reining, barrel racing, and others), the types of clients, and the location of other rehabilitation facilities are a few other items that should be determined.

(a)

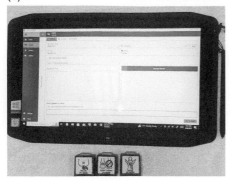

(b)

Trial:	Straight Line		
Date:	10/3/2020 at 12:15 PM		
Surface:	Soft (generic)		
Blocks:			
Attending:		Stride Settings:	Manual Window = 88%

Quantification of Asymmetry

Stride Rate: 1.3   Strides Assessed (fore/hind): 23/22

Forelimb Strides   **Hindlimb Strides**

Lameness Metrics

Ref Range for Max/Min Head (mm):	±6			Ref Range for Max/Min Pelvis (mm):	±3		
Diff Max Head (mm):	Mean:	1.6	SD: 6.2	**Diff Max Pelvis (mm):**	Mean:	1.4	SD: 3.2
Diff Min Head (mm):	Mean:	4.5	SD: 7.6	**Diff Min Pelvis (mm):**	Mean:	1.1	SD: 2.8
Ref Range for Total Diff Head (mm):	8.5						
Total Diff Head (Vector Sum) **(mm)**	4.8						
Q Score (fore): R 4.8 Imp				**Q Score (hind): R 1.4 Push / R 1.1 Imp**			

Stride Selection	**Trial AIDE**
	There is "no" evidence of LF lameness.
	There is "no" evidence of RF lameness.
	There is "no" evidence of LH lameness.
	There is "no" evidence of RH lameness.

Evaluator Notes

Generated with Lameness Locator® 20/20 by Equinosis® (5.0.8395.14460)   12 June, 2023 10:47 AM

Figure 23.2 (a) Inertial sensor system used for gait evaluation. (b) Quantitative report.

One also needs to determine if the rehabilitation service is going to be ambulatory or haul into a clinic. If it is an ambulatory service, then this will limit the type of equipment and service you can provide. Ambulatory service will be limited to those modalities that can be easily transported in a vehicle and to prescribed therapeutic exercises but is more economically feasible than a haul-in service. A "haul in" service will be able to provide a much wider range of modalities but will also be a more significant expense.

Equipment needs will depend on all the factors presented above. For an ambulatory service, equipment that should be considered includes therapeutic ultrasound, therapeutic laser, thermal therapies, shockwave therapy, and equipment to perform therapeutic monitoring. For a haul-in facility, equipment in addition to that mentioned above includes underwater treadmill, swimming pool, a cold salt therapy unit, whole body vibration, and pulsed electromagnetic field (PEMF) therapy to name a few.

The above equipment need not be all obtained initially, but future needs should be anticipated. If funds are not available to purchase an underwater treadmill, one should still plan for one in the future. The location and housing of the equipment need to be planned for. Most equipment is expensive, ranging from several hundred dollars to several thousand dollars. In addition to the purchase price of the equipment, one must account for maintenance costs. In determining the charge for a service, you must take this into account in addition to the time it takes to perform the therapy. A fee must be charged that makes the service profitable. If you have a low number of cases, then you may have to charge a significant amount in order to recoup the expenses. That is why it is extremely important to determine if the service area can support the equipment prior to purchase.

Nutrition

Nutrition is very important in the rehabilitation of the horse. Most horses that are painful and in the process of healing have specific nutritional requirements (Fleeman and Owens, 2007; Secombe and Lester, 2012). For example, horses are prone to the development of gastric ulcers. Practices that may be needed to reduce the incidence of ulceration are the feeding of a non grain based diet and alfalfa hay. An overly obese horse may only need grass hay fed at 2% of their body weight and a ration balancer. Horses that have laminitis or are prone to laminitis should be fed a low starch feed and may need to have their hay soaked in water for 30–60 minutes to leach out the fructose (Longland *et al.*, 2011). Horses that are in a catabolic state will require additional calories. This can often be met by increasing the fat content of the diet instead of increasing the concentration portion of the diet. Lastly, all horses should have clean, fresh water, and a white salt block or red mineral block.

Patient Environment and Mental Status

Many times, we focus on the injury and neglect the rest of the patient. We often have success in treating the injury but lose the use of the horse to contra-lateral limb problems, such as laminitis, breakdown of supporting structures, and angular limb problems (in the case of foals and weanlings). Providing a high plane of nutrition, a good environment and support for the other limbs are as important as the treatment of the injury. One should also not neglect the mental status of the horse. Having a companion in the barn (pony, another horse, or goat), as well as playing with toys (environmental enrichment) will go a long way in keeping the patient happy. Mental stimulation is important as many of the problems we are treating require long confinement of some type. Bedding type may need to be changed from straw to shavings or sand in the case of laminitis problems.

Therapeutic Modalities

Physiotherapy interventions that are commonly used on the horse include but are not limited to, manual therapy, thermal agents, electrotherapeutic techniques, mechanical agents, therapeutic exercise, aquatic therapy, and HBOT.

Manual therapies – include massage, stretches, joint and soft tissue mobilization, and/or chiropractic (manipulation). These are used to restore optimum joint movement by reducing adhesions, mobilizing tight joint structures, and providing enhanced joint lubrication and joint nutrition.

Stretching and massage can promote circulation, decrease muscle spasms, mobilize adhesions, and scar tissue and aid lymphatic drainage. They also can provide pain relief from tight muscles and connective tissue that are responsible for pressure or tension on nerve pathways, restore normal muscle length after injury as well as maintain normal muscle length (prevent shortening), avoid stiffness related to age or inactivity, and protect from stresses and strains. Static or passive stretching consists of stretching a muscle (or group of muscles) to its farthest point and then maintaining or holding that position (Frick, 2010). This type of stretching is the most common type used in horses as the desired motion and positioning are controlled. It requires a human assistant to perform and is not under control of the horse. It is unclear how effective stretching is in horses. No improvement in stride length was found after eight weeks of stretching in a group of normal horses (Rose *et al.*, 2009). However, they have found several significant differences in joint ROM between treatments in the

shoulder, stifle, and hock. They concluded that the frequency with which passive stretches are applied to the horse appears to have some influence on horse movement. Their research did not demonstrate consistent improvement in equine movement because of passive stretching and highlighted the possibility that stretching daily may not be appropriate and can cause delayed onset muscle soreness. They suggested that the application of stretching on a three-times-per-week basis may be safer.

The basic science rationale for massage is supported by human research indicating that massage may affect a number of physiologic systems as well as cellular and fascial components of the muscular system (Scott and Swenson, 2009; Hill and Crook, 2010). Equine therapeutic massage employs a number of techniques first developed in humans and has been reported to increase ROM and stride length, reduce activity of nociceptive pain receptors, and reduce physiologic stress responses (Scott and Swenson, 2009). There is minimal evidence on the horses that suggests that massage is of any benefit other than for promoting lymphatic drainage (Buchner and Schildboeck, 2006). One study found that massage to the caudal limb muscles significantly increased passive and active limb protraction (Hill and Crook, 2010).

Myofascial release (MFR) is the use of the hands and fingers to apply pressure to cause a release of tension in muscle or fascia. It is a form of manual therapy that involves the application of a low-load, long-duration stretch to the myofascial complex, intended to restore optimal length, decrease pain, and improve function (Ajimsha *et al.*, 2015). MFR generally involves slow and sustained pressure applied to restricted fascial layers either directly or indirectly (Ajimsha *et al.*, 2015). Direct MFR technique is thought to work directly over the restricted fascia: practitioners use knuckles or elbow or other tools to slowly sink into the fascia, and the pressure applied is a few kilograms of force to contact the restricted fascia, apply tension, or stretch the fascia (Ajimsha *et al.*, 2015). Indirect MFR involves a gentle stretch guided along the path of least resistance until free movement is achieved. The pressure applied is a few grams of force, and the hands tend to follow the direction of fascial restrictions, hold the stretch, and allow the fascia to loosen itself (Ajimsha *et al.*, 2015). The rationale for these techniques can be traced to various studies that investigated plastic, viscoelastic, and piezoelectric properties of connective tissue (Ajimsha *et al.*, 2015).

Mobilizations and manipulations are aimed at pain relief, restoration of normal joint biomechanics and nerve function, improved muscle function, and promotion of healing. They are used to treat joint dysfunctions that limit ROM by specifically addressing altered joint mechanics (Haussler, 2016). Factors that may alter joint mechanics include pain & muscle guarding, joint hypomobility (fixation), joint effusion, contractures, fibrosis, or adhesions in joint capsules or supporting ligaments and degenerative joint disease.

Passive mobilization is a passive joint movement for increasing ROM or decreasing pain (Goff, 2009). It is applied to joints and related soft tissues at varying speeds, amplitudes, or rhythms. The force is light enough that patient can stop the movement (Goff, 2009). Dynamic or active mobilization is a dynamic or active joint movement that is carried out and controlled by the patient (Goff, 2009).

Joint mobilizations and chiropractic manipulation are only to be performed by the rehabilitation veterinarian or animal physical therapist. Veterinary technicians/ nurses can perform massage, passive range of motion (PROM) exercises, and stretching techniques.

Manipulation is characterized by manual thrust delivered at high velocity in a specific direction. It incorporates a sudden, forceful thrust that is beyond the patient's control (Haussler, 2000). It is performed at the physiologic joint motion limit (elastic barrier) and into paraphysiologic space (Leach, 1994). It should only be done after receiving appropriate training.

Mobilizations have been evaluated on the horse. Most of the studies have been directed toward the axial skeleton. Clayton *et al.* found that the amount of bending in different parts of the cervical vertebral column differed among the dynamic mobilization exercises (Clayton *et al.*, 2010a, b). As the horse's chin moved further caudally, bending in the caudal cervical and thoracolumbar regions increased, suggesting that the more caudal positions may be particularly effective for activating and strengthening the core musculature that is used to bend and stabilize the horse's back (Clayton *et al.*, 2010a, b). Clayton also determined that dynamic mobilization exercises performed in cervical flexion have applications in mobilizing the cervical and thoracic intervertebral joints (Clayton *et al.*, 2010a, b). Haussler *et al.* determined that the passive vertical mobility of the trunk varied from cranial to caudal (Haussler *et al.*, 2007). At most sites, spinal manipulative therapy increased the amplitudes of dorsoventral displacement and applied force, indicative of increased vertebral flexibility, and increased tolerance to pressure in the thoracolumbar portion of the vertebral column (Haussler *et al.*, 2007). In another study, spinal manipulative therapy increased dorsoventral displacement of the trunk, which is indicative of producing increased passive spinal flexibility in actively ridden horses (Haussler *et al.*, 2010). Stubbs *et al.* determined that dynamic mobilization exercise can cause enlargement of the multifidus muscle in as little as three weeks (Stubbs *et al.*, 2011).

Based on the human literature, it has been recommended that mobilization for most injuries and post-surgery can begin within three days if careful protocols are followed (Schills and Turner, 2010). For severe ligament and tendon injuries, mobilization can begin at three weeks (Schills and Turner, 2010).

Thermal agents – This includes hot and cold applications. Heat or cold may be administered to horses using many modalities and can range from simply applying water from a hose to deep-heating ultrasound technologies.

The major physiologic benefits of cold therapy are decreases in circulation, cell metabolism, secondary tissue damage, edema, muscle spasm, and pain (Belanger, 2010a). The benefits are most effective early in the period following injury or surgery. The primary effect of cold application is to constrict blood vessels. The reduced blood flow to tissues reduces edema, hemorrhage, and extravasation of inflammatory cells. Reduced tissue metabolism inhibits the effect of inflammatory mediators and slows enzyme systems. Analgesia follows cold therapy. The viscoelasticity of soft tissues is reduced with cold therapy.

Cold therapy is indicated in acute musculoskeletal injuries or inflammation and following surgical procedures to reduce edema, slow inflammation, and reduce pain. Cold is particularly effective during the first 24–48 hours after injury.

Cold may be applied by ice–water immersion, application of ice packs, cold packs, saltwater hydrotherapy units (see Figure 23.3), and ice water-charged circulating boots.

Several studies have documented tissue effects or efficacy of cryotherapy in horses. The influence of hypertonic cold water (5–9 °C) spa bath hydrotherapy on the response of 27 horses with various lower leg injuries has been reported (Hunt, 2001). Fifteen horses with grade 2 or 3 superficial digital flexor tendon (SDFT) damage and

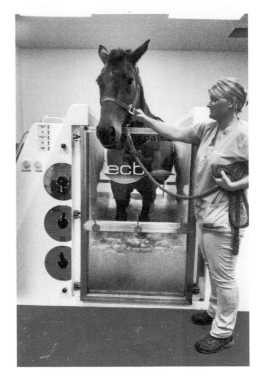

Figure 23.3 Cold salt water spa.

four with suspensory ligament injury treated for 10 minutes three times a week responded with markedly improved ultrasonographic echogenicity and fiber realignment of injured tissues. All but two of these horses, when placed back into training returned to compete successfully within six months without re-injury. Petrov *et al.* were able to reduce the core temperature of the SDFT to a minimum of 10 °C after 1 hour using a commercial compression splint with circulating coolant (Petrov *et al.*, 2003). These results indicated that topical application of cryotherapy can significantly reduce core SDFT temperature in standing horses and that the temperatures achieved in vivo during cold treatment were not detrimental to the in vitro viability of tendon cells. Cold immersion of the distal limbs is effective in reducing the severity of laminitis by decreasing the activity of laminar matrix metalloproteinases (MMP) and causing laminar vasoconstriction (van Eps and Pollitt, 2009; van Eps *et al.*, 2014). Recently, an in vitro study demonstrated that ice–water immersion led to the greatest heat loss of the methods evaluated (Marlin, 2019). In another study, a commercial dry-sleeve cryotherapy system failed to reduce the temperature of equine skin and subcutaneous tissues to a target temperature of 10–19 °C (Jacobs *et al.*, 2022). Thus, the ability to reduce the target tissue temperature to a therapeutic level is very dependent upon the method used.

The major benefits of heat therapy are increased local circulation, muscle relaxation, and increased tissue extensibility (Kaneps, 2000). By increasing blood flow tissue metabolites are mobilized, tissue oxygen levels are increased, and the metabolic rate of cells and enzyme systems are increased. Metabolic rate increases two to three times for a tissue temperature increase of 10 °C. Increased blood flow and vascular permeability promote resorption of edema. Heat application also decreases pain via the mechanisms cited earlier for cold therapy. Soft tissues may be stretched more effectively after warming. Heat is applied after acute inflammation has subsided. It is useful for reducing muscle spasms and pain because of musculoskeletal injuries. Heat therapy can be used to increase joint and tendon mobility. Heat may benefit recovery of localized soft tissue injuries by accelerating the healing response.

Superficial heat is most commonly applied using hot packs and hydrotherapy.

Deep heat may be applied using therapeutic ultrasound. The most profound physiologic effects of heat occur when tissue temperatures are raised to 40–45 °C (Kaneps, 2000). However, tissue temperatures above 45 °C may result in pain and irreversible tissue damage (Kaneps, 2000). Heating for 15–30 minutes is required to elevate deep tissue temperature to the therapeutic range. Kaneps found that tissue temperature changes due to warm water hose therapy ranged from 3.7 to 10.8 °C (Kaneps, 2000). Additionally, temperature elevation was short-lasting and dependent on the distance to the surface, with only limited effect on deep tissues more than 1.5–2 cm under the skin (Kaneps, 2000).

Utilizing therapeutic ultrasound, Montgomery *et al.* found that the SDFT and deep digital flexor tendon (DDFT) are heated to a therapeutic temperature using a frequency of 3.3 MHz and intensity of 1.0 W/cm^2. The epaxial muscles are not heated to a therapeutic temperature using a frequency of 3.3 MHz and an intensity of 1.5 W/cm^2 (Montgomery *et al.*, 2013).

Contrast therapy is characterized by alternating hot and cold cycles during a given therapeutic session. It is thought that by alternating vasoconstriction and vasodilation blood flow to the treatment area may be improved. A recent study on horses (Haussler *et al.*, 2021b) documented the ability of a contrast therapy unit to rapidly change tissue temperature down to the level of the DDFT. The authors state that therapeutic tissue temperatures were not reached due to the short timings of the cycles. Additionally, they do not know the effects on blood flow as they did not evaluate it.

Whole body cryostimulation is used in human athletes as an aid to muscle recovery. Recently, it has been investigated in horses (Bogard *et al.*, 2020). The authors used a protocol that has been used in humans. Based on infrared thermography measurements, they showed that exposing a horse for three minutes to a temperature of −140 °C does not induce sufficient skin thermal gradients in horses. They conclude that additional research should be undertaken to determine optimum protocols.

Electrical techniques – These techniques include electrical muscle and nerve stimulation, PEMF therapy, and low-level laser therapy (Schlachter and Lewis, 2016). While these have been shown to be effective in humans a recent systematic review on electrotherapy in animals failed to support the clinical effects of electrotherapies for any clinical indication in horses, dogs, or cats (Hyytiäinen *et al.*, 2022).

Neuromuscular electrical stimulation (NMES) works by making the muscle contract through motor nerve stimulation using an interrupted direct current. Of all the electrotherapy techniques this is the most appropriate, as it produces controlled motor and sensory responses both superficial and deep, while maintaining a high level of compliance by the horse (Schils, 2009). Electrical muscle stimulation improves venous and lymphatic drainage, prevents muscle atrophy, prevents the formation of unwanted adhesions, reduces scar tissue formation, builds and re-educates damaged or weakened muscle, and encourages nutrition into the affected area (see Figure 23.4).

Limited research is available on its use on the horse and it is conflicting. Berg *et al.* utilized NMES on the *m. gluteus medius* and *m. longissimus dorsi* (Bergh *et al.*, 2010). They concluded that NMES treatment was well tolerated by the horse, but their protocol did not induce significant muscle adaptations. Ravara *et al.* concluded that functional electrical stimulation (FES) is a safe rehabilitation strategy in the management of equine epaxial muscle spasms and provides clinical improvements and some structural changes of the muscle tissue at the histological level (Ravara *et al.*, 2015) (see Box 23.1). Recently, a seven-week period of dynamic mobilization exercises or NMES treatments was shown to increase the cross-sectional area (CSA) of the multifidus muscle in horses (Lucas *et al.*, 2022).

Transcutaneous electrical nerve stimulation (TENS) is primarily used for pain modulation (Belanger, 2010b). It is the application of a pulsed electrical current over the skin surface for the purpose of pain modulation (Belanger, 2010b). There

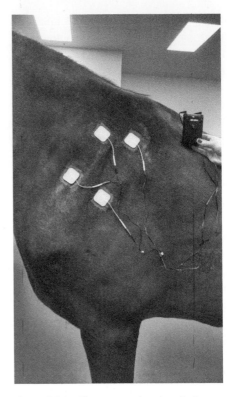

Figure 23.4 Neuromuscular electrical stimulation application for muscle strengthening.

are no scientific studies in the current literature that document effect or efficacy of the horse. In the author's experience, it has not been found to decrease the need for analgesics in horses suffering from acute laminitis.

Pulsed electromagnetic field (PEMF) therapy has been utilized to increase circulation, improve fracture healing, reduce pain and edema, and promote healing of wounds in humans and animals (Inoue *et al.*, 2002; Cinar *et al.*, 2008; Matic *et al.*, 2009; Strauch *et al.*, 2009; Rohde *et al.*, 2010; Nelson *et al.*, 2013). However, limited evidence is available on the horse that demonstrates effect or efficacy. It should be remembered that PEMF can have different intensities and frequencies depending on the unit. Biermann *et al.* (2014) evaluated the use of PEMF on back pain in polo ponies. They could not document an effect on either back pain or

---

Box 23.1   University of tennessee equine rehabilitation department's protocol for neuromuscular electrical stimulation (NEMS)

EMS utilizes (see Figure 23.4) primarily to treat or prevent muscle atrophy. The following is an example protocol for treatment of muscle atrophy:

1) Clip hair using a #40 blade where the electrodes are to be placed.
2) Clean skin with alcohol
3) Apply electrodes to the area to be treated. Most commonly this will be at the origin and insertion of the affected muscle.
4) Settings:
   - *Waveform* – Modified square wave with zero net direct current component
   - *Contraction time* – 10 seconds
   - *Relaxation time* – 30 seconds
   - *Frequency* – 30
   - *Ramp* – 3
5) Treatment protocol:
   - Once to twice daily
   - Start with 5 minutes, and then work up to 20 minutes (i.e., increase treatment

time by 2–3 minutes per day until 20–30 minutes is reached.
   - It may take a few sessions to get a good contraction
6) Suggestions:
   - Start first session with 5 minutes, and then build up successive sessions, daily, by several minutes (2–3) to get to a 20–30 minute treatment session. Helps to allow horses to eat hay during treatment for distraction.
   - You should be able to see a good contraction while it is "on," then a 10-second rest, then contraction again.
   - Only adjust intensity up when "on"
   - Can assist with "active muscle" recruitment by imposing weight shifting onto the horses involved side when the unit is "on"
   - Economical, battery-operated units may be purchased and loaned to owners to provide treatment at home if needed.

---

induced back movement. Rindler *et al.* (2014) also evaluated the effects of PEMF on the backs of actively working polo ponies. They found there was no measurable effect of PEMF on the surface temperature of horse's backs. Auer *et al.* (1983) reported beneficial effects for the repair of cortical stress fractures of metacarpal III (MC III) bones using PEMF, whereas Sanders-Shamis *et al.* (1989) did not find any significant differences in bone healing of surgically induced cortical lesions of MC III/Metatarsal III between a PEMF and control group. Watkins *et al.* (1985) found that PEMF significantly delayed maturation of the tissue formed within the defect at weeks 8 and 12 as determined by histological examination. The collagen-type transformation was also delayed by PEMF but not

significantly. Collier *et al.* (1985) found that topical treatment with a PEMF had no effect on the uptake of technetium in normal equine bone. The strongest evidence for efficacy with PEMF lies with nonunion or slow-to-heal fractures (Schlachter and Lewis, 2016). Rostad *et al.* showed that PEMF therapy has a relaxing effect evidenced by lowered heart rate immediately following treatment; however, more work is needed to determine the full effects of PEMF in performance horses (Rostad *et al.*, 2023). Dai also found a positive effect on vagal activity and relaxation in horses (Dai *et al.*, 2022). A bio-electromagnetic energy regulation therapy blanket was found to improve thoracolumbar epaxial muscle thresholds and improve postural stability both during, immediately after and one day following therapy (King *et al.*, 2022). However, no effect was found on measures of muscle tone, lameness, gait, ground reaction forces, or serum biomarkers.

Low level laser (see Figure 23.5) therapy (LLLT), which uses an intense beam of light of a single wavelength, stimulates the body's processes, activates waste removal, increases repair activity, relieves swelling, heals surface wounds, and stimulates blood and lymphatic systems (Hamblin and Demidova, 2006). It also increases serotonin, thereby achieving a calming response (Hamblin and Demidova, 2006; Kazem Shakouri *et al.*, 2009; Silver, 2009). It has been reported that laser stimulation has certain biostimulating effects such as: accelerates cell division, increases leucocytic phagocytosis, stimulates fibroblastic activity, and enhances regeneration of lymph and blood vessels (Hamblin and Demidova, 2006; Kazem Shakouri *et al.*, 2009; Silver, 2009). Studies have shown

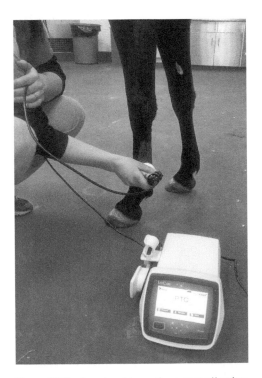

Figure 23.5 Low level laser therapy application.

that it also can cause vasodilatation (Hamblin and Demidova, 2006; Kazem Shakouri *et al.*, 2009; Silver, 2009). These effects can assist wound healing and relieve chronic pain when properly applied (Hamblin and Demidova, 2006; Kazem Shakouri *et al.*, 2009; Silver, 2009).

Lasers are divided into safety classifications in the United States by the American National Standard Institute (ANSI). Classes 1, 2, and 3a have low power output and are not used for therapeutic purposes.

Class 1 lasers or systems cannot emit accessible laser radiation more than the applicable Class 1 accessible emission limit (AEL) for any exposure times within the maximum duration inherent in the design or intended use of the laser. Class 1 lasers are exempt from all beam-hazard control measures.

Class 2 lasers are continuous wave (CW) and repetitively pulsed lasers with wavelengths between 0.4 and 0.7 μm that can emit energy more than the Class 1 AEL but do not exceed the Class 1 AEL for an emission duration of less than 0.25 seconds and have an average radiant power of 1 mW or less.

Class 3a lasers have an accessible output between 1 and 5 times; the Class 1 AEL for wavelengths shorter than 0.4 μm or longer than 0.7 μm, or less than 5 times; the Class 2 AEL for wavelengths between 0.4 and 0.7 μm.

Class 3b lasers cannot emit an average radiant power greater than 0.5 W for an exposure time equal to or greater than 0.25 seconds or 0.125 J for an exposure time less than 0.25 seconds for wavelengths between 0.18 and 0.4 μm or between 1.4 μm and 1 mm. In addition, lasers between 0.4 and 1.4 μm, exceeding the Class 3a AEL, cannot emit an average radiant power greater than 0.5 W for exposures equal to or greater than 0.25 seconds or a radiant energy greater than 0.03 J per pulse.

Class 4 lasers and laser systems exceed the Class 3b AEL.

Research on the use of LLLT in the equine is limited. Berg et al. (Bergh et al., 2007) found that minor superficial morphological changes in equine epidermis after treatment with 91 J/cm² doses of defocused CO_2 laser and severe changes with a homogeneous eosinophilic acellular zone of underlying dermis and a significantly thinner epidermis when irradiation doses of 450 J/cm² were applied. Berg also found that irradiation with defocused CO_2 laser causes a moderate to vigorous heating effect in superficial tissue and a marked increase in blood flow (Bergh, 2006). The increase in temperature was of such intensity that there was a potential risk of thermal injuries to the skin (Bergh, 2006). The results also suggest that treatment with defocused CO_2 laser is not statistically better than placebo at reducing the grade of lameness in horses with traumatic arthritis of the fetlock joint (Bergh, 2006). Ryan et al. (Ryan and Smith, 2007) found that light transmission was not affected by individual horse, coat color, or leg. However, it was associated with leg condition. They found that tendons clipped dry and clipped and cleaned with alcohol were both associated with greater transmission of light than the unprepared state. Also, the use of alcohol without clipping was not associated with an increase in light transmission. Their results suggested that, when applying laser to a subcutaneous structure in the horse, the area should be clipped and cleaned beforehand. Similarly, Duesterdieck-Zellmer et al. found that most laser energy was absorbed or scattered by the skin (Duesterdieck-Zellmer et al., 2016). A case report on 11 horses with hock pain revealed some reduction of hock pain and improvement in lameness but response to hock flexion test remained unchanged (Zielińska et al., 2023). Pluim et al. demonstrated improved healing in surgically created suspensory branch lesions following high-powered laser treatment (Pluim et al., 2021).

The most prevalent method of indicating laser therapy dosage is to measure the density of energy applied to the tissue surface. This is typically expressed in J/cm². Some variation in clinical effects can be observed; particularly at very high (>50 W) or very low (<1 W) power settings using the same J/cm² dose. The dose required for a particular condition is dependent on the equipment used and what its wave length is. Generally, the more superficial a tissue the less energy is required. In other words, the density of energy required for a wound will be less than that required for a tendon.

At the University of Tennessee's equine rehabilitation practice, the most common use of LLLT is to decrease pain and inflammation associated with musculoskeletal injuries and for wound healing. Dose recommendations and calculations have been adapted from Riegel et al. and are based on stage of injury and surface area (Riegel, 2018). Box 23.2 demonstrates an easy method of dose calculation. Table 23.1 shows dosage recommendations for locations. Box 23.3 gives guidelines as to frequency of treatments.

Radiofrequency (Figure 23.6) is electromagnetic energy that is converted to thermal energy. It produces thermal and non-thermal (mechanical) responses with physiological

---

Box 23.2 Laser dose calculation

1) A 3″ × 5″ index card is approximately 100 cm²
2) If area to be treated is the size of 1 index card then 100 is the multiplier
3) If you want 10 J/cm², the total amount of energy needed to be delivered is 1,000 J
4) Then determine how much power and how long it takes to deliver 1,000 J
5) Treat an area wider than actual injury or damage. Treat in a grid pattern & perpendicular to surface

Table 23.1 Laser dosage recommendations for locations.

Location	Dosage
Superficial tissue (i.e., skin)	1–5 J/cm^2
Superficial musculoskeletal (i.e., tendons)	8–20 J/cm^2
Deep musculoskeletal (i.e., back muscles)	15–35 J/cm^2

Box 23.3   Frequency of laser treatments

1) Case dependent
2) Post-surgical procedure
   a) one daily for two treatments
3) Acute cases
   a) Acute conditions are typically treated daily or every other day, and then at decreasing intervals until resolution of the condition
4) Chronic cases
   a) *Initially* – Treatments are administered daily until response is noted
   b) *Transitional* – Frequency of treatments gradually decreased to the minimum required to maintain clinical response
   c) *Maintenance* – Long-term treatment administered as frequently as needed to maintain clinical effect

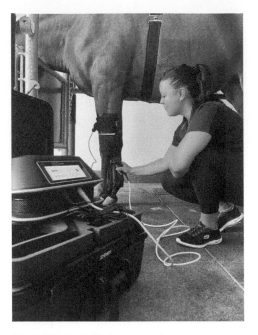

Figure 23.6   Radiofrequency therapy application. *Source:* Courtesy of Marina Rodriguez Alonso.

and therapeutic effects (Table 23.2). The purpose of the use is to significantly heat large areas of deep tissue while minimally affecting superficial tissues. The latest generation of devices produces both continuous and pulsed electromagnetic energy. These units have been determined to be relatively safe and effective in clinical use. Indications on the horse include pain relief, decreased muscle spasm, increased local blood flow,

Table 23.2   Thermal and non-thermal effects of radiofrequency therapy.

Thermal effects	Non-thermal effects
Increase in tissue temperature	Electromagnetic energy allows damaged cells to return to their normal function.
Increased blood flow	
Decreased joint stiffness	Restore normal function of damaged cells through repolarization.
Cell membrane filtration and diffusion increases	
	Increase cell growth and division
Increase in metabolism	Increases the activity of the sodium pump to remove excess sodium.
Decrease pain	
Muscle relaxation	Increase microvascular circulation
Decrease in inflammation	Bio-stimulation and Cell Regeneration

decreased joint stiffness, and increased tissue pliability, edema reduction, and stem cell stimulation (Arguelles *et al.*, 2020; Parkinson *et al.*, 2022; Hernandez-Bule *et al.*, 2014; Becero *et al.*, 2020).

Mechanical agents – These agents include therapeutic ultrasound, shockwave, and devices such as whole-body vibration units (Schlachter and Lewis, 2016).

Therapeutic ultrasound is a form of acoustic energy used to treat musculoskeletal injuries, including inflammation and wounds. It offers deep heating without excessive heating of the skin. Ultrasound can also be used to decrease pain and muscle spasms, promote wound healing, aid re-absorption of hematoma, reduce swelling, and reduce scar tissue. It increases blood flow in the area treated. It increases cell membrane permeability to ions and other substances. It blocks signal transmission in nerves. It decreases muscle spasms. It has been shown in clinical and scientific trials to increase collagen extensibility, enhance collagen remodeling, enhance collagen production, increase heat in deep tissues, increase blood flow, increase ROM, reduce pain and muscle spasm, and accelerate wound healing.

The benefits of therapeutic ultrasound have been established in human and veterinary medicine (Dyson, 1990; Heckman *et al.*, 1994; Singh *et al.*, 1997; Doan *et al.*, 1999; Saini *et al.*, 2002; Fernandes *et al.*, 2003; Maiti *et al.*, 2006; Noble *et al.*, 2007). Therapeutic effects of ultrasound are both thermal and non-thermal (biologic). Thermal (tissue heating) effects are achieved by heating tissue using non-interrupted sound waves, or *continuous ultrasound* (Porter, 2005). Thermal effects result from energy carried by ultrasonic waves being attenuated and absorbed by tissue as the waves pass through it (ter Haar, 1999). Some of the positive effects of heat produced by therapeutic ultrasound include improved extensibility of collagen, decreased pain, decreased muscle spasms, and increased blood flow (ter Haar, 1999; Levine *et al.*, 2001;

Noble *et al.*, 2007). Non-thermal (biologic) effects result from mechanical alteration of the local, cellular environment induced by the ultrasound waves. (ter Haar, 1999; Siska *et al.*, 2008). To avoid heating the treated tissue and achieve non-thermal effects, *pulsed ultrasound* is used where pulse rates interrupt the sound waves at rates of 50%, 80%, or 90% (Porter, 2005). Changes in cellular environment may lead to modifications in cellular function resulting in a shorter inflammatory phase of healing, increased vascularity at the treatment site, and enhanced proliferation of fibroblasts (ter Haar, 1999; Levine *et al.*, 2001; Pounder and Harrison, 2008; Siska *et al.*, 2008). Non-thermal ultrasound has been used as an adjunctive therapy for patients with a fracture or a tendinopathy (Saini *et al.*, 2002; Fu *et al.*, 2008; Siska *et al.*, 2008).

The increase in temperature needed to achieve the desired therapeutic effect for thermal ultrasound has been established in people (Draper *et al.*, 1995; Levine *et al.*, 2001; Demmink *et al.*, 2003). An increase in tissue temperature of 1 °C is required to increase the metabolic rate of tissue; an increase of 2–4 °C is required to lessen pain, muscle spasms, and chronic inflammation improve blood flow; and an increase ≥3 °C is required to decrease the viscoelastic properties of collagen (Draper *et al.*, 1995; Levine *et al.*, 2001; Demmink *et al.*, 2003). For people, 1-MHz ultrasound is most effective at increasing temperature at a tissue depth of 2.5–5 cm, and 3.3-MHz ultrasound is most effective at increasing temperature at a tissue depth of 1.0–2.5 cm (Draper *et al.*, 1995). Results of a study performed to evaluate the effects of 3.3-MHz ultrasound on the temperature of the thigh musculature of dogs show that using a 10-minute treatment, at an intensity of 1.0 W/cm^2, increases the temperature of tissue by 2–4 °C at depths of 1.0 and 2.0 cm. At an intensity of 1.5 W/cm^2, the temperature of tissue increases by at least 2–4 °C at depths of 1.0, 2.0, and 3.0 cm (Levine *et al.*, 2001).

Research into the use of therapeutic ultrasound is lacking. Montgomery *et al.* (Montgomery *et al.*, 2013) found that the SDFT and DDFT are heated to a therapeutic temperature using a frequency of 3.3 MHz and intensity of 1.0 W/cm^2. However, the epaxial muscles are not heated to a therapeutic temperature using a frequency of 3.3 MHz and an intensity of 1.5 W/cm^2. Adair and Levine (2019) found that a 1.0 MHz ultrasound (US) for 10 minutes in horse's epaxial muscles when clipped creates the greatest heat at 1.0 cm. The heat in the tissues at 5 cm depth is more than at 3 cm depth. Reis (2009) used a frequency of 1 MHz on pulsed mode, with an intensity of 0.5 W/cm^2 for 5 minutes treated collagenase-induced superficial flexor tendon lesions for 60 days. They found no significant difference clinically between treated and untreated limbs at either 15 or 60 days. However, there was a significant improvement in ultrasonographic evaluation at 60 days in treated limbs versus untreated. Singh *et al.* (1997) evaluated the use of ultrasound for 10 minutes per day at 1 W/cm^2 for 6 days after induction of arthritis in donkeys. They found that gross changes in the joint capsule, synovial membrane, and articular cartilage were mild in ultrasound-treated donkeys as compared to untreated controls. Low-frequency ultrasound has recently been introduced into the equine market. However, controlled scientific studies are scarce. Carrozzo *et al.* (2019) found that 20 of 23 suspensory ligament injuries improved after low-frequency ultrasound and controlled exercise.

At the University of Tennessee Equine Rehabilitation facility, therapeutic ultrasound is most commonly used for its heating effect on tendons and ligaments prior to exercise or mobilizations. The protocol used is 3.3 MHz and intensity of 1.0 W/cm^2

Extracorporeal shockwave therapy (EWST) is a non-invasive treatment that involves the delivery of high-energy sound waves, or acoustic energy, to an effected area. Shockwaves are characterized by high-pressure bars of up to 100 bar and negative pressures of 5–10 bar (McClure *et al.*, 2003). They have a rapid rise time of 30–120 ns and a short (5 µs) pulse duration (McClure *et al.*, 2003). The mechanism of action seen in tissue and its relation to the clinical effect of treatment are not fully understood. Current theories include cytokine induction, increased osteoblast activity, stimulation of nociceptors which in turn inhibits afferent pain signals, stimulation of neovascularization, induction of nitric oxide synthase, and thus bone healing/remodeling and induction of heat shock proteins (McClure *et al.*, 2000).

There are four methods for generation of sound waves: (i) piezoelectric; (ii) electromagnetic; (iii) electrohydraulic; and (iv) pneumatic ballistic. Each has its own positive and negative traits. The first three are commonly referred to as focused extracorporeal shockwave units, while the fourth is referred to as a radial extracorporeal shockwave unit. The reason for this is how the shockwave itself is generated.

EWST is generally considered safe (McClure *et al.*, 2003). No untoward effects have been noted on skin, tendons, ligaments, nerves, or bone (Boening *et al.*, 2000; McClure *et al.*, 2000; McClure *et al.*, 2003). Mild skin irritation that resolved after 24 hours has been noted with radial extracorporeal shockwave therapy (Boening *et al.*, 2000). Local analgesia, lasting upto three days has been reported, resulting in the recommendation that horses not undergo strenuous activity for a minimum of four days after treatment (McClure *et al.*, 2003). EWST is not recommended for acute injuries. Sufficient time must be allowed for inflammation to subside and in the case of tendons and ligaments the lesion to organize.

Indications claimed to be effectively treated by EWST are insertion desmopathies, navicular syndrome, dorsal spinous process impingement, arthropathies (fetlock, pastern, and hock), exostosis, constriction of the annular ligament, tendinopathies with or without calcifications, calcification of the nuchal ligament, splint bone fractures, and dorsal metacarpal disease (Boening *et al.*, 2000; Crowe *et al.*, 2002; Palmer, 2002; McClure and Weinberger, 2003; Revenaugh, 2005; Waguespack *et al.*, 2011). Khairoun *et al.* (2023) found that performing three or more ESWT on either proximal suspensory ligament desmitis or SDFT reduced lameness between the first and third treatment. However, there were no significant differences in ultrasonographic appearance. Traeger *et al.* (2020) found that three treatments of ESWT 2 weeks apart raised mechanical nociceptive thresholds over a 56-day period in horses with back pain but did not change the cross-sectional area of the multifidus muscle.

Treatment protocols vary depending on whether focused or radial EWST is used and the particular manufacturer of the unit (McClure and Weinberger, 2003). As a rule, 1,500–2,000 pulses delivered to the effected site at 10–14 day intervals for 1–4 treatments are used. Horses are rested during the treatment period and depending on the condition being treated may require and extended rest period of up to six months.

Whole body vibration therapy (see Figure 23.7) is the use of vibrating plates to induce oscillating vibrations throughout the body. It is most commonly used in human medicine to improve bone density and to improve neuromuscular function and muscle strength (Rehn *et al.*, 2006; Rauch, 2009; Slatkovska *et al.*, 2010; Von Stengel *et al.*, 2011; Chanou *et al.*, 2012; Pozo-Cruz *et al.*, 2012). However, the literature is conflicting with some reviews reporting benefit and others reporting none (Bautmans *et al.*, 2005; Cardinale, 2005; Nordlund and Thorstensson, 2006; Rehn *et al.*, 2006; Rauch, 2009; Feland *et al.*, 2010; Slatkovska *et al.*, 2010, 2011; Verschueren *et al.*, 2011; Von Stengel *et al.*, 2011; Wysocki *et al.*, 2011; Chanou *et al.*, 2012; Pozo-Cruz *et al.*, 2012; Costantino *et al.*, 2014). What is evident is that in those

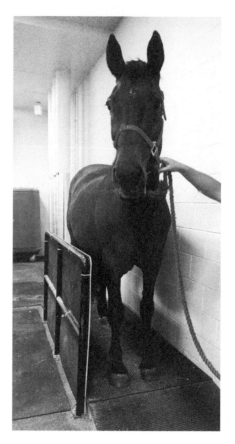

Figure 23.7 Whole body vibration.

studies that do report benefits treatments must be performed 2–3 times daily, 5–7 days per week for several months. Additionally, to see improvement in neuromuscular function or muscle strength exercises must be performed while on the plate.

While whole body vibration (WBV) has been extensively studied in humans only; recently, it has been investigated on the horse. Results of these studies have been variable with some studies showing beneficial effects, while others have shown no effect. The following is a summary of the effects of WBV on the horse:

Lab parameters
- Reduced heart rate, cortisol, and CK. No change in lactate, insulin, hematology, GGT, BUN, and creatinine (Carstanjen *et al.*, 2013)

- *Muscle* – No significant changes in BUN, AST, GGT, CK, and LA (Hyatt, 2017)

Bone mineral content
- Stalled versus exercised horses – stall confined + WBV and exercised groups had same bone mineral content (Hulak *et al.*, 2015)
- WBV was insufficient to overcome osteopenia from immobilization due to stalling and disuse (Huseman *et al.*, 2019)
- 28 days of WBV had no effect on bone mineral content, serum pyridinoline cross-links, and osteocalcin as compared to controls (Maher *et al.*, 2020)

Multifidus muscle size
- Significant increase in CSA at 30 and 60 days as compared to controls (Halsberghe *et al.*, 2017a)
- Muscle activity and warm up – no significant findings as compared to controls (Buchner *et al.*, 2017)

Hoof growth
- Conflicting as one study showed increased hoof growth (Halsberghe, 2018) and another showed no effect (Lowe *et al.*, 2017)

Lameness
- No effect on chronic lameness in horses (Halsberghe, 2017b)

Body temperature
- WBV therapy did not warm the muscles enough to increase external body temperature (Jallaq *et al.*, 2019)

Stride length
- 28 days of WBV had no effect on stride length at the trot (Maher *et al.*, 2020; Sugg, 2018)

Relaxation (qualitative observations)
- Horses appear to be more relaxed both during and after WBV (Sugg, 2018; Nowlin *et al.*, 2017)

In summary, most of the studies have been unable to document any positive effect of WBV on the horse. However, it should be noted that different WBV units or protocols were used thus making it difficult to compare results. At the University of Tennessee Equine Rehabilitation facility, whole body vibration is utilized for those horses that are confined to a stall and cannot be adequately exercised or have a limb immobilized. It is known that immobilization for several weeks causes a decrease in bone density (van Harreveld *et al.*, 2002a, b). Each case is placed on the plate for 20 minutes twice daily, 5 days per week.

Hyperbaric oxygen therapy is the delivery of oxygen to the tissues by increasing environmental oxygen levels and pressure. Minimal work has been done to evaluate HBOT in horses and that has been conflicting. Dhar *et al.* found that hyperbaric oxygen treatment resulted in a significant increase in CD90-positive cells. Horses that did not yield any cell pretreatment did so only after three HBO treatments (Dhar *et al.*, 2012). However, Holder *et al.* found that the use of HBOT after full-thickness skin grafting of uncompromised fresh and granulating wounds of horses is not indicated (Holder *et al.*, 2008). Baumwart *et al.* found that pretreatment with HBO prior to the administration of endotoxin did not offer any protection against endotoxemia (Baumwart *et al.*, 2011).

Most indications and treatment protocols have been adapted from humans and research animals. More HBOT units are now being placed in clinical practices and more information should be forthcoming. However, current clinical impressions are promising for certain conditions. The University of Tennessee Equine Rehabilitation Department is currently using HBOT for treatment of wounds, osteomyelitis, acute laminitis, and post-operative colics and has observed a more rapid improvement in these conditions verses

Table 23.3 Conditions which may benefit from hyperbaric oxygen therapy.

Thermal burns	Carbon monoxide poisoning
Smoke inhalation	Cyanide poisoning
Cerebral edema	Traumatic brain injury
Exceptional blood loss anemia	Gas gangrene – Clostridial myonecrosis
Ileus	Cranial nerve paralysis
Hypoxic encephalopathy	Soft tissue swelling
Peripheral neuropathy	Compartment syndrome
Crush injuries	Acute and chronic osteomyelitis
Cellulitis	Tendon and ligament injuries
Fracture healing – non-unions	Deep vein thrombosis
Delayed wound healing	Intra-abdominal abscess
Compromised skin flaps and grafts	Neonatal maladjustment syndrome
Meningitis	Tooth root abscess
Refractory mycoses	Myositis
Neonatal septicemia	
Chronic sinusitis	
Laminitis	

those treated without HBOT (see Table 23.3 provides a list of indications for HBOT).

HBOT is a method of increasing the amount of oxygen being delivered to the tissues. This is accomplished by placing the horse in an enclosed chamber and increasing both the percent oxygen and pressure within the chamber. Normal atmospheric pressure is 1 atmosphere absolute (ATA) which is equal to 14.7 pounds per square inch (PSI). Normal room air is approximately 21% oxygen. Most HBOT treatments are carried out under 2–3 ATAs in the presence of 70–90% oxygen (Tibbles and Edelsberg, 1996; Gill and Bell, 2004; Slovis, 2008).

The amount of oxygen delivered to the tissues is dependent on the amount of oxygen in the air that is breathed, lung function, the amount of hemoglobin in the blood, and blood pressure (Slovis, 2008). Increasing the amount of air that is breathed does not improve the amount of oxygen delivered by hemoglobin, and breathing 100% oxygen at normal atmospheric pressure only increases the amount of oxygen in the blood by a small amount (Slovis, 2008). However, the partial pressure of oxygen in

the blood is dramatically increased when breathing oxygen at two or more atmospheres of pressure. Increasing the atmospheric pressure during a treatment increases the solubility of oxygen in the body, allowing for an increased amount of oxygen to enter plasma and tissues (Slovis, 2008).

Oxygen can be considered a drug, in that not enough and too much can be detrimental to the patient. Clinical use of oxygen under pressure should not exceed 3 ATA. No benefits are derived from further increases in pressure and the risk of toxicity increases (Gill and Bell, 2004; Slovis, 2008).

HBO can increase healing of hypoxic wounds (Slovis, 2008). Fibroblasts cannot synthesize collagen without adequate oxygenation (Slovis, 2008). More rapid wound healing occurs because of accelerated angiogenesis and prevention of excessive healing (granulation tissue formation). It can improve resistance to infection and accentuate the action of some antimicrobial agents (Tibbles and Edelsberg, 1996; Leach *et al.*, 1998; Slovis, 2008).

HBO can inhibit some clostridial toxins and increases the killing ability of PMNs for *Clostridium perfringens* organisms (Slovis, 2008). It also has a direct killing effect on anaerobic organisms (Tibbles and Edelsberg, 1996).

HBO can lessen carbon monoxide toxicity and may be beneficial in animals suffering from smoke inhalation. HBO can increase osteoclastic activity. HBO may reduce hematocrit and platelet aggregation improving RBC stability. HBO improves the killing ability of neutrophils (Gill and Bell, 2004). HBO can decrease edema formation as evidenced by less edema following thermal injuries and ischemia (Tibbles and Edelsberg, 1996; Leach *et al.*, 1998; Slovis, 2008).

HBOT has complex effects on immunity, oxygen transport, and hemodynamics. The positive therapeutic effects come from a reduction in hypoxia and edema, enabling normal host responses to infection and ischemia (Gill and Bell, 2004). The normal atmospheric pressure that we live under is measured in ATAs. One ATA is the normal atmospheric pressure at sea level. This is equivalent to 14.7 pounds PSI, or 760 mm of mercury (mmHg), that we breathe. The atmospheric air is approximately 79% nitrogen and 21% oxygen, resulting in an oxygen partial pressure of about 160 mmHg.

Normal circumstances of oxygen delivery in the body are dependent on the proportion of oxygen in the air that we breathe, lung function, the amount of hemoglobin in our blood, and the body's blood pressure. Increasing the amount of air that you breathe cannot improve the amount of oxygen delivered by hemoglobin, and breathing 100% oxygen at normal atmospheric pressure will only increase the amount of oxygen dissolved in blood plasma by a small amount. The partial pressure of oxygen in the blood is dramatically increased when breathing oxygen at two or more atmospheres of pressure. Increasing the atmospheric pressure in the chamber during a treatment increases the solubility of oxygen in the body. This process allows oxygen to enter plasma and tissues more readily and promotes the formation of new cells thus further enhancing oxygen availability. Ischemic wounds and areas of infection now have new cells to increase circulation and supply lifesaving oxygen and antibiotics.

Overall HBOT is safe. The Equine Rehabilitation Department has performed hundreds of sessions with minimal issues (see Table 23.4 provides a list of contraindications). A strict protocol that includes "Go or No Go" evaluations is mandated. A checklist is utilized prior to and after therapy that includes animal evaluation as well as full assessment of the chamber function. All treatments are performed by individuals who have had advanced off-site training in HBOT. It is critical that protocols be established and personnel are adequately trained. Depending on the specific disease or injury, HBOT can be the factor that pushes the patient toward a positive outcome, when

Table 23.4 Contraindications for HBO therapy.

Absolute contraindications	Relative contraindications
Untreated pneumothorax	Chronic emphysema with CO_2 retention
Tension pneumothorax	Optic neuritis
Concurrent treatment with cis-platinum, disulfiram, or doxorubicin	History of spontaneous pneumothorax, thoracic surgery
	Seizure disorders
	High fevers
	Viral infections of the respiratory tract

standard therapeutic measures are ineffective (Geiser, 2016).

Therapeutic exercise is often used during the rehabilitation program. The amount and intensity are dependent upon the condition being treated, the extent of the damage, the time of healing, and facilities available. Types of exercise include hand walking, riding, ponying (leading a horse while riding another), mechanical walker, underwater treadmill, swimming pool, and turnout to paddock or pasture. Each exercise program is tailored to the individual and may need to be adapted several times during the rehabilitation program. The basic principle is to reduce the force and strain on injured tissue, while the normal reparative process proceeds (Davidson, 2016). Also, ground obstacles (ground poles, cavaletti's) may be incorporated to increase coordination and agility. Additionally, change in terrain may be included to target specific areas (i.e., inclines to strengthen rear limbs). The goal of therapeutic exercise is to provide a gradual return to function, improve strength and coordination, and provide mental stimulation.

Equine aquatic therapy primarily encompasses swimming and underwater treadmills. Whirlpools and recovery pools are also examples but will not be addressed in this chapter. Equine swimming pools have been available for 25–30 years; however, prior to that often ponds, lakes, or the ocean have been used. Many of the pools are located at tracks or barns. A few veterinary hospitals and equine rehab centers also have these pools. The main drawback of pools is the expense of construction and the costs of maintenance.

A cold salt water (hypertonic) spa has been reported to have anti-inflammatory, osmotic, and analgesic effects (Bender *et al.*, 2005). In horses, tendonitis and desmitis monitored ultrasonographically demonstrated reduced peritendinous and preligamentous edema, decreased inflammatory infiltration, and

improved collagen fiber alignment after the four weeks of hypertonic cold-water therapy (Hunt, 2001). The added mineral components in water provide an increased osmotic effect, which reduces soft tissue inflammation and swelling, decreases pain, and ultimately improves joint ROM. These osmotic effects can play an important role in managing soft tissue changes associated with musculoskeletal injury in horses (King, 2016).

More recently, equine underwater treadmills (see Figure 23.8) have been developed to overcome the expense of construction and maintenance of in-ground pools. These units also provide a more controlled environment than do pools with a decreased possibility of injury.

Swimming and underwater treadmills may provide several benefits. They primarily provide cardiovascular conditioning without the stresses on the musculoskeletal system (Buchner and Schildboeck, 2006). Additionally, they provide a different type

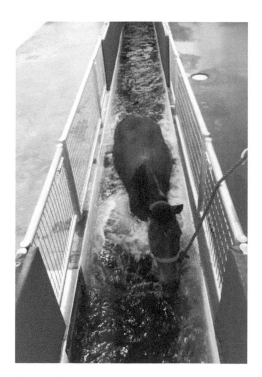

Figure 23.8 In-ground underwater treadmill.

of muscle exercise and also work different groups of muscles than when working on land. Resistance to joint movement is also a benefit that contributes to rehabilitation.

The use of swimming and the underwater treadmill in the rehabilitation of musculoskeletal injuries is becoming more common. Their use allows maintenance of cardiovascular fitness, muscle tone, and improved joint movement without undue stresses occurring on the injured limb. The reason for the decreased stresses placed on the limb is the buoyancy that the water provides. Depending on the height or depth of water, a certain amount of this depends on the amount of water in relation to the body mass of the horse. Thus, a horse that is placed in a small area will require less water to get to the level of the point of the shoulder. Because of the reduced amount of water, there is less buoyancy, thus more weight being born.

Buoyancy is the force experienced as an up-thrust, which acts in the opposite direction to the force of gravity (Monk, 2007). A body immersed in the water appears to lose weight, and the weight loss is equal to the weight of water displaced (Monk, 2007). Immersion in water allows for unweighting of tendons, ligaments, bones, and joints within the distal limb (McClintock *et al.*, 1987). There is a reduction in ground reaction forces leading to reduced concussive stresses on joints and tendons, allowing for exercise without further trauma induced by weight bearing or concussive forces (Misumi *et al.*, 1994). Reduced body weight decreases postoperative and convalescent complications. McClintock *et al.* determined the weight reduction for a horse in a floatation tank filled with saline (McClintock *et al.*, 1987). They found approximately a 10% reduction in the weight born by the limbs when the saline was at the level of the olecranon. When the saline was raised to the level of the tuber coxae there was approximately a 75% reduction in weight.

Immersion causes water displacement and increases hydrostatic pressure. Hydrostatic pressure is the sum of pressure exerted on all surfaces of a body immersed in water, for any given depth (Monk, 2007). In humans, this can cause redistribution of blood flow from the peripheral limbs due to an isotonic fluid shift from extravascular space (Yamazaki *et al.*, 2000). It can also lead to a decrease in hemoglobin and hematocrit levels within 25–60 minutes of water immersion (Yamazaki *et al.*, 2000). Hydrostatic pressure will affect lung volumes hence care needs to be taken with patients with respiratory distress or compromise (Monk, 2007).

Viscosity is the resistance of a fluid to motion (Monk, 2007). Viscosity of water increases as speed increases. This is due to increased turbulence and drag. This in turn increases the amount and intensity of work being performed. The addition of hydrojets to the pool or treadmill can increase the drag-on-limb movement. Viscosity decreases as water temperature increases (Monk, 2007). This means weaker and smaller muscles move more easily in warmer water (Monk, 2007).

Relative density and specific gravity of an object will depend on the composition of the object and will determine whether an object will float or sink (Monk, 2007). So, lean animals and heavily muscled animals have a tendency to sink and animals with a greater amount of body fat will float more easily (Monk, 2007).

Both swimming and underwater treadmill exercises are forms of aerobic exercise and help develop cardiovascular fitness. With water immersion, there is a decrease in systemic vascular resistance and the changes in total peripheral resistance are dependent on water temperature (Yamazaki *et al.*, 2000).

Following underwater treadmill exercise there is a moderate but non-significant increase in blood lactate and plasma creatine phosphokinase levels (Lindner *et al.*, 2003). Hemoglobin concentration is significantly increased as a result of the physical exercise (Voss *et al.*, 2002). Voss *et al.* concluded that underwater treadmill training, following their training protocol, represents a medium-sized aerobic workload for horses.

Swimming causes a significant increase in blood pressure (Thomas *et al.*, 1980). However, the maximum heart rate obtained while swimming is less than that obtained during ground exercise (Thomas *et al.*, 1980; Galloux *et al.*, 1994). There appears to be no relationship between heart rate and duration of swimming (Galloux *et al.*, 1994). There also appear to be increased cardiovascular benefits while working at slower speeds (Galloux *et al.*, 1994; Hobo *et al.*, 1998).

Water pressure on the horse's body during swimming prevents adequate ventilation (McClintock *et al.*, 1986a, b; Hobo *et al.*, 1998). Hobo *et al.* found an increase in respiratory rate, an increase in both inspiratory and expiratory pressure, and that the expiratory time was roughly doubled the inspiratory time (Hobo *et al.*, 1998). This suggested that a longer expiratory time may limit sudden collapse of airways by water pressure during swimming and prevent a marked decrease in air space volume, thus maintains buoyancy (Hobo *et al.*, 1998). There are no studies available on the effects of underwater treadmill exercise on the respiratory function of horses.

Walking in water at the level of the carpus or ulna resulted in a lower stride frequency and greater stride length compared to walking in water at hoof height (Scott *et al.*, 2010). Water provides a resistance to movement of the limb in the sagittal plane; so an increase in height of the flight arc may also minimize the resistance experienced in swinging the limb back and forth (Scott *et al.*, 2010). When moving in water between carpal and ulna height, the horse may find it easier to adopt a rounder flight arc by increasing flexion of the hip, stifle, and

hock joints. Water treadmill exercise may increase activity of muscles which flex the hip, flex the stifle, and protract the hindlimb (Scott *et al.*, 2010). Borgia *et al.* found no effect of water treadmill training on the properties of the gluteal and superficial digital flexor (SDF) muscles and on cardiocirculatory response to a standardized exercise test (Borgia *et al.*, 2010). However, the authors state that a more strenuous water treadmill conditioning protocol may be needed to induce a training effect in gluteal and SDF muscle and heart rate response (Borgia *et al.*, 2010).

Evaluating the effects of swimming on two-year-old thoroughbreds in race training, Misumi *et al.* found that fast-twitch, high oxidative fibers increased (Misumi *et al.*, 1995). There was an increase in aerobic capacity of muscles and a decrease in fast-twitch, low oxidative fibers. There was no change in slow-twitch fibers. They suggested that a training program, including swimming training, is seen as being useful for improvement in performance capacity since it can reduce locomotor diseases in young horses and allow for smooth progress in future training (Misumi *et al.*, 1994, 1995).

Horses use their forelimbs to regulate their lateral balance and their rear limbs function in propulsion (Galloux *et al.*, 1994). The propulsive action of the rear limbs is much exaggerated. Also, during swimming, the equine spine is lordotic. Because of the exaggerated rear limb action and lordotic back, horses with rear limb injuries or back pain should not swim.

There is an increased range of joint motion in both fore and hind limbs depending on water height. Joint angle in horses decreases as water approaches the carpus or hock. Once the level of the carpus or hock is reached, joint flexion and limb height will vary little. This may be used to target specific joints and aid in re-establishment of joint ROM after joint surgery. In dogs, there is increased flexion and ROM during swimming compared to walking in both normal and operated stifle joints post-CCL surgery (Marsolais *et al.*, 2003). The increased ROM was due to increased joint flexion. Ground treadmill walking produces greater stifle extension than swimming (Marsolais *et al.*, 2003).

Water density is 12 times greater than air (Monk, 2007). During aquatic therapy, there is increased resistance to limb or body movement and increased energy costs compared to walking at similar speeds on land due to this increased density. This provides better muscle development and muscle tone due to working against resistance and provides better balance of muscle groups working against increased resistance while maintaining a symmetrical gait (Bromiley, 2000). Additionally, underwater treadmill exercise significantly improved the horse's postural stability (King *et al.*, 2013).

Safety is a paramount importance when using swimming or an underwater treadmill. It is very important that the handlers be thoroughly familiar with the equipment and must be able to read horse's temperament. The handler should be able to anticipate and correct problems with the horse or equipment before they develop.

Swimming pools should be constructed so that two handlers can easily walk 360° around. Depth should be adequate so that the horse cannot touch the bottom. Most are 12–15 feet deep. The sides should be sloped to prevent injury. Some type of ramp system should be employed that allows easy entry and exit from the pool. The filtration system is very important. The water becomes quickly contaminated with dirt and feces, so a good filtration system is a necessity. Most horses are good swimmers but do require training. Usually, an introductory period is required with increasing time intervals in the pool. The time slowly increased to a period of approximately 15 minutes. Little research has been done on proper protocols. There has been a protocol described using a swimming test to determine the level of fitness a horse has achieved following conventional training. However, it is not very applicable for determining swimming protocols.

There are two types of underwater treadmills, in-ground and above-ground. The in-ground type allows for a greater amount of water to be used thus there is greater buoyancy. Both are variable speeds that range from 0–15 mph. This is much lower than the high-speed treadmill which can achieve speeds of 45–50 mph. Horses require training on this equipment also. Some may require sedation until they are familiar with the routine. Both units require filtration, and most can provide both heated and unheated water. These units are expensive, but the prices are becoming more reasonable.

Acclimation to water treadmill exercise requires a minimum of 2×15 minutes nonsedated acclimating runs (Nankervis and Williams, 2006). Sedation can be used to prevent horses from panicking during the first exposure but, thereafter, does not affect the time taken to acclimate.

Water temperature should be adjusted to provide maximized comfort. For active exercise and swimming use 65–82 °F. For less vigorous exercise 96–104 °F is acceptable. The least adverse physiologic effects occur at 97 °F.

Unfortunately, most of the facilities do not monitor any parameters either during or after a session. Because of this, recommended protocols are empirical. Two easy parameters that can be measured include heart rate and blood lactate levels. Heart rate can be used to monitor the level of stresses that are being placed on the cardiovascular system. Maximum heart rate of the horse is approximately 200 bpm. By using a heart rate monitor, you can set a target rate and then set a time to stay in the target range. Blood lactate is used to determine if the horse has progressed into the aerobic metabolism stage. This is a desired state to achieve adequate conditioning. Respiratory rate can also be used but is not as reliable as heart rate. Additionally, lameness evaluation should be performed at weekly intervals to determine if any musculoskeletal problem has arisen.

Summary of equine research

- High water is more strenuous than walking in low
- Walking slowly reduces FL protraction-retraction ROM and increases HL protraction-retraction ROM
- Water height has a greater impact on exercise intensity than speed
- Low-intensity exercise
- Deepwater training alters the biochemical processes and can improve the aerobic energy supply of show jumpers
- Improves joint ROM, and synovial membrane integrity
- High water causes cranial thoracic extension and thoracolumbar flexion
- No significant association between pelvic vertical displacement and water depth
- Walking on a water treadmill in high water results in a lower forelimb ROM but a higher hindlimb ROM
- Underwater treadmill training resulted in minor changes in type I muscle fiber sizes, with no effect on muscle metabolic or heart rate responses
- Increasing water depths, there are increases in flexion and rotation of the back, but decreased bending initially
- Useful for increasing the ROM of various joints
- Underwater treadmill exercise significantly improved the horses' postural stability
- Underwater treadmill speeds need to be >5.5 m/s if the effect of conditioning is to be evaluated with blood lactate

Indications for aquatic therapy include rehabilitation after injury or surgery, tendon injuries, post-arthroscopic surgery, replacement for hand walking, joint stiffness, osteoarthritis, increase in muscle development, encourage symmetric gait and back development, cardiovascular conditioning, and reconditioning after a lay-up.

Contra-indications for aquatic therapy include acute joint inflammation, skin infections, open wounds, upper limb lameness (swimming), back pain (swimming), acute myositis, cardiovascular compromise, and respiratory disease.

The following are variables that must be considered when developing a protocol for an individual patient. Of utmost importance is the disposition of the horse. There are going to be some horses that may never acclimate to aquatic therapy. In these individuals, another therapeutic plan will need to be developed.

- Injury and condition of patient
- Water level (if possible)
  - Amount of buoyancy and limb weight-bearing
  - Degree of joint flexion desired
  - Water temperature
  - Warm versus cold
- Treadmill speed
- Hydrojets – on or off (if equipped)
- Warmup period
- Duration of exercise – 5–30 minutes
- Exertion during exercise
- Frequency of exercise
- Cool down period

Sample Underwater Treadmill Protocol

See Table 23.5 is an example of an underwater treadmill program that is for a mild to moderate tendon injury. It is only begun after an ultrasound evaluation has shown significant healing has occurred and that the horse can have a significant amount of hand walking. It is important that the horse be evaluated prior to each treadmill session for any increased heat or swelling of the affected tendon or ligament. It also should be evaluated weekly for change in the degree of lameness. Ultrasonography should be

Table 23.5 Sample underwater treadmill program.

Acclimation period (days 1 and 2)

- Walk in and walk out of underwater treadmill
- Walk in unit and add 6″ of water, drain, and walk out to acclimate to sounds of unit filling
- Walk in, add water, turn on treadmill, stop treadmill, drain unit, and walk out
- May use sedation during acclimation if needed. It also helps to have a trained horse at the facility to act as a lead horse

Rehabilitation program (days 3–7)

- Water level at olecranon
  - Speed – walk at 2 mph
  - Warm up – 5 min at 2 mph
  - Duration of active walk – 5 min at 2 mph
  - Cool down – 5 min at 2 mph
  - Frequency – Once per day; five days per week
  - Outcome measures
    o Walking comfortably for 5 min duration at 2 mph
    o If successful proceed to next level

Rehabilitation program week 2

- Warm up – 5 min at 2 mph
  - Duration of active walk – 10 min at 3 mph
  - Cool down – 5 min at 2 mph
  - May begin lowering or raising water level
  - May increase speed to 2–3 mph
  - Frequency – Once per day; five days per week
  - Outcome measures
    o Walking comfortably for 10 min duration at 3 mph
    o If successful proceed to next level

Rehabilitation program week 3

- Warm up – 5 min at 2 mph
- Duration of active walk – 15 min at 4 mph
- Cool down – 5 min at 2 mph
- Adjust water level to best address specific injuries and goals
- Frequency – Once per day; five days per week
- Outcome measures
  - Walking comfortably for 15 min duration at 4 mph
- If successful proceed to next level

Rehabilitation program week 4

- Warm up – 5 min at 2 mph
- Duration of active walk – 20 min at 5 mph
- Cool down – 5 min at 2 mph
- Frequency – Once per day; five days per week
- Outcome measures
  - Walking comfortably for 20 min duration at 5 mph
  - If successful proceed to next level

Rehabilitation program week 5

- Warm up – 5 min at 2 mph
- Maximum exercise intensity of 5 mph for 20 – 30 min
- Cool down – 5 min at 2 mph
- May introduce cross-training activities
- Frequency – Once per day; 3–5 days per week;
- Outcome measures
  - Walking comfortably for at least 20 min duration at 4–5 mph

repeated at monthly intervals so that the rehabilitation program can be adjusted or terminated if necessary. Note that the ability to vary water height to any appreciable amount only applies to above-ground units. If an in-ground treadmill is used, then disregard the water height recommendation. All sessions should have a 2–5-minute warmup and 2–5-minute cool down period.

Ground exercises are exercises that are performed at hand or while being ridden. They are usually targeted at specific areas such as improvement in proprioception and coordination, strengthening of specific muscles, improving joint mobility, and improving overall body condition. There are many types of exercises that may be utilized. It is often based on the imagination of the rehabilitation veterinarian, rehabilitation physical therapist, and rehabilitation veterinary technician/nurse to develop specific exercises. One must consider the nature of the patient and injury, the equipment and facilities available, and the personnel. Many of the therapeutic exercises are inexpensive and just require time and personnel. Ursini *et al.* (2022) found that implementing ground poles can be an effective strategy to increase the activation of the multifidus muscle; however,

caution should be taken when incorporating the use of a resistance band training device as muscle work, and peak activation was significantly reduced in most locations. Walker *et al.* (2022) found that walking over poles appears to be effective at increasing joint ROM by increasing midswing flexion, without vertical excursion of the trunk, compared to normal locomotion. Shaw *et al.* (2021) found that ground poles increase in core muscle activation at the walk and trot; however, elastic resistance bands only affected the rectus abdominus muscles at the trot.

The following illustrates some different methods.

Proprioception and coordination may be improved by walking over ground poles placed in random fashion (see Figure 23.9).

Other configurations can be utilized (Paulekas and Haussler, 2009). Different surface transitions may also be utilized such as going from grass, to sand, to gravel, to water, and then to asphalt. Different obstacles and pedestals can also be utilized (Paulekas and Haussler, 2009). Improving joint mobility can be accomplished by having cavalettis arranged like spokes on a wagon wheel and having the horse step over them going in both directions (see Figure 23.10).

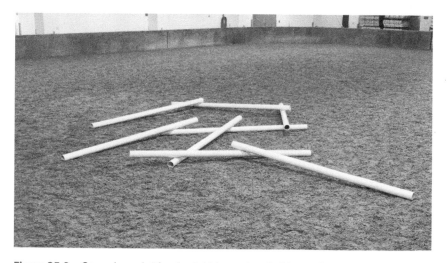

Figure 23.9 Ground cavaletti poles laid in random fashion to improve proprioception.

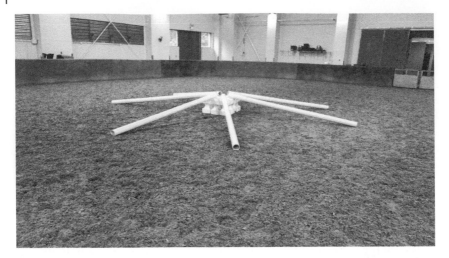

Figure 23.10 Ground cavaletti poles laid in a radius to encourage joint motion and improve coordination.

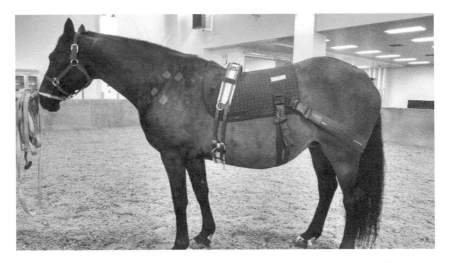

Figure 23.11 Therapeutic band application to improve core muscle strength.

Placing bracelets or weights around the pasterns can also be utilized (Clayton *et al.*, 2010a, b, 2011a, b). However, horses will become habituated to the devices (Clayton *et al.*, 2008). Core muscle stability can be improved utilizing therapeutic bands placed around the caudal limbs or abdomen (Paulekas and Haussler, 2009). These may be used at hand, lunging, or while being ridden (see Figure 23.11).

Strengthening of rear limb musculature may be accomplished by riding up and down gradual inclines or pulling a cart. This most commonly has been used as a therapy for intermittent upward fixation of the patella.

Kinesiology taping is an elastic therapeutic tape method used for treating sports injuries and a variety of other disorders. A chiropractor, Dr. Kenso Kase, developed

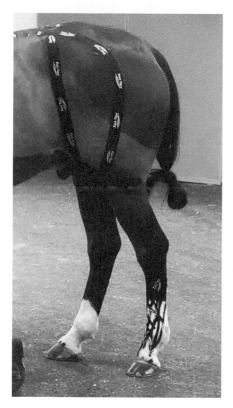

Figure 23.12 Equine Kinesiology taping.

these taping techniques in the 1970s (Williams *et al.*, 2012). It is claimed that it supports injured muscles and joints and helps relieve pain by lifting the skin and allowing improved blood and lymph flow (Williams *et al.*, 2012) (see Figure 23.12).

There is conflicting evidence in humans as to whether it is effective or not (Williams *et al.*, 2012; Montalvo *et al.*, 2014; Parreira *et al.*, 2014). Scientific evidence to support its use in the equine is scarce. Ericson *et al.* (2020) applied Kinesotape to the thoracolumbar area of horses and evaluated them at the trot. They demonstrated no effect on back flexion and extension. Likewise, Zellner *et al.* (2017) found no effect of Kinesotape on equine forelimb trajectory. Most of the effect and efficacy of Kinesiotaping is anecdotal or is based on human literature. There are courses that can be taken in the proper technique of equine kinesiology taping.

Return to Work

At some point, the rehabilitation program will end and the horse must be returned to work if possible. It is important that return to work be done gradually. While the particular injury may have healed the rest of the body may not be in condition (see Table 23.6 is an example of a conservative back-to-work plan.). We always recommend at least a 10-minute warmup and cool down period.

Table 23.6 Example back to work plan following resolution of injury.

Week	Walk	Trot	Walk	Trot	Walk
Initially start with three days of riding. After second week can be increased to five days per week if desired.					
1	20 min walking under saddle				
2	30 min walking under saddle				
3	40 min walking under saddle				
4	10 min	2 min	6 min	2 min	10 min
5	10 min	3 min	4 min	3 min	10 min
6	10 min	4 min	2 min	4 min	10 min
7	10 min	6 min	2 min	6 min	10 min

(Continued)

Table 23.6 (Continued)

Week	Walk	Trot	Canter	Walk	Trot	Walk
			Starting week 8 add canter			
8	10 min	2 min	2 min	5 min	2 min	10 min
9	10 min	3 min	2 min	4 min	3 min	10 min
10	10 min	2 min	3 min	4 min	2 min	10 min
11	10 min	4 min	4 min	4 min	4 min	10 min

Weeks 1–6: Start turning out into a paddock/round pen. Start with 2 h per day and build up to approximately 8 h by week 4. Can also be hand walked for 20–30 min, 2–3 times per day during this time if desired (in addition to walking under saddle).

Weeks 7–11: Turn out to pasture; start with 2 h per day of pasture and 6 h of paddock/round pen. Increase pasture time by 2 h weekly so that by week 11, he/she is on pasture at least 8 h per day.

Starting week 12: No restrictions in work or turn out; resume normal work over a 2–3-wk period.

Recommend re-evaluation prior to canter work and again prior to resuming regular work.

Conclusion

The equine rehabilitation veterinary technician or nurse will play an important role in carrying out the rehabilitation equine veterinarian's treatment plan and communicating that plan with the owner on a routine basis. Monitoring the patient's progress and maintaining the records will be important to track trends for the patient. Monitoring pain and advancement in achieving the therapeutic goals will be necessary to aid the rehabilitation veterinarian and physical therapist in developing plans. By understanding all aspects of equine physical rehabilitation, the equine physical rehabilitation veterinary technician or nurse will contribute to the success of bringing an injured patient back to the goals set forth by the team.

References

Adair, H.S. and Levine, D. (2019). Effects of 1-MHz ultrasound on epaxial muscle temperature in horses. *Front Vet Sci* 6 (177): 1–6.

Ajimsha, M.S., Al-Mudahka, N.R., and Al-Madzhar, J.A. (2015). Effectiveness of myofascial release: Systematic review of randomized controlled trials. *J Bodywork Movement Ther* 19 (1): 102–112.

Argüelles, D., Becero, M., Muñoz, A. et al. (2020). Accelerometric changes before and after capacitive resistive electric transfer therapy in horses with thoracolumbar pain compared to a SHAM procedure. *Animals* 10: 2305.

Auer, J.A., Burch, G.E., and Hall, P. (1983). Review of pulsing electromagnetic field therapy and its possible application to horses. *Eq Vet J* 15 (4): 354–360.

Baumwart, C.A., Doherty, T.J., Schumacher, J. et al. (2011). Effects of hyperbaric oxygen treatment on horses with experimentally induced endotoxemia. *Am J Vet Res* 72 (9): 1266–1275.

Bautmans, I., Van Hees, E., Lemper, J.-C., and Mets, T. (2005). The feasibility of whole body vibration in institutionalised elderly persons and its influence on muscle performance, balance and mobility: A randomized controlled trial. *BMC Geriatr* 5 (1): 17.

Becero, M., Saitua, A., Argüelles, D. et al. (2020). Capacitive resistive electric transfer modifies gait pattern in horses exercised on a treadmill. *BMC Vet Res* 16: 10.

Belanger, A.-Y. (2010a). Cryotherapy. In: *Therapeutic Electrophysical Agents–Evidence Behind Practice*, 2nde, 121–149. Philadelphia, PA: Lippincott Williams & Wilkens.

Belanger, A.-Y. (2010b). Transcutaneous electrical nerve stimulation therapy. In: *Therapeutic Electrophysical Agents–Evidence Behind Practice*, 277–305. Lippincott Williams & Wilkens.

Bender, T., Karagulle, Z., Balint, G.P. et al. (2005). Hydrotherapy, balneotherapy, and spa treatment in pain management. *Rheumatol Int* 25: 220–224.

Bergh, A. (2006). *Defocused CO2 Laser Irradiation in the Rehabilitation of Horses*. Sweden: Swedish University of Agricultural Sciences.

Bergh, A., Ridderstale, Y., and Ekman, S. (2007). Defocused CO2 laser on equine skin: A histological examination. *Eq Vet J* 39 (2): 114–119.

Bergh, A., NordlöF, H., and EsséN-Gustavsson, B. (2010). Evaluation of neuromuscular electrical stimulation on fibre characteristics and oxidative capacity in equine skeletal muscles. *Eq Vet J* 42: 671–675.

Biermann, N.M., Rindler, N., and Buchner, H.H.F. (2014). The effect of pulsed electromagnetic fields on back pain in polo ponies evaluated by pressure algometry and flexion testing—A randomized, double-blind, placebo-controlled trial. *J Eq Vet Sci* 34 (4): 500–507.

Boening KJ, Loeffeld S, Weitkamp K, and Matuschek S (2000) Radial extracorporeal shock wave therapy for chronic insertion desmopathy of the proximal suspensory ligament. In *Proceedings Forty-sixth Annual Convention of the AAEP*. San Antonio, TX, pp. 203–207.

Bogard, F., Bouchet, B., Murer, S. et al. (2020). Critical evaluation of whole-body cryostimulation protocol in race horses. *J Equine Vet* 88: 102944.

Borgia, L.A., Valberg, S.J., and Essen-Gustavsson, B. (2010). Differences in the metabolic properties of gluteus medius and superficial digital flexor muscles and the effect of water treadmill training in the horse. *Eq Vet J* 42 (Suppl 38): 665–670.

Bromiley M (2000) Physical therapy in equine veterinary medicine: useful or useless? *Proceedings Forty-sixth Annual Convention of the AAEP*. San Antonio, TX: pp. 94–97.

Buchner, H.H.F. and Schildboeck, U. (2006). Physiotherapy applied to the horse: A review. *Eq Vet J* 38 (6): 574–580.

Buchner, H.H.F., Zimmer, L., Haase, L. et al. (2017). Effects of whole body vibration on the horse: Actual vibration, muscle activity, and warm-up effect. *J Equine Vet* 51: 54–60.

Cardinale, M. (2005). Whole body vibration exercise: Are vibrations good for you? *Br J Sports Med* 39 (9): 585–589.

Carrozzo, U., Toniato, M., and Harrison, A. (2019). Assessment of noninvasive low-frequency ultrasound as a means of treating injuries to suspensory ligaments in horses: A research paper. *J Equine Vet* 80: 80–89.

Carstanjen, B., Balali, M., Gajewski, Z. et al. (2013). Short-term whole body vibration exercise in adult healthy horses. *Pol J Vet Sci* 16: http://content.sciendo.com/view/journals/pjvs/16/2/article-p403.xml. (accessed June 8, 2018).

Chanou, K., Gerodimos, V., Karatrantou, K., and Jamurtas, A. (2012). Whole-body vibration and rehabilitation of chronic diseases: A review of the literature. *J Sports Sci Med* 11 (2): 187.

Cinar, K., Comlekci, S., and Senol, N. (2008). Effects of a specially pulsed electric field on an animal model of wound healing. *Lasers Med Sci* 24: 735–740.

Clayton, H., White, A., Kaiser, L. et al. (2008). Short-term habituation of equine limb kinematics to tactile stimulation of the coronet. *Vet Comp Orthop Traumatol* 21: 211–214.

Clayton, H.M., Kaiser, L.J., Lavagnino, M., and Stubbs, N.C. (2010a). Dynamic mobilisations in cervical flexion: Effects on intervertebral angulations. *Eq Vet J* 42 (Suppl 38): 688–694.

Clayton, H.M., White, A.D., Kaiser, L.J. et al. (2010b). Hindlimb response to tactile stimulation of the pastern and coronet: Response to tactile stimulation. *Eq Vet Jl* 42 (3): 227–233.

Clayton, H.M., Lavagnino, M., Kaiser, L.A.J., and Stubbs, N.C. (2011a). Evaluation of biomechanical effects of four stimulation devices placed on the hind feet of trotting horses. *Am J Vet Res* 72 (11): 1489–1495.

Clayton, H.M., Lavagnino, M., Kaiser, L.J., and Stubbs, N.C. (2011b). Swing phase kinematic and kinetic response to weighting the hind pasterns: Hindlimb response to leg weights. *Eq Vet J* 43 (2): 210–215.

Collier, M.A., Loree, R.L., and Antosiewicz, P.Z. (1985). Radioisotope uptake in normal equine bone under the influence of a pulsed electromagnetic field. *Mod Vet Pract* 66 (12): 971–974.

Costantino, C., Gimigliano, R., Olvirri, S., and Gimigliano, F. (2014). Whole body vibration in sport: A critical review. *J Sports Med Phys Fitness* 54: 757–764.

Crowe O, Dyson SJ, Wright IM, *et al.* (2002) Treatment of 45 cases of chronic hindlimb proximal suspensory desmitis by radial extracorporeal shockwave therapy. In *Proceedings Forty-eigth Annual Convention of the AAEP*. Orlando, FL, 322–325.

Dai, F., Costa, E.D., Giordano, A. et al. (2022). Effects of BEMER® physical vascular therapy in horses under training. A randomized, controlled double blind study. *Res Vet Sci* 144: 108–114.

Davidson, E.J. (2016). Controlled exercise in equine rehabilitation. *Vet Clin Equine* 32: 159–165.

Demmink, J.H., Helders, P.J., Hobaek, H., and Enwemeka, C. (2003). The variation of heating depth with therapeutic ultrasound frequency in physiotherapy. *Ultrasound Med Biol* 29 (1): 113–118.

Dhar, M., Neilsen, N., Beatty, K. et al. (2012). Equine peripheral blood-derived mesenchymal stem cells: Isolation, identification, trilineage differentiation and effect of hyperbaric oxygen treatment. *Eq Vet J* 44 (5): 600–605.

Doan, N., Reher, P., Meghji, S., and Harris, M. (1999). In vitro effects of therapeutic ultrasound on cell proliferation, protein synthesis, and cytokine production by human fibroblasts, osteoblasts, and monocytes. *J Oral Maxillofac Surg* 57 (4): 409–419.

Draper, D.O., Castel, J.C., and Castel, D. (1995). Rate of temperature increase in human muscle during 1 MHz and 3 MHz continuous ultrasound. *J Ortho & Sports Phys Therap* 22 (4): 142–150.

Duesterdieck-Zellmer, K.F., Larson, M.K., Plant, T.K. et al. (2016). Ex vivo penetration of low-level laser light through equine skin and flexor tendons. *Am J Vet Res* 77: 991–999.

Dyson, M. (1990). Role of ultrasound in wound healing. In: *Wound Healing: Alternatives in Management*. Philadelphia, PA: Davis.

van Eps, A.W. and Pollitt, C.C. (2009). Equine laminitis model: Cryotherapy reduces the severity of lesions evaluated seven days after induction with oligofructose. *Eq Vet J* 41 (8): 741–746.

van Eps, A.W., Pollitt, C.C., Underwood, C. et al. (2014). Continuous digital hypothermia initiated after the onset of lameness prevents lamellar failure in the oligofructose laminitis model: Digital hypothermia initiated after lameness prevents lamellar failure. *Eq Vet J* 46 (5): 625–630.

Ericson C, Stenfeldt P, Hardeman A, and Jacobson I (2020) The Effect of Kinesiotape on Flexion-Extension of the Thoracolumbar Back in Horses at Trot 15.

Feland, J.B., Hawks, M., Hopkins, J.T. et al. (2010). Whole body vibration as an adjunct to static stretching. *Int J Sports Med* 31 (08): 584–589.

Fernandes, M.A., Alves, G.E.S., and Souza, J.C.A. (2003). Clinical, ultrasonographic and histopathological studies of two protocols of ultrasonic therapy on experimental tendonitis in horses. *Arq Brasil Med Vet Zootecn* 55 (1): 27–34.

Fleeman LM and Owens E (2007) Applied animal nutrition. In *Animal physiotherapy: assessment, treatment and rehabilitation of animals*, p. 14.

Frick, A. (2010). Stretching exercises for horses: Are they effective? *J Eq Vet Sci* 30 (1): 50–59.

Fu, S.-C., Shum, W.-T., Hung, L.-K. et al. (2008). Low-intensity pulsed ultrasound on tendon healing: A study of the effect of treatment duration and treatment initiation. *Am J Sports Med* 36 (9): 1742–1749.

Galloux, P., Goupil, X., Vial, C. et al. (1994). Heart rate and blood lactic acid concentration of the horse during swimming training. *Equine Athlete* 7 (2): 10–14.

Geiser, D.R. (2016). Hyperbaric oxygen therapy in equine rehabilitation putting the pressure on disease. *Vet Clin Equine* 32: 149–157.

Gill, A.L. and Bell, C.N.A. (2004). Hyperbaric oxygen: Its uses, mechanisms of action and outcomes. *QJ Med* 97: 385–395.

Goff, L.M. (2009). Manual therapy for the horse—A contemporary perspective. *J Eq Vet Sci* 29 (11): 799–808.

Halsberghe, B.T. (2017b). Long-term and immediate effects of whole body vibration on chronic lameness in the horse: A pilot study. *J Equine Vet* 48: 121-128.e2.

Halsberghe, B.T. (2018). Effect of two months whole body vibration on hoof growth rate in the horse: A pilot study. *Res Vet Sci* 119: 37–42.

Halsberghe, B.T., Gordon-Ross, P., and Peterson, R. (2017a). Whole body vibration affects the cross-sectional area and symmetry of them multifidus of the thoracolumbar spine in the horse. *Equine Vet Educ* 29: 493–499.

Hamblin MR and Demidova TN (2006) Mechanisms of low level light therapy. In *Biomedical Optics 2006*.

van Harreveld, P.D., Lillich, J.D., Kawcak, C.E. et al. (2002a). Clinical evaluation of the effects of immobilization followed by remobilization and exercise on the metacarpophalangeal joint in horses. *Am J Vet Res* 63 (2): 282–288.

van Harreveld, P.D., Lillich, J.D., Kawcak, C.E. et al. (2002b). Effects of immobilization followed by remobilization on mineral density, histomorphometric features, and formation of the bones of the metacarpophalangeal joint in horses. *Am J Vet Res* 63 (2): 276–281.

Haussler KK (2000) Equine chiropractic: General principles and clinical applications. In *Proceedings Forty-sixth Annual Convention of the AAEP*. San Antonio, TX, 84–93.

Haussler, K.K. (2016). Joint mobilization and manipulation for the equine athlete. *Vet Clin Equine* 32: 87–101.

Haussler, K.K., Hill, A.E., Puttlitz, C.M., and McIlwraith, C.W. (2007). Effects of vertebral mobilization and manipulation on kinematics of the thoracolumbar region. *Am J Vet Res* 68 (5): 508–516.

Haussler, K.K., Martin, C.E., and Hill, A.E. (2010). Efficacy of spinal manipulation and mobilization on trunk flexibility and stiffness in horses: A randomized clinical trial: Efficacy of spinal manipulation and mobilization. *Eq Vet J* 42: 695–702.

Haussler, K.K., King, M.R., Peck, K., and Adair, H.S. (2021a). The development of safe and effective rehabilitation protocols for horses. *Eq Vet Educ* 33: 143–151.

Haussler, K.K., Wilde, S.R., Davis, M.S. et al. (2021b). Contrast therapy: Tissue heating and cooling properties within the equine distal limb. *Equine Vet J* 53: 149–156.

Heckman, J.D., Ryaby, J.P., McCabe, J. et al. (1994). Acceleration of tibial fracture healing by non-invasive, low intensity pulsed ultrasound. *J Bone Jt Surg* 76-A (1): 26–34.

Hernandez-Bule, M.L., Paino, C.L., Trillo, M.A., and Ubeda, A. (2014). Electric stimulation at 448 kHz promotes proliferation of human mesenchymal stem cells. *Cell Physiol Biochem* 34: 1741–1755.

Hill, C. and Crook, T. (2010). The relationship between massage to the equine caudal hindlimb muscles and hindlimb protraction. *Eq Vet J* 42: 683–687.

Hobo, S., Yoshida, K., and Yoshihara, T. (1998). Characteristics of respiratory function during swimming exercise in Thoroughbreds. *J Vet Med Sci* 60 (6): 687–689.

Holder, T.E.C., Schumacher, J., Donnell, R.L. et al. (2008). Effects of hyperbaric oxygen on full-thickness meshed sheet skin grafts applied to fresh and granulating wounds in horses. *Am J Vet Res* 69: 144–147.

Hulak, E.S., Spooner, H.S., and Haffner, J.C. (2015). Influence of whole-body vibration on bone density in the stalled horse. *J Equine Vet* 35: 393.

Hunt, E.R. (2001). Response of twenty-seven horses with lower leg injuries to cold spa bath hydrotherapy. *J Eq Vet Sci* 21 (4): 188–193.

Huseman, C.J., Welsh, T.H., Suva, L.J. et al. (2019). Skeletal response to whole-body vibration in stalled, yearling horses. *J Equine Vet* 76: 46–47.

Hyatt CS (2017) Effects of Vertical Whole-Body Vibration on Select Biochemical Markers of Muscle Turnover in Yearling Horses. https://oaktrust.library.tamu.edu/handle/1969.1/165691. (Doctorial Dissertation).

Hyytiäinen, H.K., Boström, A., Asplund, K., and Bergh, A. (2022). A systematic review of complementary and alternative veterinary medicine in sport and companion animals: Electrotherapy. *Animals* 13: 64.

Inoue, N., Ohnishi, I., Chen, D. et al. (2002). Effect of pulsed electromagnetic fields (PEMF) on late-phase osteotomy gap healing in a canine tibial model. *J Orthop Res* 20 (5): 1106–1114.

Jacobs, C.C., O'Neil, E., and Prange, T. (2022). Efficacy of a commercial dry sleeve cryotherapy system for cooling the equine metacarpus. *Vet Surg* 51: 1070–1077.

Jallaq, K., Williams, T., Ware, C., and Chubb, C. (2019). Full-body vibration effects on thermography in horses. *J Equine Vet* 76: 126.

Kaneps AJ (2000) Tissue temperature response to hot and cold therapy in the metacarpal region of a horse. In *Proc of the Annual Convention of the American Association of Equine Practitioners. 46th AAEP Annual Convention*, San Antonio, TX, pp. 208–213.

Kazem Shakouri, S., Soleimanpour, J., Salekzamani, Y., and Oskuie, M.R. (2009). Effect of low-level laser therapy on the fracture healing process. *Lasers Med Sci* 25: 73–77.

Khairoun, A., Hawkins, J.F., Moore, G.E. et al. (2023). Electrohydraulic shockwave for treatment of forelimb superficial digital flexor tendinitis and proximal suspensory desmitis in horses. *J Equine Vet* 127: 104504.

King, M.R. (2016). Principles and application of hydrotherapy for equine athletes. *Vet Clin Equine* 32: 115–126.

King, M.R., Haussler, K.K., Kawcak, C.E. et al. (2013). Effect of underwater treadmill exercise on postural sway in horses with experimentally induced carpal joint osteoarthritis. *Am J Vet Res* 74 (7): 971–982.

King, M.R., Seabaugh, K.A., and Frisbie, D.D. (2022). Effects of a bio-electromagnetic energy regulation blanket on thoracolumbar epaxial muscle pain in horses. *J Equine Vet* 111: 103867.

Leach, R.A. (1994). *The Chiropractic Theories: Principles and Clinical Applications*, 3rde. Baltimore, MD: Williams & Wilkins.

Leach, R.M., Rees, P.J., and Wilmshurst, P. (1998). ABC of oxygen – Hyperbaric oxygen therapy. *B Med J* 317 (7166): 1140–1143.

Levine, D., Millis, D.L., and Mynatt, T. (2001). Effects of 3.3-MHz ultrasound on caudal thigh muscle temperature in dogs. *Vet Surg* 30 (2): 170–174.

Lindner, A., Waschle, S., and Sasse, H.H.L. (2003). Effect of exercise on a treadmill submerged in water on biochemical and physiological variables of horses. *Pferdeheilkunde* 26 (6).

Longland, A.C., Barefoot, C., and Harris, P.A. (2011). Effects of soaking on the water-soluble carbohydrate and crude protein content of hay. *Vet Rec* 168 (23): 618.

Lowe, S.J., Burk, S.V., and Birmingham, S.S.W. (2017). The effect of whole-body vibration on equine hoof growth. *J Equine Vet* 52: 41.

Lucas, R.G., Rodríguez-Hurtado, I., Álvarez, C.T., and Ortiz, G. (2022). Effectiveness of neuromuscular electrical stimulation and dynamic mobilization exercises on equine multifidus muscle cross-sectional area ☆. *J Equine Vet* 113: 103934.

Maher, K., Spooner, H., Hoffman, R., and Haffner, J. (2020). The influence of whole-body vibration on heart rate, stride length, and bone mineral content in the mature exercising horse. *Comp Exerc Physiol* 16: 403–408.

Maiti, S.K., Kumar, N., Singh, G.R. et al. (2006). Ultrasound therapy in tendinous injury healing in goats. *J Vet Med Series A* 53 (5): 249–258.

Marlin, D.J. (2019). Evaluation of the cooling efficacy of different equine leg cooling methods. *Comp Exercise Physiol* 15: 113–122.

Marsolais, G.S., McLean, S., Derrick, T., and Conzemius, M.G. (2003). Kinematic analysis of the hind limb during swimming and walking in healthy dogs and dogs with surgically corrected cranial cruciate ligament rupture. *J Am Vet Med Assoc* 222 (6): 739–743.

Matic, M., Lazetic, B., Poljacki, M. et al. (2009). Influence of different types of electromagnetic fields on skin reparatory processes in experimental animals. *Lasers Med Sci* 24 (3): 321–327.

McClintock, S.A., Hutchins, D.R., and Brownlow, M.A. (1986a). Studies on the optimal temperature of flotation tanks in the management of skeletal injuries in the horse. *Eq Vet J* 18 (6): 458–461.

McClintock, S.A., Hutchins, D.R., Laing, E.A., and Brownlow, M.A. (1986b). Pulmonary changes associated with flotation techniques in the treatment of skeletal injuries in the horse. *Eq Vet J* 18 (6): 462–466.

McClintock, S.A., Hutchins, D.R., and Brownlow, M.A. (1987). Determination of weight reduction in horses in flotation tanks. *Eq Vet J* 19 (1): 70–71.

McClure, S. and Weinberger, T. (2003). Extracorporeal shock wave therapy: Clinical applications and regulation. *Clin Tech Eq Pract* 2 (4): 358–367.

McClure S, VanSickle D, and White R (2000) Extracorporeal shock wave therapy: What is it? What does it do to equine bone. In *Proceedings Forty-sixth Annual Convention of the American Association of Equine Practioners*, San Antonio, TX, pp. 197–199.

McClure S, Sonea IM, Yeager M, *et al.* (2003) Safety of shock wave therapy in performance horses. In *Proceedings of the 49th Am Assoc Eq Pract*. New Orleans, LA, pp. 62–65.

Misumi, K., Sakamoto, H., and Shimizu, R. (1994). The validity of swimming training for two-year-old thoroughbreds. *J Vet Med Sci* 56 (2): 217–222.

Misumi, K., Sakamoto, H., and Shimizu, R. (1995). Changes in skeletal muscle composition in response to swimming training for young horses. *J Vet Med Sci* 57 (5): 959–961.

Monk, M. (2007). Principles of hydrotherapy in veterinary physiotherapy. In: *Animal Physiotherapy: Assessment, Treatment and Rehabilitation of Animals*, 187–198. Ames, IA: Blackwell Publishing.

Montalvo, A.M., Le Cara, E., and Myer, G.D. (2014). Effect of kinesiology taping on pain in individuals with musculoskeletal injuries: Systematic review and meta-analysis. *Phys Sportsmed* 42 (2): 48–57.

Montgomery, L., Elliott, S.B., and Adair, H.S. (2013). Muscle and tendon heating rates with therapeutic ultrasound in horses. *Vet Surg* 42 (3): 243–249.

Nankervis, K.J. and Williams, R.J. (2006). Heart rate responses during acclimation of horses to water treadmill exercise. *Eq Vet J* 38 (S36): 110–112.

Nelson, F.R., Zvirbulis, R., and Pilla, A.A. (2013). Non-invasive electromagnetic field therapy produces rapid and substantial pain reduction in early knee osteoarthritis: A randomized double-blind pilot study. *Rheumatol Int* 33 (8): 2169–2173.

Noble, J.G., Lee, V., and Griffith-Noble, F. (2007). Therapeutic ultrasound: The effects upon cutaneous blood flow in humans. *Ultrasound Med Biol* 33 (2): 279–285.

Nordlund, M.M. and Thorstensson, A. (2006). Strength training effects of whole-body vibration. *Scand J Med Sci Sports* 17: 12–17.

Nowlin, C.A., Nielsen, B.D., Mills, J. et al. (2017). Acute and prolonged effects of vibrating platform treatment on horses: A pilot study. *J Equine Vet* 52: 65.

Palmer SE (2002) Treatment of dorsal metacarpal disease in the thoroughbred racehorce with radial extracorporeal shock wave therapy. In *Proceedings Forty-eigth Annual Convention of the American Association of Equine Practioners*. Orlando, FL: pp. 318–321.

Parkinson, S.D., Zanotto, G.M., Maldonado, M.D. et al. (2022). The effect of capacitive-resistive electrical therapy on neck pain and dysfunction in horses. *J Equine Vet* 117: 104091.

Parreira, P., Do, C.S., Costa, L. et al. (2014). Current evidence does not support the use of Kinesio Taping in clinical practice: A systematic review. *J Physiother* 60 (1): 31–39.

Paulekas, R. and Haussler, K.K. (2009). Principles and practice of therapeutic exercise for horses. *J Eq Vet Sci* 29 (12): 870–893.

Petrov, R., MacDonald, M.H., Tesch, A.M., and Hoogmoed, L.M.V. (2003). Influence of topically applied cold treatment on core temperature and cell viability in equine superficial digital flexor tendons. *Am J Vet Res* 64 (7): 835–844.

Pluim, M., Heier, A., Plomp, S., et al. (2022). Histological tissue healing following high-power laser treatment in a model of suspensory ligament branch injury. *Equine Vet J* 54 (6): 1114–1122. https://doi.org/10.1111/evj.13556. Epub 2022 Jan 20. PMID: 35008124.

Porter, M. (2005). Equine rehabilitation therapy for joint disease. *Vet Clin N Am Eq Pract* 21 (3): 599–607.

Pounder, N.M. and Harrison, A.J. (2008). Low intensity pulsed ultrasound for fracture healing: A review of the clinical evidence and the associated biological mechanism of action. *Ultrasonics* 48 (4): 330–338.

Pozo-Cruz, B., Adsuar, J.C., Parraca, J.A. et al. (2012). Using whole-body vibration training in patients affected with common neurological diseases: A systematic literature review. *J Altern Complement Med* 18 (1): 29–41.

Prentice WE (2014) Chapter 10 Tissue Response to Injury. *Principles of Athletic Training: A Competency-Based Approach*, 15/e, McGraw-Hill Education, Columbus, OH, 265–284.

Rauch, F. (2009). Vibration therapy. *Develop Med Child Neurol* 51: 166–168.

Ravara, B., Gobbo, V., Carraro, U. et al. (2015). Functional electrical stimulation as a safe and effective treatment for equine epaxial muscle spasms: Clinical evaluations and histochemical morphometry of mitochondria in muscle biopsies. *Europ J Transl Myology* 25 (2): 109–120.

Rehn, B., Lidström, J., Skoglund, J., and Lindström, B. (2006). Effects on leg muscular performance from whole-body vibration exercise: A systematic review. *Scand J Med Sci Sports* 17: 2–11.

Reis AGMS (2009) Evaluation of therapeutic ultrasound application on equine tendinitis. *Avaliacao da aplicacao do ultrassom terapeutico em tendinites de equinos,* 148 pp.

Revenaugh, M.S. (2005). Extracorporeal shock wave therapy for treatment of osteoarthritis in the horse: Clinical applications. *Vet Clin N Am Eq Pract* 21 (3): 609–625.

Riegel, R.J. (2018). *Laser Therapy in Veterinary Medicine: Photobiomodulation.* Chichester, West Sussex, Hoboken, NJ: John Wiley & Sons Inc.

Rindler, N., Biermann, N.M., Westermann, S., and Buchner, H. (2014). The effect of pulsed electromagnetic field therapy on surface temperature of horses backs. *Wien Tierarztl Monatsschr* 101: 137–141.

Rohde, C., Chiang, A., Adipoju, O. et al. (2010). Effects of pulsed electromagnetic fields on interleukin-1β and postoperative pain: A double-blind, placebo-controlled, pilot study in breast reduction patients. *Plast Reconstr Surg* 125 (6): 1620–1629.

Rose, N.S., Northrop, A.J., Brigden, C.V., and Martin, J.H. (2009). Effects of a stretching regime on stride length and range of motion in equine trot. *Vet J* 181 (1): 53–55.

Rostad, D.R., Adair, H.S., Strickland, L.G. et al. (2023). 37 Short-term effects of a single pulsed electromagnetic field therapy session on lameness, gait quality, and stress in moderately exercising horses. *J Equine Vet* 124: 104339.

Ryan, T. and Smith, R.K.W. (2007). An investigation into the depth of penetration of low level laser therapy through the equine tendon in vivo. *Irish Vet J* 60 (5): 295.

Saini, N.S., Roy, K.S., Bansal, P.S. et al. (2002). A preliminary study on the effect of ultrasound therapy on the healing of surgically severed Achilles tendons in five dogs. *J Vet Med Series A* 49 (6): 321–328.

Sanders-Shamis, M., Bramlage, L.R., Weisbrode, S.E., and Gabel, A.A. (1989). A preliminary investigation of the effect of selected electromagnetic field devices on healing of cannon bone osteotomies in horses. *Eq Vet J* 21 (3): 201–205.

Schills SJ and Turner TA (2010) Review of early mobilization of muscle, tendon, and ligament after injury in equine rehabilitation. In *Proc of the Annual Convention of the American Association of Equine Practitioners. 56th Annual AAEP Convention*, Baltimore, MD, pp. 374–380.

Schils SJ (2009) Review of electrotherapy devices for use in veterinary medicine. In *Proceedings of the 55th Annual Convention of the American Association of Equine Practitioners, Las Vegas, Nevada, USA, 5–9 December 2009.*, pp. 68–73.

Schlachter, C. and Lewis, C. (2016). Electrophysical therapies for the equine Athlete. *Vet Clin Equine* 32: 127–147.

Scott, M. and Swenson, L.A. (2009). Evaluating the benefits of equine massage therapy: A review of the evidence and current practices. *J Eq Vet Sci* 29 (9): 687–697.

Scott, R., Nankervis, K., Stringer, C. et al. (2010). The effect of water height on stride frequency, stride length and heart rate during water treadmill exercise: Stride frequency during water treadmill exercise. *Eq Vet J* 42: 662–664.

Secombe, C.J. and Lester, G.D. (2012). The role of diet in the prevention and management of several equine diseases. *Anim Feed Sci Technol* 173 (1–2): 86–101.

Shaw, K., Ursini, T., Levine, D. et al. (2021). The effect of ground poles and elastic resistance bands on longissimus dorsi and rectus abdominus muscle activity during equine walk and trot. *J Equine Vet* 107: 103772.

Silver RJ (2009) 21st century energy medicine: Low level laser therapy. In *Proceedings N Am Vet Conf*. Orlando, FL, pp. 77–80.

Singh, K.I., Sobti, V.K., and Roy, K.S. (1997). Gross and histomorphological effects of therapeutic ultrasound (1 Watt/CM^2) in experimental acute traumatic arthritis in donkeys. *J Eq Vet Sci* 17 (3): 150–155.

Siska, P., Gruen, G., and Pape, H. (2008). External adjuncts to enhance fracture healing: What is the role of ultrasound? *Injury* 39 (10): 1095–1105.

Slatkovska, L., Alibhai, S.M.H., Beyene, J., and Cheung, A.M. (2010). Effect of whole-body vibration on BMD: A systematic review and meta-analysis. *Osteoporos Int* 21 (12): 1969–1980.

Slatkovska, L., Alibhai, S.M., Beyene, J. et al. (2011). Effect of 12 months of whole-body vibration therapy on bone density and structure in postmenopausal women: A randomized trial. *Ann Intern Med* 155 (10): 668–679.

Slovis, N. (2008). Review of equine hyperbaric medicine. *J Eq Vet Sci* 28 (12): 760–767.

Strauch, B., Herman, C., Dabb, R. et al. (2009). Evidence-based use of pulsed electromagnetic field therapy in clinical plastic surgery. *Aesthetic Surg* 29: 135–143.

Stubbs, N.C., Kaiser, L.J., Hauptman, J., and Clayton, H.M. (2011). Dynamic mobilization exercises increase cross sectional area of musculus multifidus. *Eq Vet J* 43 (5): 522–529.

Sugg SJ (2018) Effects of whole body vibration on lameness, stride length, cortisol, and other parameters in healthy horses. Ph.D. diss., Middle Tennessee State University,

Ter Haar, G. (1999). Therapeutic ultrasound. *Eur J Ultrasound* 9 (1): 3–9.

Thomas, D.P., Fregin, F., Gerber, N.H., and Ailes, N.B. (1980). Cardiorespiratory adjustments to tethered-swimming in the horse. *Pflugers Arch* 385 (1): 65–70.

Tibbles, P.M. and Edelsberg, J.S. (1996). Hyperbaric-oxygen therapy. *New Engl J Med* 334 (25): 1642.

Ursini, T., Shaw, K., Levine, D., et al. (2022). Electromyography of the multifidus muscle in horses trotting during therapeutic exercises. *Front Vet Sci 9*. https://www.frontiersin.org/articles/10.3389/ fvets.2022.844776, https://doi.org/10.3389/fvets.2022.844776.

Verschueren, S.M., Bogaerts, A., Delecluse, C. et al. (2011). The effects of whole-body vibration training and vitamin D supplementation on muscle strength, muscle mass, and bone density in institutionalized elderly women: A 6-month randomized, controlled trial. *J Bone Miner Res* 26 (1): 42–49.

Von Stengel, S., Kemmler, W., Bebenek, M. et al. (2011). Effects of whole-body vibration training on different devices on bone mineral density. *Med Sci Sports Exerc* 43 (6): 1071–1079.

Voss, B., Mohr, E., and Krzywanek, H. (2002). Effects of Aqua-treadmill Exercise on selected blood parameters and on heart-rate variability of horses. *J Vet Med Series A* 49 (3): 137–143.

Waguespack, W., Burba, D.J., Hubert, J.D. et al. (2011). Effects of extracorporeal shock wave therapy on desmitis of the accessory ligament of the deep digital flexor tendon in the horse. *Vet Surg* 40 (4): 450–456.

Walker, V.A., Tranquillle, C.A., MacKechnie-Guire, R. et al. (2022). Effect of ground and raised poles on kinematics of the walk. *J Equine Vet* 115: 104005.

Watkins, J.P., Auer, J.A., Morgan, S.J., and Gay, S. (1985). Healing of surgically created defects in the equine superficial digital flexor tendon: Effects of pulsing electomagnetic field therapy on collagen-type transformation and tissue morphologic reorganization. *Am J Vet Res* 46 (10): 2097–2103.

Williams, S., Whatman, C., Hume, P.A., and Sheerin, K. (2012). Kinesio taping in treatment and prevention of sports injuries: A meta-analysis of the evidence for its effectiveness. *Sports Med* 42 (2): 153 164.

Wysocki, A., Butler, M., Shamliyan, T., and Kane, R.L. (2011). Whole-body vibration therapy for osteoporosis: State of the science. *Ann Intern Med* 155 (10): 680–686.

Yamazaki, F., Endo, Y., Torii, R. et al. (2000). Continuous monitoring of change in hemodilution during water immersion in humans: Effect of water temperature. *Aviat Space Environ Med* 71 (6): 632–639.

Zellner, A., Bockstahler, B., and Peham, C. (2017). The effects of Kinesio Taping on the trajectory of the forelimb and the muscle activity of the Musculus brachiocephalicus and the Musculus extensor carpi radialis in horses. *PloS One* 12: e0186371.

Zielińska, P., Śniegucka, K., and Kiełbowicz, Z. (2023). A case series of 11 horses diagnosed with bone spavin treated with high intensity laser therapy (HILT). *J Equine Vet* 120: 104188.

24

Adjunctive Therapies: Veterinary Chiropractic

Robin Downing[1,2]

[1] *The Downing Center for Animal Pain Management, LLC, Windsor, CO, USA*
[2] *Affiliate Faculty, Colorado State University College of Veterinary Medicine, Fort Collins, CO, USA*

Abbreviations

DC — doctor of chiropractic
VSC — vertebral subluxation complex
SDF — segmental dysfunction
AVCA — American Veterinary Chiropractic Association
IVCA — International Veterinary Chiropractic Association
ROM — range of motion
EBM — evidence-based medicine

Introduction

Lower back pain is the leading cause of disability among American workers (Meeker and Micozzi, 2001). A study published in the British Medical Journal concluded that chiropractic adjustment out-performed hospital outpatient management for lower back pain (Meade *et al.*, 1995). Pain is the leading reason human patients seek care from chiropractic practitioners (Leach, 1994a). Pain and pain relief are central to the discipline of chiropractic (Bove and Swenson, 2001).

It makes sense to consider applying chiropractic techniques for the relief of pain in animals within the context of physical rehabilitation. Chiropractic also aims to restore normal joint range of motion (ROM). Adding incentive to the exploration and application of chiropractic care to animals are the challenges associated with assessing pain in non-verbal species and the limited pharmacologic options available for managing pain.

Physical Rehabilitation for Veterinary Technicians and Nurses, Second Edition.
Edited by Mary Ellen Goldberg and Julia E. Tomlinson.
© 2024 John Wiley & Sons, Inc. Published 2024 by John Wiley & Sons, Inc.
Companion website: www.wiley.com/go/goldberg/physicalrehabilitationvettechsandnurses

In order to better appreciate the role of the veterinary technician in the discipline of veterinary chiropractic care, it is important to have an overview understanding of chiropractic principles and practices. While chiropractic adjustments may only be performed by a veterinarian or a chiropractor trained in animal chiropractic, the veterinary technician plays a critical role in restraint and positioning of the animal patient receiving chiropractic care.

Brief History of Chiropractic Medicine

Chiropractic is a medical discipline based on spinal manipulation. The term chiropractic is derived from "cheir" or "hand" and "praxis" or "practice." Manipulation of the body and its tissues is ancient and universal. The traditional paradigm of chiropractic reflects the following core beliefs:

The body is self-regulating and self-healing

The nervous system is the master system of the body

Alterations in spinal movement adversely affect the nervous system's ability to regulate function

Correcting, managing, or minimizing the vertebral subluxation complex (VSC) via chiropractic adjustment optimizes patient health (Cleveland *et al.*, 2001)

The adaptation of chiropractic techniques for use in veterinary medicine is relatively recent (Pascoe, 2002). The American Veterinary Medical Association (AVMA) has published "Guidelines for Complementary and Alternative Veterinary Medicine" which contains the following terminology/description about chiropractic care:

> ". . .veterinary manual or manipulative therapy (similar to osteopathy, chiropractic, or physical medicine and therapy). . ."

This places chiropractic into the category of complementary care, to be used (literally) to "complement" traditional allopathic veterinary medicine and patient care. Because of its designation as a complementary medical technique, it is best to acquire informed consent from the client before beginning chiropractic treatment of an animal.

The Role of Chiropractic in Physical Rehabilitation

Chiropractic can serve as a valuable "tool in the tool chest" of the rehabilitation therapist working with animal patients. Chiropractic provides a means to maintain spinal mobility, mobility in joints of the extremities, and function in healthy athletic and working animals. In animals experiencing clinical problems like pain and lameness, chiropractic addresses spinal dysfunction, whether that dysfunction is the result of a primary pathology such as intervertebral disk disease (IVDD) or secondary to a lameness that leads to disrupted spinal biomechanics. The positive outcomes of chiropractic adjustment in animals undergoing physical rehabilitation include:

Restoration of proper spinal segmental function

Restoration of proper bony relationships

Resetting neural receptors back to healthy firing frequency

Improving overall mobility

Assisting neurologic healing

Rebalancing proper muscle tone and function

Reducing pain (Jurek, 2013)

The Vertebral Subluxation Complex (VSC)

Pathology of the spine leading to nervous system dysfunction is described as a "VSC." Unlike an orthopedic luxation where bones normally engaged in a structural relationship become disrupted or distracted (e.g., coxofemoral luxation), the VSC is a term that describes a *functional* rather than a *structural* abnormality. The VSC describes a spinal segment that is restricted from moving throughout its normal ROM. The complex describes this loss of movement within the context of one vertebra in relation to neighboring vertebrae. Gatterman specifically defines spinal subluxation as "a motion segment in which alignment, movement integrity, and/or physical function are altered though contact between the joint surfaces remains intact" (Gatterman, 1995). This is a reflection of neuromuscular dysfunction. Vertebrae that do not function properly within the spinal framework generate mechanical stress, thus accelerating the wear and tear on the surrounding spinal muscles, ligaments, discs, joints, and other spinal tissues. If left untreated, pain, inflammation, tenderness to palpation, decreased mobility, and muscle spasm/tension eventually occur. After just two weeks of immobilization in rats, degeneration of facet joint cartilage occurred in the lumbosacral joints (Yoshida, 1989).

Detailed information about chiropractic care can be found in Bergmann and Peterson (2011).

The key to appreciating the concept of the VSC and its relationship to pain is to understand the intimate relationship between structure and function. Various models of the VSC have been developed in human patients. Biped spinal biomechanics are quite different from those of quadrupeds; however, some structural and functional analogies exist between biped and quadruped skeletons, allowing for the application of chiropractic principles to four-legged patients once anatomical and motion differences are accounted for.

In order to know what to treat, the practitioner must determine which spinal segment(s) are dysfunctional and in which direction(s) motion is restricted. The chiropractic examination will always include motion palpation as a critical component in order to evaluate the relationships among spinal segments (or limb joints) as well as to identify those segments between which motion is compromised. The description of the VSC and its treatment is referred to as a "listing." The listing vernacular provides information about the place on the animal's body that will be contacted by the practitioner, the direction of reduced motion, as well as the direction in which the VSC will be adjusted or corrected. The listing vocabulary is taken from human chiropractic, specifically the Palmer-Gonstead system (Scaringe and Cooperstein, 2001), and, in acknowledgment of its origin, maintains the use of human chiropractic terminology in spite of the differences in describing analogous locations on an animal's body. One example is the use of "anterior" for "ventral" and "posterior" for "dorsal." A complete explanation of the VSC listing nomenclature is beyond the scope of this chapter.

The Chiropractic Adjustment

The fundamental chiropractic interaction between the practitioner and the patient is the adjustment. The chiropractic adjustment involves a specific, small-amplitude, high-velocity, controlled thrust to restore motion through a specific vector by moving the joint surfaces to the anatomical limit of joint play (Leach, 1994b). It is the specificity of the adjustment, in both location and direction, which differentiates the chiropractic adjustment from other less specific tissue manipulations. Sometimes during an adjustment, there will be a sound, called an "audible," caused by pressure changes in the joint (Leach, 1994b).

The chiropractic adjustment is focused on the functional spinal unit, which comprised of two adjacent vertebrae, the joints that link them, the skeletal muscles that move the joints, and the supportive structures that span the distance between them. Between the elastic barrier and the anatomical barrier is a virtual/theoretical space referred to as the "physiological space," and it is within this space that the chiropractic adjustment occurs. This is an extremely small space, which means the adjusting thrust is a very low-amplitude movement (Scaringe and Cooperstein, 2001).

The adjustment thrust is a fast, specific, and small movement applied to the affected spinal segment in the direction required to overcome the restricted motion, as diagnosed, and restore normal motion to the segment. The thrust motion stimulates mechanoreceptors and acts on the small muscles of the spinal segment (rotatory muscles), causing them to relax or reduce spasms (Sung *et al.*, 2005). Predicting or feeling for the moment of greatest relaxation takes practice and involves palpating many, many patients to train the practitioner to most effectively diagnose and adjust VSCs (Options, 2008).

Evaluation of the Animal Chiropractic Patient

The chiropractic examination should occur prior to any adjustments. An evaluation of posture and gait, vertebral and extremity palpation, motion palpation, as well as an orthopedic and neurological evaluation are part of the examination. No matter the size of the animal chiropractic patient, the principles of evaluation, diagnosis, and adjustment are the same. The cornerstone of the chiropractic examination is motion palpation. A systematic approach to palpation will reveal areas of discomfort or altered sensation along the spine and over the pelvis. A detailed description of pain

palpation in a dog is published elsewhere (Downing, 2011), but the key component for any species includes a systematic approach using pressure applied with the fleshy tissue over P3 of the first and second fingers of the palpator. If back pain is identified or if areas along the back feel tense (or less pliant) than surrounding areas, the patient may be a good candidate for chiropractic evaluation and adjustment.

As the veterinarian locates the segments that need adjustment, the animal may move away from being palpated or react negatively in some way. The soft tissues in the surrounding area may spasm under the veterinarian's fingers. The veterinarian needs to begin with light pressure and slowly increase the motion palpation as needed. The veterinary technician needs to anticipate potential discomfort while restraining the patient appropriately.

The chiropractic examination should be systematic and consistent. A habitually systematic evaluation also reduces inter-patient variability for the practitioner, as there is subjectivity involved in any physical medicine technique. Evaluation and adjustments should take place in an area large enough to accommodate the patient. A nonskid surface is necessary in order for the patient to be comfortable standing. It is also important to evaluate and adjust the patient in an area free of noise or distractions. Be aware of behavioral cues that can be interpreted by the animal as signals of aggression. In keeping with the AVMA's current recommendations, clients should not restrain their animals from the chiropractic practitioner. It is the practitioner's responsibility to keep the client safe during the chiropractic diagnosis and treatment. The animal should be monitored carefully for signs of anxiety, agitation, or aggression. It will primarily be the technician's job to keep the practitioner and client safe. If the animal cannot be reassured, the chiropractic session should be stopped until it can be resumed safely and comfortably for all.

A painful dog or cat should only be adjusted after breaking the pain cycle pharmacologically. If the patient is painful, the motion palpation prior to the adjustment will be uncomfortable for the patient, and it may be challenging to determine specifically the location and nature of the VSC, and any adjustment risks exacerbating the patient's pain. In equine patients, there are fewer pain management options, and chiropractic adjustment itself can play an important role in pain relief.

The Chiropractic Adjustment and the Veterinary Technician

Companion animals are adjusted using a one-handed technique, allowing the practitioner to use the opposite hand and arm to help stabilize the patient. Appropriate stabilization allows the practitioner to isolate the affected spinal segment for adjustment as well as to more easily take the segment into tension. In addition, appropriate stabilization of the patient ensures that most of the force of the thrust employed during the adjustment will reach the intended tissues in the VSC (Options, 2008). Appropriate stabilization without excessive restraint seems to reassure the patient, allowing them to relax into the adjustment and making the chiropractic treatment as effective as possible. Limb adjustments are accomplished by stabilizing the patient on three legs so that the chiropractor can isolate one joint at a time for adjustment. Many animal chiropractic providers report anecdotally that canine patients who are treated successfully with chiropractic adjustment appear to "enjoy" their subsequent experiences. It is a common occurrence to witness dogs

straining at the leash in order to enter the facility for their chiropractic care.

Equine chiropractic adjustment technique varies depending upon the location of the adjustment. The cervical spinal segments are adjusted using a technique in which the horse's head is positioned with one hand and the adjustment is performed with the other hand.

The thoracic and lumbar spinal segments and the pelvis are adjusted using a two handed technique, and depending upon the location and direction of the adjustment, the technician may be asked to provide stabilization on the opposite side of the horse from the practitioner.

Horse limb adjustments are performed by lifting the leg and isolating and adjusting one joint at a time.

Common sense will dictate which patients or locations on the body should not be treated with chiropractic adjustment. Examples of conditions that should NOT be treated with chiropractic include (but are not limited to):

Areas with active infection
Fractures
Acute prolapsed or ruptured intervertebral disc
Significant pain
Joint luxation (e.g., traumatic coxofemoral luxation)
Acute painful joint sprain or strain
Meningitis/encephalitis

The veterinary technician's involvement with animal chiropractic cases will depend upon the practice, the practitioner's preferences, and the specific case. In those practices where the technician has first contact with the client and patient, it will be the technician who takes the preliminary history and conducts the initial pain assessment, reporting the findings to the chiropractor before the adjustment begins. During the adjustment, the technician

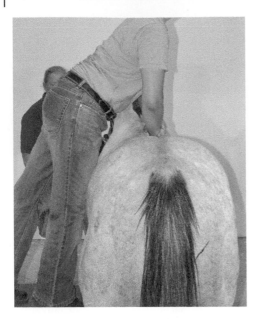

Figure 24.1 Dr. Downing adjusting an equine pelvis.

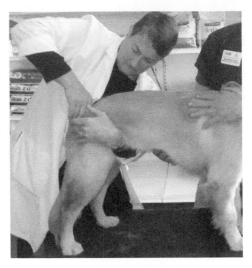

Figure 24.2 Dr. Downing performing adjustment with minimal restraint.

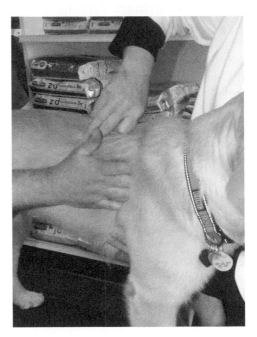

Figure 24.3 Hand position for stabilizing the thoracics during an adjustment.

provides restraint to the chiropractic patient as needed, as well as stabilization for specific adjustments.

For equine chiropractic patients, the technician will typically be positioned at the head on the same side of the horse as the chiropractor when the adjustment is along the spine or over the pelvis (see Figure 24.1).

For adjustments in the thoracic spine of the horse, the technician will provide stabilization against the dorsal spinous processes on the side opposite to the chiropractor. The precise positioning of the technician's hands, posture, and body will vary by practitioner. It is always appropriate to ask for guidance about body position when assisting with an equine chiropractic adjustment.

For canine chiropractic patients, the veterinary technician's role will vary depending on the size of the patient (see Figure 24.2).

For larger dogs, the technician will provide appropriate restraint to allow the chiropractor to isolate the segment being adjusted. During thoracic adjustments, in addition to restraining the patient, the technician will stabilize the appropriate ribs by placing the flat of the hand on the side of the ribcage opposite to the adjustment (see Figure 24.3).

For limb adjustments, the technician will help to balance the dog while chiropractor isolates and adjusts each joint. Finally, the technician will typically stabilize C1 during an occiput-C1 adjustment.

Because each practitioner has his or her own subtle variations of hand, body, and patient position during chiropractic adjustment, it is always best to seek direction in order to provide optimal assistance.

Chiropractic and Cats

While current training of veterinarians and chiropractors in animal chiropractic principles and techniques focuses on horses and dogs, all quadrupeds share many structural, functional, and biomechanical commonalities. Cats should, therefore, benefit from the application of chiropractic adjustments within the context of physical rehabilitation when they experience VSCs. Feline patients are notorious for "masking" painful conditions, making pain recognition and subsequent treatment quite challenging.

The same principles apply to diagnosing and adjusting cats using chiropractic as applied to dogs, including decreasing significant pain before adjusting in order to provide the best outcome and experience for the patient. It also means appropriate gentle handling and minimal restraint to keep the patient, assistants, and the practitioner safe. Cats may object more vigorously to restraint than the typical dog. Likewise, cats tend not to stand still for their assessments and adjustments. Cats generally require flexibility on the part of the practitioner in order to accomplish appropriate chiropractic diagnosis and treatment (see Figure 24.4).

Because of their small size, the veterinary technician's role during feline chiropractic adjustment may consist primarily of distracting the patient to minimize any objections it may have to being handled and manipulated.

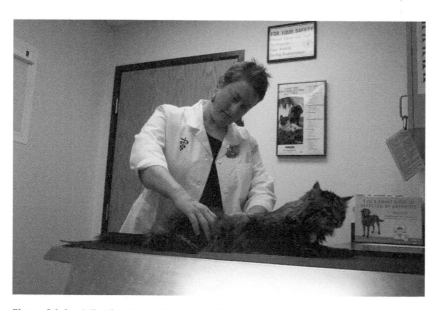

Figure 24.4 Adjusting the patient when the table can be used to stabilize the patient.

Conclusion

The need for animal–patient chiropractic studies is clear. Chiropractic care provides a reasonable strategy for complementing and enhancing the effects of pharmacological (and other) pain management strategies and restoring biomechanically sound movement and function. Physical rehabilitation is all about restoring movement, function, strength, and ability. The future position of chiropractic among accepted treatment modalities for animals undergoing physical rehabilitation will depend upon the results of rigorous clinical studies. Attention must be paid to the neurologic implications of chiropractic adjustment as well as sustaining the effects of adjustment.

While it is important for veterinary technicians to understand the principles and practices of veterinary chiropractic as they can be applied to physical rehabilitation, it is not appropriate for technicians to perform animal chiropractic adjustments. The veterinary technician is positioned to play a vital role in providing chiropractic care to companion animals, both large and small, by working hand-in-hand with those practitioners who bring the benefits of chiropractic adjustment to their patients.

References

Bergmann, T.F. and Peterson, D.H. (2011). *Chiropractic Technique: Principles and Procedures*, 3rde. St. Louis, MO: Mosby.

Bove, G. and Swenson, R. (2001). Nociceptors, pain, and chiropractic. In: *Fundamentals of Chiropractic* (ed. D. Redwood and C.S. Cleveland), 187. St. Louis: Mosby.

Cleveland, A., Phillips, R., and Clum, G. (2001). The chiropractic paradigm. In: *Fundamentals of Chiropractic* (ed. D. Redwood and C.S. Cleveland), 15–27. St. Louis: Mosby.

Downing, R. (2011). *Managing Chronic Maladaptive Pain*, 15–19. NAVC Clinician's Brief.

Gatterman, M.I. (1995). *Foundations of Chiropractic: Subluxation*, 6. St. Louis: Mosby.

Jurek, C. (2013). The role of physical manipulation (chiropractic) in canine rehabilitation. In: *Canine Sports Medicine and Rehabilitation*, 1ste, 427–446. Hoboken, NJ: John Wiley & Sons, Inc.

Leach, R.A. (1994a). Appendix B: Integrated physiological model for VSC. In: *The Chiropractic Theories: Principles and Clinical Applications*, 3rde, 373. Baltimore, 394: Williams & Wilkins.

Leach, R.A. (1994b). Manipulation terminology. In: *The Chiropractic Theories: Principles and Clinical Applications*, 3rde, 16–22. Baltimore: Williams & Wilkins.

Meade, T.W., Dyer, S., Browne, W. et al. (1995). Randomised comparison of chiropractic and hospital outpatient management for low back pain: Results from extended follow-up. *Br Med J* 311: 349–351.

Meeker, W. and Micozzi, M. (2001). Forward. In: *Fundamentals of Chiropractic* (ed. D. Redwood and C.S. Cleveland), ix–xi. St. Louis: Mosby.

Options for Animals College of Animal Chiropractic (2008) Basic animal chiropractic course notes.

Pascoe, P. (2002). Alternative methods for the control of pain. *J Am Vet Med Assoc* 221 (2): 222–229.

Scaringe, J.G. and Cooperstein, R. (2001). Chiropractic manual procedures. In:

Fundamentals of Chiropractic (ed.
D. Redwood and C.S. Cleveland), 257–291.
St. Louis: Mosby.

Sung, P.S., Kang, Y.M., and Pickar,
J.G. (2005). Effect of spinal manipulation
duration on low threshold
mechanoreceptors in lumbar paraspinal
muscles: A preliminary report. *Spine* 30
(1): 115–122.

Yoshida, M. (1989). The effect of spinal
distraction and immobilization on the facet
joint cartilage – Experimental and clinical
studies. *Nihon Seikeigeka Gakkai Zasshi*
63 (8): 789–799.

25

Acupuncture and Traditional Chinese Veterinary Medicine

Carolina Medina[1] and Mary Ellen Goldberg[2]

[1]*Elanco Animal Health Fort Lauderdale, FL, USA*

[2]*Veterinary Technician Specialist- lab animal medicine (Research anesthesia-retired), Veterinary Technician Specialist- (physical rehabilitation-retired), Veterinary Technician Specialist- (anesthesia & analgesia) – H, Veterinary Medical Technologist, Surgical Research Anesthetist-retired, Certified Canine Rehabilitation Veterinary Nurse, Certified Veterinary Pain Practitioner*

CHAPTER MENU

Traditional Chinese Veterinary Medicine (TCVM) Basics

Brief History

TCVM is a medical system that has been used in China to treat animals for about 2,000 years. TCVM emerged from its parent system, traditional Chinese medicine (TCM) that is used to treat people. Over the years, TCVM has become widely accepted in the United States and Europe. Many of the original theories are still used today; however, with advances in modern medicine, new treatment techniques have been employed. TCM is categorized into five branches: acupuncture, Chinese herbal medicine, Tui-na massage, food therapy, and Qi-gong. Due to the difference in veterinary patients, the only branch that is vastly different in TCVM is the fifth branch (Qi-gong). This branch has been termed exercise which can be considered physical rehabilitation.

Five Branches of TCVM

Acupuncture

Acupuncture is defined as the stimulation of a specific point (acupuncture point or acupoint) on the body with a specific method, resulting in physiologic effects. These physiologic effects include both systemic and local effects, as acupuncture stimulates both the central and peripheral nervous systems. Some of the systemic effects include release of endogenous substances such as beta-endorphins (Skarda *et al.*, 2002; Wu *et al.*, 1995; Han *et al.*, 1984), dynorphins, enkephalins, serotonin (Scherder and Bouma, 1993; Costa *et al.*, 1982), epinephrine, GABA, cortisol, and various hormones. Acupuncture can also improve blood flow to the pituitary axis and capillary wall enzyme concentration; release somatotropin in chronic pain; induce luteinizing hormone release which triggers ovulation; stimulate prolactin release to promote lactation; stimulate oxytocin release to induce uterine contraction; and modulate thyroid function. The local effects of acupuncture include muscle relaxation and spasm relief; release of Hageman's Factor XII which activates the clotting cascade, complement cascade, plasminogen, and kinins; degranulation of mast cells which releases histamine, heparin, and kinin protease; release of bradykinin which leads to vasodilation; and production of local prostaglandins which leads to smooth muscle relaxation (Smith, 1994; see Figure 25.1).

Chinese Herbal Medicine

Pioneer TCVM practitioners used individual (single) Chinese herbs to treat diseases. Over time, they found that combining several Chinese herbs into a formula was more effective than single herbs alone. A Chinese herbal formula contains different quantities of several herbs. A typical Chinese herbal formula contains anywhere between 4 and 15 herbs,

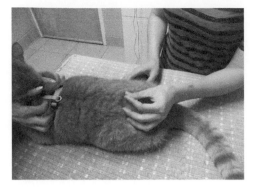

Figure 25.1   Dr. Carolina Medina placed acupuncture needles in the co-author, Mary Ellen Goldberg's cat, JimmyCat. *Source:* Ellen Goldberg (book author).

each of which has an assigned role and mechanism of action within the formula. Formulas consist primarily of plant particles, including bark, stems, roots, flowers, and/or seeds. There are a few formulas that contain minerals and animal-origin products.

Tui-na Massage

Tui-na is a form of Chinese manual therapy used for prevention and treatment of disease. It incorporates massage, acupressure, and physiotherapy techniques. It can be applied directly to acupuncture points, trigger points, and Meridians. In Chinese, Tui-na means "push-pull and lift" which is the basis of most of the techniques. Tui-na can be very useful, as it is practical to apply to most patients. It can be performed by the veterinarian and/or technician, and certain simple techniques can be taught to owners to perform at home. Like massage, Tui-na increases local circulation, which leads to vasodilatation, relaxation of the soft tissues, and pain relief.

Food Therapy

Food therapy is the use of the healing power of food and is often utilized alone or more frequently in conjunction with other TCVM therapies to treat disease. Western medicine has lately begun to understand the effect of food on healing the body, and the interaction between genes and nutrients is termed "Nutrigenomics" (Sales *et al.*, 2014). TCVM food therapy is the art and science of tailoring diet plans to individual patients, and food ingredients are chosen based on TCVM principles. Like other TCVM modalities, the goal of food therapy is to restore and maintain balance in the body. However, given its very nature, the effects of food therapy are slower-acting than modalities like acupuncture and herbal medicine. On the other hand, there are virtually no side effects when food ingredients are chosen correctly, and food therapy is a mode of treatment that can be used safely throughout a patient's lifetime.

Qi Gong

Qi gong is the human practice of aligning the body, breath, and mind for health. It is traditionally viewed as a practice to cultivate and balance Qi ("life energy"). Qi gong typically involves meditation, coordinating slow-flowing movement, deep rhythmic breathing, and a calm meditative state of mind. Since veterinary patients are incapable of practicing Qi gong, exercise in the form of physical rehabilitation is considered a suitable substitute.

Yin Yang Theory

The Yin Yang theory depicts everything as being composed of two opposing yet complementary pairs of opposites. The simplest example is the sun and the moon, in which the sun is considered Yang while the moon is considered Yin. Anything that relates to activity, brightness, or function is considered Yang, while anything that relates to inactivity, darkness, or structure is considered Yin. In regard to medicine, physiological activities belong to Yang, while nutrient substances correspond to Yin.

The Yin Yang theory is incorporated into TCVM to assist in the diagnosis and treatment of disease. Per TCVM, disease does not occur if Yin and Yang are in balance. There are four possible states of imbalance: excess Yin, excess Yang, Yin deficiency, and Yang deficiency. Excess Yin typically has an acute onset of clinical signs with a short course of disease and can present with edema, pain, and/or loose feces. Common signs of Yin deficiency include general weakness, polydipsia, and low-grade fever, and the disease state is generally chronic in nature. Excess Yang also has an acute onset of clinical signs with a short course of disease and presents with a high fever and/or hyperactivity. Yang deficiency is seen in patients with a chronic history of urinary incontinence, low back pain, limb edema, and cold extremities (Xie, 2005).

Five Element Theory

The Five Elements refer to five categories of nature: wood, fire, earth, metal, and water. There is an enhancing, inhibiting, and restraining relationship between them to maintain balance. Like the Yin Yang theory, the Five Element Theory is embodied into TCVM to assist in the diagnosis and treatment of disease. The Five Element Theory is used to describe the nature of the anatomical structures and their relationships with each other, in addition to the relationship between the patient and their environment. The liver, gallbladder, eyes (vision), tendons, ligaments, and nails belong to the Wood Element. Therefore, a patient with a cranial cruciate ligament tear is considered to have a disharmony with the Wood Element. The cardiovascular system, including the heart, pericardium, small intestines, and tongue (voice) corresponds to the Fire Element. A patient with congestive heart failure would have a disharmony with the Fire Element. The spleen, stomach, muscles, and mouth (taste) are related to the Earth Element causing a patient with gastrointestinal disease to suffer from an

Earth Element imbalance. The lungs, large intestines, skin, hair coat, pores, and nose (smell) are associated with the Metal Element. An atopic dermatitis case would be classified as a Metal Element disharmony. The kidneys, bladder, bones, reproductive system, and ears (hearing) belong to the Water Element. A patient with osteoarthritis would be categorized as having Water Element disharmony (Xie, 2005).

Acupuncture Points

Research shows that most acupuncture points are in areas of the skin with decreased electrical resistance or increased electrical conductivity (Urano and Ogasawara, 1978). This can be measured by using a point finder, acupoint detector, or an AC dermometer. In addition, it has been found that acupuncture points are closely associated with free nerve endings, veins, lymphatics, and aggregation of mast cells (Jaggar and Robinson, 2001). There are 173 major acupuncture points in horses and 361 points in people. Acupuncture points correspond to four known neural structures. Type I acupuncture points, which make up 67% of all points, are considered motor points. A motor point is the point in a muscle which, when electrical stimulation is applied, will produce a maximal contraction with minimal intensity of stimulation. Motor points are in areas where nerves enter muscles. For instance, SI-9 is located at the junction of the deltoid muscle and triceps and is supplied by axillary and radial nerves. Type II points are located on the superficial nerves in the sagittal plane of the dorsal and ventral midlines. For instance, *Bai-hui* lies in the depression between the spinous processes of the seventh lumbar and the first sacral vertebrae on dorsal midline and is supplied by the dorsal branch of the last lumbar nerve. Type III points are located at high-density loci of superficial nerves and nerve plexuses. For example, GB-34 is located where the common peroneal nerve divides into the deep and superficial branches cranial and distal to the head of the fibula. Type IV points are located at the muscle-tendon junctions where the Golgi tendon organs are located. For example, BL-57 is located at the junction between the gastrocnemius muscle and the calcanean tendon (Hwang and Egerbacher, 2001; Gunn, 1997).

Meridians

Most commonly, acupuncture points are located on Meridians. Meridians are channels or conduits of energy that connect the acupuncture points throughout the body. There are 14 major Meridians named Lung (LU) Meridian, Large Intestine (LI) Meridian, Stomach (ST) Meridian, Spleen (SP) Meridian, Heart (HT) Meridian, Small Intestine (SI) Meridian, Bladder (BL) Meridian, Kidney (KID) Meridian, Pericardium (PC) Meridian, Triple Heater (TH) Meridian, Gallbladder (GB) Meridian, Liver (LIV) Meridian, Governing Vessel (GV) Meridian, and Conception Vessel (CV) Meridian. A close correlation exists between Meridians and peripheral nerve pathways. Meridians possess bioelectric functions like peripheral nerves, and they follow along peripheral nerves. For example, the Lung Meridian follows musculocutaneous nerve, and the Pericardium Meridian follows the median nerve. A study was done to evaluate the location of Meridians in which researchers injected radioisotopes at one acupuncture point and visualized them gradually accumulating at another acupuncture point on the same Meridian. Radio signals over one acupuncture point can be picked up at another acupuncture point on the same Meridian. Meridians conduct current with flow toward the central nervous system (Smith, 1994).

Methods of Stimulation

Acupuncture can be stimulated by various means, including acupressure, dry needle, electro-acupuncture, aqua-acupuncture, moxibustion, gold implantation, pneumo-acupuncture, hemo-acupuncture, and laser acupuncture (Ferguson, 2007; Altman, 1994). Acupressure is applying firm digital pressure to an acupuncture point for a specific length of time (i.e., five minutes). This is the least invasive type of stimulation. Dry needle is the insertion of a sterile filiform needle into an acupuncture point to elicit a response. These needles are typically left in place for 15–30 minutes. Dry needle is the most commonly used technique in veterinary medicine (see Figure 25.2). Electro-acupuncture is applying electrical current to the dry needles to increase the therapeutic response (see Figure 25.3).

This modality is desirable because you can adjust the frequency and amplitude and induce a stronger stimulation than dry needle alone. Low-frequency (1–40 Hz) electro-acupuncture predominantly stimulates A-delta fibers and releases beta-endorphins and met-enkephalins (see Figure 25.4).

High-frequency (80–120 Hz) electro-acupuncture predominantly stimulates C fibers and releases dynorphins. Very high-frequency (200 Hz) electro-acupuncture

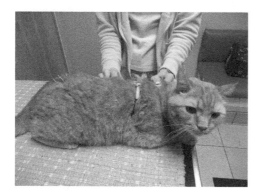

Figure 25.2 Calming point needle was placed on JimmyCat's head. *Source:* Ellen Goldberg (book author).

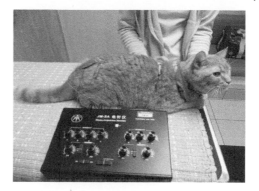

Figure 25.3 JimmyCat models electroacupuncture needles and machine. *Source:* Ellen Goldberg (book author).

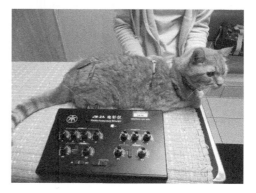

Figure 25.4 JimmyCat shows acupuncture needles attached to the electrostimulator machine. *Source:* Ellen Goldberg (book author).

predominantly stimulates serotonergic fibers and releases serotonin and epinephrine (Smith, 1994). Aqua-acupuncture is the injection of a sterile liquid (i.e., saline, vitamin B12, lidocaine, or similar) into an acupuncture point. This causes constant stimulation of the acupuncture point for an extended period (until the liquid is absorbed), and it has the added benefit of the medicinal properties of the medication used. Moxibustion is the use of a Chinese herb called *Artemesia vulgaris* that is rolled into a cigar shape and burned just above the acupuncture point without touching the skin. This is a warming technique that is therapeutic for older patients with chronic pain. Gold implantation is the injection of sterile pieces of gold, whether in a bead or wire form, into acupuncture points for permanent implantation. Gold implantation provides long-term stimulation for chronic conditions. Pneumo-acupuncture is the injection from air under the skin in the subcutaneous space to produce pressure by the air and stimulate the acupuncture points, nerves, and muscles. Pneumo-acupuncture is used solely for marked muscle atrophy. Hemo-acupuncture is the insertion of a hypodermic needle into an acupuncture point that is located on a blood vessel to draw blood. Hemo-acupuncture releases heat, toxins, and fever and can be applied like leech therapy. Laser acupuncture is the use of laser therapy to emit light to penetrate the tissues and stimulate acupuncture points. Laser acupuncture stimulates ATP production, cellular proliferation, collagen synthesis, and fibroblast activity; decreases pain; and improves circulation and wound healing.

Clinical Applications Associated with Rehabilitation – Dogs and Cats

Pain

Due to its release of endogenous opioids, acupuncture is used extensively for pain management. Acupuncture can be used as a sole agent or is more commonly practiced in conjunction with other modes of pain control as part of multimodal therapy. In rehabilitation cases, acupuncture is commonly used after therapeutic exercises or hydrotherapy. For example, a patient that is undergoing rehabilitation for a femoral head osteotomy might start with massage, laser therapy along the hips and lumbosacral junction, then exercises to encourage weight bearing and improve hip extension, followed by underwater treadmill, and finally acupuncture to alleviate pain. Acupuncture is reportedly effective for the

treatment of various painful conditions, including cervical, thoracolumbar, and lumbosacral hyperpathia, chronic lameness, and degenerative joint disease (Xie and Ortiz-Umpierre (Medina), 2006).

Musculoskeletal Disorders

The most common musculoskeletal disorders treated with acupuncture include osteoarthritis, cranial cruciate ligament rupture, hip and elbow dysplasia, tendinopathies, and fractures. Therapy can be instituted pre- or post-operative and, in many cases, used as part of medical management.

Neurologic Disorders

Acupuncture is frequently used for neurologic conditions, especially electroacupuncture to stimulate nerve function. Common applications include intervertebral disc disease, degenerative myelopathy, fibrocartilagenous embolism, polyneuropathy, cervical spondylomyelopathy, and degenerative lumbosacral stenosis.

Clinical Applications Associated with Rehabilitation – Equine

Pain

In horses, acupuncture is commonly used for painful conditions such as osteoarthritis, laminitis, back pain, tendinopathies, and colic. Performance horses commonly experience soft tissue pain due to exertion and/or overuse which can be successfully treated with 1–2 acupuncture treatments.

Musculoskeletal Disorders

Acupuncture is commonly sought out by performance horse owners and trainers as it provides pain relief without using pharmaceuticals. Musculoskeletal conditions that are effectively treated with acupuncture include osteoarthritis, laminitis, navicular syndrome, tendinopathies, and back pain. A study showed that electro-acupuncture was effective at alleviating chronic thoracolumbar pain in horses (Xie *et al.*, 2005).

Neurologic Disorders

Acupuncture can be used to treat equine neurologic conditions such as cervical spondylomyelopathy, laryngeal hemiplegia, and suprascapular neuropathy.

Safety

While acupuncture is typically considered to be a safe and minimally invasive modality, there are some conditions that warrant caution or contraindication. For example, caution must be used when treating weak, debilitated, or obtunded patients. Generally, fewer needles and less stimulation are used. It is contraindicated to needle directly into skin lesions, ulcers, scar tissue, umbilicus, tumors, or masses. Specific acupuncture points around the abdomen and lumbar area are contraindicated in pregnancy. Length of needles needs to be considered, particularly in very small patients. Electro-acupuncture wire leads should not be connected through or across a known or suspected tumor or mass. Electro-acupuncture wire leads should not be connected around or across the chests of animals with pacemakers. Electro-acupuncture should not be used in patients with a history of seizures (Xie, 2007).

Role of the Veterinary Rehabilitation Technician

See Box 25.1.

> **Box 25.1   Role of the veterinary rehabilitation technician**
>
> A) Client education
> B) Tui-na massage
> C) Acupuncture
>   1) Patient prep
>   2) Needle prep
>   3) Needle insertion – DVM only
>   4) Needle manipulation/electro-acupuncture
>   5) Withdrawal of needles

Research

The earliest scientific studies done on acupuncture focused on its analgesic effects. In the late 1970s, researchers discovered that acupuncture stimulation leads to an increased concentration of endogenous opioids in the serum and cerebral spinal fluid (Pan *et al.*, 1984; He, 1987). Other studies showed that naloxone, an opioid antagonist, blocked the effects of acupuncture and decreased the pain threshold in acupuncture subjects (Mayer *et al.*, 1977). These were the first studies showing that endogenous opioids play a role in the mechanism of action of acupuncture analgesia.

Groppetti *et al.* studied the efficacy of electro-acupuncture compared with butorphanol for post-operative pain management in dogs undergoing elective ovariohysterectomy. Twelve dogs were randomly allocated into two groups. Dogs received either electro-acupuncture (16 and 43 Hz) at BL-23, BL-25, ST-36, GB-34, LI-4, LU-9, and GV-20; or butorphanol. Intra-operative cardiovascular and respiratory parameters were recorded for both groups. Plasma β-endorphin concentrations were evaluated before surgery (baseline) and up to 24 hours later. For each dog, pain was measured using a subjective pain scoring system. Plasma β-endorphin levels in dogs receiving electro-acupuncture increased significantly against baseline values one and three hours after surgery. Moreover, the end-tidal isoflurane concentration needed for the second ovary traction was significantly lower in electro-acupuncture dogs than in control dogs. The dogs in the electro-acupuncture group experienced prolonged analgesia, over 24 hours at least, while 4 out of 6 dogs treated with butorphanol needed post-surgical ketorolac and tramadol supplementation for pain management (rescue analgesia). Their results showed supportive evidence for electro-acupuncture as a pain management technique to provide post-operative analgesia in dogs (Groppetti *et al.*, 2011).

La *et al.* investigated the effects of electro-acupuncture on nerve regeneration. The sciatic nerves (specifically at a location 5 mm above the stifle joint) of 15 rabbits were crushed by a Halsted straight mosquito hemostat with 8–11 Newton force for 60 seconds, and then the rabbits were equally divided into 3 groups. Group 1 was treated with electro-acupuncture at GB-30 and BL-40 for 25 minutes daily for 7 days. Group 2 was treated with intramuscular administration of Diclofenac 15 mg daily for 7 days. Group 3 was the control group and therefore was not treated. After treatment, the distal parts of crushed nerve were examined under light microscopy. The densities of normal myelinated fibers in $0.126 \, mm^2$ were counted, and the diameters of 20 normal myelinated fibers were measured for each rabbit. The results showed that the mean densities were 176.2 ± 5.953 in the electro-acupuncture group, 118.2 ± 10.878 in the Diclofenac group, and 101.4 ± 8.548 in the control group. The mean values were significantly different between the electro-acupuncture and Diclofenac group; highly significant difference between the electro-acupuncture and control groups; and there was no significant difference between the Diclofenac and control groups. There were more small, myelinated fibers (0–9 μm) in the electro-acupuncture group than in the Diclofenac and control groups. These results confirmed that electro-acupuncture promotes nerve regeneration (La *et al.*, 2005).

Dr. Lane and Dr. Hill performed a repeated measures therapeutic trial with 47 client-owned dogs with naturally occurring lameness that were assessed for clinical response to treatment. Treatment for musculoskeletal pain consisted of acupuncture and manual therapy. Owners were blinded to the treatment schedule and completed questionnaires to assess their dogs' comfort and mobility. Comparison between pre- and post-treatment results demonstrated that combined acupuncture and manual therapy provides immediate short-term improvement in comfort and mobility, as demonstrated by owner-observed changes in play behavior ($P = 0.015$), walking ($P < 0.001$), trotting ($P = 0.002$), jumping ($P < 0.001$), descending stairs ($P = 0.003$), rising from a lying position ($P < 0.001$), and reduced stiffness after rest ($P < 0.001$) or following exercise ($P < 0.001$). Mood and attitude also improved but did not attain statistical significance (Lane and Hill, 2016).

Silva *et al.* conducted a prospective study investigating the effects of acupuncture alone or combined with analgesics in chronic pain and quality of life assessed by owners for up to 24 weeks in 181 dogs with neurological and musculoskeletal diseases. The success rates for Helsinki chronic pain index (HCPI), quality of life assessment, and visual analog scales (VAS) for pain and locomotion were 79%, 84%, 78%, and 78% of the dogs, respectively, when both diseases and groups of treatments were combined. Dogs with musculoskeletal disorders had greater improvement in HCPI ($P = 0.003$) and VAS locomotion ($P = 0.045$) than those with neurological disorders. Use of acupuncture alone or in combination with analgesics reduced pain and improved quality of life in dogs with neurological and musculoskeletal diseases (Silva *et al.*, 2017) (see Boxes 25.2 and 25.3 for Case Studies representing the use of Acupuncture Therapy in Physical Rehabilitation).

Box 25.2 Canine case study

Jake, a 14-year-old neutered male mixed breed dog (see Figure 25.5).

History – Jake was diagnosed with hip dysplasia and osteoarthritis at 6 years of age. At that time, he was started on Rimadyl® and Cosequin®. A year later, he started rehabilitation therapy and acupuncture. He also started Adequan® injections and Duralactin® 4 years ago, as well as Amantadine and Chinese herbs 1 year ago.

Physical examination – On presentation, Jake was bright, alert, and responsive. He was lame on the right pelvic limb and had decreased range of motion of both hips and pain (4/10) on extension of both hips.

Treatment plan – Recommendations consisted of acupuncture, laser therapy, manual therapy, exercises, and hydrotherapy. Initially, therapy was performed twice a week, and currently, his maintenance schedule is once a week.

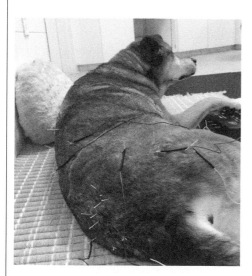

Figure 25.5 Jake from Canine Case Study undergoes acupuncture and electro-acupuncture treatment. *Source:* Deana Cappucci Lorentz.

Treatment

- Acupuncture (points varied at each visit but commonly used points are listed below)

  Dry needle – Bai hui, Shen peng, Shen jiao, ST36, GB34, LIV3, LI10, GB29, and BL40

  Electro-acupuncture – BL11, BL18, BL23, GB21, Shen shu, Jian jiao + GB30, BL54 + KID1, @ 20 Hz × 20 minutes

- Laser therapy
  - 292 Hz, 4 J/cm^2, continuous wave, 7:12 minutes, 229.624 total Joules
  - Back, hips, stifles, shoulders and carpi
- Manual therapy
  - Passive range of motion, full body massage, circles to hips, joint compressions to joints of pelvic limbs, standing compression of pelvic limb joints, and scapular glides
- Exercises
  - Rhythmic stabilization, cookie stretches, three leg standing, sit-to-stands, backward walking, and side-stepping
- Hydrotherapy
  - Underwater treadmill at 0.8–1 mph in 18 inches of water (level with the distal aspect of the greater trochanter) for 10–15 minutes or to tolerance

Outcome – Jake has been receiving multimodal therapy for his osteoarthritis for the past few years. This therapy has allowed him to have his pain level well-controlled and enjoy a good quality of life despite his debilitating osteoarthritis.

Box 25.3 Feline case study

Cricket, 13-year-old spayed female domestic shorthair (see Figures 25.6–25.8)

History – Cricket has been overweight most of her life and has been eating Hills W/D for the past 10 years. Over the past 6 months, she has had decreased mobility and has been unwilling to get on furniture, play with other cats, and go upstairs. Also, she growls at her owners when they try petting her back and hips. She had been taking Cosequin for the past 3 months.

Physical examination – On presentation Cricket was bright, alert, and responsive. She had a body condition score of 9/9 and weighed 22 pounds. She exhibited pain (5/10) in range of motion of her elbows,

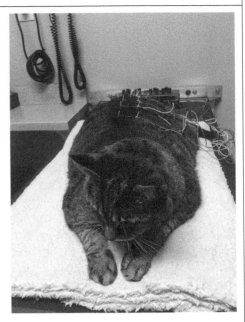

Figure 25.8 Cricket resting and dozing during acupuncture treatment. *Source:* Mary Beth Kassner.

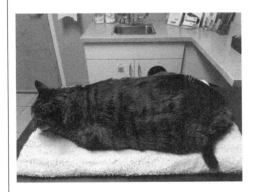

Figure 25.6 Cricket from Feline Case Study receives acupuncture treatment for obesity and pain from osteoarthritis. *Source:* Mary Beth Kassner.

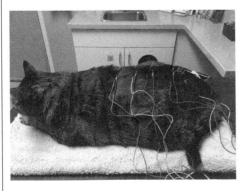

Figure 25.7 Cricket receives electro-acupuncture treatment. *Source:* Mary Beth Kassner.

hips, thoracolumbar spine, and lumbosacral junction.

Treatment plan – Recommendations consisted of continuing Cosequin, starting Gabapentin at 10 mg/kg orally every 8 hours, weekly acupuncture for 4 weeks, and switching to Hills Metabolic to promote a 10-pound weight loss.

Initial acupuncture treatment:

Dry needle – Bai hui

Electro-acupuncture – BL18, BL20, BL23, Shen jiao, BL54+Jian jiao @ 20 Hz × 20 minutes

Follow-up acupuncture treatment – (one week after initial presentation)

Dry needle – Bai hui, Shen shu, Shen peng, Shen jiao

Electro-acupuncture – BL54 + GB30, BL18, BL20, BL23, BL25 @ 20 Hz × 20 minutes

Update – Cricket is allowing her owners to pet her and jumped on their bed a few times in the past week. She is also engaging more and playing with toys.

Follow-up acupuncture treatment – (two weeks after initial presentation)

Dry needle: Bai hui

Electro-acupuncture – BL18, BL20, BL21, BL23,BL25,Shen shu @ 20 Hz × 20 minutes

Update – Cricket is engaging more with the other cats and is also jumping up on the furniture more than the previous week.

Follow-up acupuncture treatment – (three weeks after initial presentation)

Dry needle – Bai hui, Shen shu

Electro-acupuncture – Jian jiao, Shen peng, Shen jiao, BL18, BL20, BL23, BL24 @ 20 Hz × 20 minutes

Update – Cricket is much more active than in the past three weeks and is comfortable on palpation.

Outcome – Cricket has returned to doing the activities she used to enjoy doing and allows her owners to pet her without showing signs of pain. Her owners are continuing to work on weight loss and take her for acupuncture on an as-needed basis.

References

Altman, S. (1994). Techniques and instrumentation. In: *Veterinary Acupuncture: Ancient Art to Modern Medicine*, 1ste (ed. A.M. Schoen), 75–99. St. Louis, MO: Mosby, Inc.

Costa, C., Ceccherelli, F., Ambrosio, F. et al. (1982). The influence of acupuncture on blood serum levels of tryptophan in healthy volunteers subjected to ketamine anesthesia. *Acupunct Electrotherap Res* 7: 123–132.

Ferguson, B. (2007). Techniques of veterinary acupuncture and moxibustion. In: *Xie's Veterinary Acupuncture* (ed. H. Xie), 333–335. Ames, IA: Blackwell Publishing.

Groppetti, D., Pecile, A.M., Sacerdote, P. et al. (2011). Effectiveness of electroacupuncture analgesia compared with opioid administration in a dog model: A pilot study. *Br J Anaesth* 107 (4): 612–618.

Gunn, C.C. (1997). Type IV acupuncture points. *Am J Acupuncture* 5: 51–52.

Han, J.S., Xie, G.H., Zhou, Z.F. et al. (1984). Acupuncture mechanisms in rabbits studied with microinjection of antibodies against β-endorphin, enkephalin and substance P. *Neuropharmacology* 23 (1): 1–5.

He, L.F. (1987). Review article: Involvement of endogenous opioid peptides in acupuncture analgesia. *Pain* 31 (1): 99–121.

Hwang, Y.C. and Egerbacher, M. (2001). Anatomy and classification of acupoints. In: *Veterinary Acupuncture: Ancient Art to Modern Medicine*, 2nde (ed. A.M. Schoen), 19–21. St. Louis, MO: Mosby, Inc.

Jaggar, D.H. and Robinson, N.G. (2001). History of veterinary acupuncture. In: *Veterinary Acupuncture: Ancient Art to Modern Medicine*, 2nde (ed. A.M. Schoen), 4–11. St. Louis, MO: Mosby, Inc.

La, J.L., Jalai, S., and Shami, S.A. (2005). Morphological studies on crushed sciatic nerve of rabbits with electro-acupuncture or diclofenac sodium treatment. *Am J Chin Med* 33 (4): 663–669.

Lane, D. and Hill, S. (2016). Effectiveness of combined acupuncture and manual therapy relative to no treatment for canine musculoskeletal pain. *Can Vet J* 57: 407–414.

Mayer, D.J., Price, D.D., and Rafii, A. (1977). Antagonism of acupuncture analgesia in man by the narcotic antagonist naloxone. *Brain Res* 121: 368–372.

Pan, X.P. et al. (1984). Electroacupuncture analgesia and analgesic action of NAGA. *J Trad Chi Med* 4 (4): 273–278.

Sales, N.M., Pelegrini, P.B., and Goersch, M.C. (2014). Nutrigenomics: Definitions and advances of this new science. *J Nutr Metab* 2014: 202759.

Scherder, E.J.A. and Bouma, A. (1993). Possible role of the nucleus raphe dorsalis in analgesia by peripheral stimulation: Theoretical considerations. *Acupunct Electrotherap Res* 18: 195–205.

Silva, N., Luna, S., Joaquim, J. et al. (2017). Effect of acupuncture on pain and quality of life in canine neurological and musculoskeletal diseases. *Can Vet J* 58: 941–951.

Skarda, R.T., Tejwani, G.A., and Muir, W.W. (2002). Cutaneous analgesia, hemodynamic and respiratory effects, and beta-endorphin concentration in spinal fluid and plasma of horses after acupuncture and electroacupuncture. *Am J Vet Res* 63 (10): 1435–1442.

Smith, F.W.K. (1994). The neurophysiologic basis of acupuncture. In: *Veterinary Acupuncture: Ancient Art to Modern Medicine*, 1ste (ed. A.M. Schoen). Louis, MO: Mosby, Inc 35–45 4850.

Urano, K. and Ogasawara, S. (1978). A fundamental study on acupuncture point phenomena of the dog body. *Kitasato Arch Exp Med* 51: 95–109.

Wu, G.C., Zhu, J.M., and Cao, X.D. (1995). Involvement of opioid peptides of the preoptic area during electro-acupuncture analgesia. *Acupunct Electrotherap Res* 20: 1–6.

Xie, H. (2005). Traditional chinese veterinary medicine. In: *Fundamental Principles, vol. I*, 1–16, 27–28. Reddick, FL: Jing Tang.

Xie, H. (2007). *Xie's Veterinary Acupuncture*, 245–327. Ames, IA: Blackwell Publishing.

Xie, H. and Ortiz-Umpierre (Medina), C. (2006). What acupuncture can and cannot treat. *JAAHA* 42 (4): 244–248.

Xie, H., Colahan, P., and Ott, E. (2005). Evaluation of electro-acupuncture treatment of horses with signs of chronic thoracolumbar pain. *JAVMA* 227 (2): 281–286.

26

Adjunctive Therapies: Myofascial Trigger Point Therapy

Angela Stramel and Douglas Stramel

Advanced Care Veterinary Services, Carrollton, TX, USA

Introduction

Myofascial pain syndrome (MPS), described in humans as a chronic painful condition of muscle, has started to become acknowledged in the field of veterinary medicine. Muscle is the largest organ in a mammal's body (ranging from 40% in a human to 57% in a greyhound) and can be thought of as the "orphan organ" as no traditional medical specialty is designated to treat it. Until recently, it was rated to provide veterinary education on muscle dysfunction, concentrating more on muscle tears and on the bones, joints, and ligaments of the musculoskeletal system. While currently there is limited research on the development, diagnosis, and treatment of myofascial trigger points (MTrPs) in non-human animal species,

great strides are being undertaken to transpose the human techniques initially developed by MDs into the realm of veterinary patients. With the development of the American College of Veterinary Sports Medicine and Rehabilitation (ACVMSR) and its mission "advances the art and science of veterinary medicine by promoting expertise in the structural, physiological, medical and surgical needs of athletic animals and the restoration of normal form and function after injury or illness" (ACVMSR, 2015), anticipation of advancements in the study of muscle pain and dysfunction exists.

MPS, is typically thought to arise from MTrPs. The pioneers recognizing MPS were Janet Travell MD and David Simons MD, their textbook defines an MTrP as a hyperirritable spot in skeletal muscle that is associated with a hypersensitive palpable nodule in a taut band. The spot is tender when pressed, and gives rise to characteristic referred pain, motor dysfunction, and autonomic phenomena (Simons *et al.*, 1999). The three components that make up an MTrP include a sensory, a motor, and an autonomic component.

Sensory Component

MTrPs can be very painful. The pain begins as nociception in the peripheral tissues from all the normal chemical activators, including serotonin, prostaglandins, bradykinin, and substance P, among others. It is not within the scope of this chapter to go into depth of all the pain-generating substances. These substances can decrease the activation threshold of a neuron, so that the nociceptor fires more easily with less of a stimulus, potentially leading to peripheral sensitization. Sampling of tissue fluid from active MTrPs in the upper trapezius of human patients was performed. Elevated levels of protons, bradykinin, serotonin, substance P, norepinephrine, calcitonin gene-related peptide, tumor necrosis factor alpha, and interleukin-1b were detected and were significantly different compared to samples taken from areas without MTrPs (Shah *et al.*, 2005). A persistent barrage of nociceptive signals from MTrPs may eventually lead to central sensitization, a form of neural plasticity involving functional and/or structural change within the dorsal horn of the spinal cord. Central sensitization can be clinically expressed as allodynia – pain associated with typically non-painful stimuli or hyperalgesia – when an actual painful stimulus is perceived as more painful than it should.

Motor Component

MTrPs are also known as "contracture knots" due to the severe focal muscle contracture in the region of the MTrP. Contracture of the muscle fibers can compress local sensory neurons as well as compressing local blood vessels leading to a reduced supply of oxygen. MTrPs may inhibit normal motor activity in their muscle of origin or in functionally related muscles. Motor inhibition is often identified as muscle weakness and can lead to poor coordination and muscle imbalances (McPartland and Simons, 2011). Clinically, this can appear as muscle weakness without atrophy and unrelated to neurologic causes (Simons *et al.*, 1999).

Autonomic Component

The autonomic nervous system (ANS) primarily exerts control over cardiac tissue, blood vessels, visceral organs, and glands of the body. Typically, ANS responses seen in human patients with MTrPs include localized sweating, vasoconstriction or vasodilatation, and pilomotor activity (goosebumps) (McPartland and Simons, 2011). While these responses are seen frequently and are easily detectable in humans, the detection of any ANS response is rare in the veterinary patient – with pilomotor activity (pilo-erection) being the most likely event noted.

How Do MTrPs Develop

Several possible mechanisms can lead to the development of MTrPs, including low-level muscle contractions, uneven intramuscular pressure distribution, direct trauma, eccentric contraction in unconditioned muscle, and maximal or submaximal concentric contractions. The exact reason as to why these mechanisms lead to the formation of MTrPs remains unclear. The original hypothesis introduced in 1981 as *The Integrated Trigger Point Hypothesis* was dependent on an energy crisis that would result in excessive acetylcholine at the motor endplate. The excess of acetylcholine would then cause contraction of the sarcomere leading to the development of MTrPs. With advances in research, this hypothesis became *The Expanded Integrated Trigger Point Hypothesis* in 2004 (Gerwin *et al.*, 2004) (see Figure 26.1 of The Expanded MTrP Hypothesis).

Low-level muscle contractions can result in degeneration of muscle fibers. This can lead to an increase in calcium release, energy depletion, and structural damage especially to the mitochondria. During low-level muscle contractions, intramuscular pressure can lead to excessive capillary pressure causing localized hypoxia and ischemia. Direct trauma may create a vicious cycle of events wherein damage to the sarcoplasmic reticulum or the muscle cell membrane may lead to an increase of calcium concentration, subsequent activation of actin and myosin, a relative shortage of adenosine triphosphate (ATP), and an impaired calcium pump, which in turn

will increase the intracellular calcium concentration even more, completing the cycle. Eccentric and concentric exercises have been associated with hypoxia and ischemia (see Figure 26.1). However, there is currently inadequate evidence to demonstrate that these exercises are absolute precursors to the development of MTrPs (Bron and Dommerholt, 2012; Dommerholt *et al.*, 2011).

Perpetuating Factors

Perpetuation of MTrP formation in dogs appears to be most often related to mechanical stresses resulting in chronic muscle overload. Postural changes in dogs resulting from orthopedic injury, postoperative surgical trauma and pain, neuropathy, joint dysfunction, and pain related to osteoarthritis create muscle overload. Many of the same muscle-related mechanisms that lead

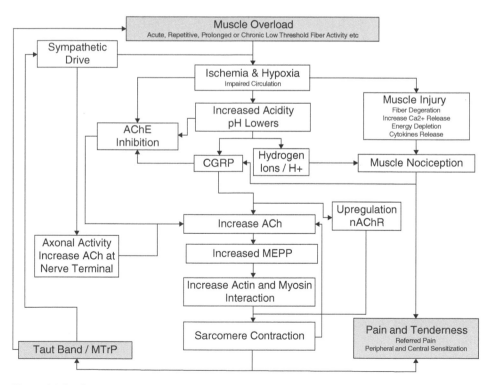

Figure 26.1 Schematic showing The Expanded Integrated Trigger Point Hypothesis.

to the development of MTPs are also perpetuating factors.

An example to illustrate this point is the canine patient with chronic osteoarthritis of the coxofemoral joints. The pain caused by the joints will cause the patient to invoke compensatory postural changes to relieve pressure on the joints, thereby activating and perpetuating MTrPs. MTrPs will readily be found in the hip flexors (e.g., iliopsoas, tensor fasciae latae, sartorius, and rectus femoris), extensors (gluteals, piriformis, semimembranosus, and semitendinosus), and adductors (gracilis, pectineus, and adductor). As the patient shifts weight cranially, thereby changing the typical 60/40 weight distribution pattern, compensatory changes will be found in the muscles of the forelimbs. The overload placed on the forelimbs can lead to the formation and presence of MTrPs; primarily in infraspinatus, triceps, teres major, and deltoids. As the patient ambulates, there will be considerable lateral flexion of the spinal muscles to avoid extensive coxofemoral flexion and extension. This can be described as a "hula type motion" when viewed from the caudal aspect of the patient. This overuse of the iliocostalis lumborum can result in the formation of MTrPs. This example of formation of trigger points secondary to joint pain not only illustrates the perpetuation that can be involved with MTrPs, but it also demonstrates the need to treat any underlying pain. If the MTrPs are cleared with treatment and any known underlying source of pain is not addressed, then the MTrPs will return and the patient will continue to suffer from myalgia as well as the underlying pain. This is just one illustration of a condition that can perpetuate MTrPs, similar findings can be found with patients suffering from shoulder injuries, antebrachial injuries, chronic medial luxating patella, and cruciate injuries among others.

In humans, MTrPs have been found from nutritional, metabolic, or systemic perpetuating factors, including the use of statin-class drugs, iron insufficiency, vitamin D insufficiency, vitamin B12 (cobalamin) insufficiency, and hormonal imbalances, such as is seen with hypothyroidism (Dommerholt and Gerwin, 2011). Hypothyroidism is the most common endocrine disorder in dogs and is associated with a variety of clinical signs; however, the veterinary literature does not mention pain resulting from hypothyroidism (Wall, 2014). However, one might pause to consider those hypothyroid dogs that suffer from myopathy and muscle weakness and closely evaluate the patient for MTrPs.

Evaluation of the Patient

Close observation of the patients prior to placing your hands on them can provide you with a lot of information and knowledge. Observing the patient at various gaits (walk, trot, and jog) or the unwillingness to move; observing position changes such as standing to sit or laying down to stand can provide the astute observer with considerable information as to which muscle or muscle groups may be involved. Video-taping the patient to analyze in slow motion can also be very beneficial. In dogs, a simple test can be performed to evaluate muscle weakness. With a dog in standing position, slowly slide the limb backward until non-weight-bearing. A slight to profound drop of the contralateral side can be indicative of muscle weakness or altered muscle firing patterns associated with MTrPs within the antigravity muscles of that limb (Wall, 2014).

MTrPs are classified as active or latent. Active MTrPs cause local or referred pain patterns while at rest, with muscle movement, or upon direct stimulation. Latent MTrPs do not trigger pain without direct stimulation (Dommerholt *et al.*, 2011). Both active and latent MTrPs are painful on compression, thereby making it virtually impossible for the veterinary examiner to know if a patient is suffering from active or latent MTrPs, so all MTrPs that are found should be addressed as a possible cause of pain and muscle dysfunction (see Figure 26.2).

Identification of taut bands and hypersensitive MTrPs within muscle is an acquired skill set that requires an understanding of these changes, skilled instruction, and repeated practice (Wall, 2014).

Without a "gold standard" of laboratory testing or diagnostic imaging to diagnose MTrPs we are heavily reliant on palpation skills. Palpation for MTrPs can be accomplished by two simple techniques. Flat palpation is the gentle but firm movement of the fingertips perpendicular to the muscle fibers being examined as they are pushed against the underlying bone (see Figure 26.3). This technique lends itself to examination of muscles such as the iliopsoas, infraspinatus, and supraspinatus.

Pincer palpation is performed by rolling the muscle perpendicular to the muscle fibers between the fingertips and thumb. This technique lends itself to the examination of muscles such as the sartorius, tensor fasciae latae, and triceps (see Figure 26.4). Once a taut band is detected, the taut band is evaluated for an area of hardness and discrete pain.

As the stimulation of an active or latent MTrP can lead to a "jump sign;" a pain response leading to vocalization or the patient trying to move away, palpation is best done with an assistant providing gentle restraint. While palpation can be performed on a standing patient, many people find it is much easier to palpate the taut bands in a relaxed muscle in a non-weight-bearing lateral recumbent position.

A "local twitch response" (LTR) may be induced during the palpation over an MTrP. The LTR is a unique spinal cord

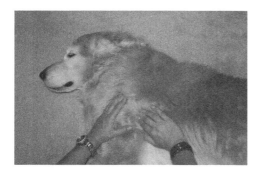

Figure 26.2 Example of Flat Palpation in a dog for the presence of MTrPs.

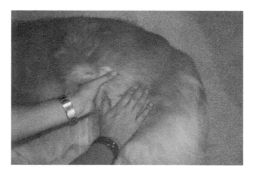

Figure 26.4 Pincer palpation on a dog.

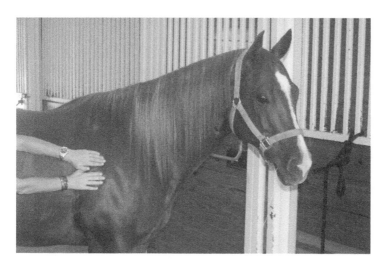

Figure 26.3 Example of flat palpation on a horse for the presence of MTrPs.

reflex resulting in a rapid contraction of the taut band following manual stimulation of the MTP. Manual stimulation can be accomplished by direct palpation or introduction of a needle. The LTR in dogs can also serve as verification of the presence of an MTrP (Wall, 2014).

The criteria for identification of MTrPs can be best summed up by: a palpable taut band, exquisite spot tenderness of a nodule in the taut band, and patient recognition of pain upon palpation of the nodule (jump sign in the veterinary patient). Confirmatory observations in the veterinary patient would be a visual or tactile identification of a local twitch response (Simons *et al.*, 1999).

Treatment of MTrPs

Therapies fall into two categories: invasive and noninvasive. At this point in time, no clinical studies have been done to evaluate the outcome or validate the effectiveness of any treatment for MTrPs in the veterinary patient. All reports are considered anecdotal and symptomatic and clinical improvement or failure of treatment is based strictly on "observation" by the clinician and the owner.

Noninvasive Therapies

Electrotherapy – Anecdotal reports from several veterinary clinicians report successful treatment of MTrPs with the Pointer Excel II™, a handheld transcutaneous electrical nerve stimulation device. The Pointer Excel II is placed on the skin over the MTrP and electrical intensity is increased until rhythmic muscle contraction is produced. Response to therapy is likely related to rapid muscle stretch that occurs with induced contraction rather than the introduction of electrotherapy (Wall, 2014).

Low level laser therapy (LLLT) – This chapter will only discuss the use of Class IIIa and IIIb lasers. As the Class IV laser (output power of greater than 500 mW) must continually be moved over the surface of the skin to prevent thermal damage, it is difficult to determine the exact J/cm^2 that would be delivered to the underlying MTrP. Class IIIa lasers produce an output power of up to 5 mW; whereas Class IIIb lasers produce an output power of up to 500 mW. During laser therapy the energy delivered is reported in Joules (J) where 1 J = 1 W/s, and the treatment area is described in cm^2; therefore, the therapeutic laser dose is described as J/cm^2. While there have been many research studies done with LLLT for the treatment of MTrPs, there is no conclusive evidence to support or deny its effectiveness (Manca *et al.*, 2014; Ilbuldu *et al.*, 2004; Altan *et al.*, 2005; Dundar *et al.*, 2007). Inadequate dosages may be the principal factor involved in the inconsistency among reports of LLLT efficacy. Until there is further research to demonstrate an effective therapeutic laser dose for the treatment of MTrPs, this modality should not be a standalone treatment procedure.

Ultrasound – Current research demonstrates that the use of conventional therapeutic ultrasound is no more effective than placebo or no treatment for MTrP pain in the neck and upper back (Manca *et al.*, 2014; Esenyel *et al.*, 2000; Lee *et al.*, 1997; Gam *et al.*, 1998).

Shockwave therapy – Current research, although limited in number of studies, is demonstrating some effectiveness for the treatment of MTrPs, and this modality will need further research to fully elucidate its role as a therapy (Moghtaderi *et al.*, 2014; Jeon *et al.*, 2012; Ji *et al.*, 2012). It is the clinical observation of the authors, that after shock wave therapy is performed on a patient with osteoarthritis of the coxofemoral joint; the number of palpable MTrPs in the tensor fasciae latae, proximal sartorius, and gluteals muscles is less after the therapy as compared to before the therapy is completed.

Manual Therapies: In humans, the evidence for manual therapies is once again not clear, as the data regarding most manual therapies is inadequate and conflicting. Most trials do not limit the number of modalities per treatment, so positive outcomes cannot be exclusively claimed by a certain therapy. Several studies reported that exercise and stretching appeared to be the effective therapy when included in treatment groups comparing active to placebo modalities (Mense and Gerwin, 2010; Rickards, 2011). Trigger point pressure release has positive research as a treatment in humans. This technique is one of the more commonly described manual techniques to address MTrPs (Llamas-Ramos *et al.*, 2014; Cagnie *et al.*, 2013; Bodes-Pardo *et al.*, 2013). Trigger point release consists of pressure progressively applied and increased over the MTrP until the fingers encounter an increase in tissue resistance (tissue barrier). This pressure is maintained until the clinician senses a relief of the taut band. At that moment, the pressure is increased again until the next increase in tissue resistance is felt. The process is repeated for three times during each session (Lewit, 1991).

Invasive Therapies

While veterinary technicians are not allowed to perform these procedures, the knowledge of the procedure and proper restrain or sedation for the procedure plays an important role as part of the animal healthcare team. Invasive procedures consist of dry needling (DN) or trigger point injections (TPI). TPI involves the use of a hypodermic needle attached to a syringe to inject a substance directly into the MTrP. Commonly used substances in the human world include lidocaine and botulinum toxin. Due to the discomfort from these injections, this procedure is not well tolerated in the veterinary patient. DN consists of the use of a filiform needle inserted into the skin and then into the deeper underlying muscle (see Figure 26.5).

The MTrP within the taut band is targeted and eliciting LTRs is essential. Once, an LTR is evoked, the needle is slightly withdrawn from the muscle, but not the skin, and can be redirected to the same MTrP until no further LTRs are evoked (see Figure 26.6). Additional MTrPs in the area can also be treated prior to the needle being completely removed from the patient. The human literature covers in depth the advantages of DN (Dommerholt and Gerwin, 2010). Treatment outcome goals would include a decrease in peripheral and central sensitization as well as improved motor function as seen with increase in muscle strength and range of motion leading to a better quality of life for the veterinary patient. A successful outcome of dry needling for the treatment of myofascial

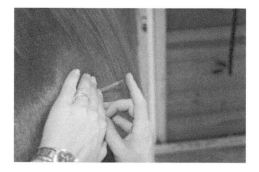

Figure 26.5 Dry Needling of a Horse for Treatment of MTrPs by Mrs. Angela Stramel.

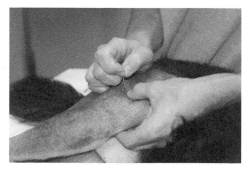

Figure 26.6 Dry Needling of a Dog for Treatment of MTrPs by Dr. Douglas Stramel.

trigger points is heavily reliant on the knowledge and skills of the veterinary clinician. One must have an in-depth knowledge of anatomy and develop keen tactile awareness and visualization of the needle pathway, as it travels through the soft tissue of the patient's body (Dommerholt and Gerwin, 2010).

Conclusions

With the awareness of myofascial trigger points affecting the veterinary patient, one can better assess those patients suffering from myalgia and having a decline in athletic performance. Knowledge that MTrPs can complicate, prolong, or delay the pain management and healing process in chronic or acute orthopedic and neurologic patients can vastly change the way patients are treated. These patients have a better outcome than those left untreated. The skill set to be able to understand, palpate, and treat MTrPs is essential for each member of the veterinary healthcare team who is interested in pain management, rehabilitation, and sports medicine.

References

ACVMSR (2015) *Our Mission*, [Online], Available: http://vsmr.org/.

Altan, L., Bingöl, U., Aykaç, M., and Yurtkuran, M. (2005). Investigation of the effect of GaAs laser therapy on cervical myofascial pain syndrome. *Rheumatol Int* 25 (1): 23–27.

Bodes-Pardo, G., Pecos-Martin, D., Gallego-Izquierdo, T., and Salom-Moreno, J. (2013). Manual treatment for cervicogenic headache and active trigger point in the sternocleidomastoid muscle: A pilot randomized clinical trial. *J Manipulative Physiol Ther* 36 (7): 403–411.

Bron, C. and Dommerholt, J. (2012). Etiology of myofascial trigger points. *Curr Pain Headache Rep* 16: 439–444.

Cagnie, B. et al. (2013). Effect of ischemic compression on trigger points in the neck and shoulder muscles in office workers: A cohort study. *J Manipulative Physiol Ther* 36 (8): 482–489.

Dommerholt, J. and Gerwin, R. (2010). Neurophysiological effects of trigger point needling therapies. In: *Diagnosis and Management of Tension Type and Cervicogenic Headache* (ed. C. Fernandez de las Penas, L. Arendt-Nielsen, and R.D. Gerwin), 247–259. Boston, MA: Jones & Bartlett.

Dommerholt, J. and Gerwin, R. (2011). Nutritional and metabolic perpetuating factors in myofascial pain. In: *Myofascial Trigger Points: Pathophysiology and Evidence-Informed Diagnosis and Management* (ed. J. Dommerholt and P. Huijbregts), 51–57. Boston, MA: Jones & Bartlett.

Dommerholt, J., Bron, C., and Franssen, J. (2011). Myofascial trigger points: An evidence-informed review. In: *Myofascial Trigger Points: Pathophysiology and Evidence-Informed Diagnosis and Management* (ed. J. Dommerholt and P. Huijbregts), 17–38. Boston, MA: Jones & Bartlett.

Dundar, U., Evcik, D., Samli, F. et al. (2007). The effect of gallium arsenide aluminum laser therapy in the management of cervical myofascial pain syndrome: A double blind, placebo-controlled study. *Clin Rheumatol* 26 (2): 930–934.

Esenyel, M., Caglar, N., and Aldemir, T. (2000). Treatment of myofascial pain. *Arch Phys Med Rehabil* 79: 48–52.

Gam, A., Warming, S., Larsen, L.H. et al. (1998). Treatment of myofascial trigger-points with ultrasound combined with massage and exercise: A randomised controlled trial. *Pain* 77: 73–79.

Gerwin, R., Dommerholt, J., and Shah, J.P. (2004). An expansion of Simon's integrated hypothesis for trigger point formation. *Curr Pain Headache Rep* 8: 468–475.

Ilbuldu, E., Cakmak, A., Disci, R., and Aydin, R. (2004). Comparison of laser, dry needling, and placebo laser treatments in myofascial pain syndrome. *Photomed Laser Surg* 22: 306–311.

Jeon, J., Jung, Y.J., Lee, J.Y. et al. (2012). The effect of extracorporeal shock wave therapy on myofascial pain syndrome. *Ann Rehabil Med* 36 (5): 665–674.

Ji, H.M., Kim, H.J., and Han, S.J. (2012). Extracorporeal shock wave therapy in myofascial pain syndrome of upper trapezius. *Ann Rehabil Med* 36 (5): 675–680.

Lee, J.C., Lin, D.T., and Hong, C.Z. (1997). The effectiveness of simultaneous thermotherapy with ultrasound and electrotherapy with combined AC and DC current on the immediate pain relief of myofascial trigger points. *Musculoskel Pain* 5: 81–90.

Lewit, K. (ed.) (1991). *Manipulative Therapy in Rehabilitation of the Locomotor System*, 3rde. Oxford: Butterworth Heinemann.

Llamas-Ramos, R., Pecos-Martín, D., Gallego-Izquierdo, T. et al. (2014). Comparison of the short-term outcomes between trigger point dry needling and trigger point manual therapy for the management of chronic mechanical neck pain: A randomized clinical trial. *J Orthop Sports Phys Ther* 44 (11): 852–861.

Manca, A., Limonta, E., Pilurzi, G., and Ginatempo, F. (2014). Ultrasound and laser as stand-alone therapies for myofascial trigger points: A randomized, double-blind, placebo controlled study. *Physiother Res Int* 19: 166–175.

McPartland, J. and Simons, D. (2011). Myofascial trigger points: Translating molecular theory into manual therapy. In: *Myofascial Trigger Points: Pathophysiology and Evidence-Informed Diagnosis and Management* (ed. J. Dommerholt and P. Huijbregts), 6–7. Boston, MA: Jones & Bartlett.

Mense, S. and Gerwin, R. (ed.) (2010). *Muscle Pain: Diagnosis and Treatment*. Berlin Heidelberg, Berlin, Germany: Springer-Verlag.

Moghtaderi, A., Samandarian, M., and Dolatkhah, N. (2014). Extracorporeal shock wave therapy of gastroc-soleus trigger points in patients with plantar fasciitis: A randomized, placebo-controlled trial. *Adv Biomed Res* 3: 99.

Rickards, L. (2011). Effectiveness of noninvasive treatments for active myofascial trigger point pain: A systematic review. In: *Myofascial Trigger Points: Pathophysiology and Evidence-Informed Diagnosis and Management* (ed. J. Dommerholt and P. Huijbregts), 129–152. Boston, MA: Jones & Bartlett.

Shah, J.P., Philips, T.M., Danoff, J.V. et al. (2005). An in vivo micoranalytical technique for measuring the local biochemical milieu of human skeletal muscle. *J Appl Physiol* 99: 1977–1984.

Simons, D.G., Travel, J.G., and Simons, L.S. (1999). Myofascial pan and dysfunction: The trigger point manual. In: *Volume 1: Upper Half Body*, 2nde (ed. J. Butler). Baltimore, MD: Williams & Wilkins.

Wall, R. (2014). Introduction to myofascial trigger points in dogs. *Topics Compan An Med* 29: 43–48.

Index

Physical Rehabilitation for Veterinary Technicians and Nurses, Second Edition.
Edited by Mary Ellen Goldberg and Julia E. Tomlinson.
© 2024 John Wiley & Sons, Inc. Published 2024 by John Wiley & Sons, Inc.
Companion website: www.wiley.com/go/goldberg/physicalrehabilitationvettechsandnurses